Infectious Diseases
of the
Female Genital Tract

**Presented as a service to the medical community
through the courtesy of
The Upjohn Company**

Representative _____

Phone Number _____

Infectious Diseases
of the
Female Genital Tract

Richard L. Sweet, M.D.

Professor and Vice-Chairman
Department of Obstetrics, Gynecology, and Reproductive Sciences
University of California School of Medicine
San Francisco, California

Ronald S. Gibbs, M.D.

Professor of Obstetrics and Gynecology
University of Texas Health Science Center
San Antonio, Texas

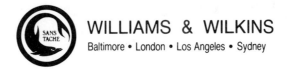

WILLIAMS & WILKINS
Baltimore • London • Los Angeles • Sydney

Editor: Carol-Lynn Brown
Associate Editor: Victoria M. Vaughn
Copy Editor: Andrea Clemente
Design: Bob Och
Illustration Planning: Lorraine Wrzosek
Production: Raymond E. Reter

Copyright ©, 1985
Williams & Wilkins
428 East Preston Street
Baltimore, MD 21202, U.S.A.

Accurate indications, adverse reactions, and dosage schedules for drugs are provided in this book, but it is possible that they may change. The reader is urged to review the package information data of the manufacturers of the medications mentioned.

Made in the United States of America

Library of Congress Cataloging in Publication Data

Sweet, Richard L.
   Infectious diseases of the female genital tract.
   Includes bibliographies and index.
   1. Generative organs, Female—Infections. 2. Generative organs, Female—Micro-biology. 3. Generative organs, Female—Diseases. I. Gibbs, Ronald S., 1943-   . II. Title. [DNLM: 1. Genital Diseases, Female.
2. Infection. WP 140 S974i]
RG218.S94 1985   618.1   84-20858
ISBN 0-683-08038-5

88 89   10 9 8 7 6 5

To our wives
Rhea and Jane
and our children
Jennifer, Suzanne, Andrew, Eric, and Stuart
whose support and understanding provided the spark and impetus
for the commitment to this work.

Preface

The field of infectious diseases as it relates to obstetrics and gynecology has undergone an immense evolution over the past two decades. Reproductive infectious diseases now encompass many specialized areas, including normal genital flora, sexually transmitted diseases, infections among nonpregnant women, perinatal infectious disease, and postoperative infection. Moreover, the volume and quality of both basic research and clinical investigation in female genital tract infections have increased tremendously.

Among the major changes in the studies of reproductive microbiology have been: (1) an interest in the pathophysiology of infectious processes; (2) the realization that many infections are polymicrobic in nature; (3) the recognition of the importance of virus, mycoplasma, chlamydia, and anaerobic microorganisms; (4) elucidation of a role for newly described organisms, such as Mobiluncus and papillomavirus; (5) the use of quantitative microbiology in reproductive tract investigations; (6) development of better diagnostic techniques for the identification of microorganisms and diseases; and (7) a virtual revolution in the availability of antimicrobial agents and in antibiotic treatment strategies.

This book is an attempt to respond to these new challenges and provide a resource for clinicians providing health care to women in the area of infectious diseases. We have provided a description of the microorganisms involved in reproductive infections and the laboratory techniques available for their isolation and/or identification. An emphasis has been placed on identifying major problem areas in infectious diseases of the female genital tract and developing a diagnostic and therapeutic approach to areas, such as the epidemic of sexually transmitted diseases, pelvic inflammatory disease, perinatal infections, premature rupture of the membranes, parasitic diseases, and prevention and treatment of postoperative infections.

Finally, we have described the multitude of antimicrobial agents available to the clinician and assessed their place in the therapeutic armamentarium of clinicians providing health care to women.

Our ultimate goal in writing this book was to provide the practicing physician with the diagnostic and therapeutic knowledge necessary to prevent the significant morbidity and occasional mortality that occurs secondary to infections in reproductive medicine.

We wish to thank Mary Bonds and Marci Yellin for their exceptional secretarial support.

Contents

CHAPTER 1

Clinical Microbiology of the Female Genital Tract

The microbiology of the female genital tract is indeed complex. In healthy women, the vagina contains 10^9 bacterial colony forming units/g of secretions. Isolates include a variety of aerobic and anaerobic bacteria, yeasts, viruses, and parasites. Influences upon these microbes include phase of the menstrual cycle, childbirth, surgery, and antibiotic therapy. The upper genital tract is usually sterile, but bacteria from the lower genital tract may ascend into the uterine cavity, fallopian tubes, or pelvic peritoneum because of menstruation, instrumentation, foreign bodies, surgery, or other predisposing factors.

This chapter presents a working knowledge of genital tract microbes for the clinician. More detailed descriptions of selected microbes are provided in later chapters.

VIRULENCE

Distinguishing "virulent" or "pathogenic" isolates from "nonvirulent" or "nonpathogenic" ones is not simple because the behavior of a given isolate is so dependent upon numbers present, host factors, and local conditions (pH, pCO_2, presence of necrosis, and foreign body). For example, although the group B streptococcus is a leading cause of maternal and neonatal septicemia, most women with genital colonization by group B streptococci suffer no consequence. On the other hand, *Staphylococcus epidermidis* is commonly considered part of the normal skin and vaginal flora, but it may also cause disease when the conditions allow; for example, *S. epidermidis* has been recognized as a cause of infective endocarditis.

In spite of such widely ranging behavior patterns, it is still practical to distinguish "high" from "low" virulence genital isolates. For practicality, the high virulence isolates are divided into aerobes and anaerobes, and each of these groups is further subdivided into gram-positive and gram-negative organisms.

AEROBIC HIGH VIRULENCE ISOLATES
Gram-Positive Cocci

The virulent organisms in this group include the aerobic streptococci and staphylococci.

STREPTOCOCCI

Many varieties have been found in the pelvis, and they have been classified by two independent schemes. In one scheme, the streptococci are distinguished by their hemolytic properties on blood agar plates. Aerobic streptococci showing partial (or green) hemolysis are termed alpha (α)-streptococci. Those showing complete (or clear) hemolysis are termed beta (β)-, and those showing no hemolysis are termed gamma (γ)-streptococci. In the other scheme, the Lancefield system, many streptococci may be classified according to surface antigens, designated by the letters A through O. In humans, streptococci of groups A, B, and D are common pathogens. Group A and B streptococci nearly always produce β-hemolysis, and group D streptococci are usually nonhemolytic (γ-streptococci) but may on occasion be either α- or β-hemolytic as well.

Group A Streptococci (*Streptococcus pyogenes*)

This organism causes pharyngeal, cutaneous, and postoperative infections. Sequelae of group A streptococcal infections may include rheumatic fever and acute glomerulonephritis. It is not generally considered to be a member of the normal vaginal flora, as it is isolated in less than 1% of asymptomatic women. Pelvic infection caused by group A streptococci may produce a characteristic clinical picture, with a high, early initial fever, chills, prostration, and diffuse tenderness. On gram stains, one sees gram-positive cocci in chains. The microorganism remains exquisitely sensitive to penicillin, and erythromycin or a cephalosporin may usually be

Table 1.1
Classification of Microorganisms Commonly Found in the Female Genital Tract

Bacteria
  Aerobes   Anaerobes

Aerobes	Anaerobes
Gram-positive cocci	Gram-positive cocci
Group A, B, D streptococci	*Peptostreptococcus* sp.
Other α- and γ-streptococci	*Peptococcus* sp.
S. aureus	
S. epidermidis[a]	
Gram-positive rods	Gram-positive rods
Lactobacilli[a]	*C. perfringens (welchii)*
Diphtheroids[a]	Other *Clostridium* sp.
	Proprionibacterium sp.[a]
	Eubacterium sp.[a]
Gram-negative cocci	Gram-negative cocci
N. gonorrhoeae	*Veillonella* sp.[a]
Gram-negative rods	Gram-negative rods
E. coli	*B. bivius*
K. pneumoniae	*B. fragilis* group
Enterobacter sp.	*B. melaninogenicus*
P. mirabilis	*B. disiens*
Other *Proteus* sp.	Other *Bacteroides* sp.
Pseudomonas aeruginosa	Fusobacterium sp.
G. vaginalis (a coccobacillus)	*Fusobacterium* sp.

Mycoplasmas
  M. hominis
  U. urealyticum (formerly T form mycoplasmas)

Intracellular bacteria
  C. trachomatis

Viruses
  Cytomegalovirus
  Herpes simplex virus

Yeasts
  C. albicans
  Other *Candida* sp.
  T. glabrata

Parasites
  T. vaginalis

[a] Species generally with low virulence.

substituted for treatment of the penicillin-allergic patient.

Group A streptococcal pelvic infections occur both in sporadic and epidemic form. Epidemics have usually been exogenous in origin, commonly resulting from nasopharyngeal carriage of the microorganism or from skin infections in hospital staff members (1). Occasionally, a mother may be the source.

Prevention of epidemics can be accomplished by placing patients with group A streptococcal infections in strict isolation and by early antibiotic treatment of hospital employees with group A streptococcal infections. Employees with positive cultures should be relieved of duty on obstetric, neonatal, and postoperative wards until their cultures become negative. When epidemics have occurred, isolation and antibiotic therapy have not always been sufficient to effect control. Additional measures such as identifying and treating all streptococcal carriers, cancellations of elective surgery, and prophylactic treatment of all patients and personnel have been necessary in some recent outbreaks.

Group B Streptococci (*Streptococcus agalactiae*)

Before the 1960s this organism was not recognized as a frequent pathogen, but has now become a major cause of sepsis among neonates and postpartum women (2). Unlike group A streptococci, group B organisms are considered part of the normal vaginal flora and are recovered in 5–35% of normal pregnant women. Isolation rates are enhanced by use of selective broth containing nalidixic acid and gentamicin. The clinical picture of group B streptococcal infection in puerperal women closely resembles group A infection. Epidemic group B streptococcal disease has not been reported among mothers, however. The neonate with group B streptococcal sepsis has usually acquired the microorganism during labor from the maternal genital tract. Even with appropriate therapy, neonatal GBS infection has a high fatality rate.

Group B streptococci are susceptible to penicillin, erythromycin, and the cephalosporin group of antibiotics. A more detailed discussion is in Chapter 13.

Group D Streptococci

This group is comprised of two subgroups: "group D enterococci" and "group D not enterococci." The former, which includes *Streptococcus faecalis* and other less common species, occurs frequently. Although these organisms cause endocarditis and urinary tract infection, their virulence in genital infections has been debatable. They are considerably less virulent than group A or B streptococci but have on occasion caused serious genital and abdominal infections (3). They are the only streptococci not sensitive to penicillin and are resistant also to cephalosporins, alone or in combination with aminoglycosides (streptomycin, kanamycin, or gentamicin), and to clindamycin, alone or in combination with aminoglycosides. Enterococci are susceptible to ampicillin, to penicillin and aminoglycoside in combination, and to vancomycin. Failure of a patient to respond to cephalosporin-aminoglycoside or clindamycin-aminoglycoside combinations may be observed when the primary pathogen is an enterococcus.

Nonenterococcal group D streptococci are commonly isolated, but are of low virulence. They are susceptible to penicillin.

Other Aerobic Streptococci

These include a variety of common bacteria which are susceptible to penicillin. Examples are α- and γ-streptococci.

STAPHYLOCOCCI

The aerobic staphylococci include *Staphylococcus epidermidis* and *Staphylococcus aureus*. *S. aureus* is isolated from 5–10% of genital tract cultures. This organism has been recognized as a cause of abdominal wound infections, breast abscesses, and nursery outbreaks of infection and has been isolated from nearly all patients with toxic shock syndrome. Most species of *S. aureus*, whether isolated in the community or in the hospital, elaborate penicillinase and are resistant to penicillin and ampicillin. Agents of choice for *S. aureus* infections are the penicillinase-resistant penicillins, such as cloxacillin, dicloxacillin, methicillin, oxacillin, and nafcillin. In the United States, very few *S. aureus* strains have developed resistance to these antibiotics, but in Europe, resistance to these agents is more common. Antibiotics for use in *S. aureus* infections in the penicillin-allergic patient are the "first generation" cephalosporins and clindamycin.

S. epidermidis is commonly isolated from the vagina and skin, but rarely causes infection.

Gram-Negative Bacilli

This group includes a large number of microorganisms with highly variable patterns of antimicrobial susceptibility. Many species have been identified, but only a few are commonly isolated from patients with pelvic infections.

ESCHERICHIA COLI

This organism is the most commonly isolated member of this group in genital tract and urine specimens. It is present in 15–90% of urinary tract infections. *E. coli* infections are usually mild but may occasionally be fulminant, as it is the microorganism most commonly identified in bacteremic obstetric and gynecologic patients (4). Its susceptibility to antibiotics varies from hospital to hospital and, probably, from service to service. Gentamicin, tobramycin, amikacin, and chloramphenicol are usually effective against more than 95% of *E. coli* species. The so-called "first generation" cephalosporin antibiotics and ampicillin are active against 60–80% of *E. coli* isolates in most hospitals, but the newer cephalosporin-like agents and newer penicillins are more active.

KLEBSIELLA SPECIES

These are found in fewer than 15% of genital tract infections, but also cause urinary tract infections and hospital-acquired pneumonia. All the cephalosporin antibiotics are highly effective against *Klebsiella*, as are the aminoglycosides and chloramphenicol. Ampicillin has little activity, but some of the newer penicillins, such as piperacillin and mezlocillin, have improved activity.

ENTEROBACTER SPECIES

Although closely related to *Klebsiella* species, these microorganisms are encountered much less frequently (<5% of genital infections). They are more resistant to antibiotics than are *Klebsiella* species. Until recently *Enterobacter* infections usually required therapy with aminoglycoside antibiotics, but some of the newer cephalosporins and newer penicillins show good activity.

PROTEUS SPECIES

These bacteria are isolated in 10–15% of genital tract infections and in a similar percent of urinary tract infections. *Proteus mirabilis*, by far the most commonly isolated species in obstetrical and gynecologic patients, is susceptible to ampicillin and the cephalosporins as well as the aminoglycosides. *Proteus vulgaris* occurs much less uncommonly. Former *Proteus* species, *Proteus morganii* and *Proteus rettgeri*, are now classified as *Morganella morganii* and *Providencia rettgeri*, respectively. These species are resistant to ampicillin and the cephalosporins, but are sensitive to the aminoglycosides and some of the newer penicillin and cephalosporin antibiotics.

PSEUDOMONAS SPECIES

Opportunistic pathogens in severe, usually hospital-acquired infections, *Pseudomonas* species are infrequently found in infections in obstetrics and gynecology, but *Pseudomonas* colonization is seen commonly in patients receiving antibiotic therapy. Antibiotics susceptibility is good to gentamicin and usually better to tobramycin and amikacin. Activity of the newer penicillins and some of the newer cephalosporins is good, and combinations of antibiotics may produce higher cure rates in serious infections.

GARDNERELLA VAGINALIS

Formerly known as *Haemophilus vaginalis* and *Corynebacterium vaginale*, *G. vaginalis* is found in vaginal cultures of nearly all women with nonspecific vaginitis, but may also be found in vaginal cultures of asymptomatic women (5). On occasion, it has been reported to cause endometritis and bacteremia. In vitro testing shows this organism is susceptible to ampicillin and tetracycline, but these agents are of limited value in curing nonspecific vaginitis. (See Chapter 6.)

OTHER GRAM-NEGATIVE BACILLI

These include microorganisms such as *Serratia, Citrobacter, Hafnia,* and *Providencia* species, all of which show resistance to commonly used antibiotics. Fortunately, these species are found rarely among obstetric-gynecologic patients, except in debilitated patients or those receiving antibiotic, immunosuppressive, or cytotoxic therapy.

Gram-Negative Cocci

In pelvic infections the only significant member of this group is *Neisseria gonorrhoeae*. *N. gonorrhoeae* may produce an asymptomatic colonization of the cervix, cervicitis, or salpingitis. Disseminated infection with septicemia, arthritis, and dermatitis occur not infrequently. It has also been recently reported as an unusual cause of amnionitis and fetal scalp abscess. Most species of *N. gonorrhoeae* remain susceptible to penicillin, tetracycline, spectinomycin, and other antibiotics. Penicillinase-producing strains of *N. gonorrhoeae* have been isolated in Southeast Asia, and a number of such isolates have been identified in the United States. Effective treatment for cervical infection with these penicillinase-producing isolates are spectinomycin, cefoxitin, and cefotaxime (6).

ANAEROBIC HIGH VIRULENCE ISOLATES

Anaerobic bacteria are likely to produce infection in the presence of traumatized or devitalized tissue and often produce a feculant odor (7).

Gram-Positive Anaerobes

ANAEROBIC STREPTOCOCCI (PEPTOSTREPTOCOCCI) AND ANAEROBIC STAPHYLOCOCCI (PEPTOCOCCI)

These strictly anaerobic cocci are isolated very commonly in the vagina and in cultures from obstetric and gynecologic infections. Penicillin is the drug of choice for infections known to be caused by peptococci and peptostreptococci, but clindamycin, metronidazole, or chloramphenicol are highly effective for the penicillin-allergic patient or for broader anaerobic activity.

CLOSTRIDIAL SPECIES

Strictly anaerobic, plump, gram-positive rods, these microorganisms may be isolated in vaginal secretions of 5–10% of asymptomatic women. The most commonly isolated species is *Clostridium perfringens* (also known as *Clostridium welchii*). Although clostridial species may produce gas gangrene (with septicemia, circulatory collapse, hemolysis, and peritonitis), they are more commonly associated with a much less disseminated infection, which responds promptly to appropriate antibiotic therapy. Simply isolating this microorganism from a pelvic site does not, therefore, indicate life-threatening infection or the need for hysterectomy. Initial therapy for clostridial infections usually consists of the administration of large doses of penicillin intravenously and close patient monitoring. If signs of extension of infection become apparent, debridement (often by transabdominal hysterectomy and bilateral salpingoophorectomy) is required. These signs include worsening clinical condition or failure to respond promptly; parametrial tenderness, crepitus or myalgia; or hypotension, falling central pressure measurements or oliguria despite adequate volume replacement. Radiographic findings of interstitial gas are uncommon and develop late in the clinical course, but an abdominal x-ray film should be obtained.

Gram-Negative Anaerobes

BACTEROIDES SPECIES

These are strictly anaerobic bacilli that produce infections which are often protracted. From recent studies of obstetric infection, the most commonly identified species is *Bacteroides bivius*, which was characterized just recently. Although the susceptibility of this species to penicillin is variable, it is sensitive to clindamycin, chloramphenicol, metronidazole, as well as many of the newer cephalosporins and newer penicillins. *Bacteroides disiens* is also isolated regularly from pelvic infections and has a susceptibility pattern similar to *B. bivius*. The *Bacteroides fragilis* group have been identified less commonly in recent studies, but still play an important role. In 1976, three subspecies of *B. fragilis* were reinstated as species. *B. fragilis thetaiotaomicron* became *B. thetaiotaomicron*; *B. fragilis vulgaris* became *B. vulgaris*; and *B. fragilis distasonis* became *B. distasonis*. Because members of this group have been recognized by clinicians for their resistance to many antibiotics and their frequent involvement in pelvic and abdominal infections, it is necessary to maintain this connotation for all these species with a simple designation. Thus, in clinical literature, these species are commonly referred to as the *B. fragilis* group. Agents of choice for the therapy of *B. fragilis* group infections are clindamycin, metronidazole, and chloramphenicol. Of the newer cephalosporins, cefoxitin and moxalactam have the best in vitro activity against the *B. fragilis* group (8). Also piperacillin, mezlocillin, and related drugs, in large parenteral doses, are also active against the vast majority of *B. fragilis* species. Newer tetracycline derivatives such as doxycycline may be more active than the older tetracycline preparations. Previously, it was presumed that *Bacteroides* species other than the *B. fragilis* were susceptible to penicillin. Recently, multiinstitutional studies in in vitro susceptibility have noted increasing resistance by *B. melaninogenicus* and others.

FUSOBACTERIA

Fusobacteria are isolated far less frequently than *Bacteroides* and are usually involved in polymicrobial infections. They appear to be less virulent than *Bacteroides* and are generally susceptible to penicillin, clindamycin, chloramphenicol, metronidazole, and many of the newer penicillins and cephalosporins.

LOW VIRULENCE ISOLATES

Included in this category are: lactobacilli, diphtheroids, *S. epidermidis*, and less commonly isolated anaerobic species such as *Propionibacterium*, *Veillonella*, and *Eubacterium* species.

Quantitatively the most abundant isolate in vaginal cultures of healthy women is lactobacillus, which plays an important role in keeping vaginal pH low (<4.5). *S. epidermidis* has been found in widely ranging percentage (12–90%) of vaginal cultures (9).

Although these organisms are commonly isolated (in combination with more virulent ones) from infected sites, they do not require specific antibiotic treatment. Similarly, they are often reported in urine cultures, but in nearly all instances represent contamination in collection or transport.

YEASTS AND ACTINOMYCES

Yeasts are commonly isolated from the vagina. *Candida albicans* is clearly the most common yeast found in vaginal cultures, but other *Candida* sp. and *Torulopsis glabrata* are seen also. *C. albicans* is responsible for 25–40% of cases and is commonly identified by direct microscopy of a KOH preparation or by culture. Vaginal candidiasis is treated topically by a number of agents or by new oral agents (such as ketoconazole). Systemic *Candida* infections in obstetric or gynecologic patients are unusual and are limited to those patients who have received protracted antibiotic or immunosuppressive therapy or who have debilitating diseases.

The genus *Actinomyces* is classified between true bacteria and molds. *Actinomyces israelii*, an anaerobic or microaerophilic organism, is a rare cause of pelvic infection but has been isolated in pelvic abscesses associated with intrauterine devices. In a representative study, *A. israelii* has been identified in 8% of IUD users but in 0% of women not using IUDs. Actinomyces are susceptible to penicillin (10).

TRICHOMONADS

Trichomonas vaginalis, a flagellated parasite, is found in vaginal secretions of approximately 6% of women and is responsible for one-quarter of cases of infectious vaginitis. *T. vaginalis* is commonly detected by direct microscopy of a wet mount of vaginal secretions. These flagellates are larger than white cells and have great motility in fresh preparations. *T. vaginalis* may also be detected on the Papanicolau smear, but the reliability of this technique is uncertain. Most authors believe that culture for *T. vaginalis* is more sensitive than the wet mount (11). Trichomoniasis is treated with metronidazole (Flagyl) or related 5-nitroimidazole derivatives.

Because this organism is transmitted sexually, partners are often treated as well.

MYCOPLASMAS

These cell wall-deficient microorganisms are distinctly different, morphologically and biochemically, from bacteria and L forms. *Mycoplasma hominis* and *Ureaplasma urealyticum* (formerly T-form mycoplasmas) are isolated with great frequency from the genital tract (12). *M. hominis* has been found in blood cultures of women with postpartum fever in studies in Boston and Seattle, and in San Antonio we isolated it more commonly in amniotic fluid from patients with intraamniotic infection. *Ureaplasma* has been implicated in chorioamnionitis, recurrent abortion, and infertility.

Culturing of mycoplasmas requires special techniques that are not available in most hospital or commercial laboratories. *M. hominis* is susceptible to tetracyclines, clindamycin, and lincomycin, whereas ureaplasmas are sensitive to tetracyclines and erythromycin.

CHLAMYDIA TRACHOMATIS

Chlamydia are intracellular bacteria, which are involved in a variety of genital and perinatal infections (13). From 2–25% of women have positive cervical cultures for *C. trachomatis*. Isolation rates of approximately 25% are found in high risk groups, such as women attending venereal disease clinics. Overall, the incidence of cervical infection in the United States would probably average 3–6%. In males, they are responsible for many instances of nongonococcal urethritis, and in females evidence of their virulence has been accumulating. Recent work from Scandinavia and the United States has strengthened their role in pelvic inflammatory disease, and especially in subsequent tubal obstruction (14). Newborns may acquire this microorganism from the maternal genital tract. If so, approximately 40% subsequently develop conjunctivitis, and 10% develop a late-onset pneumonia (13).

Tetracyclines are the antibiotics of choice in treating chlamydial infection, but erythromycin and sulfonamides may be used when alternatives are needed as in pregnancy.

VIRUSES

Only two viruses are commonly found in the female genital tract. Herpes simplex virus is well-known as a cause of an ulcerative, usually self-limited, lower genital tract infection (15).

Herpesvirus can also cause asymptomatic cervical infection. In surveys of adult females, this virus has been isolated from the genitalia in 0.02–1%.

In the past, nearly all isolates of *Herpesvirus* in the genital tract were of serologic type 2. More recently, 85% have been type 2, whereas 15% have been serotype 1, which more commonly causes oral lesions. Active maternal genital herpes infection at the time of delivery commonly leads to fulminant neonatal infection. Serologic surveys show that from 30 to 90% of reproductive age females have serum antibody to *Herpesvirus*, type 2. The most reliable method for detecting herpes infection is the culture. Clinical diagnosis and Papanicolau smear are less sensitive. Acyclovir (Zovirax) has recently become available for treatment of genital herpes infections. (Please see Chapter 13.)

Cytomegalovirus is the most common virus found in the female genital tract (15). It is found in the cervix in 3–18% of pregnant women, more commonly in indigent, young, primarous women. Serologic evidence of past infection is found in 20–70% of adults. Genital infections are asymptomatic and occur mainly in seropositive women. Cytomegalovirus may be transmitted vertically to the fetus by transplacental infection. It is estimated that 0.5–2.5% of neonates have this congenital infection, but most cases are asymptomatic. An additional 3–5% of newborns acquire cytomegalovirus during delivery. If a mother has CMV in her genital tract, there is a 30–50% chance that her neonate will acquire the virus.

CMV may be detected by culture, and several antibody tests are available. There is no known treatment for CMV infection.

CHANGES IN VAGINAL MICROFLORA

One should not conclude from this description of vaginal microflora that it is a static situation. Certainly, there are vast differences in flora between different groups of women, and interesting shifts in the flora of one particular woman from time to time.

Age

Vaginal colonization by lactobacilli appears to be less common among prepubertal girls than among menstruating women. Further, it is suggested that postmenopausal women also have a decrease in *Lactobacillus* colonization, but that

treatment with estrogens results in a higher rate of recovery of lactobacilli and probably of diphtheroids (9). Thus, there would seem to be an important interaction between vaginal colonization and hormonal milieu. Changes have been reported in other groups of bacteria with aging, but the conclusions are less uniform.

Pregnancy and Delivery

During pregnancy it has been suggested by a number of studies that there is a progressive increase in colonization by *Lactobacillus*, but changes in other bacterial groups were not well established (9). After delivery, however, dramatic changes in vaginal flora occur. There are marked increases in anaerobic species by the third postpartum day. Possible predisposing features to anaerobic vaginal colonization in postpartum women include trauma, presence of lochia and suture material, examinations in labor, and changes in hormonal levels. By the 6th week postpartum the vaginal flora is restored to a normal distribution.

Surgery

Major procedures such as hysterectomy lead to wide changes in vaginal flora including decreases in lactobacilli and diphtheroids and increases in aerobic and anaerobic gram-negative rods (predominantly *E. coli* and various *Bacteroides* species). In addition, most investigators have noted a further shift when prophylactic or therapeutic antibiotics have been used. As expected, use of antibiotics results in a decrease in susceptible flora and a corresponding increase in resistant organisms (9).

References

1. Ledger WJ, Headington JT: Group A beta-hemolytic streptococcus, an important cause of serious infections in obstetrics and gynecology. *Obstet Gynecol* 39:474, 1972.
2. Baker CJ: Summary of the workshop on perinatal infections due to group B streptococci. *J Infect Dis* 136:137, 1977.
3. Garrison RN, Fry DE, Berberich S, et al: Enterococcal bacteremia, clinical implications and determinants of death. *Ann Surg* 196:43, 1982.
4. Blanco JD, Gibbs RS, Castaneda YS: Bacteremia in obstetrics: clinical course. *Obstet Gynecol* 58:621, 1981.
5. Pheifer TA, Forsyth PS, Durfee MA, et al: Nonspecific vaginitis, role of *Haemophilus vaginalis* and treatment with metronidazole. *N Engl J Med* 298:1429, 1978.
6. Sexually transmitted diseases treatment guide-

lines 1982. *MMWR* 31:375, 1982.

7. Sweet RL: Anaerobic infections of the female genital tract. *Am J Obstet Gynecol* 122:891, 1975.

8. Tally FP, Cuchural GJ, Jacobus NV, et al: Susceptibility of the *Bacteroides fragilis* group in the United States. *Antimicrob Agents Chemother* 23:536, 1983.

9. Larsen B, Galask RP: Vaginal microbial flora: practical and theoretic relevance. *Oobstet Gynceol* 55:100(s), 1980.

10. Hager WD, Douglas B, Majumudar B: Pelvic colonization with actinomyces in women using intrauterine contraceptive devices. *Am J Obstet Gynecol* 135:680, 1979.

11. Spence MR, Hollander DH, Smith J, et al: The clinical and laboratory diagnosis of *Trichomonas vaginalis* infection. *Sex Transm Dis* 7:168, 1980.

12. Taylor-Robinson D, McCormack: The genital mycoplasmas. *N Engl J Med* 302:1003, 1063, 1980.

13. Schachter J: Chlamydial infections. *N Engl J Med* 298:428, 1978.

14. Sweet RL: Chlamydial salpingitis and infertility. *Fertil Steril* 38:530, 1982.

15. Amstey MS: Maternal viral infection with adverse results: cytomegalovirus and herpes virus. *Semin Perinatol* 1:1, 1977.

CHAPTER 2

Use of the Microbiology Laboratory in Infectious Diseases

Several factors have contributed to an increasing communication gap between clinicians and the microbiology laboratory (1). Firstly, the introduction of potent antimicrobial agents with their dramatic favorable impact upon mortality due to infection in obstetrics and gynecology has lulled clinicians into complacency. Secondly, the trend to centralize laboratory facilities made it difficult for: (a) clinicians to work with laboratory personnel; (b) for the central microbiology laboratory to meet the needs for obtaining and transporting specimens; and (c) for the laboratory to recover and identify the tremendous variety of microorganisms now recognized to be human pathogens. Thirdly, as academic microbiology departments have focused on basic research involving molecular biology, medical students may graduate with minimal background in clinical microbiology and infectious disease. Lastly, the virtual explosion in knowledge and technology related to the field of microbiology has widened the gap between the reality of microbiology laboratory capabilities and the clinicians understanding of these capabilities and their application to patient care.

This chapter will review the role played by the microbiology laboratory in clinical medicine, describe the proper collection of specimens, and emphasize the important role clinicians must take in providing the laboratory with appropriate specimens in a timely manner and adequate patient information to enable the laboratory to perform its job.

The basic purpose of the microbiology laboratory is to isolate and identify microorganisms that cause clinical disease (2). However, the laboratory must be capable of dealing with a wide variety of specimens from a multitude of clinical infection sites and which require a diversity of collection-transports systems. Physicians look to the laboratory not only to assist them in the diagnosis and treatment of infec-

tious diseases, but expect the laboratory to: (a) produce clinically useful results rapidly; (b) establish rapid reporting systems; (c) provide guidelines for proper specimen collection and transport; and (d) instigate interpretive reporting for unusual microorganisms, normal flora, and monitoring of therapeutic response.

As for the physician, she (he) must provide the laboratory with pertinent patient information, perform appropriate specimen collection, ensure that specimens are transported properly and promptly to the laboratory, and request isolation of suspected pathogenic organisms. In addition, it is incumbent upon the clinician to not inundate the laboratory with requests for routine examinations. Most importantly, the physician must be prepared to interpret and act upon results provided by the laboratory.

Finally, physicians must also be cognizant of problems that exist for the laboratory in their attempt to provide timely results. Culture methodology relies upon isolation of living organisms, and this requires time (generally measured in days). Microbiology, unfortunately, is not a standardized art, and each microorganism has its own requirements for growth. Also, different microbiology laboratories have variable capabilities for isolating microorganisms, especially those, such as anaerobic bacteria, *Chlamydia trachomatis*, mycoplasmas, and viral agents, which require sophisticated technology and experienced technicians.

Washington has suggested general guidelines for the collection of clinical specimens from infected patients (2). The specimen that is submitted should be obtained from the site of infection and be representative of the infection process. An adequate quantity of material must be obtained to enable the laboratory to perform a complete examination. The clinician must be scrupulously careful to avoid contamination of the specimen by microorganisms that are indigenous to skin and/or mucous membranes (i.e., oral cavity, vagina, or bowel). Once a specimen is obtained, it should be promptly forwarded to the laboratory. Finally, it is crucial that specimens for culture be obtained prior to institution of antimicrobial treatment.

INFECTIONS OF THE LOWER FEMALE GENITAL TRACT

Clinically important infections of the lower genital tract in women fall into four major categories (see Table 2.1). Symptoms of urethritis may be associated with urinary tract infections or with actual urethral infection. The major etiologic agents for urethritis are the sexually transmitted agents *Neisseria gonorrhoeae* and *C. trachomatis*. To obtain an appropriate urethral specimen, a sterile calcium alginate swab (Calgiswab) is inserted 2–3 cm into the urethral orifice, twirled slowly, and allowed to remain for 10–15 sec. Direct smear of an urethral specimen can be made for *N. gonorrhoeae*; either methylene blue or gram stain can be used. Methylene blue is quicker and as accurate as the gram stain for identifying the typical intracellular diplococci of the gonococcus. Unlike the cervix, direct smears for GC from the urethra have a high degree of sensitivity and specificity (3). Direct smear for detection of *C. trachomatis* intracellular inclusions from the lower genital tract is fraught with a high degree of inaccuracy and is not recommended. In the future, availability of fluorescent tagged monoclonal antibody direct smears for *C. trachomatis* will allow for rapid, accurate diagnosis of chlamydial urethritis.

N. gonorrhoeae is a fastidious organism that requires an enriched medium, high humidity, and increased CO_2 tension for its optimal growth. The most common selective media is modified Thayer-Martin which contains vancomycin, colistin, nystatin, and trimethoprim to prevent growth of fungi and non-*Neisseria* bacteria. The urethral swab is directly streaked onto the selective media which is placed in either a CO_2 incubator or in a candle jar placed in an incubator. The plates are examined daily for 3 days. Any colonies should be gram-stained to identify gram-negative diplococci and tested for oxidase production to confirm the presence of *N. gonorrhoeae*. Commercially available transport media and systems are available such as Transgrow, Amies, Neigon, JEMBEC, or MICROCULT, but their sensitivity is less than Thayer-Martin media unless they reach the laboratory rapidly (less than 24 hr) (3, 4). For isolation of *C. trachomatis* an adequate specimen requires the presence of cellular material from the epithelium because *C. trachomatis* is an obligate intracellular organism. The calcium alginate swab is placed into a transport system containing a minimal essential media with broad spectrum antibiotics and antifungal agents. Once the media is inoculated, it should be refrigerated at 4°C until taken to the laboratory; if more than 72 hr will lapse before the specimen can be brought to the laboratory, the transport media should be frozen at −20°C (5, 6).

It is now recognized that cervicitis is a true clinical entity. More specifically, mucopurulent endocervicitis has been described as the analagous entity to male urethritis (7). Similarly, *N. gonorrhoeae* and *C. trachomatis* are the major etiologic agents of endocervicitis. Unlike urethral specimens, direct smears for *N. gonorrhoeae* from the cervix lack specificity and sensitivity. Thus, diagnosis of *N. gonorrhoeae* infection of the cervix (symptomatic or asymptomatic) requires isolation and identification of the gonococcus by culture methods as described for urethritis. A single endocervical swab will result in recovery of approximately 90% of *N. gonorrhoeae*, while either two consecutive endocervical swabs or a endocervical plus anal culture will recover over 99% of *N. gonorrhoeae*.

In obtaining specimens for *Chlamydia* it is critical that epithelial cells also be obtained. Preliminary studies by Tam and coworkers suggested that use of fluorescent tagged monoclonal antibodies will allow direct smear identification of *C. trachomatis* infection of the cervix (8). The third pathogen capable of producing cervicitis is herpes simplex virus (HSV). Unlike *N. gonorrhoeae* or *C. trachomatis* HSV involves the ec-

Table 2.1
Causative Agents in Lower Genital Tract Infection of Women

Infection	Etiologic agent
Urethritis	*N. gonorrhoeae*
	C. trachomatis
Cervicitis	*N. gonorrhoeae*
	C. trachomatis
	Herpes simplex virus
Vaginitis	*T. vaginales*
	C. albicans
	G. vaginalis/anaerobes
Vulvitis	Herpes simplex virus
	C. albicans

tocervix as well as the endocervix. Identification of HSV is best accomplished with culture isolation of the viral agent in cell culture. The specimen is placed in a viral transport media such as Hanks or Earle's balanced salt solution which are supplemented with broad spectrum antimicrobials to kill bacteria and fungi. Optimally, specimens for viral isolation should be taken immediately to the laboratory after collection. If a delay of greater than 24 hr is anticipated, the specimen should be frozen; for less than 24 hr delay refrigeration is sufficient. Demonstration of multinucleated giant cells on cytologic specimens from the cervix is diagnostic of HSV infection, but negative smears do not rule out HSV infection.

The most common infectious disease seen by obstetrician-gynecologists is vaginitis. Fortunately, the etiologic agent responsible for the symptoms and/or signs of vaginitis can be identified rapidly in the office or clinic by use of simple, inexpensive methodology. The diagnosis of trichimoniasis is generally made by demonstration of motile *Trichimonas vaginalis* organisms on a wet mount preparation; microscopic examination of wet mounts detects nearly 90% of trichimonas vaginitis. Culture such as Diamond's media is available and will detect 100% of *T. vaginalis. Candida albicans* infection is usually made by identifying the presence of pseudohyphae on a 10% KOH preparation or methylene blue stain. Culture is available, although generally not necessary; Nickerson's media is the most sensitive. The diagnosis of nonspecific vaginitis (vaginosis) due to a synergistic *Gardnerella vaginalis* anaerobic bacteria infection does not require culture methodology. In fact, nearly 60% of normal healthy women have *G. vaginalis* as part of their normal vaginal flora. The criteria for diagnosis of NSV include demonstration of: (a) a homogeneous vaginal discharge; (b) vaginal pH more than 4.5; (c) presence of "clue" cells (squamous epithelial cells to whose border are adhered *G. vaginalis*); and (d) release of a "fishy" amine odor on addition of 10% KOH to vaginal secretions (9). Culture of *G. vaginalis* is best accomplished with use of a selective and differential media, Columbia CNA agar base supplemented with 2 mg amphotericin B/ml (10). Holmes and coworkers have reported on the use of gas-liquid chromotography to identify the presence of short-chained organic acids which are produced by the anaerobic bacteria that are associated with nonspecific vaginosis (9).

INFECTIONS OF THE UPPER GENITAL TRACT

As discussed in depth in Chapter 9, infections involving the upper genital tract (i.e., uterus, fallopian tubes, ovaries, and pelvic peritoneal cavity) are typically of mixed anaerobic-aerobic bacterial etiology (11). Pelvic inflammatory disease (PID) is also associated with sexually transmitted organisms, especially *N. gonorrhoeae, C. trachomatis*, and possibly *Mycoplasma hominis* (12). Table 2.2 lists the more common type of soft tissue pelvic infections encountered in clinical practice, the appropriate site from which to obtain specimen(s), and the microorganisms assumed to be pathogens at these sites.

Because the pathogens involved in upper genital tract infections generally arise from the normal flora of the vagina and cervix (except *N. gonorrhoeae, C. trachomatis*, and group A β-hemolytic *Streptococcus*) microbiological isolation attempts must bypass the heavy bacterial colonization of the lower female genital tract (11). In addition, anaerobic bacteria are such prevalent pathogens in pelvic infections that microbiologic methodology should be employed that is appropriate for the recovery of anaerobic bacteria.

In patients with endomyometritis following delivery (vaginal or cesarean) or abortion, the appropriate specimen for culture is an endometrial aspirate. This is best obtained with the use of a telescoping double plastic cannula with an inner wire brush (13) which nicely prevents contamination with the vaginal and cervical flora. The cervix is an inappropriate site from which to obtain specimens for anaerobic and facultative bacteria because it has both a rich microflora of anaerobes and aerobes and does not accurately reflect the pathogens present in the upper genital tract. Patients with acute pelvic inflammatory disease should have their cervix cultured for *N. gonorrhoeae* and *C. trachomatis* as described above in the section on lower genital tract infection. Specimens from the endometrial aspirate are submitted for isolation of anaerobic and facultative bacteria, *C. trachomatis* and *N. gonorrhoeae*.

The ideal site for specimens in acute PID is the fallopian tube. To obtain cultures from the tube requires the use of laparoscopy. Thus, it is limited due to logistical and economic concerns. If laparoscopy is performed, cultures should be obtained from the fallopian tubes and cul de sac for anaerobic and facultative bacteria, *N. gon-*

Table 2.2
Appropriate Microbiologic Specimens from Soft Tissue Infections of the Female Upper Genital Tract

Type of infection	Appropriate site for specimen	Microorganisms cultured for
Endomyometritis	Endometrial/aspirate	Anaerobic bacteria Facultative bacteria
Pelvic inflammatory disease	Endocervix	N. gonorrhoeae C. trachomatis
	Fallopian tube by lapscope	N. gonorrhoeae
	Culdocentesis	C. trachomatis
	Endometrial aspirate	Anaerobes Facultatives ? M. hominis
Post hysterectomy pelvic cellulitis	Peritoneal cavity Fluid (culdocentesis)	Anaerobes Facultatives
Pelvic abscesses	Aspirate of abscess contents or ideally a piece of tissue from the abscess wall	Anaerobes Facultatives

orrhoeae and C. trachomatis. Culdocentesis has been widely employed to obtain peritoneal fluid as a specimen which is processed for anaerobic and facultative bacteria, N. gonorrhoeae, and C. trachomatis. While better than cervical cultures, culdocentesis is limited because of a high degree of vaginal contamination (14). Recently, we have utilized endometrial aspirates to obtain specimens for culture of anaerobic and facultative bacteria, N. gonorrhoeae and C. trachomatis from the upper genital tract of patients with acute PID (12). The endometrial aspirate is both a more accurate reflection of the microbiologic etiology of PID and better tolerated by the patients (12). Patients with posthysterectomy pelvic cellulitis should have specimens obtained from the peritoneal cavity. This is best accomplished via culdocentesis and submitted for anaerobic and facultative cultures. Similarly, the appropriate specimen in patients with a pelvic abscess is purulent material which has been aspirated from the abscess (either in the operating room or percutaneously) and evaluated for anaerobic and facultative bacteria and, in the case of tuboovarian abscess, N. gonorrhoeae. In fact, the ideal specimen from an abscess for culture attempts is tissue obtained from the abscess wall at the time of surgery.

Because of the presence of anaerobic bacteria the collection and transport of the specimens obtained from the upper genital tract require special methodology to ensure their survival. Fluid or pus aspirated into a syringe is the preferred method of specimen collection; there

is no place for using swabs to obtain specimens for anaerobic culture when fluid is available. Transport media are available such as trypticase soy broth or thioglycolate broth. The use of transport media is convenient and easy but is associated with a false-negative rate of 40%. The preferred method is to utilize anaerobically sterilized, prereduced cultures, such as CO_2-filled tubes or gas packs. The simplest approach is use of a capped syringe from which air has been expelled. A single specimen will suffice for anaerobic and facultative organisms; the latter grow anaerobically as well as under aerobic conditions. The use of anaerobic tubes or a syringe requires prompt transport to the laboratory.

The gram stain is an important clinical tool in the management of upper genital tract infections. It allows for prompt identification of bacterial pathogens and provides a quality control mechanism on the culture techniques being used, especially as related to recovery of anaerobes. The presence of bacteria on the gram-stained smear in the face of negative cultures should raise concerns as to the adequacy of the anaerobic methodology being used for collection of specimens and/or the laboratories capability to grow and identify anaerobic bacteria.

URINARY TRACT INFECTIONS

Infections involving the urinary tract are among the most common infections seen by obstetrician-gynecologists in their practice. Thus, it is important to understand the methods available for proper collection and handling of urine specimens for microbiologic evaluation (1). While the absolute criteria for the diagnosis of urinary tract infection (UTI), in both symptomatic and asymptomatic patients, rests on the presence of a positive culture from a properly collected and handled urine specimen that has not been contaminated by vulvo/vaginal bacteria, immediate microscopic examination of urine sediment may often be helpful (1).

Because of the desire to limit the use of catheterization, a midstream, clean catch urine has become the most widely obtained specimen for both culture and microscopic evaluation of urine. It is important that the patient be properly instructed in how to obtain a midstream, clean catch urine specimen. At least a 4-h period should have elapsed since the last voiding. An alternative method, favored by some urologists, is suprapubic bladder aspiration. However, this method is not commonly employed by obstetrician-gynecologists.

Kass popularized the use of quantitative urine cultures and established the criterion of $\geq 10^5$ bacteria/ml for the diagnosis of UTI (16). This criterion is reliable for acute pyelonephritis and asymptomatic bacteriuria. Moreover, in women two consecutive cultures with $\geq 10^5$ bacteria/ml are required for the diagnosis of asymptomatic bacteriuria. However, Stamm and co-workers have demonstrated that a criterion of $\geq 10^5$ bacteria/ml is unreliable in association with acute bacterial cystitis (17). They noted a 50% false-negativity with a single specimen using this criterion. In patients with acute cystitis, a midstream clean catch urine with $\geq 10^2$ bacteria/ml is the appropriate criterion (17).

Urine is an excellent culture medium at room temperature. In such conditions, bacteria in urine double every 45 min. A 6 hr delay at room temperature will result in 10^3 bacteria/ml increasing to 10^5 bacteria/ml. Thus, it is imperative that the urine specimen be promptly transported to the laboratory; or if more than 1–2 hr delay will occur, the urine should be refrigerated.

Among the rapid methods available to detect $\geq 10^5$ bacteria/ml, microscopic exam of a urine specimen is most commonly employed. A gram stain of well mixed, unspun urine which demonstrates 2 bacteria per high power field has a 90% correlation with results of quantitative cultures. In addition, it allows for determination of the adequacy of the specimen by demonstrating absence of epithelial cells. In contradistinction, demonstration of pyuria (more than 5 WBC/HPF of centrifuged specimen) has variable sensitivity (pyuria is present in 90% of symptomatic UTIs, but only 50% of asymptomatic bacteriuria) and poor specificity (17).

Many chemical methods have been introduced to detect significant bacteriuria in urine specimens (17). These include the Griess test, tetrazolium reduction, glucose oxidase, and catalase. The best of the chemical tests is the Griess test, which measures conversion of nitrate to nitrite. However, it is valid only for gram-negative bacteria, is useful only if positive, and has a false-negative rate of nearly 50%. It is commercially available as N-multistix (Ames), Microstix-3 (Ames), Chemstrip-8 (Bio Dynamics), or Bac-U-Dip (Warner/Chilcott).

In office practice, especially for routine screening of prenatal patients, a multitude of office urine culture kits are available. Basically there are three categories of culture kits: (a) Dipstrip with culture pads (Microstix-3); (b) coated shell, coated tube, or agar cup (Testuria, Speri-Test, Bactercult); and (c) Dipslide (Uricult, Medical Technology Corp), Dipchex (York Scientific). Of these the Dipslide is the most versatile and easiest to use. Most importantly, it is the most accurate, with a 99% correlation with standardized quantitative culture techniques. Thus, it permits inexpensive culture both prior to therapy and as a test of cure. Any organism isolated remains viable for several weeks and is available to be sent to laboratory for identification and susceptibility testing, if necessary.

BACTEREMIA

Fortunately, bacteremia is not a common occurrence in patients with infection on obstetric and gynecologic services. However, bacteremia represents a serious and potentially life-threatening complication of pelvic infections. Thus, it is important to recognize the presence of bacteremia. In order to optimize the ability to diagnose bacteremia, clinicians must be cognizant of the clinical determinants of positive blood cultures.

Most bacteremias are intermittent and usually precede the onset of fever and chills. An exception is intravascular sources such as endocarditis in which bacteremias are continuous. The sensitivity of most media used in blood culture attempts is 2–3 organisms per ml. However, the magnitude for bacteremia is low. Adults with endocarditis or gram-negative bacteremia generally have 10–100 colony-forming units (CFU)/ml (20, 21). Previous antibiotic therapy (even up to 2 weeks prior) may completely or partially suppress growth of bacteria giving false-negative results.

The two major variables in detection of bacteremia are timing of blood cultures and the volume of blood collected. In endocarditis, where bacteremia is continuous, two cultures (from separate venipunctures) at one time is usually adequate. Soft tissue pelvic infections are associated with intermittent bacteremias. In such bacteremias, Washington has demonstrated that the sensitivity of a single culture is 80% (21). Two separate cultures drawn at least 1 hr apart have an 89% sensitivity, and three separate cultures drawn at least one hour apart have a 99% sensitivity. The volume of blood is probably the single most important determinant on the appropriateness of a blood culture specimen (22). A 30-ml sample is associated with a 50% increase in positive results as compared to a 10-ml sample as is drawn by most laboratories.

It is crucial to differentiate the presence of true pathogens from contaminants in interpretation of blood culture results. With pathogenic organisms numerous cultures are positive, and less than 3 days is required for detection of organisms. Pathogenic organisms include gram-negative bacilli, *Staphylococcus aureus*, *Streptococcus faecalis*, group viridans streptococci if multiple, anaerobes, fungi, and yeasts. On the other hand, contaminants are characterized by a single positive culture and greater than 3 days is required for detection of organisms. Typical contaminants in blood cultures include *Corynebacterium* species, *Proprionibacterium* species, group viridans streptococci (single culture), and *Staphylococcus epidermidis*. To prevent such contamination, the venipuncture site must be carefully disinfected prior to obtaining the blood culture. This is crucial because these commensals may be involved in infections of implanted prosthetic material.

Although the incidence of bacteremia arising from soft tissue pelvic infections is relatively low (19), blood cultures are a valuable diagnostic tool in evaluating such infections. A positive culture demonstrating bacteremia identifies a subgroup of patients with severe pelvic infections and who may require more lengthy courses of therapy.

ANTIMICROBIAL SUSCEPTIBILITY TESTS

Antimicrobial agents are among the most commonly used drugs in clinical practice, both office- and hospital-based. Surprisingly, a great deal of confusion exists among clinicians concerning utilization and interpretation of antimicrobial susceptibility testing by the laboratory.

The most common antibiotic test performed in general hospital laboratories has been disc susceptibility. Proper interpretation of disc susceptibility tests depends upon the clinician's understanding the mechanics and the underlying scientific basis of the test (1). The Bauer-Kirby disc diffusion was established as a standardized, reliable, and inexpensive test to evaluate the susceptibility of clinical isolates to antimicrobial agents. The zone sizes are interpreted as susceptible, intermediate, or resistant based on serum levels of antibiotics and according to published criteria based on standard procedures. Disc susceptibility testing was designed for microorganisms which grow rapidly on Mueller-Hinton agar such as staphylococci, Enterobacteriaceae, and *Pseudomonas*. It is not reliable for anaerobic bacteria.

The most accurate measurements of antimicrobial susceptibility are tube dilution tests, which actually are the standards utilized to determine the accuracy of the disc susceptibility tests. However, because they are expensive and time-consuming, the tube dilution tests have not completely replaced disc susceptibility testing. In many major medical centers dilution testing is becoming the primary tool for antimicrobial susceptibility testing. For dilution testing, increasing concentrations of antimicrobial agents are added to either agar or broth, and the medium is then inoculated with the bacterial microorganism to be tested. The minimum inhibitory concentration (MIC) is the lowest concentration of an antibiotic which will inhibit the growth of an organism. These dilution procedures have been made practical for clinical medicine by the use of inocula replicators and microdilution techniques. Interpretation of MIC values requires an understanding of the pharmacokinetics of antimicrobial agents (2). Generally, a microorganism is considered susceptible when the MIC is one half to one quarter of the safely attainable peak serum level of the antimicrobial agent. Susceptibility depends on the drug level at the site of infection. Sensitive levels are present if the peak drug level divided by the MIC equals 2.5 or greater. Intermediate levels are in the 1.5–2.5 range, and resistant levels are less than 1.5. Finally, MIC determination is more versatile, and drug dosage can be adjusted to achieve necessary concentration in various body fluids. Determination of MICs is indicated for: (a) slow growing, fastidious, or anaerobic organisms; (b) to establish activity of potentially toxic agents with intermediate levels of activity when resistance is present to safer drugs; and (c) to test urinary isolates determined to be resistant by disc diffusion tests.

Bactericidal tests are also available. The mean bactericidal concentration (MBC) is the lowest or minimal concentration of an antimicrobial agent that kills 99.9–100% of the test inoculum. There are few clinical indications for determining the MBC (2). Generally, it is used for isolates recovered from serious infections in sites or patients with limited humoral and cellular immunologic capabilities; examples include endocarditis, meningitis, and/or osteomyelitis.

An increasing number of bacterial organisms have acquired the ability to produce β-lactamase enzymes, which precludes therapy with penicillin, ampicillin, and first generation cephalosporins. β-lactamases can be produced by S. aureus, N. gonorrhoeae, H. influenzae, Enterobacteriaceae, and B. fragilis. In appropriate clinical settings, the microbiology laboratory must be capable of testing for β-lactamase enzymes.

Assay of antimicrobial levels is available in many hospitals. The laboratory can determine the amount of antimicrobial agent present in body fluids (e.g., blood, CSF). In general, only patients receiving aminoglycosides (gentamicin, tobramycin, or amikacin) with their narrow therapeutic range are evaluated for antibiotic levels.

SEROLOGY

Serology is useful for diagnosing infectious diseases that are caused by microorganisms which are not easily or quickly recovered by culture. There are two basic approaches to serologic testing: antigen detection and antibody detection. Antigen detection is generally rapid and accurate. It is performed on a specimen of infected tissue (biopsy or body fluid). Antigen detection is useful for many pathogens which are difficult or impossible to culture in the laboratory. Examples include herpes simplex, rotavirus, Legionnaire's disease, and syphilis. Monoclonal antibody technology has stimulated a tremendous explosion of current investigative efforts, and a multitude of new antigen detection tests should be available in the future (e.g., herpes simplex virus, C. trachomatis, N. gonorrhoeae, mycoplasmas).

Serologic tests based on antibody detection

Table 2.3
Infectious Diseases Which Are Commonly Diagnosed by Antibody Response

Single specimen usually adequate	Paired specimens usually required
Amoebic liver abscess	Mycoplasma pneumonias
Brurellosis	Chlamydial diseases
Coccidioidom	Meningoencephalitis
Echinococcal cyst	Cytomegalovirus
Hepatitis A (IgM)	Histoplasmosis
Hepatitis B (IgM and anti-HBCAg)	Legionnaires disease
Anti H-B	Rubeola
Malaria	Mumps
EBV mononucleosis	Rickettsial disease
Group A β-hemolytic streptococci	Rubella
Trichinosis	Tularemia
Neonatal chlamydia pneumonia	Yellow fever

(Table 2.3) generally are slower and less precise than those based on antigen detection. There are frequent cross-reactions between antibodies of the various organisms. A single specimen which measures IgM antibody may be diagnostic. However, most available tests measure IgG and thus cannot differentiate past from present infection. A convalescent specimen is obtained 14–21 days after the initial specimen and must show a 4-fold rise in antibody titer.

The use of serology in the diagnosis of syphilis is fully described in Chapter 3. Initial evaluation involves the use of nontreponemal tests (VDRL, RPR). They are nonspecific and are associated with many false-positives. In addition, they are insensitive in acute primary syphilis, with 25% still negative 2 weeks after the chancre appeared. The major clinical use of the nontreponemal tests is screening, because they are quick and inexpensive. Quantitative titers can be used to evaluate therapy. The FTA-Abs test is the first test to become positive and may stay positive for life. There are rare and transient false-positives (mononucleosis, herpes, hepatitis, LGV, and collagen vascular disease). Its primary clinical use is to confirm positive VDRL or RPR. However, it is expensive and technically difficult. The microhemagglutination assay for T. pallidum (MHA-TP) is easier to perform and less expensive. It has replaced the FTA in many centers.

References

1. Ledger WJ: *Infection in the Female.* Philadelphia, Lea & Febiger, 1977.
2. Washington JA III: The clinician and the microbiology laboratory: bacteria, fungi, and parasites. In Mandel GL, Douglas RG, Bennett JE (eds): *Principles and Practice of Infectious Diseases.* New York, John Wiley & Sons, 1979.
3. Riccardi NB, Felman YM: Laboratory diagnosis in the problem of suspected gonococcal infection. *JAMA* 242:2703–2705, 1979.
4. Spence MR, Guzick DS, Katta RA: The isolation of *Neisseria gonorrhoeae*: a comparison of three culture transport systems. *Sex Transm Dis* 10:138–140, 1983.
5. Kallings I, Mardh P-A: Sampling and specimen handling in the diagnosis of genital *Chlamydia trachomatis* infection. *Scand J Infect Dis* 32(Suppl):21–24, 1982.
6. Sweet RL, Landers DV, Schachter J: Chlamydial infections in obstetrics and gynecology. *Clin Obstet Gynecol* 26:143–164, 1983.
7. Brunham RC, Paavonen J, Stevens CE, et al: Mucopurulent cervicitis—the ignored counterpart in women of urethritis in men. *N Engl J Med* 311:1–6, 1984.
8. Tam MR, Stamm WE, Handsfield HH, et al: Culture independent diagnosis of *Chlamydia trachomatis* using monoclonal antibodies. *N Engl J Med* 310:1146–1150, 1984.
9. Holmes KK: Nonspecific vaginosis. *Scand J InfectDis* 26(Suppl):110, 1981.
10. Totten PA, Amsel, Holmes KK: Selective differential agar medium for isolation of *G. vaginalis*. In *Abstracts of the 80th Annual Meeting of the American Society for Microbiology*, Miami Beach, May, 1980. Abst. 310, Washington, DC, American Society for Microbiology.
11. Sweet RL: Treatment of mixed aerobic-anaerobic infections of the female genital tract. *J Antimicrob Chemother* 8(Suppl D):105–114, 1981.
12. Sweet RL, Schachter J, Robbie MO: Failure of beta-lactam antibiotics to eradicate *Chlamydia trachomatis* from the endometrium of patients with acute salpingitis despite apparent clinical cure. *JAMA* 250:1641–2645, 1983.
13. Knuppel RA, Scerbo JC, Mitchell GW, et al: Quantitative transcervical uterine culture with a new device. *Obstet Gynecol* 57:243–248, 1981.
14. Sweet RL, Draper DL, Schachter J, et al: Microbiology and pathogenesis of acute salpingitis as determined by laparoscopy: what's the appropriate site to sample? *Am J Obstet Gynecol* 138:985–989, 1980.
15. Kass EH: Asymptomatic infections of the urinary tract. *Trans Assoc Am Physicians* 69:56, 1956.
16. Stamm WE, Counts GW, Running KR, et al: Diagnosis of coliform infection in acutely dysuric women. *N Engl J Med* 307:463–468, 1982.
17. Kunin CM: *Detection, Prevention and Management of Urinary Tract Infections*, ed 3. Philadelphia, Lea & Febiger, 1979.
18. Ledger WJ, Norman M, Gee C, Lewis WP: Bacteremia on an obstetric-gynecologic service. *Am J Obstet Gynecol* 121:205–212, 1975.
19. Werner AS: Studies on the bacteremia of bacterial endocarditis. *JAMA* 202:130–134, 1967.
20. Kreger BE: Gram negative bacteremia. III. Reassessment of etiology and ecology in 612 patients. *Am J Med* 68:332–343, 1980.
21. Washington JA (ed): *The Detection of Septicemia.* Boca Raton, FL, CRC Press, 1978.
22. Ilstrup DM, Washington JA: The importance of volume of blood cultured in the detection of bacteremia and fungemia. *Diagn Microbiol Infect Dis* 1:107–110, 1983.

CHAPTER 3

Sexually Transmitted Diseases

During the past two decades there has been a virtual revolution in the field of sexually transmitted diseases. The recognition that we are in the midst of an epidemic of sexually transmitted diseases (STD) has focused increased attention on STD and led to an expanded spectrum and scope of STD. From the classic five venereal diseases of gonorrhea, syphilis, chancroid, lymphogranuloma venereum, and granuloma inguinale, the number of STD agents has grown to over 20 (Table 3.1). In addition, the spectrum of STD includes such diseases as nongonococcal urethritis, epididymitis, vaginitis, cervicitis, pelvic inflammatory disease, infertility, perinatal infections, hepatitis, enteric infections, arthritis syndromes, genital oncogenesis, and immunologic disorders such as AIDs (Table 3.2).

These newly recognized additional STDs do not reflect the emergence of new pathogens nor only the current liberation of sexual attitudes. Rather, the recognition of the epidemic nature of *Chlamydia*, herpes simplex, hepatitis B, and other "new" STD is the result of major technological advances in our ability to recover and identify these organisms and application of sophisticated epidemiologic techniques which have revealed the distribution and determinants of STD in the population.

GONORRHEA

Gonorrhea, which is caused by the gram-negative diplococcus, *Neisseria gonorrhoeae*, is the most commonly reported communicable disease in the United States (1). Man is the only natural host for *N. gonorrhoeae*. Because the organism has a predilection for columnar or pseudostratified epithelium, it is most commonly found in the urogenital tract (2). *N. gonorrhoeae* is a fastidious organism with specific nutrient and environmental needs. Its growth is optimal at pH 7.4, temperature 35.5°C, and a 2–10% CO_2 atmosphere. The virulence of *N. gonorrhoeae* is associated with specific colony types (4). Of the Kellogg colony types 1 through 4, only 1 and 2

which contain pili are capable of producing infection. The pili appear to facilitate attachment of gonococci to epithelial surfaces (5). James and Swanson noted that colony phenotype was also important (6). They reported that transparent colonies are more characteristic in cultures from the endocervix than the male urethra, especially at the time of menses. Draper et al noted that transparent gonococcal colonies were the virulent form obtained from the fallopian tubes of PID patients (7). It is estimated that approximately 3 million cases occur annually in the United States. In men the gonococcus is a major etiologic agent for urethritis, proctitis, epididymitis, and prostatitis. Among nonpregnant women *N. gonorrhoeae* is an important cause of urethritis, cervicitis, and pelvic inflammatory disease (8). Pharyngeal gonorrhea and disseminated gonorrhea occur in men and women. Infection with *N. gonorrhoeae* in pregnancy is also a major concern. Gonorrheal ophthalmia neonatorum has long been recognized as a major consequence of maternal infection. More recently an association between maternal gonococcal infection and disseminated gonococcal infection, amniotic infection syndrome, and perinatal complications such as premature ruptured membranes, chorioamnionitis, prematurity, intrauterine growth retardation, neonatal sepsis, and postpartum endometritis has been recognized.

Epidemiology

N. gonorrhoeae infects both males and females; the primary site of involvement is the genitourinary tract. In males, the infection is usually an acute symptomatic urethritis. Female infection is often asymptomatic, and the primary site of involvement is the endocervical canal and the transition zone of the cervix. Recently it has been recognized that women with endocervical gonorrhea frequently are symptomatic, and most commonly they present

Table 3.1
Sexually Transmitted Pathogens

Bacterial agents	Viral agents
N. gonorrhoeae	Herpes simplex virus
C. trachomatis	Hepatitis B virus
M. hominis	Cytomegalovirus
U. urealyticum	Human papilloma virus
T. pallidum	Molluscum contagiosum virus
G. vaginalis	
H. ducreyi	Protozoan agents
Shigella	T. vaginalis
Campylobacter	E. histolytica
Group B Streptococcus	G. lamblia
Fungal agents	Ectoparasites
C. albicans	P. pubis
	S. scabiei

Table 3.2
Major Sexually Transmitted Diseases

Syndrome/complication	STD agent(s)
Pelvic inflammatory disease	N. gonorrhoeae, C. trachomatis, M. hominis (?)
Infertility	N. gonorrhoeae, C. trachomatis, M. hominis (?), U. ureaplasma (?)
Ectopic pregnancy	N. gonorrhoeae, C. trachomatis, M. hominis (?)
Female lower genital tract infection:	
Vulvitis	C. albicans, herpes simplex virus
Vaginitis	C. albicans, T. vaginalis, G. vaginalis
Cervicitis	N. gonorrhoeae, C. trachomatis, herpes simplex virus
Urethritis	N. gonorrhoeae, C. trachomatis
Pregnancy associated:	
Chorioamnionitis	N. gonorrhoeae, M. hominis, group B Streptococcus
Spontaneous abortion/fetal wastage	Herpes simplex virus, T. pallidum
Prematurity/PROM	Group B Streptococcus (?), U. urealyticum (?), C. trachomatis (?), N. gonorrhoeae (?), T. pallidum, HSV
Postpartum endometritis	Group B Streptococcus, N. gonorrhoeae, M. hominis (?), C. trachomatis (?)
Congenital/perinatal infections:	
TORCH syndrome	CMV, HSV, T. pallidum
Sepsis/death	Group B streptococcus, HSV, CMV, T. pallidum
Conjunctivitis	C. trachomatis, N. gonorrhoeae
Pneumonia	C. trachomatis, group B Streptococcus, T. pallidum, CMV(?)
Neurologic impairment	CMV, HSV, T. pallidum, group B Streptococcus
Male genital tract:	
Urethritis	N. gonorrhoeae, C. trachomatis, U. urealyticum (?)
Epididymitis	C. trachomatis, N. gonorrhoeae
Proctitis	N. gonorrhoeae, HSV, C. trachomatis
Genital ulceration	HSV, T. pallidum, H. ducreyi, C. granulomatis, C. trachomatis (LGV)
Hepatitis	Hepatitis B virus, C. trachomatis (?), CMV
Acute arthritis	N. gonorrhoeae, C. trachomatis (?)
Enterocolitis	G. lamblia, E. histolytica, Shigella, Campylobacter

with vaginal discharge, dysuria, and abnormal uterine bleeding (3). In addition, it has been established that a significant reservoir of asymptomatic men with urethral gonorrhea exists.

The current epidemic of gonorrhea commenced in 1957 and reached its peak in 1975 with nearly a 300% increase in gonorrhea cases between 1966 and 1975. Since then gonorrhea rates leveled off and began to fall slightly at an average rate of approximately 1% per year (2, 9) (see Fig. 3.1). During 1983, United States gonorrhea cases were down nearly 7%. Although decreasing, the level of gonorrhea in 1983 remained at major epidemic levels. Of special concern is the increasing rate of gonorrhea among the young age group (15- to 19-year old). Indeed, for the first time, gonorrhea in 5- to 14-year-old children exceeded the combined reported prevalence of measles, mumps, and rubella (9). Many factors contribute to this epidemic, including changes in sexual mores, contraceptive techniques, adequate reporting systems, an increased population mobility, and a large reservoir of asymptomatic patients (males and females) harboring the gonococcus. Over 80% of the reported gonorrhea cases in the United States occur in individuals in the 15- to 29-year-old age group. Although the heaviest concentration is in the 20- to 24-year-old age group, an ever increasing number of adolescents are infected. While gonorrhea in the total population predominates in males by a factor of 1.5:1, among young teenagers this trend is reversed and females predominate.

In the United States between 1973 and 1981, an average of 7.5 million women have been screened annually in non-STD clinic settings with an average gonorrhea detection rate of 2.7%. National surveys have demonstrated that the prevalence rate for gonorrhea among females varies from 1 to 2% for private physician visits to nearly 5% in hospital-based gynecology clinics (1). The incidence of gonorrhea in pregnancy has been reported to range from 0.5 to 7%. Rates as high as 25% have been documented in females attending STD clinics (1).

Risk factors for the acquisition of gonococcal infection have been described. The major deter-

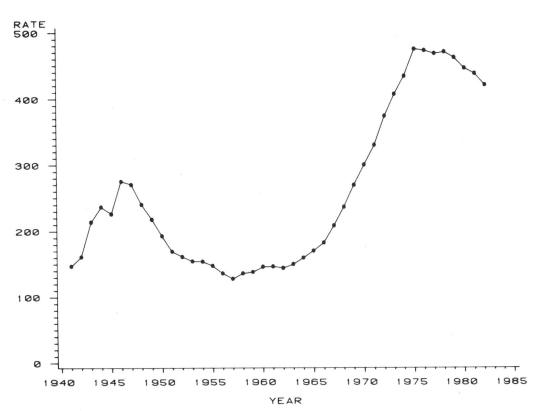

Figure 3.1. Gonorrhea. Reported civilian cases per 100,000 population by year, United States, 1941–1982. (From Centers for Disease Control: Annual summary 1982: reported morbidity and mortality in the United States. *MMWR* 31:29, 1983.)

minant for acquisition of gonorrhea is the prevalence of the disease in the sexual partners. While an association between the number of different sex partners and the risk of acquiring gonorrhea has been shown (10, 11) by some investigators, others have failed to confirm this relationship (12–13). Recently, Ross (14) reported an increased risk of gonorrhea existed only if the number of sexual partners exceeded two per month. Young age is an additional risk factor. The age group 15 through 24 years old has the highest prevalence of gonorrhea. Most likely this is due to the increased number of sex partners, failure to use barrier contraceptive methods which protect against STD, and the risk-taking behavior patterns of teenagers. Socioeconomic status also has been felt to influence the risk of acquiring gonorrhea. However, as noted by Spence, this factor, like that of race or ethnicity, may well reflect a skewing of the data because gonorrhea is most likely to be reported by clinics where nonwhites and the poor seek health care (2).

Transmission of gonorrhea is almost entirely by sexual contact. The female is at greater risk of infection than the male. While it is estimated that a male having a single sexual encounter with a gonorrhea-infected female will become infected 20–25% of the time, the risk of transmission from male to female is estimated at 80–90% (15). A short incubation time of 3–5 days occurs.

Since their identification in 1976, penicillinase-producing *N. gonorrhoeae* (PPNG) strains have steadily increased in frequency in the United States. From the 190 cases in 1977 the number of reported PPNG cases rose to 4507 in 1982, an increase of over 2000%. Approximately 0.5% of gonorrhea infections in the United States are due to PPNG. Although PPNG strains have been reported from at least 43 states, more than 40% have occurred in California. Other high prevalence states include Hawaii, Florida, and New York.

The prevalence of pharyngeal gonococcal infection is to a large degree dependent upon patterns of sexual activity. Bro-Jorgensen and Jensen reported, in an STD clinic, that the prevalence of pharyngeal gonorrhea was 10, 7, and 25% among women, heterosexual males, and homosexual males, respectively (16). Approximately half of the patients with pharyngeal gonorrhea have the pharynx as the only positive site for *N. gonorrhoeae*. The mode of infection is generally associated with the practice of fel-latio; cunnilingus and mouth to mouth kissing are less likely modes of transmission.

CLINICAL MANIFESTATIONS OF MALE UNCOMPLICATED GONORRHEA

N. gonorrhoeae infection in males most often presents as acute urethritis with complaints of urethral discharge and/or burning or discomfort with urination. In the male homosexual population proctitis is also a very common presentation for gonococcal infection.

Recent information has indicated that while the majority of gonococcal infections in men are symptomatic, there exists a pool of asymptomatic male carriers of *N. gonorrhoeae*. In particular, male partners of women with gonococcal PID have a high asymptomatic carrier rate (R.L. Sweet, unpublished data). Although the incidence of asymptomatic cases among all men with gonorrhea is low, they represent a substantial reservoir of gonococcal infection and play a major role in transmission of the gonococcus.

UNCOMPLICATED ANOGENITAL GONORRHEA IN FEMALES

Uncomplicated anogenital gonorrhea in women may involve the endocervix, urethra, Skene's glands, Bartholin's glands, and/or anus; the most commonly infected site is the endocervix. Gonococcal infection of the vagina is rare except in prepubertal and postmenopausal patients. At one time uncomplicated anogenital gonorrhea in females was considered an asymptomatic disease. It is now recognized that although the majority of women harboring *N. gonorrhoeae* are asymptomatic, a large share of women with anogenital gonorrhea are symptomatic.

Curran et al reported that positive gonococcal cultures were obtained at a higher rate from women with symptoms and/or signs of genital tract disease (i.e., abnormal uterine bleeding, dysuria and/or frequency, vaginal discharge, or cervicitis) (3). Similarly, Weisner suggested that between 40–60% of women who have gonorrhea develop some symptoms (17). In 15–20% of women with uncomplicated anogenital gonorrhea, upper genital tract infection (PID) occurs (8). Gonococcal associated PID tends to occur at the end of or just after menstruation. A detailed description of PID and the role of *N. gonorrhoeae* in its etiology and pathogenesis is reviewed in Chapter 4. The cervix infected with

N. gonorrhoeae can appear healthy or reveal an inflamed cervical canal with ectopy and a mucopurulent exudate. In general those signs of gonococcal cervicitis are indistinguishable from other causes of cervicitis, and thus an absolute diagnosis of gonococcal cervicitis requires confirmatory laboratory tests.

Gonococcal infections in pregnant patients are most commonly asymptomatic. The two most common symptoms are vaginal discharge and dysuria. On examination an endocervicitis may be present with erythema and a mucopurulent discharge. Pelvic inflammatory disease may occur during pregnancy, but it is very rare. If routine screening for *N. gonorrhoeae* is not employed during pelvic examinations, the presence of lower genital tract complaints or signs such as abnormal bleeding, discharge, dysuria, mucopurulent endocervicitis, and/or pelvic discomfort should suggest that cultures be obtained to determine if the gonococcus is present.

NONGENITAL GONOCOCCAL SYNDROMES

Nongenital tract gonococcal disease may result from direct or contiguous spread and by bloodstream dissemination. The direct or contiguous spread route occurs for epididymitis, prostatitis, anorectal infection, perihepatitis (Fitz-Hugh-Curtis syndrome), conjunctivitis, and pharyngeal gonococcal infection.

Anorectal gonococcal infection is relatively common among homosexual men, but also 36–44% of women with cervical gonorrhea will have positive anorectal cultures (18). Although penile-anal contact is responsible for approximately three-fourths of anorectal gonorrhea in women, extension of *N. gonorrhoeae* to the anorectum from infected vaginal secretions can occur in women without penile-anal contact (19).

The majority of patients with pharyngeal gonococcal infection are asymptomatic. In patients with symptomatic pharyngeal gonococcus (GC) a mild sore throat and erythema are usually present. However, oral ulcerative lesions and exudate of the pharynx and tonsils may occur.

Rarely, *N. gonorrhoeae* causes conjunctivitis in adults. This usually is the result of direct sexual contact or indirect via contaminated hands, amniotic fluid at delivery, or accidental inoculation in the laboratory with clinical isolates. The typical presentation for gonococcal conjunctivitis is an acute onset of purulent conjunctivitis with extensive inflammation and copious purulent secretions.

DISSEMINATED GONOCOCCAL INFECTIONS

Disseminated gonococcal infection (DGI) occurs when gonococcal bacteremia produces extragenital manifestations of gonococcal infection. The prevalence of DGI among total gonorrhea cases ranges from 0.1 to 0.3%, with females predominating over men by about 4:1 (20, 21). The majority of women with DGI develop symptoms either during pregnancy, especially the third trimester, or within 7 days from the onset of menstruation. Only certain strains of *N. gonorrhoeae* have a predisposition to disseminate. In general they are strains that are highly antibiotic-sensitive (22), resistant to bactericidal activity of human serum (23), and have a unique nutritional requirement for arginine, hypoxanthine, and uracil (i.e., $Arg^- Hyx^- Ura^-$ auxotype) (24). In addition complement deficiencies have been demonstrated to be associated with an increased risk for DGI (25).

Disseminated gonococcal infection manifests two stages: an early bacteremic stage and an arthritis stage. The bacteremic stage is characterized by chills, fever, typical skin lesions, and asymmetric involvement. The bacteremic stage is associated with a dermatitis which is characterized by a variety of skin lesions of gonococcal emboli. These lesions appear initially as small vesicles which become pustules and develop a hemorrhagic base. The center becomes necrotic. These lesions occur on any body region, but are most frequently present on the volar aspects of the upper extremities, the hands, and the digits. These skin lesions resolve spontaneously without residual scarring. Blood cultures are positive for *N. gonorrhoeae* in half of the patients cultured during the bacteremic stage. Bacterial endocarditis occasionally ensues. Joint symptoms are frequently present during this stage, as well as in the septic arthritis phase.

The septic arthritis stage is characterized by a purulent synovial effusion. The knees, ankles, and wrist joints are most commonly involved. Blood cultures during this stage are usually sterile. Gonococci may be isolated from the septic joint during this stage. Since the introduction of penicillin, gonococcal endocarditis and meningitis have been rarely seen complications of DGI.

NEONATAL GONOCOCCAL OPHTHALMIA

Gonococcal ophthalmia neonatorum has been recognized since 1881. Prior to the introduction by Crede of silver nitrate prophylaxis, ophthalmia neonatorum occurred in approximately 10%

of infants born in the United States. Introduction of eye prophylaxis resulted in a rapid reduction in this rate. However, the resurgence of gonorrhea over the past 2 decades has led to a reappearance of gonococcal conjunctivitis in newborns, which is the most common clinical manifestation of *N. gonorrhoeae* in the newborn.

Most newborns who are infected with gonorrhea acquire it during passage through an infected cervical canal. Gonococcal ophthalmia usually is manifested within 4 days after birth, but incubation periods up to 21 days have been reported. A frank purulent conjunctivitis occurs which usually affects both eyes. Untreated gonococcal ophthalmia can rapidly progress to corneal ulceration, resulting in corneal scarring and blindness.

GONOCOCCAL INFECTION IN PREGNANCY AND THE NEONATE

In recent years, postabortal gonococcal endometritis and salpingitis have been recognized with increasing frequency after pregnancy termination. Patients undergoing therapeutic abortion who have untreated endocervical gonorrhea are at increased risk for developing postabortion endometritis (26).

The effects of gonorrheal infection on both mother and fetus have not been fully appreciated until recently (27–30). The amniotic infection syndrome is an additional manifestation of gonococcal infection in pregnancy. This entity presents with placental, fetal membrane, and umbilical cord inflammation which occurs after PROM and which is associated with a positive oral gastric aspirate for *N. gonorrhoeae*, leukocytosis, neonatal infection, and maternal fever. This syndrome is characterized by premature rupture of membranes, premature delivery, and a high infant morbidity and/or mortality.

Recent studies (27–29) have identified an association between untreated maternal endocervical gonorrhea and perinatal complications, including an increased incidence of premature rupture of membranes, preterm delivery, chorioamnionitis, neonatal sepsis, and maternal postpartum sepsis. In addition, a higher incidence of intrauterine growth retardation has been observed in gravid women with gonococcal infection.

Handsfield and colleagues noted that maternal gonococcal infection in the third trimester was associated with an increased risk for PROM, prematurity, chorioamnionitis, fetal infection, neonatal sepsis, and maternal infection postpartum (28). Similarly, Edwards and co-workers demonstrated that GC-positive pregnancy women had an increased incidence of chorioamnionitis, perinatal infections, and intrauterine growth retardation (29). Such investigations demonstrate the need to screen pregnant women (especially among populations at high risk for STD) for *N. gonorrhoeae*. Because almost all patients with gonococcal infection during pregnancy are asymptomatic, we recommend routine cultures for *N. gonorrhoeae* at the initial prenatal visit and early in the third trimester.

Diagnosis

In males the diagnosis of gonococcal urethritis relies for the most part on presumptive evidence. In men with urethral discharge and dysuria, the gram stain of the urethral exudate is considered diagnostic for *N. gonorrhoeae* when gram-negative diplococci are seen within polymorphonuclear leukocytes (31). However, the predictive accuracy of the gram stain is markedly influenced by the experience of the technician interpreting urethral smears. The majority of women with gonorrhea (pregnant and nonpregnant) are asymptomatic. Thus, the diagnosis of these infections depends upon sampling of potential infected sites. The major site of primary infection in women is the endocervix. The anal canal, urethra, and pharyngeal cavity are important sites to consider, as well. Unfortunately, microscopic examination of a gram-stained specimen from the infected site produces a diagnosis of gonorrhea in only 60% of women compared with 95% of men. In women the diagnosis of *N. gonorrhoeae* infection requires isolation of the organism by culture. Ideally, all sexually active women should be screened at every opportunity (i.e., annual routine pelvic examinations, presenting with gynecologic complaints). Obviously this would be a major logistic and economic burden, especially in patient populations with low rates (<1%) of gonorrhea. At a minimum, certain at risk patient groups should be routinely screened. These include partners of men with gonorrhea or urethritis, women with symptoms and signs referred to the lower genital tract, patients with known other STDs, patients with multiple sexual partners, and patients with pelvic inflammatory disease. All pregnant women should have a culture for *N. gonorrhoeae* obtained during their initial prenatal visit. In patients at high risk for gonorrheal infection, cultures should be repeated in the third trimester.

Clinical isolation is best performed using a

selective media for *N. gonorrhoeae*, such as Thayer-Martin medium containing the antibiotics vancomycin, colistin, and nystatin, which inhibits the growth of contaminating organisms present in the same body sites as the gonococcus. Culture remains the sine qua non for diagnosing endocervical gonorrhea. The proper collection, handling, and processing of culture specimens is crucial to obtaining accurate results. A dry, sterile cotton-tipped swab is inserted into the endocervical canal, moved from side to side, and allowed to remain for 15–30 sec for absorption of organisms to the swab. The specimen is then plated onto selective media for *Neisseria* sp. (i.e., Thayer-Martin or New York City). Following inoculation this media should be placed in a carbon dioxide incubator or candle jar to provide an adequate concentration of carbon dioxide. A modification of this medium is the addition of trimethoprim to prevent *Proteus* contamination. When culture facilities are not readily available, a holding or transport medium should be used. Goodhart and co-workers recently reviewed the results with these various systems (32). Transport via holding media such as Aime's, Culturette, or Stuart's was associated with a 10–79% loss of isolates after 24 hr. Use of an environmental chamber (JEMBEC) for transport led to a 7–22% loss of isolates after 1 day and 4–55% loss after 3 days (i.e., over a weekend). Transgrow medium is a modification of the Thayer-Martin selective medium, which is available to clinicians in a bottle sealed under carbon dioxide tension. After inoculation of the specimen onto the Transgrow medium, the bottle is resealed and transported (or mailed) to an appropriate laboratory. However, delays in transport significantly decrease the reliability of this system, and in general Transgrow has not proven to be practical.

The diagnosis of a *N. gonorrhoeae* infection is made by identification of the organism with a typical growth on selective media, a positive oxidase reaction, and a gram-negative diplococcal morphology on gram stain of the isolated colonies. Fermentation reactions may be also performed which take advantage of the ability of the gonococcus to ferment glucose, but not sucrose or maltose.

For optimal yield of *N. gonorrhoeae*, either two consecutive endocervical specimens or a combination of an endocervical and an anal specimen should be obtained. A single endocervical swab will miss approximately 10% of gonococcal infection. Gonococcal pharyngitis is more frequently encountered in females. Although these cases often present with clinical symptoms similar to other types of pharyngitis, the disease may be asymptomatic. In patients with sore throat or with history of oral-genital contact, cultures should be obtained from the tonsillar area and from the pharynx behind the uvula. The limitations of the gram stain and the time delay associated with culture for *N. gonorrhoeae* has led to a search for methods to provide rapid and accurate diagnosis of *N. gonorrhoeae* infection. Serodiagnosis for gonorrhea has been disappointing because of persistence of antibody due to previous gonococcal disease. The Gonozyme test is a solid-phase enzyme immunoassay for detecting gonococcal antigens in urethral and/or endocervical specimens (33). However, its requirement for numerous steps, multiple reagents, a prolonged time (i.e., >1 hr), and need for a spectrophotometer may limit its usefulness. Jaffe and colleagues evaluated the Genetic Transformation Test (a method to detect gonococcal DNA) and noted it to be comparable to culture in accuracy (34). This test requires mailing of specimens to special laboratories resulting in long delays. Although the most reliable method for diagnosis of *N. gonorrhoeae* remains culture, antigen detection techniques which are very sensitive and specific will probably be the diagnostic approach of the near future.

Treatment

UNCOMPLICATED GONORRHEA

N. gonorrhoeae is sensitive to a large number of antimicrobial agents including penicillins, tetracyclines, cephalosporins, erythromycin, aminoglycosides, and aminocyclitols (35). The guidelines for treatment of uncomplicated and complicated gonococcal disease have been recently updated by the Centers for Disease Control (35). Both men and nonpregnant women with uncomplicated gonococcal infection are treated with the same drug regimens (Table 3.3). Gonococcal strains which are susceptible to penicillin are successfully eradicated by single dose therapy with aqueous procaine penicillin, ampicillin, or amoxicillin. Either tetracycline hydrochloride or doxycycline are effective multiple-day approaches for gonococcal therapy. The single dose approach with one of the penicillins has the advantage of low cost and excellent compliance; however, it is inadequate therapy for *Chlamydia trachomatis* which coexists in 20–40% of men with gonococcal urethritis and 30–

Table 3.3
Centers for Disease Control Recommended Regimens for Treatment of Uncomplicated Anogenital Gonorrhea in Adults, 1982

1. Single dose regimens:
    Tetracycline HCl: 500 mg by mouth, 4 times a day for 7 days (Doxycycline (100 mg by mouth twice a day for 7 days) may be substituted)

    or

    Amoxicillin/ampicillin: amoxicillin (3.0 g) or ampicillin (3.5 g) either with 1.0 g probenecid by mouth

    or

    Aqueous procaine penicillin G: 4.8 million units intramuscularly at 2 sites with 1.0 g probenecid by mouth
2. Combined regimen
    Amoxicillin/ampicillin: amoxicillin (3.0 g) or ampicillin (3.5 g) either with 1 g probenecid by mouth

    plus

    Tetracycline HCl: 500 mg, by mouth, 4 times a day for 7 days. (Doxycycline (100 mg, by mouth, twice a day for 7 days) may be substituted)
3. Treatment failures on nonspectinomycin regimens
    Spectinomycin: 2.0 g IM
4. Penicillinase-producing *N. gonorrhoeae*
    Spectinomycin: 2.0 g IM
    Alternate regimens:
    Cefoxitin (2.0 g IM) plus oral probenecid (1.0 g)

    or

    Cefotaxime (1.0 g IM)

50% of women with gonococcal cervicitis (36). While the multiple day tetracycline regimens are effective against coexisting chlamydial infection, they require patient compliance for success. If such compliance is lacking the emergence of tetracycline-resistant gonococcal strains and/or asymptomatic carriers of GC are encouraged. In order to address the problems of coexisting chlamydial infection and patient compliance, the CDC has suggested use of a combination regimen (Table 3.3) which consists of a single dose of one of the penicillins plus a 7-day treatment course with a tetracycline. Both tetracycline hydrochloride and doxycycline are equally effective. Doxycycline has the advantages of twice a day dosing, reliable absorption with simultaneous food intake, and milder gastrointestinal side effects. However, doxycycline is much more expensive than tetracycline, and this limits its availability to a large segment of the population that receives their care through publicly funded programs. In addition, all patients treated for gonorrhea should have a serologic test for syphilis and where available a culture (or chlamydial antigen detection screening) for *C. trachomatis*.

The treatment for pregnant women with un-complicated gonococcal infection is similar to that in nonpregnant women with the exception that tetracycline should not be used in pregnancy. Both asymptomatic and symptomatic infections should be treated. For pregnant women the drug regimens of choice are ampicillin (3.5 g by mouth) or amoxicillin (3.0 g by mouth) each with probenecid (1 g). Pregnant women who are allergic to penicillin should be treated with spectinomycin (2.0 g intramuscularly (IM)). Erythromycin is effective against *N. gonorrhoeae* in only two-thirds to 75% of cases and should not be used as a single agent to treat *N. gonorrhoeae* in penicillin-allergic pregnant women. However, erythromycin, 500 mg by mouth 4 times daily for 7 days can be added to one of the single dose penicillin regimens to treat coexistent chlamydial infection in pregnancy. Many pregnant women will not tolerate the 500-mg dose, and a regimen of erythromycin, 250 mg by mouth 4 times daily for 14 days, can be used.

Follow-up cultures should be obtained 4–7 days after completion of therapy. In women this should include both an endocervical and a rectal culture for the gonococcus. Many of the resistant *N. gonorrhoeae* and thus treatment failures are found in the rectal culture. Patients treated with either one of the penicillin regimens, tetracyclines or a combined penicillin-tetracycline regimen and in whom gonorrhea persists posttreatment, should receive 2.0 g of spectinomycin IM. Continued gonococcal infection after treatment is usually due to either reinfection or infection with a PPNG strain. The CDC recommends that for recurrent gonorrhea after treatment all isolates should be tested for penicillinase production. Spectinomycin-resistant PPNG strains have now been isolated. Patients with positive cultures (PPNG isolates) after spectinomycin therapy should be treated with cefoxitin (2.0 g IM) plus 1.0 g probenecid or cefotaxime (1.0 g IM) without probenecid.

In addition, it is important that sexual partners of patients with gonorrhea be examined, cultured, and treated (prior to culture results). Treatment should be with one of the CDC regimens for uncomplicated gonorrhea, preferably with treatment for coexistent chlamydial infection.

Attempts are underway to develop gonococcal vaccines based on providing immunity against a variety of virulence factors such as pili, outer-membrane proteins, capsular polysaccharide, and lipopolysaccharide (37). To data these efforts have been unsuccessful.

COMPLICATED GONORRHEA

Treatment of complicated (upper- or extragenital) gonococcal infection depends on the anatomic location, the severity of the disease, and the clinical response. Basically, the same antibiotics are used as for uncomplicated gonorrhea, but the doses are different.

DISSEMINATED GONORRHEA

The organisms causing disseminated gonorrhea are very sensitive to penicillin, more than the organisms causing uncomplicated disease. Penicillin is the drug of choice for non-PPNG strains associated with DGI. The current CDC recommendations and alternate drugs are listed in Table 3.4. Cefoxitin or cefotaxime is suggested for PPNG strains. Outpatient therapy of DGI is appropriate, and hospitalization is reserved for patients who are unreliable, have uncertain diagnosis, have purulent joint effusions, or life-threatening complications such as endocarditis or meningitis. Whether pregnant patients with DGI should be hospitalized for bed rest and close observations for the occurrence of preterm labor or intrauterine infection has not been established. Until further information is available, our policy has been to treat pregnant women on an inpatient basis.

PHARYNGEAL GONORRHEA

The preferred treatment for pharyngeal gonorrhea is procaine penicillin (4.8 million units IM) plus 1 g probenecid by mouth or tetracycline (500 mg by mouth 4 times daily for 7 days).

Table 3.4
Centers for Disease Control Recommended Regimens for Treatment of Complicated Extragenital Gonorrhea

---

1. Disseminated gonococcal infection

    Aqueous crystalline penicillin G: 10 million units intravenously, per day until improvement occurs, followed by amoxicillin (500 mg) or ampicillin (500 mg), by mouth, 4 times a day to complete at least 7 days

    or

    Tetracycline HCl: 500 mg, by mouth, 4 times a day for at least 7 days

    or

    Cefoxitin/cefotaxime: cefoxitin (1.0 g) or cefoxatime (500 mg), either given 4 times a day IV for at least 7 days

    or

    Erythromycin: 500 mg, by mouth, 4 times a day for at least 7 days

2. Pharyngeal gonorrhea

    Aqueous procaine penicillin G: 4.8 million units intramuscularly at 2 sites with 1 g probenecid by mouth

    or

    Tetracycline HCl: 500 mg by mouth, 4 times a day for 7 days

    Pharyngeal gonococcal infection due to PPNG

    A daily single dose of 9 tablets of trimethoprim/sulfamethoxazole (80 mg/400 mg) for 5 days.

Neither spectinomycin nor ampicillin or amoxicillin regimens are effective for the treatment of pharyngeal gonococcal disease. Nonpregnant patients with pharyngeal infection caused by PPNG should be treated with sulfamethoxazole/trimethoprim (9 tablets daily for 5 days).

The pregnant patient who is allergic to penicillin and has pharyngeal gonorrhea is a treatment problem. Spence has recommended that such patients should have skin testing to document the penicillin allergy, and if she is truly allergic, erythromycin (500 mg by mouth, 4 times daily for 7 days) can be prescribed (2). These patients require careful follow-up because of the high failure rates associated with erythromycin.

GONOCOCCAL PELVIC INFLAMMATORY DISEASE

Approximately 25–50% of patients with PID have gonococci isolated from their cervix. Treatment of PID is discussed in detail in Chapter 4. The penicillins, tetracyclines, cephalosporins, and aminoglycosides are effective against the non-PPNG gonococcus associated with PID. Concomitant therapy should be included that is effective against *C. trachomatis*. Current CDC recommendations for PID therapy stress combination regimens that provide efficacy against *N. gonorrhoeae*, *C. trachomatis*, and anaerobic bacteria (including penicillin-resistant anaerobes).

GONOCOCCAL OPHTHALMIA

Gonococcal ophthalmia is usually an infection of the neonate. However, the gonococcus can and does cause adult conjunctivitis. The CDC recommends that neonates with gonococcal ophthalmia be hospitalized and isolated for 24 hr after initiation of therapy (35). Aqueous crystalline penicillin G (50,000 units/kg/day, intravenously, in 2 doses for 7 days) is the therapy of choice. Eyes should be irrigated immediately with saline or buffered ophthalmic solutions and then irrigated at hourly intervals until the discharge is eliminated. Topical antibiotic preparations alone are neither sufficient nor required when appropriate systemic antibiotic therapy is given. Adults with gonococcal conjunctivitis should receive treatment with intravenous penicillin G (10 million units/day for 5 days). If PPNG is involved, cefoxitin 1 g four times a day or cefotaxime 0.5 g four times a day is appropriate.

Prevention

The increasing frequency of asymptomatic gonorrheal infection in women makes screening for *N. gonorrhoeae* during the antepartum period an important aspect of prevention of the perinatal morbidity associated with this organism. Additionally, the use of silver nitrate 1% or ophthalmic ointments or drops containing tetracycline or erythromycin should be instilled into the conjunctiva of newborns to protect against gonococcal conjunctivitis. It seems reasonable to promote the use of erythromycin or tetracycline as local agents because they will also help prevent chlamydial newborn conjunctivitis.

Most important to any prevention effort is the treatment of sexual contacts. Even those without symptoms must be treated if the cycle of infection is to be halted.

Hopefully the efforts to develop gonococcal vaccines will bear fruit. Of particular interest are the attempts to develop vaccine(s) for the prevention of gonococcal PID and its associated legacy of infertility and ectopic pregnancies.

SYPHILIS

Syphilis is a chronic infectious process due to the spirochete *Treponema pallidum*. It has been recognized for several centuries that primary, secondary, or early latent syphilis in pregnant women caused infection of the fetus, with resultant stillbirths, prematurities, congenital abnormalities, and active disease at birth. Because of this significant morbidity, great emphasis has been placed on routine screening of all pregnant women for the presence of syphilis. Acquisition is generally through sexual contact. Individuals with primary, secondary, or early latent (up to 1 yr) syphilis are capable of transmitting syphilis to susceptible hosts. *T. pallidum* is capable of penetrating intact skin or mucosal surfaces. Subsequently, the chancre (the primary lesion) appears at the site of entry of the spirochetes. The chancre, if untreated, resolves within 3–6 weeks and is followed by a secondary stage. Secondary syphilis is a generalized disease with dermatologic manifestations, lymphadenopathy, and spirochetemia, which lasts 2–6 weeks. This stage is also self-limiting, and with resolution of the secondary stage, the patient enters the latent phase in which there are no clinical manifestations of disease. Without therapy approximately one-third of patients develop tertiary syphilis with progressive damage to the central nervous system, cardiovascular system, musculoskeletal system, or other parenchyma.

T. pallidum is a strict anaerobic spirochete. The organism has never been grown in vitro in the laboratory. However, it can be grown in laboratory animals, especially rabbits. Because no in vitro system for culture of *T. pallidum* is available, diagnostic efforts must rely on direct smears and/or serologic tests.

Epidemiology

The total number of cases of syphilis in the United States progressively decreased from the 1940s until 1957. In 1958 the trend reversed and the number of reported cases of primary and secondary syphilis (the best indicator of incidence trends) has been steadily increasing (1) (Fig. 3.2). There were approximately 34,000 reported cases of primary and secondary syphilis in the United States during 1982 (1); it is estimated that 3 unreported cases exist for every reported case. Therefore, about 136,000 cases of primary and secondary syphilis occur annually in the United States. Although much of this increase in cases of primary and secondary syphilis has occurred in the male homosexual population (2), an increasing rate has also been observed in heterosexuals, including pregnant women. The incidence of congenital syphilis cases has followed a similar pattern. A low point of 200 cases occurred in 1958, but approximately 350 cases of congenital syphilis are currently reported annually in the United States.

Clinical Manifestations

Following exposure to syphilis there is an incubation period ranging from 10 to 90 days before the primary lesion, the chancre, appears (Fig. 3.3). The chancre arises at the spirochete point of entry and is a painless, ulcerated lesion with a raised border and an indurated base. Most commonly the "hard" chancre of syphilis appears in the genital area. In men the lesion is easily apparent, and syphilis is often diagnosed in its primary stage in men. Although chancres on the female external genitalia are easily recognized, more commonly the lesion is on the cervix or in the vagina and not recognized. Thus

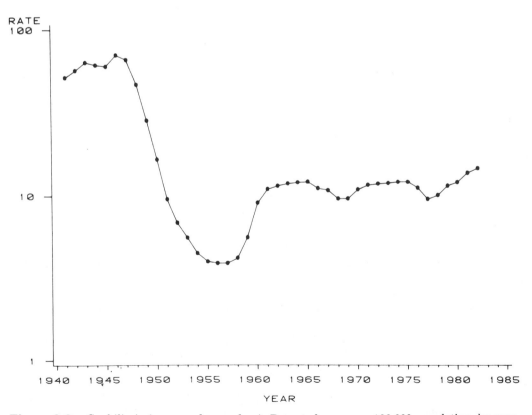

Figure 3.2. Syphilis (primary and secondary). Reported cases per 100,000 population, by year, United States, 1941–1982. (From Centers for Disease Control: Annual summary 1982. Reported morbidity and mortality in the United States. *MMWR* 31:77, 1983.)

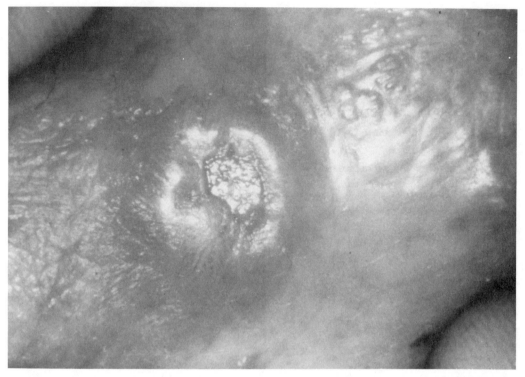

Figure 3.3.   Primary chancre of syphilis with smooth raised border and "clean," nonnecrotic base.

the chancre often escapes detection in women, and it is unusual to diagnose the primary stage of syphilis in females. Extragenital sites for chancres include the anus, mouth, oropharynx, and nipple. Although the chancre of syphilis has many typical characteristics, the appearance of syphilytic lesions is often atypical, and clinicians should have a high index of suspicion for all genital ulcerative lesions (Table 3.5). Painless inguinal lymphadenopathy is frequently present. The primary chancre, even without treatment, spontaneously disappears in 2–6 weeks.

Following resolution of the primary stage, the patient enters the secondary or bacteremia stage of syphilis. During the secondary stage of syphilis, which occurs 6 weeks to 6 months after the primary inoculation, there is involvement of all major organ systems by *T. pallidum*. However, clinically, the secondary stage presents primarily with skin and mucous membrane lesions. These clinical manifestations of secondary syphilis include a generalized maculopapular rash involving the palms and soles, mucous patches, condyloma latum, and generalized lymphadenopathy. Chapel recently reported on

the clinical findings in 105 cases of secondary syphilis (3). The maculopapular lesions were most common (70%) with the palms and soles being the most common site (50%). Mucosal lesions were noted in 21%, and lymphadenopathy was seen in 85%. Surprisingly, Chapel reported that over 40% of these cases had a history of pruritis.

These findings of secondary syphilis spontaneously clear within 2–6 weeks, and the latent stage of syphillis is entered, in which there is no apparent clinical disease. In about 25% of such patients the early latent phase (less than 2 yr) may be associated with an exacerbation of secondary syphilis in which the mucocutaneous lesions are infectious. The majority of relapses occur within the 1st year. The late latent stage (greater than 2 yr) is not infectious by sexual transmission, but the spirochete may still be transplacentally transmitted to the fetus.

If treatment is not provided, one-third of patients progress and develop tertiary syphilis with involvement of the cardiovascular, central nervous, or musculoskeletal systems, and/or involvement of various organ systems with gummas (late benign tertiary syphilis) (4, 5). The

Table 3.5
Differential Diagnosis of Genital Ulcers

Syphilis
Herpes simplex genitalis
Chancroid
Lymphogranuloma venereum
Granuloma inguinale
Superinfection of genital warts, scabies, or
    molluscum contagiosum
Trauma
Malignancy
Erythema multiforme
Behcet's syndrome

cardiovascular manifestations of tertiary syphilis include aortic aneurysm and aortic insufficiency. In the central nervous system tertiary disease produces general paresis, tabes dorsalis, optic atrophy, meningovascular syphilis; the Argyll-Robertson pupil (does not react to light but accommodates) is virtually pathognomonic of tertiary syphilis.

CONGENITAL SYPHILIS

In the past, syphilis was felt to invade the fetus via transplacental infection only after 16 weeks of gestation, because it was believed that spirochetes were unable to penetrate Langerhan's layer of the placenta. However, recent work has documented that *T. pallidum* can be transferred across the placenta and infect the fetus as early as 6 weeks of gestation. Clinical manifestations are not apparent until after 16 weeks gestation when the fetus develops immunocompetence. Thus the risk to the fetus is present throughout pregnancy. The degree of risk to the fetus or neonate is related to the quantity of spirochetes in the maternal bloodstream and correlates with the maternal stage of syphilis (7, 8). Women with primary or secondary syphilis are more likely to transmit infection to their offspring, than are those with latent disease. Fiumara and co-workers (8) reported that with untreated primary or secondary syphilis, there was a 50% probability of congenital syphilis, and half the infants were stillborn, neonatal deaths, or premature; there were almost no normal full-term infants among mothers with untreated primary or secondary syphilis. With early latent syphilis a 40% risk for congenital syphilis was present; 20% premature, 16% stillbirth, and 4% neonatal death. This risk decreased to 10% in mothers with late syphilis, and in this group there was no increase in prematures or perinatal deaths. In addition, the

manifestations of congenital syphilis are usually less severe in association with long-standing maternal disease than with early syphilis (less than 1 yr duration).

The clinical spectrum in fetal infection includes stillbirths, neonatal death, clinically apparent congenital syphilis during the early months of life (early congenital syphilis), and development of the classic stigmata of late congenital syphilis (8). Prematurity and stillbirths are frequent when the mother has early syphilis (less than 1 yr duration). However, at the present, pregnant women diagnosed as having syphilis are usually asymptomatic in the latent stage and have had the disease for greater than a 1 yr duration. Consequently, most infants with early congenital syphilis are asymptomatic at birth and do not develop evidence of active disease for 10 days–2 weeks. Chancres do not occur unless the disease is acquired at the time of passage through the birth canal. The characteristic manifestations of early congenital syphilis (onset less than 2 yr of age) include a maculopapular rash that may progress to desquamation or vesicular and bullae formation, snuffles (a flu-like syndrome associated with a nasal discharge), mucous patches in the oral-pharyngeal cavity, hepatosplenomegaly, jaundice, lymphadenopathy, pseudoparalysis of Parrot due to osteochondritis, chorioretinitis, and iritis (8). Both cutaneous and mucous lesions contain spirochetes that can be seen on darkfield exam.

Untreated or incompletely treated early congenital syphilis will progress to the classic manifestations of late congenital syphilis. These include Hutchinsonian teeth, mulberry molars, interstitial keratitis, eighth nerve deafness, saddle nose, rhagades, saber shins, neurologic manifestations (mental retardation, hydrocephalus, general paresis, optic nerve atrophy, and Clutton's joints.

Diagnosis

The most specific method for diagnosing syphilis is by demonstration of *T. pallidum* on dark-field examination of fresh specimens from the lesions of infected individuals. This methodology is only applicable to the lesions of primary or secondary syphilis. A specimen for darkfield exam should be obtained from any lesion suspected as being a chancre or manifestation of secondary syphilis. To obtain the specimen the lesion is cleaned with normal saline, and after drying, it is abraded with cotton gauze until minimal bleeding is initiated. Then by applying pressure to the lesion clear serum is expressed, which is applied to a slide. A cover slip is placed over the serum and sealed at its periphery with petroleum jelly. Specimens for dark-field exam should be evaluated promptly. However, the majority of men and nearly all women who are diagnosed as having syphilis are usually asymptomatic and in the latent stage. Thus, the diagnosis is most often based on serologic testing. The serologic tests are classified into two types; nonspecific tests for reagin-type antibodies and specific antitreponemal antibody tests (9). Nonspecific antibody tests for syphilis available today include the VDRL and the rapid plasma reagin test (RPR). These are used as screening tests. All pregnant women should be screened at their initial prenatal visit with one of these nontreponemal tests. High risk patients should be rescreened at 32–34 weeks of gestation. Treponema-specific tests are employed for confirming the diagnosis of syphilis in patients that have reactive VDRL or RPR tests. These tests include the *T. pallidum* immobilization (TPI) test, the fluorescent treponemal antibody absorption (FTA-ABS) test, or the micro hemagglutination assay (MHA) test.

It is important to recognize that when the syphilitic chancre first appears, both the nonspecific antibody tests (VDRL and RPR) and the treponemaspecific tests (FTA-ABS and MHA) may be nonreactive. Therefore, lesion(s) of syphilitic chancre(s) should be sampled for a dark-field exam. The presence of spirochetes on this exam is the sine qua non for the diagnosis of primary syphilis. During the next several weeks, after the chancre appears, these serum tests become positive; by 4–6 weeks 100% of patients with primary syphilis have positive nonspecific and specific treponemal serum tests. The FTA-ABS test becomes positive slightly earlier than the VDRL. Both serum tests will be positive during the secondary and latent stages of syphilis

Pregnant women with a reactive nontreponemal test should promptly have a quantitative nontreponemal test (usually the VDRL) and a confirmatory treponemal test such as the FTA-ABS performed. False-positive reactions can occur with all of these tests but are uncommon with the specific antitreponemal tests. Common causes of false-positive nontreponemal tests include viral infections, autoimmune diseases (systemic lupus, sarcoidosis, rheumatoid arthritis), narcotics abuse, and pregnancy. The false-positive tests with nontreponemal tests are most

often only weak or borderline reactions. In pregnancy, it is best to consider positive FTA-ABS or TPI tests to be truly positive in order to maximize treatment of the fetus at risk.

Controversy has arisen over whether all patients (including pregnant women) who are asymptomatic but have a positive serologic diagnosis of syphilis should have a spinal tap for the detection of asymptomatic neurosyphilis. The spinal tap ensures proper treatment of neurosyphilis (see section of treatment). If a spinal tap is not performed the patient should be treated as if asymptomatic neurosyphilis is present, which requires a series of injections. Cerebrospinal fluid demonstrating pleocytosis, elevated protein concentrations, and a reactive VDRL is diagnostic of active neurosyphilis. Several studies have suggested that the VDRL is relatively insensitive for the detection of neurosyphilis and recommend that the FTA-ABS or TPHA test be done on CSF specimens (10, 11). Jones and Harris have demonstrated that this approach is also appropriate for pregnant patients with early syphilis (12).

The diagnosis of reinfection or persistence of active syphilis can be made in patients previously known to have syphilis by following the titer of the quantitative VDRL. With successful therapy the VDRL titer should decrease and become negligible within 6–12 months in early syphilis and 12–18 months with late syphilis of more than 1 yr duration. A rising titer would indicate a need for further diagnostic measures such as a spinal tap and appropriate treatment.

Congenital syphilis is easily diagnosed in the clinically apparent case where a jaundiced, hydropic baby with florid disease and a large, edematous placenta are delivered and laboratory studies confirm the presence of the disease. However, the vast majority of infected newborns are asymptomatic at birth, but have a positive nonspecific test for syphilis in the cord blood. The problem is attempting to determine whether this is merely IgG antibody passively transferred from the mother or whether it is IgM antibody indicative of a fetal infection. The FTA-ABS also is an IgG antibody and crosses the placenta. An IgM FTA-ABS test has been developed; however, there are problems with the test related to separating the IgM from the IgG, and only specialized laboratories can perform this test. If an infant's seropositivity is due to passive transfer of maternal IgG antibodies, a progressive decrease in the VDRL titer occurs, and the titer becomes negative within 3 months of delivery. Any infant with a reactive VDRL but no clinical evidence of syphilis should be followed with serial monthly quantitative VDRL tests for at least 9 months. A rising titer indicates active disease and need for therapy. Infected infants may be both asymptomatic and the serum VDRL may be normal if maternal infection occurred late in pregnancy.

Treatment

All patients with a history of sexual contact with a person with documented syphilis or either a positive dark-field exam or serologic evidence of syphilis with a specific treponemal test should be treated. In addition, those in whom the diagnosis cannot be ruled out with certainty or in those with previous treatment who have evidence of reinfection such as dark-field positive lesions or a four-fold rise in titer of a quantitative nontreponemal test should receive appropriate treatment.

Penicillin is the drug of choice for the treatment of syphilis. Alternative drugs include tetracycline and erythromycin. Tetracycline should not be used in pregnancy; erythromycin estolate, also, is not recommended for use in pregnancy because of potential hepatotoxicity in the mother and adverse effects on the fetus. Erythromycin base or erythromycin stearate can be used to treat pregnant women who are allergic to penicillin. The treatment schedules for syphilis recommended by the Centers for Disease Control (1982) are presented in Table 3.6. While *T. pallidum* has remained sensitive to low levels of penicillin (0.03 μg/ml is treponemicidal), its long replication time (>30 hr) necessitates that low levels of penicillin be maintained for periods of 1–2 weeks (4). The efficacy of nonpenicillin regimens have not been as fully evaluated as the penicillin regimens. For the penicillin-allergic patient who cannot tolerate tetracycline, the CDC suggests two options. If compliance and serologic follow-up can be assured, erythromycin can be administered at a dose appropriate for the stage of syphilis (Table 3.6). If compliance and serologic follow-up cannot be assured, consideration should be given to hospitalization and penicillin desensitization.

At all stages of pregnancy, patients with syphilis should receive penicillin parenterally, in dosage appropriate for duration of disease, as recommended for nonpregnant patients. Pregnant patients who are allergic to penicillin should receive erythromycin as indicated by duration of disease. Failures have been reported with erythromycin treatment of syphilis, and this agent crosses the placenta poorly with resultant low levels being achieved in the fetus. It has been suggested that the newborn of a mother who received erythromycin therapy for syphilis be treated as if no treatment had been given. An alternative including ampicillin, cephalosporins, streptomycin, and chloramphenicol has been used in the treatment of syphilis. However, these agents are less efficacious than penicillin.

The treatment of neurosyphilis remains controversial. The CDC suggests that CSF examination should be done for patients with clinical symptoms or signs consistent with neurosyphilis. CSF examination is encouraged for all other patients with syphilis of greater than 1 yr duration to exclude asymptomatic neurosyphilis. The lack of detectable penicillin in CSF after use of benzathine penicillin suggests that documented neurosyphilis requires either aqueous procaine penicillin or aqueous crystalloid penicillin treatment (14).

Therapy should be monitored with serial quantitative VDRL titers at 3, 6, 9, 12 months after therapy for early syphilis. Patients with syphilis of more than 1 yr duration should also have repeat titers at 18 and 24 months posttherapy. During pregnancy quantitative VDRL should be assessed monthly. Those who show a four-fold rise should be retreated.

Congenital syphilis is unusual if the mother received adequate treatment with penicillin during pregnancy. Infants should be treated if maternal treatment was inadequate, unknown, with drugs other than penicillin, or if adequate follow-up of the infant is not possible. Any child suspected of having congenital syphilis should have a spinal tap prior to treatment. If the spinal fluid is normal, a single intramuscular injection of benzathine penicillin G (50,000 units/kg) should be given. If the spinal fluid is abnormal or unexamined, the infant should receive aqueous crystalline penicillin G (50,000 units/kg daily for 10 days).

CHANCROID

Chancroid, commonly referred to as "soft" chancre, is one of the ulcerative genital diseases caused by sexually trasmitted organisms (Table 3.5). The causative agent of chancroid is *Hemophilus ducreyi*. This bacterium is a small, nonmotile, gram-negative rod which has a characteristic "chaining" appearance on gram stain.

Table 3.6
Centers for Disease Control Recommended Treatment of Syphilis (1982)

Early syphilis (primary, secondary, latent syphilis of ≤1 year's duration)
1. Recommended regimen
   Benzathine penicillin G: 2.4 million units total, IM, at a single session
2. Penicillin-allergic patients
   Tetracycline HCl: 500 mg, by mouth, 4 times a day for 15 days

or

   Erythromycin: 500 mg, by mouth, 4 times a day for 15 days

Syphilis of more than one year's duration
1. Recommended regimen
   Benzathine penicillin G: 2.4 million units, IM, once a week for 3 successive weeks (total 7.2
   million units)
2. Penicillin-allergic patients
   Tetracycline HCl: 500 mg, by mouth, 4 times a day for 30 days

or

   Erythromycin: 500 mg, by mouth, 4 times a day for 30 days

Syphilis in pregnancy
1. Recommended regimens
   For patients who are not allergic to penicillin, penicillin should be used in dosage schedule
   appropriate for the stage of syphilis as recommended for nonpregnant patients.
2. Penicillin-allergic patients
   If compliance and serologic follow-up can be assured, administer erythrocmycin in dosages
   appropriate for the stage of syphilis.
   If compliance and follow-up cannot be assured, consider hospitalization and penicillin desensitization.

Neurosyphilis
   Aqueous crystalline penicillin G: 12–24 million units, IV, per day for 10 days, followed by
   benzathine penicillin G, 2.4 million units, IM, weekly for 3 doses

or

   Aqueous procaine penicillin G: 2.4 million units, IM, daily plus probenecid (500 mg by mouth, 4
   times a day, for 10 days) followed by benzathine pencillin G, 2.4 million units, IM, weekly for
   3 doses

or

   Benzathine penicillin G: 2.4 million units, IM, weekly for 3 doses.

It is a facultative anaerobe with fastidious growth requirements (1).

Epidemiology

Chancroid is relatively rare in the United States. It is most common in tropical, developing countries of the world. While less than 1400 cases were reported in the United States during 1982 (2), worldwide chancroid is estimated to be more common than syphilis (1), and there are limited areas where it has been more common than gonorrhea (3, 4). However, the nearly 1400 cases in the United States during 1982 was a significant increase from the 850 cases in 1981 (2).

The disease is described most commonly in men, especially young sexually active males who have a history of recent contact with prostitutes (1, 5). Ronald et al reported that, in their population in Winnipeg, 80% of chancroid cases admitted to an average of two previous STD episodes, and 30% had concomitant gonorrhea (1). In addition to their greater prevalence, males are more frequently symptomatic. Asymptomatic women with lesions of chancroid are rarely seen. Whether the presence of asymptomatic lesions in the female are the explanation for their perceived lower frequency of chancroid is not proven but probable. In addition, the extent females play as a reservoir for *H. ducreyi* and as carriers in the spread of chancroid is not clear (1).

Clinical Presentation

The lesions of chancroid are generally limited to genital sites that tend to be traumatized during sexual intercourse. In men they are most commonly found on the internal surface of the prepuce and the frenulum and on the labia, clitoris, and fourchette in women. Trauma facilitates the entry of *H. ducreyi*, which, unlike *T. pallidum*, is incapable of invading intact skin or mucosal surfaces (1, 3).

The incubation period of chancroid is 3–5 days. At the site of entry, a small papule develops which is surrounded by a zone of erythema. Within 2–3 days the lesion becomes pustular or vesiculopustular and ulcerates. The classic ulcer of chancroid is superficial and shallow with a ragged edge (Fig. 3.4). The chancre is surrounded by an inflammatory red halo. The base of the ulcer is covered with a necrotic exudate. Unlike the nontender syphilitic chancre, the chancre of chancroid is painful and tender. In addition it is not indurated (i.e., "soft"). Multiple ulcers are the rule and appear to represent autoinoculation.

In approximately 50% of cases a bubo devel-ops. The bubo appears 7–10 days after the initial lesion and is characterized by acute, painful, tender, inflammatory inguinal adenopathy. The bubo is unilateral in about two-thirds of cases and is unilocular. If untreated the bubo will rupture, forming a large ulcer in the inguinal area.

Diagnosis

The diagnosis of chancroid relies on gram-stained smears, culture, and clinical characteristics of the lesion(s). A gram stain of the exudate from the lesion or an aspirate of the bubo may reveal the presence of gram-negative rods which tend to form chains (Fig. 3.5). The sensitivity of the gram-stain from lesion or bubo is only 50% (6). A definitive laboratory diagnosis of chancroid depends on the isolation of *H. ducreyi* from the lesion or bubo. However, the organism is fastidious, and isolation of *H. ducreyi* is not routinely performed in most general clinical microbiology laboratories. Thus in many instances the diagnosis of chancroid is based upon clinical findings and exclusion of the other causes of genital ulcers (i.e., herpes simplex vi-

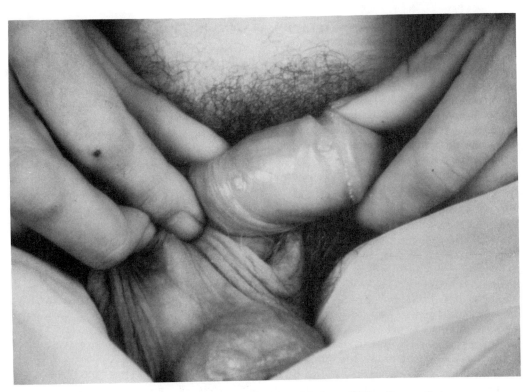

Figure 3.4. Chancre of chancroid with red halo and "dirty" necrotic base.

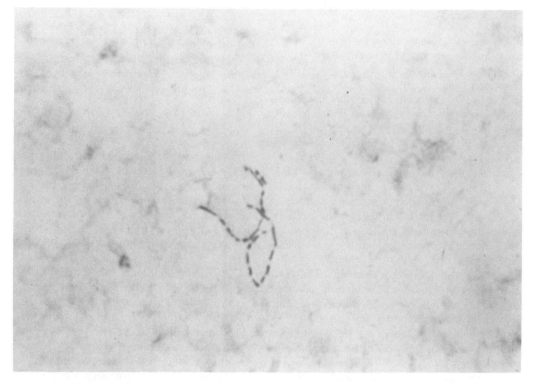

Figure 3.5. The "school of fish" appearance of *H. ducreyii* on gram stain.

rus, syphilis, lymphogranuloma venereum). Ideally, an attempt should be made to make a definite diagnosis by identifying the causative agent. Hammond has recently described the use of a blood-free selective medium consisting of gonococcal medium base, enriched with 1% hemoglobin and Isovitalox, and to which vancomycin (3 g/ml) is added; this has been a significant help in the laboratory diagnosis of chancroid (6).

Treatment

Although sulfonamides and tetracyclines have been the mainstay in the treatment of chancroid for many years, frequent reports of clinical resistance have occurred recently (4). Currently the drug of choice for treatment of chancroid is trimethoprim (160 mg)-sulfamethoxazole (800 mg) twice a day for 10 days. Erythromycin (500 mg by mouth 4 times a day for 10 days) is an effective alternative and is the treatment of choice for pregnant women with chancroid. Sexual partners must also be treated with similar regimens (2, 5).

Fluctuant nodes should be aspirated to prevent rupture, since suppuration may occur despite antimicrobial therapy.

LYMPHOGRANULOMA VENEREUM

Lymphogranuloma venereum (LGV) is a sexually transmitted disease caused by *C. trachomatis* serotypes L_1, L_2, and L_3 (1). These LGV strains of *Chlamydia* are easily differentiated from other *C. trachomatis* strains by antigenic structure and because they are much more invasive in tissue culture systems (2). The disease is manifested by both generalized systemic symptoms and a wide spectrum of anogenital lesions, lymphadenopathy, and gross devastation of perineal tissue (2). LGV is uncommon in the United States. It usually presents as inguinal adenopathy, since the painless genital ulcer stage of the disease often goes unnoticed.

Epidemiology

Although LGV is worldwide in distribution, it most commonly occurs in tropical areas. South America, the West Indies, West and East Africa, Southeast Asia, and India have the greatest prevalence of LGV (3). Approximately 350 cases/yr are reported in the United States, and the majority of these are in men (4). Schachter suggested this sex differential is due to patterns of pelvic lymph drainage which in women results in deep iliac adenopathy which is not apparent, rather than the inguinal adenopathy seen commonly in men (4).

Clinical Presentation

The clinical presentation of LGV is divided into primary, secondary, and tertiary stages. Following an incubation time that ranges from 4 to 21 days, the primary lesion develops in the genital area. In the male the primary lesion usually occurs on the coronal sulcus, while in females the site is usually the posterior aspect of the vulva. This primary lesion is vesicular or papular and painless; it may ulcerate but heals within a few days without scarring. The primary lesion generally is not appreciated or recognized by patients. An exception is primary rectal LGV which manifests as proctitis with diarrhea, discharge, and ulceration (5).

The secondary stage of inguinal adenopathy develops 1–4 weeks after the primary lesion. This stage of inguinal adenopathy is the most frequent clinical manifestation of LGV (2). The adenopathy is usually unilateral and begins as firm, discrete, multiple nodes which are slightly tender. Over the next week or two a more exten-

sive adenitis commences as the nodes become matted together and become adherent to the subcutaneous tissue and overlying skin. The skin often is discolored, and the lesion becomes very painful. The horizontal group of superficial inguinal nodes is most commonly involved, but the femoral nodes may also. If both groups become involved, the inguinal ligament creates a groove between the node groups, producing the "groove sign" which occurs in 10–20% of LGV cases (Fig. 3.6). The matted mass proceeds to suppurate, and multiple draining sinuses arise from the necrotic lymph nodes. Systemic symptoms such as fever, myalgias, headache, and arthralgias are common during the secondary stage (6).

The tertiary stage involves the external genitalia and anorectal areas. It is characterized by progressive tissue destruction and extensive scarring. Especially in women, this phase of disease may be the initial clinical manifestation for which the patient seeks care. This stage may present as hypertrophic ulceration and elephantiasis. Hypertrophic lesions are more common among women, but elephantiasis occurs in both men and women. Sinuses, fistula tracts and ultimately strictures may occur in the vulva, per-

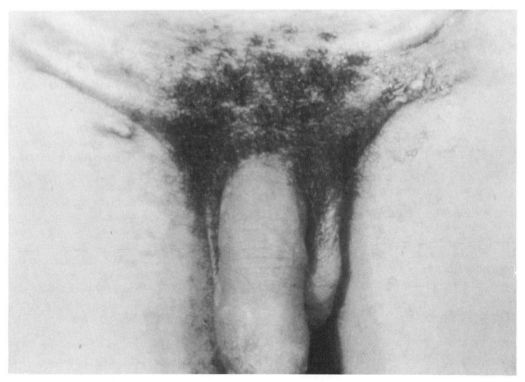

Figure 3.6. The grooved nodes (saddle nodes) which are characteristic for lymphogranuloma venereum due to the L_1, L_2, L_3 strains of *C. trachomatis.*

ineum, and/or rectum. Anorectal involvement is more common in women and homosexual males. Proctitis is present early in the disease course and presents with passage of blood, mucus, and pus per rectum. Stricture formation follows within a few months to 10 yr (2).

Diagnosis

LGV occurs with multiple, variable presentations, and no single pathognomonic lesion exists. Thus diagnosis solely on clinical grounds is, at best, difficult. The diagnosis of LGV can be made by isolation of the chlamydial organism or with use of serology. Schachter and co-workers reported that aspiration and culture of pus from fluctuant nodes was positive in approximately 50% of cases (7). With the introduction of monoclonal antibodies to *Chlamydia* into clinical practice, direct smears of nodal aspirates may become the test of choice.

The most commonly used diagnostic test for LGV, at present, is the compliment fixation test for *Chlamydia* group antibodies. This test is very sensitive, and titers greater than 1:64 are considered diagnostic. However, CF titers are present with mucosal infections due to other chlamydial subgroups, although usually at lower titers (8). The microimmunofluorescence test of Wang and Grayston can be used for typing isolates of *Chlamydia*.

The Frei intradermal test was for many years the backbone of diagnostic efforts for LGV. A positive Frei is not evidence of active infection but only indicates previous LGV infection.

Treatment

As recommended by the CDC, tetracycline (500 mg 4 times a day) is the therapy of choice for LGV (9). The duration of treatment required is at least 2 weeks, and some authorities suggest a 3–4 week course. Alternative regimens include: (a) doxycycline (100 mg, by mouth, twice a day); (b) erythromycin (500 mg, by mouth, 4 times a day); or (c) sulfamethoxazole (1.0 g, by mouth, twice a day) (or other sulfonamides in equivalent doses). These alternative regimens also are given for at least 2 weeks. Fluctuant inguinal nodes should be aspirated to prevent sinus tract formation. Incision and drainage or surgical extirpation of nodes is contraindicated, as such intervention will delay healing and may further obstruct lymphatic drainage. Late sequelae such as strictures and/or fistula may require surgical intervention (9).

GRANULOMA INGUINALE (DONOVANOSIS)

Granuloma inguinale (donovanosis) is caused by *Calymmatobacterium granulomatis*. This organism is a gram-negative, nonmotile, nonsporing, encapsulated rod and is grouped with Enterobacteriaceae because it cross-reacts with *Klebsiella* and *Escherichia coli* (1, 2). These Donovan bodies characterize this infection (Fig. 3.7). While *C. granulomatis* does not grow on cell-free media, it has been cultured in chicken embryonic yolk sac (1).

Epidemiology

Donovanosis is most common in New Guinea, India, the Caribbean, and other tropical areas. The disease is very rare in temperate climates, and less than 100 cases are reported annually in the United States (1).

The variable incubation time and initial subtle clinical findings have confused the epidemiology of donovanosis (2). Although it is generally believed that donovanosis is a sexually transmitted disease, its exact mode of transmission is still not clearly understood. Young children and very old adults without sexual activity develop the infection.

The sexually transmitted hypothesis is supported by a variety of evidence (2, 3). They include: (a) The majority of lesions occur on the genitalia; (b) The disease occurs most frequently in the sexually active age group; (c) There is almost always a history of sexual exposure before the appearance of the ulcer; (d) Other STD are present among donovanosis patients; and (e) donovanosis has been proven to exist in more than 50% of the sex partners of patients with the disease. An alternative hypothesis has been championed by Goldberg (4) which suggests that donovanosis is not necessarily an STD, and the habitat of *C. granulomatis* is the intestinal tract. The transmission can be nonsexual as well as sexual, and autoinoculation associated with trauma may be a more important mode of transmission than sexual activity. He points to the antigenic similarity between *C. granulomatis* and Enterobacteriaceae and the occasional cases that occur in the very young or elderly patients with recent sexual activity for support of the second concept.

Clinical Presentation

Donovanosis is a low-grade chronic infection whose communicability is low, and repeated

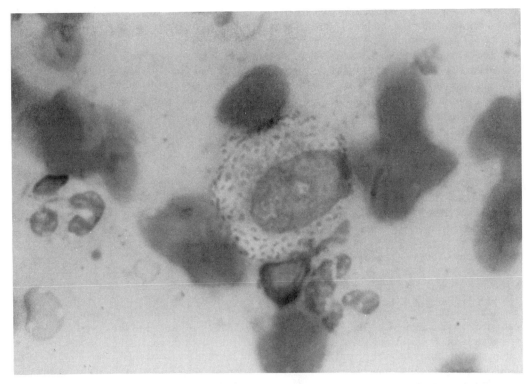

Figure 3.7. *C. granulomatis* (commonly known as Donovan body), the etiologic agent of granuloma inguinale.

close physical contact seems to be necessary for transmission (2). The incubation period varies from a few days to a few months (1). The disease has a very insidious onset, and the earliest lesion presents as a papule or nodule which is painless and often not noticed by patients. The sites commonly involved are genital, inguinocrural, perianal, and oral regions. The epithelium overlying the lesion subsequently ulcerates, producing an enlarging granulomatous beefy red, velvety ulcer. If untreated, the lesions may spread to involve the inguinal regions, producing the "pseudobubo." However, despite extensive disease there is a characteristic absence of adenopathy in the inguinal region. The pseudobubo is a subcutaneous granulomatous process rather than adenopathy. Rarely lymphatic obstruction and fibrosis occur.

Diagnosis

The diagnosis of donovanosis is usually made on clinical grounds because of the characteristic granulomatous process. Diagnosis may be confirmed by a stained smear of a crushed tissue preparation or biopsy of the lesion. The smear is stained with Giemsa or Wright stain. Dono-

van bodies in the smear or biopsy must be demonstrated to make a certain diagnosis. Neither culture nor serologic tests are available for donovanosis.

Treatment

Initially, treatment was with streptomycin, but currently, tetracycline (500 mg, four times a day, for 3 weeks) is the treatment of choice. Treatment should be continued until all lesions are healed. Chloramphenicol (500 mg, three times a day for 2 weeks) has been shown to be very effective (5).

ECTOPARASITES

Scabies

Human scabies is caused by an insect, *Sarcoptes scabiei*. This mite is 400 μm long and has four pairs of legs; the front two have suckers, while the rear two end in bristles (1). The female is more often seen and is larger. *S. scabiei* moves briskly across the skin at 2.5 cm/min and can travel from the neck to the wrist in a few hours (1).

The adult female excavates a burrow in the

skin. It is here that fertilization takes place and makes her fertile for life. Following fertilization the female emerges and excavates a new burrow which she extends by 0.5–5 mm a day as she begins laying 2 to 3 eggs per day. The eggs hatch in 3–4 days, and the larva emerge from the burrow and dig into adjacent skin where three moultings occur before adulthood is achieved. The mite lives for about 30 days.

EPIDEMIOLOGY

Scabies is common throughout the world and appears to increase in prevalence in 30-yr cycles (2). It is commoner in men than women and in whites than blacks.

Scabies is now considered a sexually transmitted disease, and close and prolonged contact with an infested person is a prerequisite for transmission. The disease is also spread by nonsexual contact; close person to person contact as with crowded living conditions or sharing a bed can be responsible. The role of fomites in transmission is possible, but the risk with contaminated clothing and bed linen is small (3). Unlike most STD which may be spread by brief sexual encounters, scabies is more likely to be contacted by sharing a night in bed (4).

CLINICAL PRESENTATION

Scabies manifests itself with a pruritic, pleomorphic rash that has an insidious onset and a characteristic pattern of involvement that includes wrists, finger webs, elbows, axillae, genitals, and buttocks (1). Initial infestations are clinically latent for 4–6 weeks following acquisition of scabies. Patients report a gradual onset of pruritis and rash. With repeat infestations the onset of symptoms is relatively prompt.

Pruritis is the predominant symptom and may be intense. Typically, the itching is worst at night. The physical findings in scabies include the presence of the burrows, a papular erythematous rash, and persistent pruritic nodules (1). The burrows are 5–10 mm long, and the organism may be seen as a tiny brown and white speck at the inner end.

DIAGNOSIS

The burrow of scabies is pathognomonic. However, they are not apparent in many cases of scabies infestation. Confirmation of the diagnosis is made by identifying the mite, eggs, or fecal pellets from burrows on microscopic ex-amination. Fresh lesions should be used for obtaining mites.

Scabies is called the great imitator because patients can present with a variety of lesions. Thus many dermatologic conditions must be considered in the differential diagnosis (1–4). These include: eczema, acute urticaria, impetigo, erythrasma, insect bites, neurodermatitis, and dermatitis herpetiformis. However, the history of insidious onset and the presence of nocturnal pruritis, pleomorphic lesions, and the characteristic distribution of lesions should strongly suggest scabies.

TREATMENT

Successful treatment of scabies necessitates correct application of an effective scabicide to the patient, sexual contacts, and family members. The Centers for Disease Control recommend lindane (1%) cream or lotion (Kwell) as the treatment of choice for scabies (5). The medication is applied to the entire skin surface from the neck down. Lindane should be left on the skin for 8 hr and then washed off. Because of concern over central nervous system toxicity, it has been suggested that in children and infants a 6-hr application is sufficient (6). The patient should be instructed that continued lesions and pruritis may occur, even though the mites and eggs have been killed. However, if no clinical improvement is noted a reapplication after 1 week is indicated. Lindane is not recommended for pregnant nor lactating women.

Alternative therapies include crotamiton (10%) cream or lotion (Eurax) applied to the entire body from the neck down nightly for 2 nights and washed off thoroughly 24 hr after the second application, and sulfur (6%) in petrolatum applied to the entire body from the neck down nightly for 3 nights. At the conclusion of therapy, the patient's underwear, night clothes, sheets and pillowcases should be washed at at least 50°C for 10 min.

Pediculosis Pubis

Phthirus pubis, the crab louse, is the responsible etiologic agent for pediculosis pubis. Similar to other STD, this infestation has also been increasing. Infestation by the crab (or pubic) louse should be considered in any patient complaining of groin irritation or pruritis. The organism is 1–2 mm long, grey, tough skinned, and square in shape. It has six pairs of legs of which the last two pairs are adapted for grasping suitable spaced hairs. Crab lice move relatively slowly, about 10 cm/day (1–3).

Twenty-four hours after mating, the female begins to lay eggs at a rate of 3/day. The eggs are attached to a hair near its root. After an incubation time of 7 days, a nymph is hatched which proceeds through 3 molts over the next 13–17 days. Once the louse reaches sexual maturity, the adult expectancy of life is 3–4 weeks (1).

EPIDEMIOLOGY

Although acquisition of *P. pubis* is nearly always through sexual contact, it may be spread through fomites. Pediculosis pubis is more contagious than any other STD, with a 95% chance of contracting the disease with a single sexual encounter (2). Pediculosis pubis is most commonly encountered during adolescence and young adulthood; from ages 15–19 it is more common in females, while after 20 males are more commonly infected (3).

CLINICAL PRESENTATION

The incubation time of pediculosis is 30 days. Patients present with irritation and/or pruritis secondary to bites. The intense itching is believed to be due to allergic sensitization (2). On occasion patients may see the crab louse moving over the skin. Distribution involves the pubic, perineal, and perianal regions.

DIAGNOSIS

Visualization of lice, larvae, and nits with use of a magnifying glass is diagnostic for pediculosis pubis. Microscopic examination will reveal the typical crab-like morphology.

TREATMENT

The treatment of choice for pediculosis pubis is lindane (1%) lotion or cream (Kwell). It should be applied in a thin layer to the infested and adjacent hairy areas and thoroughly washed off after 8 hr. Lindane (1%) shampoo is available and is more convenient; it can be lathered and left on for 4 min and then rinsed off. It has been associated with CNS toxicity and blood dyscrasias and thus should be used with caution in infants, pregnant women, and lactating women. Alternatives suggested by the CDC are pyrethrins and piperonyl butoxide which are applied

to the infested and adjacent hairy areas and washed off after 10 min (4). Following either treatment, combing the infested areas with a fine-toothed comb facilitates removal of remaining lice and nits.

Retreatment is indicated after 7 days if lice are found or eggs are observed at the hair-skin junction. Clothing or bed linen that may have been contaminated within the last 2 days should be washed and dried on hot cycle or dry cleaned. All sexual partners, family members, and close contacts must be treated at the same time, even if asymptomatic.

MOLLUSCUM CONTAGIOSUM

Molluscum contagiosum is a viral skin infection of children and young adults. The Molluscum contagiosum virus is a pox virus containing double-stranded DNA. Like other pox viruses its life cycle consists of cytoplasmic replication, prominent inclusion bodies, and cytopathic hyperplasia (1). Characteristic small, firm, umbilicated papules occur on the extremities or trunk and in sexually transmitted cases in the genital area. Examination of infected cells reveal the pathognomonic molluscum bodies which are ovoid accumulations of maturing virons (2).

Epidemiology

Molluscum contagiosum is transmitted by skin to skin contact, fomites, and autoinoculation. The incubation period ranges from 2 to 7 weeks. As noted by Brown and associates there are two major forms of molluscum contagiosum (1). The childhood disease which affects the face, trunk, and limbs is transmitted by skin contact and fomites. Disease affecting young adults is sexually transmitted, occurs in the genital area, and is acquired by skin contact during sexual intercourse. Cases of molluscum contagiosum appear to be increasing in frequency in the United States and United Kingdom (1, 3).

Clinical Presentation

Molluscum contagiosum affects normal skin rather than mucous membranes. The characteristic dome-shaped papules with central umbilication develop slowly and remain stable for long periods of time. Lesions are multiple, but generally less than 20.

The disease is usually asymptomatic, but on occasion pruritis may be present. The usual life of a lesion is less than 2 months, but they can last for several years. Most usual is for the crop of molluscum contagiosum lesions to be self-limited and of a 6- to 9-month duration (1).

Diagnosis

Examination reveals the characteristic smooth, light-colored papules with an umbilicated center. They are usually multiple and have the distribution noted above for either childhood disease or sexually transmitted forms. To confirm the diagnosis, if it is in doubt, microscopic examination can be performed. Either the lesion can be squeezed to express the white caseous material from its core or the lesion may be curetted off. The specimen is then crushed on a slide and stained with gram, Wright, or Giemsa stain. The cells will reveal the pathognomonic large intracytoplasmic molluscum bodies (2).

Treatment

Molluscum contagiosum is a benign and self-limited disease. The goal of treatment is to prevent spread of disease; secondarily it is for cosmetic reasons. Several alternative therapies are available (1). A small superficial incision in the top of the lesion may be made, and the contents are then removed with a comedo extractor. Curetting off the lesion can be done. For multiple lesions freezing with liquid nitrogen has been successful. Sexual partners should be examined and treated as well.

CONDYLOMA ACUMINATUM

Condyloma acuminata, often called genital or venereal warts, are benign epithelial tumors of the genitalia, perineum, and anus caused by a type of human papillomavirus (HPV). Since the work of Barrett and co-workers, the sexual route of transmission has been generally accepted (1). In addition, vertical transmission from mother to infant during parturition also may occur (2).

The human papillomavirus (HPV) is 55 nm in diameter, and its genetic material is contained within double-stranded DNA which has a molecular weight of 5×10^6 daltons (3). Recent technical advances in molecular biology have resulted in the identification of at least 15 papillomavirus types (4). In 1980, Gissman and zur Hausen (5) identified HPV-6 as the virus associated with condyloma acuminata. HPV-1 has also been found in condyloma acuminata (6).

Epidemiology

The sexual transmission of HPV which are associated with condyloma acuminatum is well established. The lesions occur in the urogenital and anorectal areas. Young, sexually active adolescents and adults are the highest prevalence group for genital warts. Oriel described an infectivity rate of about 65% among sexual contacts (7). Women are affected with an equal frequency as are men.

Condyloma acuminata appear to be occurring at epidemic proportions. The CDC estimated that the number of consultations for condyloma acuminatum by office-based private physicians in the United States increased over 450% in the past 15 yr (8). Moreover, in 1981 there were three times as many office visits for condyloma acuminatum as there were for genital herpes.

CLINICAL PRESENTATION

Condyloma acuminata occur in the urogenital and/or anorectal regions. They are pedunculated or broad based, pink to grey soft fleshy excrescenses which occur singly or in clusters. The lesions vary in size from pinhead to large cauliflower-like masses. Condyloma acuminata are generally not symptomatic, but may be friable and bleed easily. The morphologic appearance of genital warts is similar whether they involve the penis, urethra, perineum, anus, rectum, vulva, or vagina. Lesions on the cervix may be flat and endophytic (9).

In heterosexual males, the penis is the most common site for condyloma acuminatum. Perianal and intraanal condyloma occur in patients who engage in anal intercourse (homosexual males or heterosexual females). Condyloma acuminata in women are generally located on the external genitalia and perineal regions. They also occur in the vagina and on the cervix. The typical appearance of condyloma is not present for cervical lesions which have recently been described as flat and endophytic condyloma that can only be recognized with the aid of a colposcope (9). In fact, a high proportion of cervical lesions previously classified as CIN grade 1 or 2 are now considered to be this variant of condyloma acuminatum.

Diagnosis

Other than the atypical cervical lesions, most condyloma are so characteristic in appearance that the diagnosis is generally made on clinical grounds alone. If lesions appear atypical or the diagnosis is uncertain, biopsy should be obtained. As noted above, colposcopy may be required for the diagnosis of the flat condyloma acuminatum involving the cervix.

Histologically, condyloma acuminata are characterized by papillated epidermal hyperplasia, parakeratosis, koilocytes, occasional nonatypical mitotic figures, and increased numbers of dilated and tortuous capillaries.

Treatment

Topical podophyllin treatment of condyloma acuminata is considered the drug of choice. The USP podophyllin topical solution is 25% podophyllum resin and benzoin in alcohol. As noted by the CDC the treatment of condyloma acuminata has not been well studied, and no treatment is completely satisfactory (8).

For lesions on the external genitalia or the perianal area the CDC recommends that podophyllin 10–25% in compound tincture of benzoin be carefully applied to the lesions, avoiding normal tissue. Within 4 hr the medication should be washed off. For persistent lesions, weekly applications can be used; after 4 weeks alternative therapy should be considered. Alternative therapies include cryotherapy, electrosurgery, or surgical removal. Laser therapy and topical 5-fluorouracil have been advocated by some.

Vaginal condyloma acuminata may be treated as are lesions on the external genitalia. However, if podophyllin is used for vaginal lesions, care must be taken to ensure that the treated area is dried before removing the speculum. In general, the use of podophyllin for cervical warts is not recommended. Cryotherapy or possibly laser therapy is appropriate.

For anorectal warts the use of podophyllin is discouraged. The use of cryotherapy, electrosurgery, or surgical removal are generally recommended.

The management of condyloma acuminata in pregnancy presents a problem. The drug podophyllin has strong antimitotic activity and may be teratogenic. During pregnancy lesions are profuse and vascular, which predisposes for systemic absorption of podophyllin. The application of podophyllin is contraindicated in pregnancy because absorption of the resin may be harmful to mother and/or fetus. Cases have been reported in which fetal death and/or maternal neuropathy have occurred with use of podophyllin in gravid women (10). The best approach to treatment in pregnancy is excision of lesions, electrocautery, or cryosurgery.

An association between maternal condyloma acuminata and the development of neonatal laryngeal papillomas has been reported (11). Greater efforts should be made to eradicate condyloma acuminata prior to labor and delivery. Whether cesarean section is indicated in mothers with persistent or recurrent condyloma acuminata when labor commences is not clear and must await future study.

TRICHOMONIASIS

Trichomonas vaginalis is one of the most prevalent parasites in humans and is transmitted primarily via sexual intercourse. In the United States *T. vaginalis* is found in from about 10% of normal healthy women to nearly 50% in patients attending STD clinics. It has been estimated that some 180 million infections/yr occur worldwide, with approximately 2.5 million in the United States (1). Since 1963, metronidazole has been the only systemic trichimonicidal agent available in the United States. For discussion of the epidemiology, clinical findings, diagnosis, and treatment of *T. vaginalis* infection see the detailed discussion of trichomoniasis in Chapter 6.

GAY BOWEL SYNDROME

In 1977 Sohn and Robilotti coined the phrase "gay bowel syndrome" to describe the variety of anal, rectal, and colon diseases found in homosexual men (1). Homosexual men are at risk for these infections as a result of analingus, anal intercourse, and/or fellatio following anal intercourse. The proctitis component of "gay bowel syndrome" is discussed under its etiologic categories—i.e., herpes simplex virus, *Chlamydia* and LGV, gonorrhea, and syphilis. Enteritis is characterized by abdominal pain, bloating, nausea, cramping, and diarrhea, occasionally bloody. These diseases of the small intestine and colon occur as a result of infection with organisms that are usually transmitted by the fecal-oral route. They are the consequence of analingus or fellatio following anal intercourse with an infected partner. The major enteric bacterial pathogens (*Shigella* sp. and *Campylobacter* sp.) and protozoa (*Entamoeba histolytica* and *Giardia lamblia*) are involved in this syndrome.

Entamoeba histolytica

During the 1970s studies in New York City and San Francisco demonstrated the occurrence of amebiasis in gay men (1, 2). Cases of amebiasis have continued to increase to an estimated greater than 700 annually (3).

Infections with *E. histolytica* are often asymptomatic. However, the cysts excreted in the feces of asymptomatic carriers are infectious when ingested. Symptomatic amebiasis ranges from mild diarrhea to severe dysentary. Infection can spread from the intestine to produce liver abscesses and less commonly involve the lungs, pleura, or pericardium.

Diagnosis depends on demonstrating *E. histolytica* in stool specimens or on rectal biopsy. In patients with active intestinal or extraintestinal infection serologic tests are helpful.

For symptomatic patients the regimen of choice is metronidazole (750 mg, by mouth, 3 times a day for 5–10 days) plus either iodoguinol (diidohydroxyguin) (650 mg, by mouth, 3 times a day for 20 days) or diloxanide furate (500 mg, by mouth, 3 times a day for 10 days). An alternative regimen is paromomycin (25–30 mg/kg/day in 3 divided doses for 7 days) (3). Asymptomatic carriers with passage of amebic cysts should receive either iodoquinol (650 mg, by mouth, 3 times a day for 20 days) or diloxanide furoate (500 mg, by mouth, 3 times a day for 10 days).

Giardiasis

The disease giardiasis is caused by the parasitic organism *Giardia lamblia*. Similar to amebiasis, *G. lamblia* infection is now recognized as a sexually transmitted form of enteritis among male homosexuals (1, 2). The major mode of transmission is via analingus or fellatio following anal intercourse. Quinn and co-workers demonstrated that *G. lamblia* was present in 14% of homosexual men with symptomatic enteritis as compared to 4% of asymptomatic controls (3).

The proximal small bowel is the primary site of giardial infection, and thus signs of proctitis are absent. Upper gastrointestinal findings with epigastric pain, nausea, vomiting, and foul sulfuric eructation are present. The classical history for giardiasis is abrupt onset of explosive diarrhea, distention, and flatulence, and over several days development of a chronic illness in which low grade symptoms persist for months with weight loss (4).

Diagnosis is made by stool examination for cysts or trophozoites. If repeated stool specimens are negative in suspected cases, jejunal biopsy and aspiration can be performed to identify cysts or trophozoites.

The drug of choice for symptomatic and asymptomatic infection is quinacrine (100 mg, by mouth, 3 times a day for 7 days) (5). An alternative choice is metronidazole (250 mg, by mouth, 3 times a day for 7 days). The CDC recommends that for coexistent amebiasis and giardiasis, metronidazole in the higher dose as recommended for amebiasis is preferred.

Campylobacter

Campylobacter jejuni is now recognized as a pathogen in cases of enteritis. Blaser and Reller have suggested that this organism is a more frequent cause of bacterial diarrhea than salmonella or shigella (1). Quinn and co-workers documented the frequency and importance of *C. jejuni* in homosexual men with proctitis and colitis (2).

Campylobacter enteritis presents with sudden onset of abdominal pain and fever followed within 24 hr by diarrhea. Bloody diarrhea is present in about half the cases, and the majority have eight loose stools per day. Constitutional symptoms such as malaise, anorexia, headache, arthralgias, and myalgias occur in many patients.

The diagnosis is based upon recovery of *C. jejuni* from a stool specimen. The treatment of choice is erythromycin (500 mg, by mouth, 4 times a day for 7 days) (3).

Shigella

Dritz and Back described an epidemic of shigellosis in San Francisco's male homosexual population in the mid-1970s (1) and demonstrated the sexually transmitted nature of the disease. Quinn et al found shigellosis in 3% of intestinal infections in homosexual men (2).

The clinical presentation of shigellosis may vary from a mild, self-limited illness to a systemic, life-threatening infection. It begins insidiously or abruptly, following a 24- to 48-hr incubation period, with fever, abdominal cramps, and diarrhea. In mild cases it resolves completely, but may progress to dysentery with severe cramps, tenesmus, and bloody mucoid rectal discharges.

Treatment consists of correcting fluid and

electrolyte losses. Opiate or anticholinergic antidiarrheal drugs are to be avoided; they prolong symptoms and delay clearance of the organism and/or enterotoxin. Formerly ampicillin (500 mg, by mouth, four times a day for 7 days) was the regimen of choice. The CDC currently recommends trimethoprim/sulfamethoxazole, double strength tablets (160/800 mg) by mouth, twice daily for 7 days (3).

HEPATITIS B

Hepatitis B (formerly serum hepatitis) is caused by hepatitis B virus (HBV). The CDC estimates that 200,000 new cases of HBV occur annually in the United States (1). Of these cases approximately 5% are hospitalized. Based on CDC estimates, there are nearly one million carriers of HBV surface antigen (HBsAg) in the United States, and 25% of these carriers develop chronic active hepatitis which may progress to cirrhosis. Worldwide it is estimated that there are 150 million carriers of HBsAg. In addition, an undefined small percentage of these carriers will develop liver cancer (1).

HBV is a complex DNA virus consisting of an inner nuclear core, containing the double stranded DNA with hepatitis core antigen (HBcAg), which is completely enveloped by HBsAg. Once infected an immune response is manifested, by most patients, which clears the infection. This response includes antibodies to the core antigen (Anti-HBc) and surface antigen (Anti-HBs). Unfortunately, the CDC estimates that 6–10% of patients with acute HBV infection do not eliminate the virus and become chronic carriers with persistent HBs-Ag levels. More recently an additional antigen, the e antigen (HBe antigen) has been identified. It correlates with high levels of HBsAg, and its presence identifies patients that are at greater risk to develop chronic liver disease and those who are highly contagious and at greater risk for transmitting HBV (via sexual or vertical transmission).

The role of HBV in maternal infection and its effect on the fetus and neonate are detailed in Chapter 13. In this section only the role of HBV as a sexually transmitted disease agent will be discussed.

Fass proposed that HBV could be sexually transmitted in 1974 (2). Confirmation of this hypothesis was accomplished through a series of investigations which demonstrated that patients attending STD clinics had a significantly increased incidence of prior exposure to HBV than did controls (3–5). Studies in homosexual men revealed a 40–75% incidence of prior exposure to HBV (5–7). Further evidence for sexual transmission of HBV was provided by studies revealing higher levels of anti-HBs among prostitutes than controls (8, 9). Reiner and co-workers noted the presence of HBsAg in lesions of the rectal mucosa of male homosexuals who had HBsAg in their blood and suggested that these asymptomatic punctate bleeding sites are the source for HBV transmission with anal intercourse (10). In addition, HBsAg has been demonstrated in semen and saliva.

Clinical Presentation

The incubation time for hepatitis B is 30–130 days. Following the incubation period there is usually a prodromal phase with anorexia, nausea and vomiting, fever, malaise, headache, and abdominal pain. In hepatitis B this prodrome tends to be vague and insidious and lasts from several days to several weeks. As these symptoms abate jaundice appears. Most cases resolve without sequelae, except for the nearly 10% of patients with hepatitis B who develop chronic disease, 7% develop chronic persistent hepatitis, and 3% chronic active hepatitis. The jaundice period lasts from a few weeks to several months with HBV. Among homosexual men clinical hepatitis is unusual.

Diagnosis

Specific diagnosis of hepatitis B depends upon laboratory confirmation. HBsAg is the primary diagnostic tool for identifying HBV. It is present in the blood 30–50 days after exposure and 7–21 days prior to the onset of jaundice. HBsAg may disappear with onset of jaundice, or it may persist for several weeks. Chronic carriers of HBsAg occur in 1% of patients in the United States. This rate is higher among homosexual men. Hepatitis Be antigen appears early in the disease and persists for days to weeks; in some cases it lasts indefinitely. When HBeAg is present the patient is likely to be infectious.

Treatment and Prevention

No specific treatment exists for hepatitis B. Prevention is the best management. Initially, only passive immunization with either recent lots of immune globulin or preferentially hepatitis B immune globulin (HBIG) was available. Subsequent recommendations from CDC suggest giving HBIG (0.06 mg/kg) to susceptible individuals (i.e., no antibodies to HBsAg or HBcAg) exposed to HBsAg-positive blood (1). One dose is given immediately, and a second dose is given in 1 month's time.

Active immunization to HBV by means of an HBV vaccine is now available. Three doses (20 g/1.0 ml) are required at time 0, 1 month, and 6 months. In clinical trials among male homosexuals the vaccine has been shown to be very effective (11, 12). The vaccine has also been effective in preventing neonatal acquisition (13) and in protecting medical workers at high risk (14).

As of June, 1984, the Immunization Practices Advisory Committee for the CDC proposed new recommendations for postexposure prophylaxis of hepatitis B (15). These updated recommendations were the result of studies demonstrating the high efficacy of HB vaccine combined with HBIG in preventing chronic HB infection in infants of HBsAg-positive mothers. Passive immunization with HBIG has been partially effective in preventing clinical HB following needlestick accidents (16) and sexual exposure to acute HB (17). However, HBIG alone is only 75% effective and is expensive, costing over $150.00 per adult dose (two doses required) (15). Studies have demonstrated that simultaneous HBIG administration does not interfere with the immune response to HB vaccine and that the combination of HB vaccine and one dose of HBIG results in immediate and sustained high levels of anti-HBs (18). Moreover, Beasley and co-workers demonstrated that such a combination approach was highly effective in preventing HBV carrier state in infants born to HBeAg-positive mothers (19). Thus the CDC recommends that for needlestick, ocular, or mucous-membrane exposure to blood known to contain HBsAg, a single dose of HBIG (0.06 ml/kg or 5.0 ml for adults) should be given as soon as possible after exposure and within 24 hr if possible. HB vaccine 1 ml (20 g) should be given IM at a separate site simultaneously with HBIG and the second and third doses (20 g) given at 1 month and 6 months (15). In addition, the CDC recommends a single dose of HBIG (0.06 ml/kg or 5 ml for adults) be given to susceptible individuals who have had sexual contact with an HBsAg-positive person(s) if the HBIG can be given with 14 days of the last sexual contact (15).

GENITAL MYCOPLASMAS

The clinically significant genital tract mycoplasmas include *Mycoplasma hominis* and *Ureaplasma urealyticum* (formerly T-mycoplasma).

As these organisms are discussed thoroughly in Chapter 7, they will only be briefly reviewed here.

M. hominis and *U. urealyticum* are common genital organisms that have been associated with a variety of clinical conditions, including nongonococcal urethritis (1), nonspecific vaginitis (2), pelvic inflammatory disease (3–5), spontaneous abortion and stillbirths (6), premature birth and low birth weight (7, 8), chorioamnionitis (9, 10), and postpartum infections (11, 12). However, mycoplasmas are part of the normal genital tract flora of many sexually active men and women who have no obvious clinical disease or abnormalities (13). Thus any pathogenic role in human disease that is ascribed to the genital mycoplasmas must be assessed with this epidemiologic background in mind.

Colonization with *M. hominis* and *U. urealyticum* correlates with onset of sexual activity and increases directly with the number of sexual partners (13). A wide range in the recovery rate has been reported for *U. urealyticum* (40–95%) and for *M. hominis* (15–72%) among sexually active women. In men a similar pattern occurs but at a lower rate (*M. hominis*, 14% and *U. urealyticum*, 45%) (14). A newly described mycoplasma, *Mycoplasma genitalium* has been proposed as a human pathogen for the genital tract (15, 16).

The clinical manifestations, diagnostic features, and management of mycoplasma infections are described in Chapter 7.

CHLAMYDIA TRACHOMATIS

C. trachomatis has emerged as one of the most common (perhaps the most common) sexually transmitted organisms. *Chlamydia* is discussed in detail in Chapter 8, and its role in sexually transmitted diseases will be only briefly reviewed in this section.

Human strains of *C. trachomatis* have been differentiated into 15 serotypes. Serotypes L_1, L_2, L_3 cause lymphogranuloma venereum and A, B, Ba, and C are the pathogens in trachoma. The remaining serotypes (D through K) are the agents associated with sexually transmitted genital tract infections and vertically transmitted infections from mother to fetus or neonate (1).

C. trachomatis has been implicated in an expanded spectrum of diseases. Chlamydia is the major etiologic agent for nongonococcal urethritis (2), postgonococcal urethritis (1), and epididymitis in young men (3). Among women *C. trachomatis* has been associated with mucopurulent endocervicitis (4), endometritis (5, 6), pelvic inflammatory disease (7, 8), infertility due to tubal factors (9, 10), and the acute urethral syndrome (11). In pregnant women vertical transmission resulting in chlamydial conjunctivitis and/or pneumonia is well documented (12). A role for *C. trachomatis* in postpartum infections (13), premature labor and delivery (14, 15), ruptured membranes (14, 15), and perinatal mortality (14, 15) is controversial and not established.

The epidemiology, clinical presentation, diagnosis, and treatment of chlamydial infection is described in Chapter 8 and will not be discussed here.

HERPES SIMPLEX VIRUS

Genital herpes is a sexually transmitted disease caused by herpes simplex virus types 1 and 2 (HSV-1 and HSV-2). HSV contains an inner core of double-stranded DNA surrounded by a glycoprotein envelope. The two types of HSV are distinguished by biochemical, immunologic, and serologic methods. Although HSV-2 infections are found primarily in the genital area, approximately 15% of primary genital herpes infections are caused by HSV-1 (1). The use of restrictive endonuclease cleavage of the HSV DNA has led to the recognition that there are multiple specific strains of HSV-1 and HSV-2, rather than only the two types. Herpes is discussed in detail in Chapter 13, especially in reference to perinatal effects of HSV. In this section the STD aspects of HSV will be emphasized.

Epidemiology

Estimates from the CDC demonstrate that from 1966 to 1979 there was a nine-fold increase to 260,000 physician visits for genital herpes (2). It is estimated that 500,000 new cases of genital HSV infection occur annually in the United States, with the prevalence of genital HSV disease being 20 million cases (3). Based on the work of Corey et al (4) and Chuang et al (5) it seems apparent that genital herpes occurs in a slightly older, more educated, married and white population. Not surprisingly, Corey et al recently noted a significant progressive increase in the number of neonatal HSV infections between 1966 and 1981 (6); case rates increased from 2.6 per 100,000 live births to 11.9 per 100,000 live births.

Genital herpes is a recurrent disease, and the frequency of recurrence is three to four-fold higher in HSV-2 versus HSV-1 infections. Unfortunately nearly one-fourth of recurrences are asymptomatic viral excretors (4). Baker summarized the epidemiology of HSV as follows: (a) It is a sexually transmitted disease; (b) HSV is endemic in the United States; (c) the incidence is approximately 1–2% of the population; (d) 50–80% of adults have antibodies to HSV-1 or HSV-2; (e) the highest frequency of HSV occurs in the 15- to 29-year-old age group; and (f) HSV is associated with the presence of other STDs (3).

Presence of cervical HSV infection is in large part determined by the type of HSV infection. HSV cervical shedding occurs in 80–86% of women with primary genital infection, 65% of nonprimary first episode HSV-2 infections, and about 12% of recurrent genital HSV (4).

While the role of HSV as a STD and its serious implications for the neonate are generally accepted, considerable controversy exists over the role (if any) HSV plays in the etiology of cervical carcinoma (7, 8).

Corey has summarized two hypothesis for triggering of recurrent episodes of HSV (1). The "ganglion trigger" theory states that a stimulus affects the latently infected ganglion cells in such a way that productive viral replication associated with axonal flow of virus down the peripheral nerve occurs, invasion of skin occurs, and the characteristic vesicular lesions develop. The alternative "skin trigger" hypothesis states that virus is produced frequently by the ganglion, reaching the skin every few days. The body's immune defenses normally eliminate the microfoci of infection; if local immunosuppression occurs there is enough viral production to cause the vesicular lesions of HSV.

Clinical Presentation

The clinical manifestations of genital HSV occur as three distinct syndromes (4). First episode primary genital herpes is the initial genital HSV infection in an individual without circulating antibodies to HSV-1 or HSV-2. Approximately 75% of susceptible sexual partners of patients actively shedding HSV develop HSV infection (9). First episode primary HSV is associated with severe local symptoms with multiple painful lesions which progress from vesicles to an ulcerative stage, inguinal adenopathy, and systemic effects such as fever, malaise, myalgias, headache, and nausea.

First-episode nonprimary genital herpes is the initial clinical episode of genital HSV in patients with circulating antibodies to HSV-1 and HSV-2. It has a clinical course which is similar to that seen in recurrent genital herpes. Recurrent disease occurs more frequently following initial HSV-2 infection than HSV-1. Mild local symptoms usually occur and last about half as long as primary first episode HSV infection. Only a few lesions occur, and systemic manifestations are absent. In addition, the duration of viral shedding is shorter, and the likelihood of concomitant cervical HSV shedding is less than with primary disease.

Diagnosis

In the majority of HSV genital infections the diagnosis is made clinically and is based on the presence of the characteristic herpetic lesions. Laboratory procedures will confirm the diagnosis. At present, viral culture for HSV is the most reliable diagnostic test. Attempts have been made to develop rapid diagnostic tests such as indirect immunoperoxidase and direct immunofluorescence.

Cytologic testing is associated with a high percentage of false-negative readings. A positive cytologic find of typical viral giant cells is useful. Serologic studies on paired acute and convalescent bloods are only useful in identifying first episode primary HSV genital infection and cannot verify the presence of active viral shedding in recurrent genital herpes. Corey and Holmes maintain that isolation of HSV in tissue culture is the most sensitive and specific test for confirming active HSV infection. Cytologic and antigen detection techniques are roughly 50 and 70% as sensitive, respectively, as culture (10).

Treatment

Acyclovir remains the only compound demonstrated by controlled trials to be effective in the treatment of genital HSV infection (10). Initially, topical acyclovir was shown to be effective in reducing local symptoms and signs of first episode primary HSV infections (11). More recently, intravenous acyclovir (5 mg/kg dose at 8 hourly intervals for 5 days) has been very effective in first episode primary HSV by decreasing the duration of viral shedding, local and systemic symptoms, and accelerating the rate of lesion healing (12). Oral acyclovir (200 mg, 5 times per day for 10 days) significantly reduced the duration of viral shedding, accelerated healing time, and reduced the duration and severity of symptoms in first episode primary herpes (13). Use of oral acyclovir as a prophylactic agent to prevent recurrent HSV genital

infections has been reported (14). However, the preventive effect was seen only while the drug was continuously taken; once oral acyclovir was stopped, recurrences resumed (14).

Recently, Straus et al (15) and Douglas et al (16) have demonstrated in placebo controlled, double-blind studies that oral acyclovir suppresses genital herpes in patients with frequent recurrent HSV disease. However, oral acyclovir does not influence the long-term natural history of the disease (16), and concerns over inducing drug resistance and long-term safety of acyclovir require additional study (15).

CYTOMEGALOVIRUS

Cytomegalovirus (CMV) is a member of the *Herpesvirus* family. It is a DNA virus which is capable of producing recurrent and/or latent infection (1, 2). Initially, CMV was associated with fulminant neonatal infection characterized by jaundice, thrombocytopenia, purpura, hepatosplenomegaly, and central nervous system involvement (2). Subsequently, CMV has been recognized as a fairly common cause of subclinical congenital infection (3). More recently, CMV has been implicated as a sexually transmitted agent (4, 5). The impact of CMV as a perinatal infection is discussed in Chapter 13 and will not be described here. In this section the role of CMV as a STD will be examined. Sexual transmission of CMV was suggested by studies which recovered CMV from both semen (4) and cervical secretions (5).

CMV has been described as an ubiquitous virus because of its widespread occurrence (6). The prevalence of antibody to CMV suggesting past CMV infection varies according to the population studied and geographic area from 20 to 100% (7, 8). In the United States and Western industrialized nations adult populations have antibody levels in the 20–80% range (8), while higher antibody rates occur in the underdeveloped nations and among lower socioeconomic groups (7). Interestingly, Luby and Shasby reported that women have higher prevalence rates of anti-CMV antibodies than men (9). In addition, women attending STD clinics have a higher prevalence of CMV antibodies than comparison control populations (5, 10, 11). Similarly, these studies noted that in the STD population the isolation rate from cervical secretions was higher than in control patients (5, 10, 11). Handsfield and co-workers reported the isolation of CMV from three of six sexual partners of women with positive CMV cultures; among the 16 control women, none of their partners had recovery of CMV (11). In particular, as noted by Knox et al, young sexually active females in the 11- to 14-year age group had the highest prevalence of cervical CMV (15 %), and the rate of positive cultures decreased with age to be negligible over the age of 30 yr (12). Further evidence for the sexual transmission of CMV comes from the work of Drew and colleagues in homosexual men (13). They noted that homosexual men had an antibody prevalence rate of 94% compared to a 54% rate in heterosexual men attending the same STD clinic. Whereas none of the heterosexual men had CMV cultured from the urethra, 14 of 190 homosexual men had CMV recovered from the urethra.

The optimum method for detecting active infection is isolation of CMV (2). Specimens for viral isolation include urine, urethra, cervix, or nasopharynx. CMV is grown in human fibroblast cell culture and identified by the presence of typical cytopathic effects. Several methods of serologic testing are available. These include complement fixation, indirect fluorescent antibody, enzyme-linked immunosorbent assays, and monoclonal antibodies (14).

Therapy of severe CMV infections has been studied with adenosine arabinoside (15) and interferon (16) without much success. More recently, clinical trials with acyclovir have also been attempted (17). However, these treatment modalities have not been attempted in patients with CMV carriage in their cervix or urethra but without severe clinical infection. Starr and coworkers have demonstrated that an attenuated life CMV vaccine produced evidence of both cellular and humoral immunity (18). Only large scale trials will ultimately determine if CMV vaccine(s) can prevent CMV infection and/or acquisition.

References

Gonorrhea

1. U.S. Department of Health and Human Services Public Health Service (1981). STD Fact Sheet, Edition 35: Basic Statistics on the Sexually Transmitted Disease Problems in the United States. HHS Publication No. (CDC) 81-8195.
2. Spence MR: Gonorrhea. *Clin Obstet Gynecol* 25:111–124, 1983.
3. Curran JW, Rendtorff RC, Chandler RW, et al: Female gonorrhea: its relationship to abnormal uterine bleeding, urinary tract symptoms and cervicitis. *Obstet Gynecol* 45:195–198, 1975.
4. Kellogg DS Jr, Peacock WL Jr, Deacon WE, et al: *Neisseria gonorrhoeae*. I. Virulence genetically linked to clonal variation. *J Bacteriol* 85:1274–1279, 1963.
5. Ward ME, Watt DJ, Robertson JN: The human fallopian tube: a laboratory model for gonococcal infection. *J Infect Dis* 129:650–659, 1974.
6. James JF, Swanson J: Studies on gonococcus infection. XIII. Occurrence of color/opacity colonial variant in clinical cultures. *Infect Immun* 19:332–340, 1978.
7. Draper DL, James JF, Brooks GF, Sweet RL: Comparison of virulence markers of peritoneal-fallopian tube and endocervical *Neisseria gonorrhoeae* isolates from women with acute salpingitis. *Infect Immun* 27:882–888, 1980.
8. Sweet RL: Acute salpingitis: diagnosis and management. *J Reprod Med* 19:21–30, 1977.
9. Centers for Disease Control: Annual summary 1982: reported morbidity and mortality in the United States. *MMWR* 31:29–33, 1983.
10. Darrow WW, Barrett D, Jay K, Young A: The gay report on sexually transmitted diseases. *Am J Public Health* 71:1004–1011, 1981.
11. Cooper DL, Bernstein GS, Ivler D, et al: Gonorrhea screening program in a women's hospital outpatient department: results and analysis of risk factors. *J Am Vener Dis Assoc* 3:71–75, 1976.
12. Darrow WW: Social stratification, sexual behavior and the sexually transmitted diseases. *Sex Transm Dis* 6:228–230, 1979.
13. Noble, RC, Kirk NM, Siegal WA, et al: Recidivism among patients with gonococcal infection presenting to a venereal disease clinic. *Sex Transm Dis* 4:39–43, 1977.
14. Ross MV: Social factors in homosexually acquired venereal disease: comparison between Sweden and Australia. *Br J Vener Dis* 58:263–268, 1982.
15. Dans PE: Gonococcal anogenital infection. *Clin Obstet Gynecol* 18:103–119, 1975.
16. Bro-Jorgensen A, Jensen T: Gonococcal pharyngeal infections. Report of 110 cases. *Br J Vener Dis* 49: 491–499, 1973.
17. Weisner PJ: Gonorrhea. *Cutis* 27:249–254, 1981.
18. Klein EJ, Fisher LS, Chow AW, Guze LB: Anorectal gonococcal infection. *Ann Intern Med* 86:340–346, 1977.
19. Pariser H, Marino AF: Gonorrhea—frequently unrecognized reservoirs. *South Med J* 63:198–201, 1970.
20. Holmes KK, Counts GW, Beaty HN: Disseminated gonococcal infection. *Ann Intern Med* 74:979–993, 1971.
21. Suleiman SA, Grimes EM, Jones HS: Disseminated gonococcal infections. *Obstet Gynecol* 61:48–51, 1983.
22. Weisner PH, Handsfield HH, Holmes KK: Antibiotic resistance of gonococci causing disseminated infection. *N Engl J Med* 288:1221–1222, 1973.
23. Schoolnick GK, Buchanan TM, Holmes KK: Gonococci causing disseminated gonococcal infection are resistant to bactericidal action of normal human sera. *J Clin Invest* 58:1163–1173, 1976.
24. Knapp JS, Holmes KK: Disseminated gonococcal infections caused by *Neisseria gonorrhoeae* with unique nutritional requirements. *J Infect Dis* 1132:204–208, 1975.
25. Peterson BH, Lee TJ, Snyderman R, Brooks GF:

Neisseria meningitis and *Neisseria gonorrhoeae* bacteremia associated with C_6, C_7, C_8 deficiency. *Ann Intern Med* 90:917–920, 1979.

26. Burkman RT, Tonascia JA, Atienza MF, et al: Untreated endocervical gonorrhea and endometritis following abortion. *Am J Obstet Gynecol* 126:648–651, 1976.

27. Sarrel PM, Pruett KA: Symptomatic gonorrhea during pregnancy. *Obstet Gynecol* 32:670–673, 1968.

28. Handsfield HH, Hodson A, Holmes KK: Neonatal gonococcal infection. I. Orogastric contamination with *Neisseria gonorrhoeae*. *JAMA* 225:6977–701, 1973.

29. Edwards LE, Barrada MI, Hamann AA, Hakanson EY: Gonorrhea in pregnancy. *Am J Obstet Gynecol* 132:637–641, 1978.

30. Holmes KK: Gonococcal infection. In Remington JS, Klein JO (eds): *Infectious Diseases of the Fetus and Newborn Infant*. Philadelphia, WB Saunders, 1983, pp 616–636.

31. Handsfield HH: Gonorrhea and nongonococcal urethritis—recent advances. *Med Clin North Am* 62:925–943, 1978.

32. Goodhart GL, Kramer M, Zaidi AA: Characteristics of defaulters in treatment for infection with *Neisseria gonorrhoeae*. *J Infect Dis* 140:649–651, 1979.

33. Aardom HA, DeHoop D, Iserief COA, et al: Detection of *Neisseria gonorrhoeae* antigen by a solid phase enzyme immunoassay. *Br J Vener Dis* 58:359–362, 1982.

34. Jaffe HW, Kraus SJ, Edwards TA, et al: Diagnosis of gonorrhea using a genetic transformation test on mailed clinical specimens. *Infect Dis* 146:275–279, 1982.

35. Sexually transmitted diseases treatment guidelines 1982. MMWR 31(Suppl):37–42, 1982.

36. Sweet RL, Schachter J, Landers DV: Chlamydial infections in obstetrics and gynecology. *Gynecol* 26:143–164, 1983.

37. Robbins JB: Problems posed by potential gonococcal vaccines viewed from the vantage point of a control agency. *Br J Vener Dis* 53:170–172, 1977.

Syphilis

1. Centers for Disease Control: Annual summary 1982: reported morbidity and mortality in the United States. *MMWR* 31:77–82, 1983.

2. Centers for Disease Control: Syphilis trends in the United States. *MMWR* 31:441–444, 1981.

3. Chapel TA: The signs and symptoms of 2° syphilis. *Sex Transm Dis* 7:161–164, 1980.

4. Charles D: Syphilis. *Clin Obstet Gynecol* 26:125–137, 1983.

5. Youmans JB: Syphilis and other venereal diseases. *Med Clin North Am* 48:571–824, 1964.

6. Harter CA, Benirschke K: Fetal syphilis in the first trimester. *Am J Obstet Gynecol* 124:705–711, 1976.

7. Ingall D, Musher D: Syphilis. In Reminton JS, Klein JO (eds): *Infectious Diseases of the Fetus and Newborn Infant*. Philadelphia, WB Saunders, 1983, pp 335–374.

8. Fiumara NJ, Fleming WL, Downing JG, Good FL: The incidence of prenatal syphilis at the Boston City Hospital. *N Engl J Med* 247:48–52, 1952.

9. Sequeira PJL: Serological diagnosis of untreated syphilis: importance of the differences in THA, TPHA and VDRL test titers. *Br J Vener Dis* 59:145–150, 1983.

10. Lugar A, Schmidt BL, Steyrer K, et al: Diagnosis of neurosyphilis by examination of the cerebrospinal fluid. *Br J Vener Dis* 57:232–237, 1981.

11. McGeeney T, Yount F, Hinthorn DR, Liu C: Utility of the FTA-ABS test of cerebrospinal fluid in the diagnosis of neurosyphilis. *Sex Transm Dis* 6:195–198, 1979.

12. Jones JE, Harris RE: Diagnostic evaluation of syphilis during pregnancy. *Obstet Gynecol* 54:611, 1979.

13. Sexually transmitted diseases treatment guidelines 1982. *MMWR* 31(Suppl), 1982.

14. Polnikorn N, Witoonpanich R, Vorachit M, et al: Penicillin concentrates in cerebrospinal fluid after different regimens for syphilis. *Br J Vener Dis* 56:363, 1980.

Chancroid

1. Ronald AR, Wilt JC, Albritton WL: Haemophilus ducreyi. In Holmes KK, Mardh P-A (eds): *International Perspectives on Neglected Sexually Transmitted Diseases*. Washington, DC, Hemisphere Publishing Corp, 1983, pp 93–102.

2. Centers for Disease Control: Annual summary 1982. *MMWR* 31:173–175, 1982.

3. Gaisin A, Heaton CL: Chancroid: alias the soft chancre. *Int J Dermatol* 14:188–197, 1975.

4. Marmar JL: The management of resistant chancroid in Vietnam. *J Urol* 107:807–808, 1972.

5. Centers for Disease Control: Chancroid California. *MMWR* 31:173–175, 1982.

6. Hammond GW, Chang JL, Wilt JC, Ronald AR: Comparison of specimen collection and laboratory techniques for isolation of *Haemophilus ducreyi. J Clin Microbiol* 7:39–43, 1978.

Lymphogranuloma Venereum

1. Grayston JT, Wang SP: New knowledge of chlamydiae and the diseases they cause. *J Infect Dis* 132:87–105, 1975.

2. Osoba AO: Lymphogranuloma venereum. In Holmes KK, Mardh P-A (eds): *International Perspectives on Neglected Sexually Transmitted Diseases*. Washington, DC, Hemisphere Publishing Corp, 1983, pp 193–204.

3. Willcox RR: International aspects of the venereal diseases and nonvenereal treponematoses. *Clin Obstet Gynecol* 18:207–222, 1975.

4. Schachter J: Lymphogranuloma venereum and other nonocular *Chlamydia trachomatis*. In Hobson D, Holmes KK (eds): *Nongonococcal Urethritis and Related Infections*. Washington, DC, American Society for Microbiology, 1977, pp 91–97.

5. Bolan RK, Sands M, Schachter J, et al: Lymphogranuloma venereum and acute ulcerative proctitis. *Am J Med* 72:703–706, 1982.

6. Hart G: Chancroid, Donovanosis and Lymphogranuloma Venereum. U.S. Department of Health and Human Services Publication 1982; No. (CDC) 82-8302.

7. Schachter J, Smith DE, Dawson CR, et al: Lymphogranuloma venereum. I. Comparison of the Frei test, complement fixation test and isolation

of the agent. *J Infect Dis* 120:372–375, 1969.
8. Schachter J: Chlamydial infections. *N Engl J Med* 298:428–435, 490–495, 540–549, 1978.
9. Centers for Disease Control: Sexually transmitted disease, treatment guidelines 1982. *MMWR* 31(Suppl):505–545, 1982.

Granuloma Inguinale

1. Kuberski T: Granuloma inguilnale (donovanosis). *Sex Transm Dis* 7:29–36, 1980.
2. Sowmini CN: Donovanosis. In Holmes KK, Mardh P-A (eds): *International Perspectives on Neglected Sexually Transmitted Diseases*. Washington, DC, Hemisphere Publishing Corp, 1983, pp 205–217.
3. Lal S, Nicholas C: Epidemiological and clinical features in 165 cases of granuloma inguinale. *Br J Vener Dis* 46:461–463, 1970.
4. Goldberg J: Studies on granuloma inguinale, VI and VIII. *Br J Vener Dis* 40:137–145, 1964.
5. Lal S, Garg BR: Further evidence of the efficacy of the co-trimoxazole in granuloma inguinale. *Br J Vener Dis* 56:412–413, 1980.

Scabies

1. Oriel JD: Ectoparasites. In Holmes KK, Mardh P-A (eds): *International Perspectives on Neglected Sexually Transmitted Diseases*. Washington, DC, Hemisphere Publishing Corp., 1983, pp 131–138.
2. Orkin M: Resurgence of scabies. *JAMA* 217:593–597, 1971.
3. Cohen HB: Scabies continues. *Int J Dermatol* 21:134–135, 1982.
4. Orkin M, Maibach H: Scabies, a current pandemic. *Postgrad Med* 66:53–65, 1979.
5. Centers for Disease Control: Sexually transmitted disease, treatment guidelines, 1982. *MMWR* 31(Suppl):55–56.
6. Kramer MS: Toxicity of 1% gamma benzene hexachloride (GBH): an operational assessment. *Cutis*, September Suppl:20–25, 1981.

Pediculosis Pubis

1. Oriel JD: Ectoparasites. In Holmes KK, Mardh R-A (eds): *International Perspectives on Neglected Sexually Transmitted Diseases*. Washington, DC, Hemisphere Publishing Corp, 1983, pp 131–138.
2. Felman YM, Nikitas JA: Pediculosis pubis. *Cutis* 25:482, 487–489, 559, 1980.
3. Fisher I, Morton RS: Pthirus pubis infestation. *Br J Vener Dis* 46:326–329, 1970.
4. Centers for Disease Control: Sexually transmitted disease treatment guidelines 1982. *MMWR* 31(Suppl):56.

Molluscum Contagiosum

1. Brown ST, Nalley JF, Kraos SJ: Molluscum contagiosum. *Sex Transm Dis* 8:227–234, 1981.
2. Kwitten J: Molluscum contagiosum: some new histologic observations. *Mt Sinai J Med NY* 47:583–588, 1980.
3. Chief Medical Officer of the Department of Health and Social Security: Extract from the Annual Report for the year 1978: Sexually transmitted diseases. *Br J Vener Dis* 56:178–181, 1980.

Condyloma Acuminatum

1. Barrett TJ, Silbar JD, McGinley JP: Genital warts—a venereal disease. *JAMA* 154:333–334, 1954.
2. Felman YM, Nikitas JA: Condyloma acuminata. *NY State J Med* 79:1747–1749, 1979.
3. Coggin JR, zur Hausen H: Workshop on papillomaviruses and cancer. *Cancer Res* 39:545–546, 1979.
4. Lutzner MA: The human papilloma viruses: a review. *Arch Dermatol* 119:631–635, 1983.
5. Gissman L, zur Hausen H: Partial characterization of viral DNA from human genital warts (condyloma acuminata). *Int J Cancer* 25:605–609, 1980.
6. Staguet MJ, Viac J, Bustamante R, Thivolet J: Human papillomavirus type I purified from human genital warts. *Dermatologica* 162:213–219, 1981.
7. Oriel JD: Natural history of genital warts. *Br J Vener Dis* 47:1–13, 1971.
8. Centers for Disease Control: Condyloma acuminatum—United States, 1966–1981. *MMWR* 32:306–308, 1983.
9. Meisels A, Fortin R, Roy M: Condylomatous lesions of the cervix. II. Cytologic, colposcopic and histopathologic study. *Acta Cytol* 21:379–390, 1977.
10. Chamberlain MJ, Reynolds AL, Yeoman WB: Toxic effects of podophyllin. Application in pregnancy. *Br Med J* 3:391–392, 1972.
11. Cook TA, Cohn AM, Brunchwig JP, et al: Wart viruses and laryngeal papillomas. *Lancet* 1:782–783, 1973.

Trichomonas vaginalis

1. Lossick JG: Treatment of *Trichomonas vaginalis* infections. *Rev Infect Dis* 4(Suppl):801–818, 1982.

Gay Bowel Syndrome

1. Sohn N, Robilotti JG: The gay bowel syndrome. A review of colonic and rectal conditions in 200 male homosexuals. *Am J Gastroenterol* 67:478–484, 1977.

Entamoeba histolytica

1. Schmerin MH, Gelston A, Jones TC: Amebiasis. An increasing problem among homosexuals in New York City. *JAMA* 238:1386–1387, 1977.
2. Pearce RB: Intestinal protozoal infections and AIDS. *Lancet* 2:51, 1983.
3. Centers for Disease Control: Sexually transmitted diseases treatment guidelines 1982. *MMWR* 31(Suppl):56–58, 1982.

Giardiasis

1. Mildvan D, Gelb AM, William D: Venereal transmission of enteric pathogens in male homosexuals. *JAMA* 238:1387–1389, 1977.
2. Schmerin MJ, Jones TC, Klein H: Giardiasis: association with homosexuality. *Ann Intern Med* 88:801–803, 1978.
3. Quinn TC, Stamm WE, Goodell SE, et al: The polymicrobial origin of intestinal infections in

homosexual men. *N Engl J Med* 309:576–582, 1983.

4. Wolfe MS: Giardiasis. *N Engl J Med* 298:319–321, 1978.
5. Centers for Disease Control. Sexually transmitted diseases treatment guidelines 1982. *MMWR* 31(Suppl):58, 1982.

Campylobacter

1. Blaser MJ, Reller LB: Campylobacter enteritis. *N Engl J Med* 305:1444–1452, 1981.
2. Quinn TC, Stamm WE, Goodell SE, et al: The polymicrobial origin of intestinal infections in homosexual men. *N Engl J Med* 309:576–582, 1983.
3. Centers for Disease Control: Sexually transmitted diseases treatment guidelines 1982. *MMWR* 31 (Suppl):57, 1982.

Shigella

1. Dritz SK, Back AF: Shigella enteritis venereally transmitted. *N Engl J Med* 291:1194, 1974.
2. Quinn TC, Stamm WE, Goodell SE, et al: The polymicrobial origin of intestinal infections in homosexual men. *N Engl J Med* 309:576–582, 1983.
3. Centers for Disease Control. Sexually transmitted diseases treatment schedules 1982. *MMWR* 31(Suppl):57, 1984.

Hepatitis B

1. Centers for Disease Control: Inactivated hepatitis B virus vaccine. Recommendations of the Immunization Practices Advisory Committee. *Ann Intern Med* 97:379–383, 1982.
2. Fass RJ: Sexual transmission of viral hepatitis? *JAMA* 230:861–862, 1974.
3. Hentzer B, Skinhoj P, Hoybye G, et al: Viral hepatitis in a venereal clinic population. *Scand J Infect Dis* 12:245–249, 1980.
4. Szmuness W, Much MI, Prince AM, et al: On the role of sexual behavior in the spread of hepatitis B infection. *Ann Intern Med* 83:489–495, 1975.
5. Dieetzman DE, Harnisch JP, Ray CG, et al: Hepatitis B surface antigen (HBsAg) and antibody to HBsAg. Prevalence in homosexual and heterosexual men. *JAMA* 238:2625–2626, 1977.
6. Murphy BL, Schreeder MJ, Maynard JE, et al: Serologic testing for hepatitis B in male homosexuals. Special emphasis on hepatitis Be antigen and antibody by radioimmunoassay. *J Clin Microbiol* 11:301–303, 1980.
7. Hoybye G, Skinhoj P, Hentzer B, et al: An epidemic of acute viral hepatitis in male homosexuals. *Scand J Infect Dis* 12:241–244, 1980.
8. Frosner GG, Buchholz HM, Gerth HJ: Prevalence of hepatitis B antibody in prostitutes. *Am J Epidemiol* 102:241–250, 1975.
9. Papaevangelou G, Trichopoulos D, Kremastinou T, Papoutsakis G: Prevalence of hepatitis B antigen and antibody in prostitutes. *Br Med J* 2:256–258, 1974.
10. Reiner NE, Judson FN, Bond WW, et al: Asymptomatic rectal mucosal lesions and hepatitis B surface antigen at sites of sexual contact in homosexual men with persistent hepatitis B virus infection. *Ann Intern Med* 96:170–173, 1982.

11. Szmuness W, Stevens CE, Harley EJ, et al: Hepatitis B vaccine. Demonstration of efficacy in a controlled clinical trial in a high-risk population in the United States. *N Engl J Med* 303:833–841, 1980.
12. Francis DP, Hadler SC, Thompson SE, et al: The prevention of hepatitis B with vaccine. Report of the Centers for Disease Control. Multicenter efficacy trial among homosexual men. *Ann Intern Med* 97:362–366, 1982.
13. Maupas P, Barin F, Chiron J-P, et al: Efficacy of hepatitis B vaccine in prevention of early HBsAg carrier state in children. *Lancet* 1:289–292, 1981.
14. Szmuness W, Stevens CE, Harley EJ, et al: Hepatitis B vaccine in medical staff of hemodialysis units. *N Engl J Med* 307:1481–1486, 1982.
15. Centers for Disease Control: Postexposure prophylaxis of hepatitis B. *MMWR* 33:285–290, 1984.
16. Seeff LB, Wright EC, Zimmerman HJ, et al: Type B hepatitis after needle-stick exposure: prevention with hepatitis B immune globulin. Final report of the Veterans Administration Cooperative Study. *Ann Intern Med* 88:285–293, 1978.
17. Redecker AG, Mosley JW, Gocke DJ, et al: Hepatitis B immune globulin as a prophylactic measure for spouses exposed to acute type B hepatitis. *N Engl J Med* 293:1055–1059, 1975.
18. Szmuness W, Stevens CE, Oleszko WR, Goodman A: Passive-active immunization against hepatitis B: immunogenicity studies in adult Americans. *Lancet* 1:575–577, 1981.
19. Beasley RP, Hwang LY, Lee GC, et al: Prevention of perinatally transmitted hepatitis B virus infections with hepatitis B immune globulin and hepatitis B vaccine. *Lancet* 2:1099–1102, 1983.

Mycoplasmas

1. Oriel JD: Role of genital mycoplasmas in nongonococcal urethritis and prostatis. *Sex Transm Dis* 10(Suppl):263–270, 1983.
2. Paavonen J, Miettinen A, Stevens CE, et al: *Mycoplasma hominis* in nonspecific vaginitis. *Sex Transm Dis* 10(Suppl):271–275, 1983.
3. Mardh P-A, Westrom L: Tubal and cervical cultures in acute salpingitis with special reference to *Mycoplasma hominis* and T-strain mycoplasmas. *Br J Vener Dis* 46:179–186, 1970.
4. Eschenbach DA, Buchanan T, Pollock HM, et al: Polymicrobial etiology of acute pelvic inflammatory disease. *N Engl J Med* 293:166–171, 1975.
5. Sweet RL, Draper DL, Schachter J, et al: Microbiology and pathogenesis of acute salpingitis as determined by laparoscopy: what is the appropriate site to sample? *Am J Obstet Gynecol* 138:985–989, 1980.
6. Harwick HJ, Purcell RH, Iuppa JB, et al: *Mycoplasma hominis* and abortion. *J Infect Dis* 121:260–268, 1970.
7. Braun P, Lee Y-H, Klein JO, et al: Birth weight and genital mycoplasmas in pregnancy. *N Engl J Med* 284:167–171, 1971.
8. Kass EH, McCormack WM, Lin J-S, et al: Genital mycoplasmas as a cause of excess premature delivery. *Trans Assoc Am Phys* 94:261–266, 1981.
9. Shurin PA, Alpert S, Rosner B, et al: Chorioamnionitis and colonization of the newborn infant with genital mycoplasmas. *N Engl J Med* 293:5–8, 1975.

10. Blanco JD, Gibbs RS, Malherbe H, et al: A controlled study of genital mycoplasmas in amniotic fluid from patients with intra-amniotic infection. *J Infect Dis* 147:650–653, 1983.
11. McCormack WM, Lee Y-H, Lin J-S, Rankin JS: Genital mycoplasmas in postpartum infection. *J Infect Dis* 127:193–196, 1973.
12. Lamey JR, Eschenbach DA, Mitchell SM, et al: Isolation of mycoplasmas and bacteria from the blood of postpartum women. *Am J Obstet Gynecol* 143:104–111, 1982.
13. McCormack WM: Epidemiology of *Mycoplasma hominis*. *Sex Trans Dis* 10:261–262, 1983.
14. Taylor-Robinson D, McCormack WM: The genital mycoplasmas. *N Engl J Med* 302:1003–1010, 1063–1067, 1980.
15. Møller BR, Taylor-Robinson D, Furr PM: Serological evidence implicating *Mycoplasma genitalium* in pelvic inflammatory disease. *Lancet* 1:1102–1103, 1984.
16. Tully JG, Cole RM, Taylor-Robinson D, Rose DL: A newly discovered mycoplasma in the human urogenital tract, *Lancet* 1:1288–1291, 1981.

Chlamydia trachomatis

1. Schachter J: Chlamydial infections. *N Engl J Med* 298:428–435, 490–495, 540–549, 1978.
2. Holmes KK, Handsfield HH, Wang S-P, et al: Etiology of nongonococcal urethritis. *N Engl J Med* 292:1199–1206, 1975.
3. Berger RE, Alexander ER, Monda GD, et al: *Chlamydia trachomatis* as a cause of "idiopathic" epididymitis. *N Engl J Med* 298:301–304, 1978.
4. Tait IA, Rees E, Hobson D, et al: Chlamydial infection of the cervix in contacts of men with nongonococcal urethritis. *Br J Vener Dis* 56:37–45, 1980.
5. Mardh P-A, Moller BR, Ingerselv HJ, et al: Endometritis caused by *Chlamydia trachomatis*. *Br J Vener Dis* 57:191–195, 1981.
6. Gump DW, Dickstein S, Gibson M: Endometritis related to *Chlamydia trachomatis* infection. *Ann Intern Med* 95:61–63, 1981.
7. Mardh P-A, Ripa KT, Svensson L, Westrom L: *Chlamydia trachomatis* in patients with acute salpingitis. *N Engl J Med* 296:1377–1379, 1977.
8. Sweet RL, Schachter J, Robbie MO: Failure of B-lactam antibiotics to eradicate *Chlamydia trachomatis* in the endometrium despite apparent clinical cure of acute salpingitis. *JAMA* 250:2641–2645, 1983.
9. Jones RB, Ardery BR, Hui SL, et al: Correlation between serum antichlamydial antibodies and tubal factors as a cause of infertility. *Fertil Steril* 38:553–555, 1982.
10. Gump DW, Gibson M, Ashikaga T: Evidence of prior pelvic inflammatory disease and its relationship to *Chlamydia trachomatis* antibody and intrauterine contraception devices in infertile women. *Am J Obstet Gynecol* 146:153–159, 1983.
11. Stamm WE, Wagner KF, Ansel R, et al: Causes of the acute urethral syndrome in women. *N Engl J Med* 303:409–415, 1980.
12. Schachter J, Grossman M: Chlamydia. In Remington J, Klien JO (eds): *Infections of the Fetus and Newborn*. Philadelphia, WB Saunders, 1983.
13. Wager GP, Martin DH, Koutsky L, et al: Puerperal infectious morbidity: relationship to route of delivery and to antepartum *Chlamydia trachomatis* infection. *Am J Obstet Gynecol* 138:1028–1033, 1980.
14. Martin DH, Koutsky L, Eschenbach DA, et al: Prematurity and perinatal mortality in pregnancies complicated by maternal *Chlamydia trachomatis* infections. *JAMA* 247:1585–1588, 1982.
15. Harrison HR, Alexander ER, Weinstein L, et al: Cervical *Chlamydia trachomatis* and mycoplasmal infections in pregnancy. Epidemiology and outcomes. *JAMA* 250:1721–1727, 1983.

Herpes Simplex Virus

1. Corey L: Herpes simplex virus. In Holmes KK, Mardh P-A (eds): *International Perspectives on Neglected Sexually Transmitted Diseases*. Washington, DC, Hemisphere Publishing Corp, 1983, pp 63–82.
2. Centers for Disease Control: Genital herpes, United States 1966–1979. *MMWR* 31:137–139, 1982.
3. Baker DA: Herpes virus. *Clin Obstet Gynecol* 26:165–172, 1983.
4. Corey L, Adams HG, Brown ZA, Holmes KK: Genital herpes simplex virus infections: clinical manifestations, course and complications. *Ann Intern Med* 98:958–972, 1983.
5. Chuang T-Y, Su WPD, Perry HO, et al: Incidence and trend of herpes progenitalis. *Mayo Clin Proc* 58:436–441, 1983.
6. Sullivan-Bolyai J, Hull HF, Wilson C, Corey L: Neonatal herpes simplex infection in King County, Washington. Increasing incidence and epidemiological correlates. *JAMA* 250:3059–3062, 1983.
7. Cassai E, Rotola A, Meneguzzi G, et al: Herpes simplex virus and human cancer. I. Relationship between human cervical tumors and herpes simplex type 2. *Eur J Cancer* 17:685–693, 1981.
8. Fish EN, Tobin SM, Cooter NBE, Papsin ER: Update on the relationship of herpes virus hominis type II to carcinoma of the cervix. *Obstet Gynecol* 59:220–224, 1982.
9. Nahmias AJ, Roizman B: Infection with herpes simplex viruses 1 and 2. *N Engl J Med* 289:667, 1973.
10. Corey L, Holmes KK: Genital herpes simplex virus infections: current concepts in diagnosis, therapy, and prevention. *Ann Intern Med* 98:973–983, 1983.
11. Corey L, Benedetti JK, Critchlow CW, et al: Double-blind controlled trial of topical acyclovir in genital herpes simplex virus infections. *Am J Med* 73:326–334, 1982.
12. Corey L, Fife KH, Benedetti JK, et al: Intravenous acyclovir for the treatment of primary genital herpes. *Ann Intern Med* 98:958–972, 1983.
13. Bryson YJ, Dillon M, Lovett M, et al: Treatment of first episodes of genital herpes simplex virus infection with oral acyclovir. *N Engl J Med* 308:916, 1983.
14. Douglas J, Critchlow D, Benedetti J, et al: Trial of prophylactic oral acyclovir for frequent recurrences of genital herpes: efficacy and long-term follow-up. Twenty-third Interscience Conference on Antimicrobial Agents and Chemotherapy, October, 1983, Las Vegas, abstract no. 561.
15. Straus SE, Takiff HE, Seidlin M, et al: Suppres-

sion of frequently recurring genital herpes. A placebo-controlled double-blind trial of oral acyclovir. *N Engl J Med* 310:1545–1550, 1984.

16. Douglas JM, Critchlow C, Benedetti J, et al: A double-blind study of oral acyclovir for suppression of recurrences of genital herpes simplex virus infection. *N Engl J Med* 310:1551–1556, 1984.

Cytomegalovirus

1. Stinski MF, Thomsen DR, Wathen MW: Structure and function of the cytomegalovirus genome. In Nahmias AJ, Dowdle WR, Schinazi RF (eds): *The Human Herpes-Viruses*. New York, Elsevier, 1981, pp 72–84.
2. Weller TH: The cytomegaloviruses: ubiquitous agents with protean clinical manifestations. *N Engl J Med* 285:203–244, 267–274, 1971.
3. Hanshaw JB: Cytomegalovirus. In Remington JS, Klein JO (eds): *Infectious Diseases of the Fetus and Newborn*. Philadelphia, WB Saunders, 1983.
4. Land DJ, Kummer JF: Demonstration of cytomegalovirus in semen. *N Engl J Med* 287:756–758, 1972.
5. Jordan MC, Rosseau WE, Noble GR, et al: Association of cervical cytomegalovirus with venereal disease. *N Engl J Med* 288:923–934, 1973.
6. Lang DJ: Cytomegalovirus. In Holmes KK, Mardh P-A (eds): *International Perspectives on Neglected Sexually Transmitted Diseases*. Washington, DC, Hemisphere Publishing Corp, 1983.
7. Krech U: Compliment-fixing antibodies against cytomegalovirus in different parts of the world. *Bull WHO* 49:103–106, 1973.
8. Gold E, Nankervis GA: Cytomegalovirus. In Evans AS (ed): *Viral Infections of Humans: Epidemiology and Control*. New York, Plenum Medical Book Co, 1976.

9. Luby JP, Shasby DM: A sex difference in the prevalence of antibodies to cytomegalovirus. *JAMA* 222:1290–1291, 1972.
10. Willmott FE: Cytomegalovirus in female patients attending a VD clinic. *Br J Vener Dis* 51:278–280, 1975.
11. Hansfield HH, Chandler SC, Caine VA, et al: Sexual transmission of cytomegalovirus. Presented at 1st Sexually Transmitted Diseases World Congress, San Juan, Puerto Rico, Nov 15–21, 1981.
12. Knox GE, Pass RF, Reynolds DW, et al: Comparative prevalence of subclinical cytomegalovirus and herpes simplex virus infections in the genital and urinary tracts of low-income urban women. *J Infect Dis* 140:419–422, 1979.
13. Drew WL, Mintz L, Miner RC, et al: Prevalence of cytomegalovirus infections in homosexual men. *J Infect Dis* 143:188–192, 1981.
14. Chou S, Merigan TC: Rapid detection and quantitation of human cytomegalovirus in urine through DNA hybridization. *N Engl J Med* 308:921–925, 1983.
15. Ch'ien LT, Cannon NJ, Whitley RJ, et al: Effect of adenine-arabinoside on cytomegalovirus infection. *J Infect Dis* 130:32–39, 1974.
16. Emodi G, O'Reilly R, Muller A, et al: Effect of human exogenous interferon in cytomegalovirus infection. *J Infect Dis* 133S:199–204, 1976.
17. Balfour HH, Bean B, Mitchell CD, et al: Acyclovir in immunocompromised patients with cytomegalovirus disease: a controlled trial in one institution. *Am J Med* 73:241–248, 1982.
18. Starr SE, Glazer JP, Freidman HM, et al: Specific cellular and humoral immunity after immunization with live Towne Strain cytomegalovirus. *J Infect Dis* 143:585–589, 1981.

CHAPTER 4

Pelvic Inflammatory Disease

As a result of the liberalization of attitudes toward sexuality, earlier onset of sexual activity, and increased sexual activity, the United States is currently in the midst of an epidemic of sexually transmitted diseases. Sexually transmitted diseases, especially gonorrhea, have been reported at epidemic proportions in the United States since the mid-1960s. Between 1950 and 1975 the incidence of reported gonorrhea in the total United States population has tripled to its hyperendemic rate of over 1 million cases reported annually. Because of underreporting, it is estimated that over 3 million cases occur each year in the United States. In addition, *Chlamydia* has become recognized as an even more common sexually transmitted disease; and recent estimates suggest that over 3–5 million cases of chlamydial infection occur annually in this country. Of even greater concern has been the recognition that this STD epidemic has been associated in women with a secondary epidemic of acute pelvic inflammatory disease (PID) and ultimately a tertiary epidemic of infertility due to tubal factors and ectopic pregnancies. Acute pelvic inflammatory disease is the acute clinical syndrome attributed to ascending spread of microorganisms from the vagina and endocervix to the endometrium, fallopian tubes, and/or contiguous structures.

Both as a result of this epidemic and the widespread use of the intrauterine contraceptive device, the incidence of acute salpingitis has also increased (1, 2, 3). For women, acute salpingitis is the most common important complication of sexually transmitted pathogens. Incidence estimates are based largely on data from the National Disease and Therapeutic Index, The National Ambulatory Medical Care Survey, The Hospital Discharge Survey, and from projections of gonorrhea disease statistics, since actual reporting to health departments is not required. An estimated 1 million women a year are treated for acute salpingitis in the United States (4). Approximately, 250,000–300,000 women are hospitalized each year with a diagnosis of salpingitis or PID. Over 2.5 million physician visits occur annually in the United States for acute salpingitis, and an estimated 150,000 surgical procedures are performed annually for complications of acute salpingitis (5, 6).

Washington and co-workers recently assessed trends in hospitalization for PID in the United States for 1975 to 1981 (6). Their analysis was based on data from the Hospital Discharge Survey conducted by the National Center for Health Statistics. They reported that both the estimated number and rate of hospitalization for PID among women age 15–44 yr rose slightly. During this period of time, an estimated average of 267,200 women were admitted to hospitals per year for PID, and the hospitalization rate averaged 5.3 per 1000 women (an increase from the 4.9 per 1000 women rate for 1970–1975). The age group 20–24 yr had the highest average rate (7.0 per 1000), followed by the 25- to 29-yr-old group (6.7 per 1000). However, the data were calculated using as the denominator all women, rather than only sexually active women. Undoubtedly, if only sexually active women were analyzed, the age group 15–19 yr would have the highest rate, and the rate of hospitalization for PID would be inversely related to age. Washington et al also noted that nonwhite women had an average rate of hospitalization for PID that was 2.5 times higher than that for white women (10.6 versus 4.3 per 1000). However, this relative risk had decreased from the 1970 to 1975 figure of 3.3. The concomitant increase in the annual rate of hospitalization for PID and the decline in relative risk for nonwhite women compared to white women during the years 1975 to 1981 reveal that the overall rise in rates is almost entirely due to increases among young white women during this time period. These authors put forth several reasons to explain this increased rate of hospitalization for PID. Possibly, but very unlikely, the severity of PID has worsened. More probably, physicians are more likely to hospitalize patients with PID because of the spreading recognition of unacceptably high failure rates associated with outpatient therapy. Finally, it simply appears that more women are experiencing PID. Most likely this is the result of the increase in nongonococcal putative agents such as *Chlamydia trachomatis*, a liberalized sexual behavior by young women which exposes them to an increased risk of acquiring PID, and a shift away from contraceptive methods that protect against sexually transmitted diseases and PID.

Curran has estimated that the direct cost of treating salpingitis in the United States is nearly 700 million dollars annually and that the total annual cost of this disease is close to 3 billion dollars (4). Not only are the economic consequences of salpingitis significant, but major medical problems result as well. One fourth of all women who have had acute salpingitis will experience one or more long-term sequelae. The most common and most important is involuntary infertility which occurs in approximately 20% (3, 7). Ectopic pregnancies are increased six- to ten-fold (3). Other important sequelae associated with salpingitis include chronic pelvic pain, dyspareunia, pelvic adhesions and inflammatory residua, which often lead to surgical intervention. Such complications are estimated to occur in 15–20% of cases.

In order to prevent the significant economic and medical sequelae of pelvic inflammatory disease, methods of prevention and treatment must be developed, which are based on the microbiologic etiology of the disease. Unfortunately there are several major problems which complicate the attempt to elucidate this etiology. Among these are the fact that the clinical criteria for diagnosis are vaguely defined and have not been standardized among the various studies in the literature. Secondly, the fallopian tubes, which are the site of infection, are inaccessible for routine microbiologic studies. In addition, the microbiologic methodology used in many of the investigations have focused on *Neisseria gonorrhoeae* and have not attempted to recover all the potential organisms which may be responsible for acute salpingitis, such as *C. trachomatis*, *Herpes virus*, genital tract mycoplasmas, anaerobic bacteria, and/or facultative bacteria.

ETIOLOGY

Risk Factors

Several predisposing factors to developing acute pelvic inflammatory disease have been identified. Women who have had previous episodes of gonococcal pelvic inflammatory disease are more likely to have recurrent infections (8, 9). It is generally accepted that this statement applies to all etiologic classes of acute salpingitis. The exact mechanism for this increased susceptibility has not been delineated. Perhaps, as the result of acute salpingitis, the fallopian tube loses some of its natural protective mechanisms against microorganisms. Gregg and coworkers have demonstrated that the gonococcus produces a lipopolysaccharide toxin that destroys fallopian tube cilia (10) and Draper et al, utilizing scanning electron microscopy, noted that there is loss of the normal fallopian tube endothelial architecture following acute salpingitis (11).

A second predisposing factor is sexual activity with multiple partners. Women with multiple sexual partners have a 4.6 times increased risk to develop acute salpingitis, compared to women with monogamous sexual relationships (9). This risk exists for women with multiple consorts over a short time span, approximately 3–6 months. With multiple partners, the risk of being exposed to a sexually transmitted organisms is increased.

The intrauterine device (IUD) is a third predisposing factor (1, 9, 12–17). It has been estimated that IUD users have a three- to five-fold increased risk to develop acute salpingitis. Initially no particular IUD was implicated as having a statistically significant increased risk above the other brands. However, Kaufman reported that compared to nonusers Dalkon Shield users had a 13-fold increased risk, Lippe's Loop and Safety-coil users had an 8-fold increased risk, and Cooper 7 users had a 4-fold increased risk in developing acute salpingitis (12). In addition, the overall risk for salpingitis doubled at 5-years of continuous use in the Kaufman study. More recently, Lee and co-workers have demonstrated that women wearing Dalkon Shield IUDs were at statistically significant increased risk to develop acute pelvic inflammatory disease (17). Compared to the risk in women using no contraception, the relative risk of PID in women using the Dalkon Shield was 8.3. This represented a five-fold increase in risk compared to women using other types of IUDs. Moreover, the risk to Dalkon Shield wearers continued to progressively increase in proportion to duration of use. This phenomenon was not seen with other IUDs whose risk peaked at 4 months postinsertion. Animal model investigations have suggested that the multifilament string in the

Dalkon Shield is a major contributing factor to the increased risk for PID (18, 19). The second factor is the ability of the shield itself to interfere with the normal intrauterine host defense mechanisms. Because of its large contact area with the endometrial surface, the shield is more likely to alter these defenses, cause endometrial abrasion and ulceration, and initiate what Burnhill (20) has termed the syndrome of progressive endometritis which leads to acute pelvic inflammatory disease.

The role of parity in IUD-associated acute salpingitis remains controversial. Some investigators have found that nulligravid women have an increased risk (1, 16); while Osser and colleagues reported no such association (14). In addition, IUD users less than 20 yr of age are reported to be at greater risk when compared to an older aged population (1, 15).

In contrast, most studies have shown that oral contraceptives (BCPs) provide protection against acute salpingitis (1, 14, 15, 17, 21). The mechanism for such protection remains speculative. Perhaps the effect of BCPs on cervical mucus precludes the ascension of vaginal and cervical microorganisms up into the upper genital tract. Women using BCPs have a shorter duration of menses and less flow; this could result in a shorter "window" for microorganisms to gain access to the uterus and/or fallopian tubes. Svennson and co-workers have recently reported that, in addition to protecting against PID, the use of BCPs both ameliorated PID if it occurred and was associated with a better prognosis for future fertility than was seen in women with acute PID using other contraceptive methods or none (21).

Finally, adolescent females are at significant risk to develop acute salpingitis. Westrom (3) reported that nearly 70% of females with acute salpingitis were younger than 25 yr of age, 33% experienced their first infection before the age of 19, and 75% were nulliparous. The risk for developing acute pelvic inflammatory disease in the sexually active adolescent is estimated to be 1:8; the risk decreases to 1:80 in females 24 yr or older. Based on current trends, Westrom has estimated that by the year 2000, 50% of the women who turned 15 yr old in 1970 will have had at least one episode of acute salpingitis (3). He predicted that among these young women, 10% will be sterile, and 3% will have had an ectopic pregnancy as a result of acute salpingitis. It has been suggested that the adolescent population is at greater risk because this population has a high prevalence of sexually transmitted diseases, has multiple sexual partners, and tends not to use contraceptives—many of which (i.e., BCP, diaphragms, condoms) protect against the development of acute pelvic inflammatory disease.

Microbial Etiology

In the United States, nontuberculous acute salpingitis was traditionally separated into gonococcal and nongonococcal disease. This division was based solely on the recovery of *N. gonorrhoeae* from the endocervix of patients with acute salpingitis. Studies utilizing endocervical cultures have implicated the gonococcus as the causative agent in 33–81% of the cases of acute salpingitis (2, 9, 22–31). However, it has become apparent that the presence of pathogenic microorganisms in the endocervix is not absolute proof that such microorganisms are causally associated with upper genital tract infections such as salpingitis. Investigations utilizing transvaginal culdocentesis and laparoscopy to obtain culture specimens from the peritoneal fluid or fallopian tube exudate have shown a poor correlation between the cervical and intraabdominal cultures. Despite isolation from the endocervix of patients with acute salpingitis, *N. gonorrhoeae* was recovered from only 6–70% of the peritoneal and/or tubal cultures (23, 28, 29, 32, 33, 34, 35, 36). Recent investigations utilizing culdocentesis and appropriate anaerobic culture techniques have resulted in the isolation of a variety of aerobic and anaerobic bacteria from the peritoneal fluid of patients with acute salpingitis (22, 23, 28, 29, 30, 33, 35, 37). The most frequent organisms recovered in these studies were *N. gonorrhoeae* and anaerobic bacteria, including *Peptostreptococcus*, *Peptococcus*, and *Bacteroides* species. A characteristic pattern evolved from these studies (Table 4.1). There is a high prevalence of *N. gonorrhoeae* in the cervix of these patients. Approximately one-third of the cases had *N. gonorrhoeae* as the only organism recovered from an intraabdominal site. An additional third of the patients had a mixture of *N. gonorrhoeae* plus mixed anaerobic and aerobic bacteria (predominantly anaerobes). The final one-third to one-half of the patients did not have *N. gonorrhoeae*, but only a mixture of anaerobic and aerobic bacteria were recovered from the abdominal cavity. These culdocentesis studies have demonstrated that the etiology of acute salpingitis is polymicrobic in nature and have brought into question the exact role of *N. gonorrhoeae* in the pathogenesis of acute pelvic inflammatory disease. Cunningham et al (22),

Table 4.1
Isolation of *N. Gonorrhoeae*, Anaerobes, and Aerobes from Culdocentesis Aspirates in Acute Pelvic Inflammatory Disease

Study	Number of patients	Endocervical *N. gonorrhoeae* (%)	Culdocentesis		
			N. gonorrhoeae only (%)	*N. gonorrhoeae* plus anaerobes and aerobes (%)	Anaerobes and aerobes only (%)
Cunningham et al (22)	104	56 (54)	12 (22)	18 (32)	26 (46)
Thompson et al (30)	30	24 (80)	5 (21)	5 (21)	14 (58)
Eschenbach et al (23)	54	21 (39)	6 (28)	1 (5)	5 (24)
Monif et al (35)	17	16 (94)	5 (31)	5 (31)	6 (38)
Sweet et al (37)	26	13 (50)	4 (31)	4 (31)	4 (31)
Chow et al (33)	20	13 (65)		1 (5)	18 (95)

Chow et al (33), and Monif et al (35) have postulated that the gonococcus initiates acute pelvic inflammatory disease and produces tissue damage and changes in the local environment, which in turn allow access to the upper genital tract for anaerobic and aerobic organisms from the vaginal and cervical flora. On the other hand, McCormack et al (38), Eschenbach (9), and Sweet et al (29) have suggested that not all pelvic inflammatory disease follows gonococcal infection and that, in fact, acute pelvic inflammatory disease initially has a polymicrobial etiology.

However, these investigations utilized transvaginal culdocentesis to obtain peritoneal fluid. It is not clear that microorganisms obtained from cul-de-sac fluid, aspirated transvaginally, are representative of the microorganisms present in the fallopian tube. A preliminary study by Sweet et al demonstrated a discrepancy between culdocentesis and fallopian tube isolates from females with acute salpingitis (37). Culdocentesis specimens yielded greater numbers of bacteria common to the vaginal flora than did the fallopian tube isolates. A subsequent study included ten patients utilizing cultures from the fallopian tube, the cul-de-sac contained via laparoscopy, and the cul-de-sac obtained via transvaginal culdocentesis (29). Although close agreement between fallopian tube exudate and the cul-de-sac aspirate via laparoscopy was found there was a poor correlation with the culdocentesis results, suggesting that contamination may occur during transvaginal culdocentesis.

The optimum microbiologic information for elucidating the etiology of acute salpingitis would be obtained using specimens obtained directly from the site of infection—the fallopian tubes. Sweet and co-workers have reported their results with the use of laparoscopy to obtain fallopian tube specimens in a preliminary study

of 39 patients (29). These results are presented in Table 4.2. Although nearly 50% of the patients had *N. gonorrhoeae* recovered from the endocervix, the gonococcus was isolated from the fallopian tube in 8 of 35 patients (23%). Of the salpingitis patients with endocervical *N. gonorrhoeae*, only 42% had the gonococcus recovered from the fallopian tube. Anaerobic bacteria were the most frequent fallopian tube isolates from these females with acute salpingitis. Anaerobes were recovered in ten cases (29%); *Peptostreptococcus* and *Peptococcus* species were the most prevalent anaerobes. In this initial work *Ureaplasma urealyticum* was rarely recovered from the fallopian tube, while no isolates of *Mycoplasma hominis* or *C. trachomatis* were obtained. Recently, Sweet et al described the microbiologic results of cultures obtained from the upper genital tract (endometrial aspirates and/or fallopian tube specimens) of an additional 74 hospitalized women with acute salpingitis (Table 4.3) (39). *N. gonorrhoeae* and *C. trachomatis* were recovered from 39 and 24%, respectively. However, nongonococcal, nonchlamydial bacteria were the most frequently recovered organisms. Again, anaerobic bacteria were the predominant isolates and were present in 57 (92%) of the 62 patients with nongonococcal (NG) nonchlamydial (NC) bacteria. Overall, an average of 7 microorganisms were recovered from the upper genital tract of these women with acute salpingitis. The NG, NC organisms identified are noted in Table 4.4. The most common included *Bacteroides* species, *Bacteroides bivius*, anaerobic cocci, *Gardnerella vaginalis*, group B streptococcus, and *Escherichia coli*. Sweet has noted (R.L. Sweet, unpublished data) that isolates obtained from the endometrial cavity more closely mirror those in the fallopian tube than those obtained via culdocentesis.

Table 4.2
Distribution of Microorganisms Isolated from Women with Acute Pelvic Inflammatory disease at San Francisco General Hospital (Based on Data from Reference 29)

Microorganisms	Fallopian tube (N = 35)		Culdocentesis (N = 35)		Endocervix (N = 35)	
	No.	%	No.	%	No.	%
N. gonorrhoeae	8	(23)	11	(31)	19	(49)
N. gonorrhoeae only	6	(17)	3	(8.5)		
N. gonorrhoeae in combination with other bacteria	2	(6)	8	(23)		
Aerobic bacteria only	1	(3)	1	(3)		
Anaerobic bacteria	10	(29)	20	(57)		
Anaerobes only	3	(8.5)	5	(14)		
Mixed anaerobes/aerobes	7	(20)	15	(43)		
M. hominis	0		1	(3)	28	(80)
U. urealyticum	3	(8.5)	6	(17)	21	(60)
C. trachomatis	0		0		2	(5)
No growth	13	(37)	9	(26)		

Table 4.3
Microbiologic Results from Hospitalized Patients with Acute Salpingitis at San Francisco General Hospital

Organisms	No. of patients positive/No. of patients cultured	% positive
N. gonorrhoeae	29/74	39
C. trachomatis	17/71	24
Nongonococcal/nonchlamydial bacteria	62/74	84
Aerobes only	5/62	8
Anaerobes only	7/62	11
Anaerobes and aerobes	50/62	81
Total isolated		
432 bacteria, 7/patient		
273 anaerobes, 4.4/patient		
161 aerobes, 2.6/patient		

Table 4.4
Nongonococcal Nonchlamydial Bacteria Recovered from the Upper Genital Tract of Patients with Acute Salpingitis at San Francisco General Hospital (N = 74)

Bacteroides species	48	G. vaginalis	30
B. bivius	35	E. coli	18
Peptococcus asaccharolyticus	38	Nonhemolytic streptococci	16
Peptococcus prevotii	16	Group B streptococci	16
Peptostreptococcus anaerobius	24	Coagulase-negative staphylococci	22
Veillonella parvula	19		

The studies, demonstrating the isolation of a variety of bacteria other than *N. gonorrhoeae* from several different intraabdominal sites, most notably the fallopian tubes, provide support for the concept of the polymicrobial etiology of acute salpingitis. This has led to a reevaluation of the role of the gonococcus in the pathogenesis of acute salpingitis. It was a common belief that as the duration of symptoms increased, the microflora of the fallopian tube changed from *N. gonorrhoeae* (the initiator of disease and tubal destruction) to the secondary invaders, such as the facultative and anaerobic bacterial flora from the lower genital tract. This concept was initially proposed in 1921 by Curtis, who found *N. gonorrhoeae* only in cases which showed microscopic evidence of active inflammation at operation, but not in patients that had been afebrile for 14 days (40). Curtis concluded that gonococci survived only a short time in the fallopian tube. Lip and Burgoyne also noted that the isolation of *N. gonorrhoeae* is dependent on the stage of infection (28). They were unable to isolate the gonococcus if symptoms had been present for 7 days or more. Therefore, it is possible that acute salpingitis patients admitted to the hospital after several days of symptoms have already passed through an initial stage, in which *N. gonorrhoeae* participates as a primary pathogen, after which they progressed to a mixed aerobic/anaerobic infection involving secondary invading pathogens from the cervix and vagina. Using fallopian tube isolates, Sweet et al were able to demonstrate that 70% of the patients presenting within the initial 24 hr of the onset of symptoms had *N. gonorrhoeae* present (36). Anaerobic bacteria, especially *Peptostreptococci* and *Peptococci*, were present in the tubes within the initial 24 hr of symptoms as well. If symptoms had been present for greater than 24 hr, there appeared to be a shift in the bacteria isolated from the fallopian tube: anaerobic bacteria and ureaplasma became predominant. If symptoms had been present for greater than 48 hr, we could recover the gonococcus from only 19% of patients (p < 0.001). Direct cultures from the fallopian tube failed to confirm the initial concept that anaerobes would be secondary invaders. In patients presenting with less than 24 hr of symptomatology, mixtures of anaerobic and aerobic bacteria were recovered in 37% of the patients. This ability to recover anaerobes from the fallopian tube persisted during subsequent duration of the disease. In a small number of patients (3) anaerobic bacteria were the most common fallopian tube isolates within the first 24 hr of onset of symptoms: neither *N. gonorrhoeae* nor *C. trachomatis* were isolated from the tubes or cervix of these patients. Therefore, it appears that nongonococcal, nonchlamydial bacteria from the cervix and vagina may also be present early in the disease process. If the gonococcus were the initiator, we would expect an inverse relationship between the frequency of isolation of *N. gonorrhoeae* and anaerobic bacteria; this relationship does not seem to exist.

Several explanations have been offered for the relatively infrequent isolation of *N. gonorrhoeae*

isolates from intraperitoneal specimens. Eschenbach and Holmes suggested that the low recovery rate of the gonococcus only demonstrated difficulties in recovering the organism from pus (8). They noted that recovery of *N. gonorrhoeae* required the presence of large numbers of organisms. A second explanation for the failure to isolate *N. gonorrhoeae* in purulent exudate from the fallopian tube may be that the gonococcus has the ability to attach and invade the epithelial cells of the fallopian tube and, therefore, may not be available in the tubal exudate. Studdiford et al were able to isolate *N. gonorrhoeae* from tubal tissue in 67% of cases, despite their inability to recover the organism from the purulent exudate in these patients (41). A similar finding was reported by Tronca et al with disseminated gonorrhoeae. The gonococcus could be isolated from tissue obtained by skin biopsy, but not from the purulent exudate in the skin pustule (42).

In addition, investigations by Cunningham et al (22) and Sweet et al (29, 36) showed that approximately one-third of cultures from culde-sac aspirates and fallopian tube exudates from women with acute salpingitis are sterile. Several reasons have been used to explain this high frequency of sterile cultures: (a) Repeated episodes cause inflammation and scar formation, resulting in tubal obstruction which could prevent passage of the organisms within the tubal lumen into the abdominal cavities; (b) Organisms other than the gonococcus may be intracellular and not in the tubal exudate; (c) Salpingitis may be a latent infection due to an infectious agent (such as *Chlamydia*) bound to tissue or living intracellularly and, therefore, not accessible by aspiration; (d) Salpingitis may represent an autoimmune process initiated only by an infectious agent such as *Mycoplasma* or *Chlamydia*, and tubal destruction may then occur secondary to a complex antibody/antigen interaction; or (e) Appropriate culture methodology was not used to detect suggested causative microorganisms, such as genital tract mycoplasmas, chlamydia, and viruses.

In addition to *N. gonorrhoeae* and anaerobic and aerobic bacteria, other microorganisms have been implicated as etiologic agents in acute salpingitis. The genital tract mycoplasmas, *M. hominis* and *U. urealyticum*, have been suggested as potential pathogens in the etiology of acute salpingitis. Although *M. hominis* and *U. urealyticum* have been frequently recovered from the lower genital tract of women with salpingitis, no difference exists between the rates of isolation from the cervices of these patients and in sexually active control patients (23, 43). Moreover, the genital tract mycoplasmas have been recovered infrequently from the peritoneal cavity and/or fallopian tube of patients with salpingitis. Mardh and Westrom reported that *M. hominis* was recovered from the fallopian tubes in 4 of 52 cases of PID and *U. urealyticum* in two cases (44). Speculation as to a role of genital mycoplasmas in the etiology of PID has focused predominantly on *M. hominis.* For *M. hominis* Mardh and Westrom (44) reported a cervical isolation rate of 52%; Eschenbach et al (23) recovered *M. hominis* from lower genital tracts of 145 (72%) of 204 women with acute PID and Møller et al (49) recovered it from 91 (55%) of 166 PID cases. Although Sweet and co-workers in their laparoscopy studies recovered *M. hominis* from the endocervix in 80% of acute salpingitis patients, and *U. urealyticum* in 60%, no isolates of *M. hominis* were found in the fallopian tube, and in only 8.5% of cases (3 of 35) was *U. urealyticum* recovered from the fallopian tube (29). Similarly, Mardh and Westrom (44) and Eschenbach et al (23) were able to recover genital mycoplasmas from the fallopian tube in only 2–8% of pelvic inflammatory disease patients, despite a 60–81% rate of recovery from the cervix and/or vagina. Serologic studies have also suggested a role for *M. hominis* in the etiology of acute PID (23, 43–45). In these studies antibodies to *M. hominis* were present in from one-fourth to one-half of women with acute PID. In addition to the low recovery rate from the fallopian tube, in vitro studies with fallopian tube explant systems have suggested that mycoplasmas may be commensals rather than pathogens in acute salpingitis. Taylor-Robinson and Carney reported that despite proliferation of *M. hominis*, there was no apparent tubal damage produced (46). This is in contradistinction to the circumstance when *N. gonorrhoeae* is placed in a similar system and extensive epithelial damage occurs and the tubal epithelium is completely destroyed within 7 days. More recently Hare and Barnes have noted that the use of *Bacteroides fragilis* in the tubal explant system resulted in tubal destruction and epithelial destruction within 72–96 hr (47). However, it is important to recognize that the in vitro fallopian tube explant system precludes the immune response and host defense mechanisms which may be important in the pathogenesis of acute salpingitis (48). Møller and co-

workers using the Grivet monkey model reported that *M. hominis* produces a parametritis rather than an acute salpingitis, and this could possibly explain the failure to recover mycoplasmas except in a few cases from the fallopian tubes (49). Using scanning electron microscopy, Mardh et al showed that *M. hominis* induced pathologic swelling in fallopian tube cilia in organ culture systems (50). Although results obtained with serologic studies and cervical isolation approaches are suggestive, the role of the genital tract mycoplasmas in the etiology of acute salpingitis remains unclear; and elucidation of this role will require studies utilizing laparoscopy to obtain specimens directly from the fallopian tube.

Recently, *C. trachomatis* has received considerable attention as an etiologic agent in acute salpingitis. *C. trachomatis* is currently recognized as one of the most common sexually transmitted pathogens. It is estimated that nearly 3 million cases occur annually in the United States (51). This organism is responsible for a significant proportion of nongonococcal urethritis and acute epididymitis in men under the age of 35 and is found in association with cervicitis in women (51). Historically the association of chlamydial infection with postpartum pelvic inflammatory disease has been recognized since the 1930s, when pelvic inflammatory disease developed postpartum in mothers of neonates with inclusion conjunctivitis.

There is also more recent evidence that *C. trachomatis* is associated with acute salpingitis (Table 4.5). In Scandanavia, *C. Trachomatis* has been recovered from the cervix in from 22 to 47% of women with a diagnosis of acute salpingitis (52, 53, 54–62). More important have been the results obtained from the fallopian tube cultures of women undergoing laparoscopy. Initially *C. trachomatis* was isolated from the fallopian tubes in 2 (9%) of 22 women with acute salpingitis laparoscoped by Eilard et al (52). Subsequently, Mardh and colleagues were able to recover *C. trachomatis* from the fallopian tubes of 6 of 20 (30%) patients with acute salpingitis at laparoscopy (53). In the seven women with chlamydia in the cervix and in whom laparoscopy was performed, six had *C. trachomatis* recovered from the fallopian tube. Scandinavian studies utilizing serologic surveillance have suggested that *C. trachomatis* is associated with 23–62% of acute salpingitis cases (52, 54–61). Treharne et al noted high acute phase chlamydial antibody titers (1:64) in 62% of 143 women with

Table 4.5
Chlamydia trachomatis in Acute Pelvic Inflammatory Disease

Study	No. of patients	Isolation rate of *C. trachomatis*		Four-fold rise in serum antibodies (%)
		Endocervix (%)	Upper genital and peritoneal cavity (%)	
Eilard et al (52)	22	6 (27)	2 (9)[a]	5 (23)
Mardh et al (53)	53	19 (37)	6/20 (30)[a]	
Treharne et al (54)	143			88 (62)[b]
Paavonen et al (55)	106	27 (26)		19/72 (26)
Paavonen (56)	228	68 (30)		32/167 (19)
Mardh et al (57)	60	23 (38)		24/60 (40)
Ripa et al (58)	206	52/156 (33)		118 (57)[c]
Gjonnaess et al (59)	56	26 (46)	5/42 (12)[a]	26/52 (46)
Moller et al (60)	166	37 (22)		34 (21)
Osser and Persson (61)	111	52 (47)		37/72 (51)
Eschenbach et al (23)	100	20 (20)	1/54 (2)[d]	15/74 (20)
Sweet et al (29)	37	2 (5)	0[a]	5/22 (23)
Thompson et al (30)	30	3 (10)	3 (10)[e]	
Sweet et al (39)	71	10 (14)	17 (24)[f]	

[a] Fallopian tube.
[b] Chlamydial IgG ≥1:64; 23% had IgM ≥ 1:8.
[c] Chlamydial IgG ≥1:64; four-fold rise in 28/80 (35%).
[d] Culdocentesis.
[e] Exudate from fallopian tube.
[f] Fallopian tube and/or endometrial cavity.

acute salpingitis and that these antibody titers were correlated with the severity of tubal inflammation clinically graded at laparoscopy (54). The highest geometric mean titers were present in those patients with the severest disease at laparoscopy. Paavonen et al, in Finland, reported that 26% of patients showed serial conversion in a single antichlamydial immunofluorescent test (55).

Interestingly, the Scandinavian investigators have noted an association between chlamydia and age. Paavonen showed that 60% of women with acute salpingitis and endocervical chlamydia were less than 20 yr of age (55). Using serology, Treharne et al noted that *C. trachomatis* was associated with more than half of all cases of acute salpingitis occurring in women less than 25 yr of age (53).

Initial investigations in the United States failed to confirm that chlamydia was a major putative agent in acute salpingitis. Eschenbach and co-workers recovered *C. trachomatis* from the peritoneal cavity in only 1 of 54 cases, despite a 20% isolation rate of this organism from the cervix (23). Thompson et al showed that 10% of women with acute salpingitis had chlamydia isolated from the culdocentesis aspirates (30). In the only laparoscopy study performed in the United States, Sweet and co-workers

failed to recover *C. trachomatis* from the fallopian tube exudate in 37 patients (29); chlamydia was recovered from the cervix in 5% of their cases. Serologic data obtained from studies in the United States show a four-fold rise in chlamydial antibodies in approximately 20% of acute cases (23, 29). Thus, until recently, most evidence in support of chlamydia as a major factor in acute salpingitis in the United States was indirect and derived from endocervical isolation and immunologic studies. The conflicting findings from Scandinavia and the United States were felt to be due to several factors. In Sweden specimens for chlamydial cultures were obtained via biopsy or needle aspiration of the fallopian tube; in the United States studies had utilized cultures from peritoneal fluid and/or tubal exudate. *C. trachomatis* is an intracellular organism, and, thus, fresh infected cells, such as obtained via biopsy, may be necessary to recover the organism. Secondly, in the United States *N. gonorrhoeae* is much more commonly recovered from salpingitis patients than in Sweden and may mask the role of chlamydia. Thirdly, the patient population studied may be different; the Swedish investigators studied women with a milder disease than is usually admitted to hospitals and studied in the United States. In fact, it has been suggested by Svensson and colleagues that patients with milder pelvic inflammatory disease are more likely to have *C. trachomatis* as the causative agent (62). These investigators noted that the women with *C. trachomatis* as the causative agent were more likely to be afebrile and have longer standing disease of milder type than women with gonococcal or nongonococcal, nonchlamydial disease. Paradoxically though, at laparoscopy those women with *C. trachomatis* infection based on serologic data had the most severe fallopian tube involvement and the highest estimated erythrocyte sedimentation rates (ESR) (62). This Scandinavian group of investigators have noted that patients with anaerobes recovered were more likely to be febrile, appeared to have more severe clinical symptoms and signs, and were prone to have associated inflammatory adnexal masses (L. Westrom, personal communication, 1982).

Recent information further suggests that chlamydia may play a possible role in infertility due to tubal obstruction and salpingitis (63–69). Punnonen et al reported an association of both prevalence of antibody and increased geometric mean titers against *C. trachomatis* in patients with infertility due to tubal obstruction, as compared to infertility patients with normal hysterosalpingograms and pregnant women (63). In infertility patients with abnormal hysterosalpingogram (HSG) 21 of 23 (91%) had antibody against *C. trachomatis* as compared to 52 of 105 (50%) infertile patients with normal HSG and 20 of 68 (29%) pregnant women. Henry-Souchet et al reported the recovery of *C. trachomatis* in 12 of 46 (26%) women with infertility and tubal obstruction, using direct fallopian tube and peritoneal adhesion cultures at the time of laparoscopy or laparotomy (64). These investigators have also documented serologic evidence for the association of *C. trachomatis* with high rates of tubal obstruction in infertility. Several recent studies (65–69) have confirmed as association between infertility due solely or in part to tubal factors and the presence of antibodies to *C. trachomatis*. Although very suggestive for a direct etiologic role in tubal infertility for *C. trachomatis*, these seroepidemiologic studies do not prove causation.

Further evidence that supports the role of *C. trachomatis* in acute salpingitis has been animal model work, which has demonstrated the ability of chlamydia to produce acute salpingitis. Several in vitro and in vivo models have been developed to study the possible role of chlamydia in salpingitis. Utilizing the human fallopian tube organ model, Hutchinson et al found that although *C. trachomatis* would infect cells and replicate, it caused no tissue damage (70). As in all in vitro models, the organ is divorced from the immunologic response system which could be a factor in the tissue destruction associated with acute salpingitis. Consequently, in vivo animal models have been employed to study the pathogenesis of chlamydia in acute salpingitis. Ripa et al, in a Grivet monkey model, have shown that *C. trachomatis* causes an ascending salpingitis similar to that seen with *N. gonorrhoeae* (71). In an immunosuppressed guinea pig model, White et al have demonstrated the pathogenesis of the GPIC agent in acute salpingitis (72). Sweet et al have demonstrated that the guinea pig inclusion conjunctivitis (GPIC agent) can produce an acute salpingitis in a guinea pig animal model (73). In this nonimmunosuppressed guinea pig model the GPIC agent, when directly inoculated in the uterine horn, resulted in an acute self-limited salpingitis. More recently, Swenson et al (74) and Swenson and Schachter (75) in a mouse model have shown that the mouse pneumonia biovar of *C. trachomatis* when inoculated into the ovarian bursa resulted in acute salpingitis, hydrosalpinges, and infertility.

Perihepatitis is the presence of acute right upper quadrant pain and tenderness in association with acute salpingitis. More commonly this entity is known as the Fitz-Hugh-Curtis syndrome. Usually the symptoms and signs of this syndrome are preceded by the clinical onset of acute pelvic inflammatory disease. On occasion, though, the right upper quadrant findings occur before the symptoms and signs of pelvic inflammatory disease become apparent. Differentiation from acute cholecystitis may be difficult in such instances. Initially this syndrome was ascribed as a complication of gonococcal salpingitis. It was estimated that 1–10% of patients with gonococcal salpingitis developed perihepatitis (Fitz-Hugh-Curtis syndrome) (76, 77). *N. gonorrhoeae* has been rarely isolated from the peritoneal cavity of women with this syndrome (76). Perihepatitis with the Fitz-Hugh-Curtis syndrome has recently been found to be associated with *C. trachomatis* infection in women with acute salpingitis. Wolner-Hanssen et al have isolated *C. trachomatis* and have shown serologic changes consistent with chlamydial infection in four patients with Fitz-Hugh-Curtis syndrome (78). In addition, Wang and co-workers in Seattle reported serologic evidence for *C. tra-*

chomatis in patients with perihepatitis and acute salpingitis; both prevalence of antibodies to *C. trachomatis* and geometric mean titers of antibody correlated with the presence of Fitz-Hugh-Curtis syndrome (79). Additional studies have confirmed an association between the Fitz-Hugh-Curtis syndrome and evidence of chlamydial infection (80–83). The bulk of this data is serological with use of the microimmunofluorescence antibody against *C. trachomatis.*

Recent studies have demonstrated a definite role for *C. trachomatis* as an etiologic agent for acute salpingitis in the United States and Canada. This is particularly true in the milder forms of the disease in which patients are often afebrile and present with minimal tenderness and pain. Bowie, in studies of a venereal disease clinic population in Vancouver, reported that women diagnosed to have acute pelvic inflammatory disease had *C. trachomatis* recovered from their cervix significantly more often than women attending the clinic who did not have pelvic inflammatory disease (84). In this report *C. trachomatis* was recovered from the cervix in 50% of women diagnosed as having acute PID, compared to 20% of women attending the STD clinic who did not have acute PID. More pertinent has been the recent direct evidence provided by Sweet and co-workers utilizing specimens obtained from the upper genital tract (endometrial cavity and/or fallopian tubes) of hospitalized women with acute salpingitis (39). These investigators recovered *C. trachomatis* from 17 (24%) of 71 of these patients. Confirmation of a major role for *C. trachomatis* in the etiology of acute salpingitis has been provided by Eschenbach and colleagues (85). Thus, clinicians must appreciate that current evidence strongly supports a putative role for *C. trachomatis* in acute salpingitis. This has major implications for clinical management as will be discussed in a subsequent section.

PATHOGENESIS

Sexual transmission of the gonococcus and *C. trachomatis* has been well described. In gonococcal salpingitis the usual route of infection is thought to be direct canalicular spread of the organism from the endocervix, along the endometrial surface to the tubal mucosa, leading to endosalpingitis. Factors which determine whether the gonococcus is localized in the endocervix or gains access to the uterus and tubes are unknown. Approximately 10–17% of females who acquire endocervical gonorrhoeae will develop upper genital tract infection (2, 8). Although not as well described, chlamydial salpingitis is also believed to be the result of intracanalicular spread from the endocervix via the endometrium to the fallopian tube (39). Westrom has reported that approximately 10% of women with endocervical *C. trachomatis* develop chlamydial salpingitis (L. Westrom, personal communication, 1982).

The menstrual cycle may influence the environment of the lower genital tract and play a significant role in the breakdown of local host mechanisms which normally prevent the ascent of microorganisms from the endocervix. Sixty-six to 77% of the patients with gonococcal salpingitis present at the end of, or just after, the menstrual period (8, 38, 86). In our preliminary laparoscopic study, a more dramatic relationship between the menses and gonococcal salpingitis has been noted (37). Although the recovery of the gonococcus from the cervix was most frequent within the first 7 days of the menstrual cycle, it was recovered from the cervix throughout the menstrual cycle. On the other hand, the gonococcus was isolated from the fallopian tubes only within the first 7 days after the onset of menses. Previously, it has been postulated that during the menstrual period the loss of the cervical mucous plug allows microorganisms from the endocervix and vagina to gain access to the endometrial cavity. Additionally, the endometrium, which may offer local protection against bacterial invasion, has been sloughed. Menstrual blood from the endometrial cavity is an excellent culture media. It had been postulated that the gonococci either migrate into the fallopian tubes or are carried there with refluxed menstrual blood. Another possible mechanism which has been suggested by Toth et al may be the transport of gonococci via sperm attachment to the fallopian tubes (87). Carney and Taylor-Robinson utilizing human tube organ cultures have shown that as gonococci reach the endosalpinx they become attached to mucosal epithelial cells, penetrate the epithelial cells, and cause cell destruction (88). Within 2–7 days, ciliary motility is lost in fallopian tube organ cultures inoculated with *N. gonorrhoeae.* Recently, Gregg et al have reported on the production of an endotoxin by the gonococcus which damages ciliated cells in human fallopian tube organ culture systems (10). Destruction of the endosalpinx results in the production of a purulent exudate. In the early stages of the disease, the tubal lumen is open, and the purulent material exudes from the fimbriated end of the tubé, resulting in pelvic peritonitis. As a result of the peritoneal inflammation, contiguous pelvic structures such as the ovary, omentum sigmoid, small bowel, broad ligament, and cecum become involved in the process. In an attempt to protect the upper abdomen and wall off the source of peritoneal contamination, the fimbriated end of the tube may become blocked with the resultant development of an acute pyosalpinx. If the ovary becomes involved in the infectious process, the result is a tuboovarian abscess (TOA).

The realization that only 10–17% of women with endocervical gonorrhea developed upper genital tract disease and the finding by Sweet in his laparoscope study that the gonococcus could only be recovered from the fallopian tube in women during the first 7 days of the menstrual cycle suggested that inherent properties of the gonococcal organism may determine its ability to produce upper genital tract disease. It has been postulated that there are different strains of gonococci and that a particular strain or strains may be the virulent one for the development of salpingitis. This concept holds for disseminated gonorrhea in which the strain producing disseminated disease varies by microbiologic susceptibility patterns and auxotypes from the organism causing asymptomatic lower genital tract disease. Sweet and co-workers studied several potential virulence factors in paired fallopian tube-peritoneal cavity and endocervical isolates of N. gonorrhoeae obtained from acute salpingitis patients undergoing laparoscopy. Specifically, auxotypes (nutritional requirements), antimicrobial susceptibility, serum bactericidal activity, and colony phenotype were studied (89, 90). Similar to the finding with disseminated gonorrhea, the gonococci recovered from women with salpingitis had significantly different auxotypes and antimicrobial susceptibility patterns compared to those in uncomplicated anogenital disease. In contradistinction to the findings with disseminated gonorrhea, the gonococci causing acute salpingitis were relatively more resistant to multiple antimicrobial agents, and the auxotype pattern most associated with acute salpingitis was the prototrophic pattern (i.e., no extra amino acids required for growth), whereas it was the arginine hypoxanthine and uracil auxotype pattern which was associated with uncomplicated lower genital tract gonorrhea. However, there was no difference among paired peritoneal cavity/cervical isolates of N. gonorrhoeae recovered from

salpingitis patients relative to auxotypes and antimicrobial susceptibility patterns. The potential virulence factor which was significantly different in the paired fallopian tube endocervical gonorrhea specimens was colony phenotype (89). The organisms in the fallopian tube of women with acute salpingitis tended to be the transparent colony phenotype, whereas those present in the cervix of the same women tended to be opaque. In previous studies, women cultured during the menstrual cycle except during the time of the menses had a preponderance of opaque organisms isolated with a peak at the time of ovulation. The organisms usually recovered from the male urethra are heavily opaque, and the organisms recovered from women on oral contraceptives are opaque (women on oral contraceptives appear to be protected against the development of upper genital tract disease if they acquire gonorrhea). Thus, epidemiologically and clinically it appears that the transparent colony phenotypes may well be the virulent form of the gonococcus in the pathogenesis of acute salpingitis. To test this hypothesis, human fallopian tube and cervical organ culture explant systems were used to evaluate endocervical and fallopian tube attachment. At both the endocervix and fallopian tubes it is the transparent colony phenotype of N. gonorrhoeae which attaches more avidly to human fallopian tube tissue than their opaque colony phenotype counterparts (91). It appears that something in the cervical milieu, hormones, pH, or an unidentified factor, may either select out the transparent colony phenotype or selectively drive the gonococci from opaque to transparent forms. The basic difference between the opaque and transparent colony phenotypes are proteins present in the outer cell membrane of the organism. A great deal of current investigation is underway evaluating these outer membrane proteins. Of future importance to the clinician is the work of Buchanan and associates utilizing principal outer membrane proteins to serotype the gonococcus (92). These investigators have reported the presence of nine serotypes of gonococci. They have noted that three of the serotypes (1, 2, and 8) are responsible for nearly 75% of gonococcal salpingitis. In addition, these investigators reported that reinfection with a similar serotype of gonococci results in cervical infection but not in fallopian tube infection, whereas reinfection with gonococci of a different serotype results in both cervical and fallopian tube infection. This finding suggests the presence of immunity of the fallopian tube site among previously infected women. Based on these findings, this group is actively pursuing a vaccine to prevent gonococcal salpingitis based on the principal outer membrane proteins.

It is generally held that chlamydial salpingitis, similar to the situation in gonococcal salpingitis, results from the intracanalicular spread of *C. trachomatis* from the endocervix across the endometrium to the fallopian tube (39, 93). Ripa et al have shown that *C. trachomatis* in a Grivet monkey model gains access to the fallopian tube mucosa as an ascending intracanalicular infection from the endocervix (71). Toth et al have demonstrated that *C. trachomatis* attach to sperm and suggested that sperm may well be the vector that facilitates spread of microorganisms including chlamydia into the upper genital tract (87). Recently, an association between chlamydial salpingitis and menstruation, similar to that for *N. gonorrhoeae*, has been noted (R.L. Sweet, unpublished data). Thus, it appears that the pathogenesis of chlamydial salpingitis parallels that seen in gonococcal disease.

Very little of the pathogenesis in nongonococcal, nonchlamydial salpingitis has been elucidated. Recent reports have shown that salpingitis is a polymicrobial infection, and the organisms implicated include aerobic and anaerobic bacteria and genital tract mycoplasmas, especially *M. hominis*. The mechanisms by which these microorganisms gain access to the upper genital tract are not known. Mycoplasmas can reach the adnexa from the cervix and the endometrium by lymphatic spread via the parametrial tissues and broad ligament, resulting in parasalpingitis and parametritis (47). Whether such a pathogenic mechanism exists in humans is not proven, and the role of *M. hominis* and *U. urealyticum* as putative agents in acute salpingitis remains unclear.

The cervix and vagina of healthy women have been shown to contain a multitude of aerobic and anaerobic bacteria (94). How these organisms gain access to the upper genital tract is not known. As postulated for *N. gonorrhoeae*, they may reach the fallopian tube in menstrual blood reflex or attach to sperm and then are carried to the fallopian tubes. Eschenbach has suggested that there may be a critical number of organisms needed to overwhelm local host defense mechanisms in the cervix, thereby allowing an infection to ascend to the upper genital tract (9). Possibly there is a continuum from the entity of nonspecific vaginitis, which has

recently been shown to be associated with high colony counts of anaerobic bacteria in a synergistic infection with *Gardnerella vaginalis* and nongonococcal nonchlamydial bacterial salpingitis. Such a scenario is suggested by the microbiology results presented by Sweet and co-workers (39). These investigators recovered *G. vaginalis* from the upper genital tract in 30 (40%) of 74 hospitalized women with acute salpingitis. This organism was nearly always found in association with anaerobic bacteria, particularly *Bacteroides* species, *Bacteroides bivius*, and anaerobic cocci. A hypothesis that requires confirmation is that the synergistic infection with anaerobes and *G. vaginalis* may be a third (in addition to *N. gonorrhoeae* and *C. trachomatis*) instance in which a lower genital tract infection ascends into the upper genital tract and produces acute salpingitis. Even if such a hypothesis is not confirmed, it is apparent that nongonococcal nonchlamydial bacteria are involved in the etiology and pathogenesis of acute salpingitis (23, 39). Moreover, the nongonococcal, nonchlamydial organisms can cause acute salpingitis without antecedent infection with *N. gonorrhoeae* and/or *C. trachomatis*. Although not identified yet, some alteration in the normal cervical defense mechanism that precludes microorganisms from the cervix and vagina gaining access to the upper genital tract most probably does exist. This is a fertile area which requires investigation.

The pathogenic mechanism of IUD-associated salpingitis is different from that seen with the gonococcus or chlamydia. When the IUD was reintroduced into clinical practice in 1959 it was postulated that infection would occur only at the time of insertion, with a break in sterile technique or the introduction of pathogenic bacteria. More recently, it has become apparent that the device alters the host defense mechanisms within the uterine cavity. In addition, recent studies have shown that the IUD string is a wick for bacteria to ascend to the lower uterine segment (18, 19). In these studies the lower uterine segment has become colonized in patients wearing IUDs with strings, whereas it has not become colonized in those wearing IUDs without strings. This combination of the wicking effect for bacteria from the lower genital tract and the presence of a foreign body interfering with local host defense mechanisms seems to set the stage in the uterine cavity for the development of endometritis. These patients usually present with intermenstrual bleeding and crampy abdominal pain. Histologically there are submucosal microabscesses beneath the area of the IUD placement. Once an endometritis is established, the pathogenesis of infection is similar to that seen with postabortion or postpartum infections. Bacteria ascend the lymphatics in the parametrial tissue and broad ligament to reach the tube and adnexa producing a perisalpingitis. It has been suggested that women with acute salpingitis in association with the IUD are at increased risk for the development of adnexal abscesses (95). In addition, it was felt that these infections tend to be unilateral compared to gonococcal disease, which tends to be bilateral. Recently, Landers and Sweet (96) reported that 70% of their series of 232 tuboovarian abscesses were unilateral; this was true for IUD and non-IUD users. Thus, it appears there is not an association between IUD use and unilateral adnexal infection.

DIAGNOSIS

Acute salpingitis presents with a broad spectrum of clinical manifestations, including lower abdominal pain, purulent cervical discharge, cervical motion tenderness, adnexal tenderness, as well as fever and leukocytosis. However, these traditionally accepted symptoms and signs are based upon unconfirmed clinical observations. Laparoscopy has shown that the diagnosis of acute salpingitis based on these clinically accepted criteria is often inaccurate and unsatisfactory (27). Insistence upon such rigid criteria as fever, leukocytosis, elevated ESR, and adnexal masses may result in a greater number of cases of salpingitis being misdiagnosed or inappropriately treated. In 1969, Jacobson and Westrom challenged the accepted clinical diagnosis of acute salpingitis with their objective data based on laparoscopic visualization (27). Of 814 women laparoscoped for presumed diagnosis of acute salpingitis, only 512 (65%) had visual confirmation of the diagnosis: 184 (23%) had normal pelvic findings, and 98 (12%) and other pelvic pathology, including acute appendicitis, endometriosis, ruptured ovarian cysts, or ectopic pregnancy. Evaluation of the symptoms and the signs in the laparoscopic study of Westrom and Jacobson failed to identify clinical factors that can reliably differentiate between patients with acute salpingitis and a visually normal group. A comparison of symptoms presented by the patients with a normal pelvis, as opposed to those with confirmed salpingitis at laparoscopy, revealed no significant difference in the incidence

of lower abdominal pain, increased vaginal discharge, irregular bleeding, urinary symptoms, or gastrointestinal symptoms. The only significant difference noted was a history of fever and chills in patients with documented salpingitis. However, only 40% of the patients with laparoscopically confirmed salpingitis give a history of fever and chills (Table 4.6). Evaluation of the clinical signs or laboratory data upon admission did reveal significant increases in the incidence of adnexal tenderness, elevated ESR, fever, and abnormal vaginal discharge in patients with visually confirmed salpingitis (Table 4.7). However, the overlap between the visually normal and the acute salpingitis group was so large that it precluded reliance upon these factors to differentiate the individual patient with acute salpingitis from the patient with the normal pelvis. Only 30% of patients with visually confirmed acute salpingitis had a documented fever. In fact, only 20% of the patients who were confirmed visually to have acute salpingitis had a combination of the classically described signs and symptoms of pelvic pain, purulent cervical discharge, cervical motion tenderness, adnexal tenderness, fever, leukocytosis, and elevated ESR. It seems apparent that the clinical pattern of acute salpingitis is to a great extent similar to that of other pathologic processes in the pelvis. In an interesting investigation, Wolner-Hanssen et al reported on the laparoscopy findings in 104 women who presented with pelvic pain, adnexal tenderness, and *C. trachomatis* isolation from the cervix (97). Despite such a triad of findings, 28 (27%) of the women had no laparoscopic evidence of acute salpingitis. Although the women documented to have salpingitis were significantly more likely to have had pelvic pain of longer duration, irregular bleeding, and an elevated ESR, none of these findings were of a high predictive value. Moreover, there was no statistical difference noted between the women with and without salpingitis for the presence of a temperature more than or equal to 38°C or a white blood cell count more than 10,000 WBC/mm³. Thus, if clinicians rigidly insist on the conventionally accepted criteria, many women with acute salpingitis will be either incorrectly diagnosed or inadequately treated, and thus will be predisposed to the medical and economic sequelae associated with this disease.

In the Jacobson and Westrom study an additional 91 acute salpingitis cases were detected at laparoscopy with presumed diagnoses other than salpingitis. Many of these women lacked the

Table 4.6
Frequency of Symptoms among Women with Acute Pelvic Inflammatory Disease (PID)[a]

Symptoms	Acute pelvic inflammatory disease (N = 622) (%)	Pelvis normal on laparoscopy (N = 184) (%)	p
Lower abdominal pain	585 (94.0)	173 (94.0)	NS
Increased vaginal discharge	340 (54.6)	104 (56.5)	NS
History of fever or chills	257 (41.0)	36 (19.6)	0.001
Irregular bleeding	221 (35.5)	79 (42.9)	NS
Urinary symptoms	116 (18.6)	37 (20.1)	NS
Gastrointestinal symptoms	64 (10.3)	17 (9.2)	NS

[a] Adapted from Jacobson L, Westrom L: Objectivized diagnosis of acute pelvic inflammatory disease. *Am J Obstet Gynecol* 105:1088, 1969.

Table 4.7
Objective Findings on Admission in Patients with Acute Pelvic Inflammatory Disease (PID)[a]

Clinical findings	Acute PID (N = 591) (%)	Normal pelvis on laparoscopy (N = 184) (%)	p
Adnexal tenderness	573 (97.0)	160 (87.0)	0.05
Increase ESR	473 (76.0)	97 (53.0)	0.001
Abnormal vaginal discharge	394 (63.7)	74 (40.2)	0.001
Fever	205 (33.0)	26 (14.0)	0.001

[a] Adapted from Jacobson L, Westrom L: Objectivized diagnosis of acute pelvic inflammatory disease. *Am J Obstet Gynecol* 105:1088, 1969.

classical abdominal pain and adnexal tenderness on bimanual exam. This group may represent what Rees and Annels have termed "subclinical disease," which may be fairly common (98). Because definitive diagnosis in treatment may be delayed or absent, such women may be at greater risk for infertility in future years than the more clearly recognizable acutely ill women with obvious disease.

In summary, laparoscopic studies have shown that: (a) The clinical diagnosis of acute salpingitis is often inaccurate; (b) Acute salpingitis is frequently found in patients undergoing laparoscopy for other causes of acute pelvic pain; (c) The laparoscope is a safe way to make the visual diagnosis; (d) Laparoscopy is an excellent means of obtaining cultures directly from the tube.

Recognizing that laparoscopy is currently the only way to make an absolute diagnosis of acute salpingitis, it is logistically and economically impractical for all patients suspected to have the diagnosis of acute salpingitis to undergo diagnostic laparoscopy in the United States. Because of the impracticality of universal laparoscopy in the diagnosis of acute salpingitis and with recognition that the presence of increasing numbers of signs and/or symptoms and/or laboratory data suggestive of acute salpingitis increase

the accuracy of the clinical diagnosis, an attempt has been made to standardize the diagnosis of salpingitis. The criteria presented in Table 4.8 have been proposed for making the diagnosis of salpingitis based on clinical grounds. All patients should have the initial three findings. Rebound tenderness is not required because rebound may not be present early in the disease process until there is purulent exudate spilled into the peritoneal cavity and pelvic peritonitis develops. However, because these findings are all subjective and based on pain and tenderness, one of the six additional findings which suggest all subjective and based on pain and tenderness, one of the six additional findings which suggest the presence of acute inflammation should also be present. An additional finding which may prove useful would be the presence of WBC on a cervical smear.

Recently, Westrom et al have suggested that the determination of nonpancreatic isoamylases in peritoneal fluid and serum was helpful in confirming a diagnosis of acute salpingitis (100). The quotient of the activities of the nonpancreatic isoamylases derived from peritoneal fluid and serum was determined (P/S). In healthy women, specific nonpancreatic isoamylases were demonstrable in peritoneal fluid at compara-

Table 4.8
Criteria for the Diagnosis of Acute Salpingitis[a]

All three must be present
1. History of lower abdominal pain and the presence of lower abdominal tenderness; with or without evidence of rebound.
2. Cervical motion tenderness.
3. Adnexal tenderness.

One of these must be present
1. Temperature >38°C.
2. Leukocytosis >10,500 WBC/mm^3
3. A culdocentesis which yields peritoneal fluid containing white blood cells and bacteria.
4. Presence of an inflammatory mass noted on pelvic examination or sonography.
5. Elevated ESR.
6. A gram stain from the endocervix revealing gram-negative intracellular diplococci suggestive of *N. gonorrhoeae* or a monoclonal directed smear from endocervical secretions revealing *C. trachomatis.*

[a] Adapted from Hager WD, et al: Criteria for diagnosis and grading of salpingitis. *Obstet Gynecol* 61:113–114, 1983.

tively high values but were diminished or totally absent in cases of acute salpingitis. Therefore, the P/S was low in patients with salpingitis and high in healthy women or women with only lower genital tract disease and normal fallopian tubes, as evaluated by laparoscopy. These findings require substantiation; if confirmed, a fairly simple method for clinicians to increase accuracy for the diagnosis of acute salpingitis would be available. However, the time required to perform such a laboratory test negates against its clinical usefulness. This statement also applies to attempts to use C-reactive protein measurement as an aide in the diagnosis of acute salpingitis.

Procedures such as sonography and culdocentesis may not be readily available to physicians in general practice. Thus, the clinician may still have to base the diagnosis on observation for the classical signs and careful history taking. Until more large scale, controlled, prospective studies are conducted which utilize laparoscopy for visual and microbiologic confirmation, the diagnosis and treatment of acute salpingitis will remain unsatisfactory.

In general, the diagnosis of tuboovarian abscesses has been based on clinical findings, i.e., pelvic examination revealing a tender pelvic mass in association with the signs and symptoms of pelvic inflammatory disease. The diagnosis of tuboovarian abscesses based on physical examination has been questioned because of the difficulty in evaluating the bimanual examination in women with acute pelvic peritonitis. Differentiating a tuboovarian abscess from acute salpingitis with bowel adhesed to the adnexa is difficult. Recently, sonography and CT scan

have been suggested as methods to increase diagnostic accuracy (96). Sonography may prove to be an accurate replacement for documenting the presence of an abscess by surgically draining the purulent material. However, the routine use of sonography in patients with acute salpingitis does not seem indicated. Rather, if the patient is not able to be adequately examined because of tenderness and pain to exclude an adnexal mass or there is a lack of response to antimicrobial therapy in the initial 48–72 hr of therapy then sonography may be indicated to evaluate the possibility of an inflammatory mass being present. The diagnosis of tuboovarian abscess is described in greater detail in Chapter 12.

TREATMENT

It is important to recognize that the therapeutic goals in the management of acute salpingitis are prevention of infertility and the chronic residua of infection. Before the advent of antibiotics, many cases of acute salpingitis managed by conservative supportive therapy resolved spontaneously and without sequelae (23, 40, 101). Curtis stated that 85% of acute salpingitis patients improved without surgery, whereas 15% had prolonged or progressive symptoms that led to surgical intervention (40, 101). In a review of 1,262 patients, Holtz noted a 9% incidence of persistent severe symptoms, a 6% incidence of pyrexia present for greater than 2 months, and a 1.3% incidence of mortality (24). Antibiotics have been reported to have decreased the sequelae of salpingitis, such as abscesses and infertility (102). Studies from Scandinavia in the late

1950s and early 1960s suggested that the advent of antibiotics had improved the prognosis for acute salpingitis; mortality had been eliminated; the frequency of ruptured pelvic abscesses and persistent masses requiring surgery decreased, and the subsequent fertility rate improved (25, 102, 103). In the preantibiotic era, Holtz reported a 22.8% pregnancy rate in patients with gonococcal salpingitis (24). These early studies noted that the use of antibiotics for the treatment of gonococcal salpingitis resulted in crude pregnancy rates of 39–51% (24, 25). If patients with gonococcal salpingitis who are voluntarily infertile or in whom surgical intervention precluded conception are excluded, corrected pregnancy rates of 67–84% were reported (24, 25). Antibiotic treatment in cases of nongonococcal salpingitis resulted in crude pregnancy rates of 25–44% and corrected pregnancy rates of 60–81% (24, 103, 104).

While on the surface it appears that antimicrobial therapy has improved the prognosis for fertility significantly, the results are far from satisfactory. The higher pregnancy rates after antibiotic treatment are corrected rates that have excluded patients for whom the infection resulted in surgical intervention that prevented future fertility. Exclusion of such patients may preclude a fair assessment, for the true prognosis for fertility rates were similar in the group treated with antibiotics and in the control group treated with bed rest and supportive therapy only (104).

More recently, in a long-term longitudinal study of women with laparoscope-confirmed salpingitis, Westrom has documented that, despite antibiotic therapy, patients with at least one episode of acute salpingitis have a 21% rate of involuntary infertility, as compared to the control population rate of 3% (7). In addition, in this report of the 88 patients with involuntary infertility, 72 (81%) had tubal blockage on hysterosalpingogram or repeat laparoscopy, and 54 (61%) required a subsequent surgical procedure. In addition, despite the antibiotic treatment, there was a six-fold increase in the incidence of ectopic pregnancies in the salpingitis patients. Of particular importance in the Swedish long-term studies was the finding that the prognosis for infertility is directly related to the number of episodes of salpingitis. With a single episode, the risk of infertility is approximately 11%, rising to 34% with two episodes, and to 54% after three or more episodes of disease (3).

Another major finding in the Swedish lapa-

roscopy studies was that those patients with gonococcal salpingitis had a better prognosis for fertility than did those with nongonococcal disease (7). A probable explanation for this finding is that patients with gonococcal disease present with the classically described picture of acute salpingitis with a high fever, leukocytosis, and purulent discharge from the cervix in addition to the findings of pelvic pain and tenderness. Clinicians relying on the usually accepted criteria for diagnosis of acute salpingitis results in gonococcal disease being more likely to be diagnosed and treated earlier and more often than nongonococcal disease. More importantly, the patients with gonococcal disease meet most physicians' criteria for admission to the hospital and are, thus, admitted early in their disease course and treated with intravenous antibiotic regimens which have been designed to treat the gonococcus. Thus, it should not be surprising that these patients with gonococcal disease who are diagnosed and treated appropriately have a better prognosis for fertility. It is those patients with nongonococcal disease who often present with milder symptoms, do not get diagnosed and treated, and have the poorer prognosis for future fertility. Whether any particular nongonococcal pathogen such as chlamydia, mycoplasmas, or anaerobic bacteria carry a worse prognosis for future fertility is not clear at this time. Westrom and colleagues have suggested that patients with chlamydial salpingitis (determined by presence of serologic confirmation of C. trachomatis with significant rises in antibody titer or by recovery of C. trachomatis from the fallopian tube) are more likely to have severe inflammatory involvement of the fallopian and have the worst prognosis for future fertility (3, 7). Recently, however, this same Swedish group of investigators reported that, based on the results of cervical cultures, there was no difference in the involuntary infertility rate among women with chlamydial salpingitis, gonococcal salpingitis, chlamydial and gonococcal salpingitis, and nonchlamydial, nongonococcal salpingitis; the rates of infertility were 22.7, 23.5, 20, and 22%, respectively (21). Although animal model work of intraabdominal sepsis suggests that anaerobic bacteria resistant to penicillins and first generation cephalosporins such as B. fragilis are important in the pathogenesis of intraabdominal abscesses, whether this model is applicable to the situation of acute salpingitis and the development of tuboovarian abscesses is not clear. Hare and Barnes demonstrated that in the fallopian tube organ explant system, *B. fragilis* produced rapid and complete destruction of the fallopian tube mucosa (45).

Early diagnosis and treatment are crucial to the preservation of future fertility. Several investigations have shown that the effectiveness of therapy in preventing infertility depends on the interval between the onset of symptoms and the institution of treatment (25, 102, 104). These follow-up investigations which utilized hysterosalpingogram and/or laparoscopy have documented that in women treated early in the course of acute salpingitis, tubal patency remains unimpaired in a significant number of women. Viberg reported that none of the patients treated within 2 days of the onset of symptoms was involuntarily infertile, and all had patent fallopian tubes on hysterosalpingogram (104). On the other hand, if treatment had been instituted on day 7 or later, only 70% of patients were shown to have tubal patency. These findings again stress the importance of not relying on the strict criteria for the diagnosis of acute salpingitis that have existed in the past and of the necessity to institute early treatment based on a more flexible and realistic approach to the diagnosis.

The failure of antibiotics to prevent the sequelae of acute salpingitis may reflect the emphasis on gonorrhea as an etiologic agent and the lack of antimicrobial regimens that provide coverage for the polymicrobic etiology of acute salpingitis, including chlamydia and anaerobic bacteria. If antibiotic therapy is to be effective and prevent the sequelae of salpingitis, it must be instituted early in the disease process and an antibiotic regimen must be utilized that takes into account the polymicrobial nature of the etiology of acute salpingitis. The major pathogens include *C. trachomatis*, anaerobic bacteria (especially the resistant *Bacteroides* species), and aerobic streptococci (including group B). Whether *B. fragilis*, an anaerobe usually resistant to penicillins and first generation cephalosporins, must be covered is not clear at this time. Although Eschenbach and co-workers recovered *B. fragilis* from culdocentesis specimens obtained from patients with acute salpingitis and demonstrated the presence of antibody to the *B. fragilis* capsule, most investigations have not recovered *B. fragilis* except rarely (22, 29, 33, 35). Weinstein and co-workers developed an animal model that identifies a biphasic disease process in intraabdominal infections (107). The initial stage is one of peritonitis and sepsis associated with aerobic or facultative organisms such as *E. coli* and a high mortality rate. The surviving animals enter a secondary phase characterized by the development of intraabdominal abscesses in which anaerobic organisms and especially *B. fragilis* predominate. In order to prevent both stages of this biphasic infectious process, it was necessary to institute an antibiotic regimen that was effective against both components of this mixed aerobic/anaerobic infection (108). Either a single agent or a combination of agents which covered *B. fragilis* was necessary in order to prevent the abscess stage. The relevance of this study to pelvic infection seems apparent. Acute salpingitis is analogous to the peritonitis stage, and the abscess stage is represented by pyosalpinx or tuboovarian abscesses. Whether employment of antimicrobial regimens that cover *B. fragilis* would either prevent TOAs or enhance the prognosis for future fertility is not known.

Controversy has arisen over the issue of outpatient treatment with oral antibiotics versus inpatient treatment with parenteral antibiotics in patients with acute salpingitis. There are no data available to evaluate the need for hospital versus ambulatory management of acute salpingitis. For economic and logistic reasons only 25–30% of cases are hospitalized in the United States; the majority remain outpatients during treatment. The Center for Disease Control has published recommended treatment schedules for both ambulatory and hospitalized patients with acute salpingitis (109). These recommendations are shown in Table 4.9. These current recommended treatment regimens are based on the premise that it is appropriate to cover all the major etiologic agents involved in acute salpingitis, including *N. gonorrhoeae*, *C. trachomatis*, anaerobes including anaerobic cocci and *Bacteroides*, and gram-negative enterics such as *E. coli*. The need to cover these major etilogic groups is best demonstrated by the consistent 10–13% infertility rate reported by Westrom et al in a group of just over 600 first episodes of laparoscoped confirmed PID treated with regimens on an inpatient basis that failed to provide such broad spectrum coverage (110).

The prior CDC recommendations for outpatient treatment had been evaluated in two prospective trials. These studies compared tetracycline (500 mg four times a day for 10 days) with procaine penicillin (4.8 million units IM with 1.0 g probenecid by mouth) followed by ampicillin (500 mg four times a day for 10 days). Cun-

Table 4.9
Centers for Disease Control Recommended Treatment Schedules for Acute Pelvic Inflammatory Disease—1982

Ambulatory treatment
  Cefoxitin (2.0 g IM)
    or
  Amoxicillin (3.0 g by mouth)
    or   } along with probenecid by mouth
  Ampicillin (3.5 g by mouth)
    or
  Aqueous procaine penicillin G (4.8 mU IM)
    Followed by
  Doxycycline (100 mg by mouth), 4 times a day for 10–14 days)
    or
  Tetracycline HCl (500 mg by mouth, 4 times a day for 10–14 days)

In hospital treatment
1. Cefoxitin (2.0 g IV, 4 times a day)
     plus
   Doxycycline (100 mg IV, twice a day)
   Continue drugs IV for at least 4 days and at least 48 hr after patient defervesces. Continue doxycycline (100 mg by mouth twice a day) after discharge from the hospital to complete 10–14 days of therapy.
2. Clindamycin (600 mg IV, 4 times a day)
     plus
   Gentamicin or tobramycin (2.0 mg/kg IV, followed by 1.5 mg/kg IV, 3 times a day) in patients with normal renal function
   Continue drugs IV for at least 4 days and at least 48 hr after patient defervesces. Continue clindamycin (450 mg by mouth, 4 times a day) after discharge from the hospital to complete 10–14 days of therapy.
3. Metronidazole (1.0 g IV, twice a day)
     plus
   Doxycycline (100 mg IV twice a day)
   Continue drugs IV for at least 4 days and at least 48 hr after patient defervesces. Then continue both drugs at same dosage orally to complete 10–14 days of therapy.

ningham and colleagues reported excellent initial response and no difference in cure rates between the ampicillin regimen and the tetracycline regimen (34). However, the report by Thompson and colleagues which involved a six-hospital collaborative study comparing the older 1979 ambulatory regimens recommended by the Center for Disease Control was more pessimistic (111). In the 240 patients with salpingitis and a positive gonococcal culture from the endocervix, 33 (13.8%) were treatment failures. No statistically significant difference existed between the effectiveness of the penicillin-ampicillin and the tetracycline regimens. In nongonococcal salpingitis the overall failure rate reached 17%; 59 of 345 did not respond to treatment; again, there was not a statistically significant difference between the two regimens. The major drawback to this study was the lack of either culdocentesis or laparoscopy performance of culture. This study produced two important conclusions.

Firstly, such high failure rates are unacceptable when the potential end point is infertility due to tubal obstruction. Secondly, it seriously questioned the adequacy of single agent therapy in the management of acute salpingitis and indeed the appropriateness of ambulatory therapy. No prospective data exist which addresses the issue of the clinical efficacy of outpatient versus inpatient therapy of acute salpingitis. Whether the 1982 recommendations for ambulatory therapy will prove to be effective in producing initial clinical response and in preventing subsequent complications such as infertility and ectopic pregnancy is not known. The answer must await large scale prospective studies which include sufficiently long duration of posttreatment follow-up to allow for an assessment of the impact on fertility, ectopic pregnancy, and the need for surgical intervention.

The clinician who diagnoses acute salpingitis in the office or emergency room is faced with the question of hospitalization. There is no satisfactory answer to this dilemma, and the controversy between ambulatory and hospital management still wages. Indications for hospitalization of acute salpingitis patients have been suggested and are listed in Table 4.10. We feel it is important to admit patients who have not responded promptly to ambulatory therapy; it is crucial to reevaluate patients within 48 hours to determine the effectiveness of ambulatory therapy and, if no response has been obtained, then admission should be promptly instituted with parenteral antibiotics to hopefully prevent the sequelae of salpingitis. Of special note should be the finding that patients with suspected or diagnosed inflammatory adnexal masses, such as pyosalpinx or tuboovarian abscesses, should be hospitalized for parenteral therapy. We recommend that women wearing IUDs should be treated on an inpatient basis, because of the high coexistent rate of adnexal inflammatory masses. In addition, it is suggested that all adolescents with salpingitis should be hospitalized. The latter suggestion is based on the high noncompliance rate among the adolescent population, especially with the use of multiple doses in therapy. It has also been proposed that patients undergoing their first episode of acute salpingitis be treated as inpatients, with hopes to optimize the prevention of damage to the reproductive system.

The previous CDC recommendation for inpatient treatment of acute salpingitis included either a regimen of penicillin G(10–20 million units IV per day), followed by ampicillin (500 mg IV four times a day for 10 days) or a regimen of tetracycline (500 mg IV four times a day followed by 500 mg orally for a total of 10 days).

Similar to the outpatient recommendations, these previous CDC recommendations for in-

Table 4.10
Criteria for Hospitalization of Patients with Acute Pelvic Inflammatory Disease

1. Question all acute pelvic inflammatory disease cases
2. Suspected pelvic or tuboovarian abscess
3. Pregnancy
4. Temperature >38°C
5. Uncertain diagnosis
6. Nausea and vomiting precluding oral medications
7. Upper peritoneal signs
8. Failure to respond to oral antibiotics within 48 hr

patient therapy were based on the premise that *N. gonorrhoeae* was the major etiologic agent in acute salpingitis and provided poor coverage against *B. fragilis* and many strains of gram-negative enteric bacteria. In Table 4.9 the current CDC recommendations (as of August 1982) for treatment of hospitalized patients with acute salpingitis are listed. In general, these recommendations were an attempt to provide treatment regimens that are active against the broadest range of the multiple pathogens associated with acute pelvic inflammatory disease. Thus, these regimens attempt to cover *N. gonorrhoeae*, *C. trachomatis*, anaerobic bacteria (including *Bacteroides* and anaerobic cocci), facultative gram-negative rods, and *M. hominis*. In addition, Sweet et al have demonstrated that facultative streptococci, such as group B streptococcus, are also frequently isolated from the upper genital tract in acute pelvic inflammatory disease, and these organisms should also be covered (39).

As can be seen in Table 4.9, the major emphasis has been to use combinations of agents to cover the multitude of microorganisms involved in the polymicrobial etiology of acute PID. It is important to recognize that the combination regimens recommended by the CDC have not undergone clinical prospective comparative trials and essentially were based on theoretic calculations of putative agents and in vitro antimicrobial susceptibility patterns. The relative in vitro activities of these regimens is presented in Table 4.11. The cefoxitin plus doxycycline regimen appears to provide coverage against all the major pathogen groups. Doxycycline is active against both *N. gonorrhoeae* and *C. trachomatis*. The cefoxitin covers *N. gonorrhoeae* (including penicillinase producing strains), gram-positive aerobes, gram-negative aerobes, and penicillin-sensitive and nonpenicillin-sensitive anaerobes. While the clindamycin plus aminoglycoside combination provides excellent activity against anaerobes (clindamycin), gram-negative aerobes (aminoglycoside), and gram-positive aerobes (clindamycin), it does not provide optimal activity against *C. trachomatis* and *N. gonorrhoeae*. In vitro studies have demonstrated that clindamycin is effective against approximately 90% of *C. trachomatis* strains (112); its efficacy in clinical cases of chlamydial salpingitis has not been demonstrated. Although neither clindamycin nor aminoglycosides are the agent of choice against *N. gonorrhoeae* they are both effective against nonpenicillinase producing strains (90). The metronidazole plus doxycycline regimen

Table 4.11
Sensitivity of Pathogens Associated with Acute Salpingitis

	N. gonorrhoeae		C. trachomatis	Gram + aerobes	Entero-bacteriaceae	Penicillin-sensitive anaerobes	Penicillin-resistant anaerobes
	Non-PPNG	PPNG					
Cefoxitin/doxycycline	+	+	+	+	+	+	+
Clindamycin/ aminoglycoside	+		?	+	+	+	+
Metronidazole/ doxycycline	+		+		±	+	+

provides excellent activity against anaerobes and *C. trachomatis*. Activity against penicillinase producing *N. gonorrhoeae*, some gram-negative rods, and gram-positive aerobes is not optimal. The relative efficacy of these regimens has not been evaluated in clinical trials.

The emergence of penicillinase-producing *N. gonorrhoeae* (PPNG) has produced a major problem. If β-lactamase-producing gonococci are suspected in acute salpingitis patients' outpatient therapy is spectinomycin (2.0 g IM × 3 days). PPNG strains resistant to spectinomycin have been reported and are discussed in detail in Chapter 3. For hospitalized patients the antibiotic of choice against the β-lactamase-producing gonococci has been cefoxitin (2 g IV every 6 hr). More recently the third generation cephalosporin, cefotaxime, has also been noted to be very active against *N. gonorrhoeae*, including β-lactamase-producing strains.

Unfortunately, no microbiologically controlled prospective studies comparing the various antibiotic regimens have been performed. Such studies are urgently needed to determine whether all potential pathogens must be covered by antimicrobial therapy. In addition, controversy exists between the efficacy of outpatient oral antibiotic treatment regimens which do not take into account the polymicrobial nature of the disease in contrast to inpatient parenteral antibiotics, which are broad based and cover most suspected organisms. No well controlled study to date has compared short- and long-term outcomes of outpatient versus inpatient regimens. To ensure the best possible prognosis for future fertility and prevent other serious long-term sequelae, it is our belief that vigorous inpatient parenteral treatment coupled with careful outpatient follow-up is essential.

Appropriate management of acute PID includes examination and treatment of the sexual partners of women with acute PID. These partners should be treated with one of the regimens for uncomplicated gonorrhea and chlamydial in-

fection (i.e., ampicillin (3. 5 g) plus probenecid (1 g) followed by doxycycline (100 mg twice a day for 7 days). The importance of treating sexual partners cannot be overstressed. In a surveillance study of gonococcal PID in San Francisco, 13% of male partners screened were asymptomatic urethral carriers of *N. gonorrhoeae* (R.L. Sweet, unpublished data). Eschenbach reported that 25% of gonococcal PID cases were readmitted to the hospital with a subsequent episode of PID within 10 weeks of initial treatment (8). Women with acute PID return to the same social mileau they were in prior to treatment, and if the large pool of male partners with asymptomatic *N. gonorrhoeae* and *C. trachomatis* is not treated, they will be exposed to a risk for additional episodes of PID.

Tuboovarian abscess is a complication of acute salpingitis and develops when infected material from the fallopian tubes spills into the adjacent ovary and gains access to the ovary. The resulting mass may be unilateral or bilateral and associated with a subacute or chronic disease. It is estimated that palpable adnexal swelling is found in 25% of acute salpingitis, representing acute adnexal inflammation or a tuboovarian abscess. The actual incidence of tuboovarian abscess formation is estimated between 7–16% (96, 113, 119). A detailed description of the management of TOAs is presented in Chapter 12. This will be briefly reviewed here. Although treated by radical gynecologic surgery as primary management by some (115), initial treatment of tuboovarian abscess when there is no suspicion of rupture more appropriately, includes hospitalization and vigorous medical management with broad spectrum antibiotic regimens that include coverage of *B. fragilis*, *N. gonorrhoeae*, anaerobic gram-positive cocci, and gram-negative facultative organisms (96, 116, 117). In patients with suspected tuboovarian abscesses, antibiotic therapy should include a drug that is effective against *B. fragilis*, because of the high prevalence of this anaerobe in association with pelvic abscesses. All three CDC-recommended regimens for hospitalized patients with acute PID contain antimicrobial agents that are effective against *B. fragilis* and penetrate into and are active inside abscesses (118). We believe that conservative medical therapy for tuboovarian abscesses is appropriate in lieu of suspicion for a ruptured tuboovarian abscess, which is a surgical emergency. Ruptured TOAs are reported to occur in from 3 to 15% of tuboovarian abscesses and represent a surgical emergency (113, 115, 119). Aggressive surgical intervention with hysterectomy and bilateral salpingoophorectomy following spontaneous rupture of tuboovarian abscesses results in over 95% recovery rate. Franklin et al (116), Ginsberg et al (117), and Landers and Sweet (96) reported that the conservative medical approach to the treatment of tuboovarian abscesses was associated with a 70% response rate. However, if patients do not begin to improve within 48–72 hr of institution of antimicrobial therapy, surgical intervention is undertaken conserving as much of the reproductive system as possible. Our preference is transabdominal laparotomy rather than vaginal colpotomy. If when we enter the abdominal cavity the infection is limited to one adnexal area, unilateral salpingoophorectomy is performed and the contralateral fallopian tube and ovary preserved. In addition, the uterus is also left. In this way we hope to preserve future reproductive potential. Irrigation of the pelvic cavity is performed with copious amounts of saline, but no antibiotic solution is added to the irrigant. Closed suction drainage is brought out through the vagina. The final step in the operative management of these patients is utilization of a delayed primary closure of the abdominal wound, with permanent suture being placed in the fascia, and the remainder of the wound is left open. If the wound is clean, the incision is reapproximated on the 4th day postoperatively. The use of the delayed primary approach will significantly decrease the incidence of postoperative wound infections. Recently, it has been proposed that with the use of CT scan and real time sonography, percutaneous aspiration and drainage of intraabdominal abscesses may be possible (120). Experience with this technique in the pelvis is limited. It is an appealing concept, but requires clinical evaluation.

In acute salpingitis, the purulent and inflammatory reaction in the pelvis is often severe, with subsequent adhesions, sterility, and chronic pain. To prevent these sequelae, the concomitant use of steroids has been advocated. However, Falk, in a prospective investigation, reported that the use of steroids in the treatment of acute salpingitis produced no difference in the end result as judged by hysterosalpingogram findings, fertility, or the findings at subsequent laparoscopy (25). Whether the use of a higher dose steroid regimen similar to that employed in the therapy of septic shock would be beneficial is speculative. In addition, the role of antiprostaglandin agents should be evaluated in future investigations as potential aides in preventing the adhesions and scarring that occur subsequent to episodes of acute PID.

SUMMARY

Prevention of the significant medical and economic sequelae of acute salpingitis relies on the institution of appropriate treatment regimens, which are based on the true microbiologic etiology of acute salpingitis and cognizant of the polymicrobic nature of this etiology. The clinician must maintain a high index of suspicion for acute salpingitis, in order that early diagnosis and treatment can be made. We believe that hospitalization and utilization of parenteral antimicrobial therapy will be of greatest benefit to the patient. This therapy should include combination agents that provide coverage for *N. gonorrhoeae, C. trachomatis,* anaerobes (including *Bacteroides* and anaerobic cocci), gram-negative aerobic rods, and gram-positive aerobes (including group B streptococcus). Finally, it is crucial to prevent repeat reinfection by seeking out the sexual partners of women with acute salpingitis and treating them for sexually transmitted diseases. In this way, the recurrent infections, which lead to the poor prognosis for fertility can be circumvented.

References

1. Eschenbach DA, Harnisch JP, Holmes KK: Pathogenesis of acute pelvic inflammatory disease: role of contraception and other risk factors. *Am J Obstet Gynecol* 128:838, 1977.
2. Sweet RL: Diagnosis and treatment of acute salpingitis. *J Reprod Med* 19:21, 1977.
3. Westrom L: Incidence, prevalence, and trends of acute pelvic inflammatory disease and its consequences in industrialized countries. *Am J Obstet Gynecol* 138:880, 1980.
4. Curran JW: Economic consequences of pelvic inflammatory disease in the United States. *Am J Obstet Gynecol* 138:848, 1980.
5. Jones OG, Saida AA, St. John RK: Frequency and distribution of salpingitis and pelvic inflammatory disease in short stay hospitals in the

United States. *Am J Obstet Gynecol* 138:905, 1980.

6. Washington AE, Cates W, Zadi AA: Hospitalizations for pelvic inflammatory disease. Epidemiology and trends in the United States, 1975 to 1981. *JAMA* 251:2529–2533, 1984.
7. Westrom L: Effect of acute pelvic inflammatory disease on fertility. *Am J Obstet Gynecol* 122:876, 1975.
8. Eschenbach DA, Holmes KK: Acute pelvic inflammatory disease: current concepts of pathogenesis, etiology, and management. *Clin Obstet Gynecol* 18:35, 1975.
9. Eschenbach DA: Epidemiology and diagnosis of acute pelvic inflammatory disease. *Obstet Gynecol* 55:142(S), 1980.
10. Gregg CR, Melly MA, McGee ZA: Gonococcal lipopolysaccharide: a toxin for human fallopian tube mucosa. *Am J Obstet Gynecol* 138:981, 1980.
11. Draper DL, Donegan EA, James JF, et al: In vitro modeling of acute salpingitis caused by *Neisseria gonorrhoeae*. *Am J Obstet Gynecol* 138:996–1002, 1980.
12. Kaufman DW, Shapiro S, Rosenberg L, et al: Intrauterine contraceptive device use and pelvic inflammatory disease. *Am J Obstet Gynecol* 136:159, 1980.
13. Ory HW: A review of the association between intrauterine devices and acute pelvic inflammatory disease. *J Reprod Med* 20:200, 1978.
14. Osser S, Gullberg B, Lieholm P, Sjoberg NO: Risk of pelvic inflammatory disease among intrauterine device users irrespective of previous pregnancy. *Lancet* 1:386, 1980.
15. Senanayake P, Kramer DG: Contraception and the etiology of pelvic inflammatory disease: new perspectives. *Am J Obstet Gynecol* 138:852, 1980.
16. Westrom L, Bengtsson LP, Mardh P-A: The risk of pelvic inflammatory disease in women using intrauterine contraceptive devices as compared to non-users. *Lancet* 2:221, 1976.
17. Lee NC, Rubin GL, Ory AW, Burkman RT: Type of intrauterine device and the risk of pelvic inflammatory disease. *Obstet Gynecol* 62:1–6, 1983.
18. Sparks RA, Purrier BG, Watt PJ, Elstein M: Bacteriological colonization of uterine cavity; role of tailed intrauterine contraceptive devices. *Br Med J* 282:1189–1191, 1981.
19. Skangalis M, Mahoney CJ, O'Leary WM: Microbial presence in the uterine cavity as affected by varieties of intrauterine contraceptive devices. *Fertil Steril* 37:263–269, 1982.
20. Burnhill MS: Syndrome of progressive endometritis associated with intrauterine contraceptive devices. *Adv Planned Parent* 8:144–150, 1973.
21. Svensson L, Mardh P-A, Westrom L: Infertility after acute salpingitis with special reference to *Chlamydia trachomatis*. *Fertil Steril* 40:322–329, 1983.
22. Cunningham FG, Hauth JC, Gilstrap LC, Herbert WNP, Kappus S: The bacterial pathogenesis of acute pelvic inflammatory disease. *Obstet Gynecol* 52:161, 1978.
23. Eschenbach DA, Buchanan T, Pollock HM, et al: Polymicrobial etiology of acute pelvic inflammatory disease. *N Engl J Med* 293:166, 1975.
24. Holtz F: Klinische studien uber die nicht tuber-

kulose salpingoophoritis. *Acta Obstet Gynecol* 10(S):5, 1930.
25. Falk V: Treatment of acute nontuberculous salpingitis with antibiotics alone and in combination with glucocorticoids. *Acta Obstet Gynecol Scand* 44(S-16):65, 1965.
26. Hundley JM, Diehl WK, Baggott JW: Bacteriologic studies in salpingitis with special reference to gonococcal viability. *Am J Obstet Gynecol* 60:97, 1950.
27. Jacobson L, Westrom L: Objectivized diagnosis of acute pelvic inflammatory disease. *Am J Obstet Gynecol* 105:1088, 1969.
28. Lip J, Burgoyne X: Cervical and peritoneal bacterial flora associated with salpingitis. *Obstet Gynecol* 28:561, 1966.
29. Sweet RL, Draper DL, Schachter J, et al: Microbiology and pathogenesis of acute salpingitis as determined by laparoscopy: what is the appropriate site to sample? *Am J Obstet Gynecol* 138:985, 1980.
30. Thompson SE, Hager WD, Wong KH, et al: The microbiology and therapy of acute pelvic inflammatory disease in hospitalized patients. *Am J Obstet Gynecol* 136:179, 1980.
31. Rendtorff RC, Curran JC, Chandler RW, et al: Economic consequences of gonorrhea in women. *J Am Vener Dis Assoc* 1:40, 1974.
32. Andrews FT: Notes on causes of salpingitis. *Am J Obstet Gynecol* 49:177, 1940.
33. Chow AW, Malkasian KL, Marshall Jr, et al: The bacteriology of acute pelvic inflammatory disease. *Am J Obstet Gynecol* 122:876, 1975.
34. Cunningham FG, Hauth JC, Strong JD, et al: Evaluation of tetracycline or penicillin and ampicillin for the treatment of acute pelvic inflammatory disease. *N Engl J Med* 296:1380, 1977.
35. Monif GRG, Welkos SL, Baer H, et al: Cul de sac isolates from patients with endometritis, salpingitis, peritonitis and gonococcal endocervicitis. *Am J Obstet Gynecol* 126:158, 1976.
36. Sweet RL, Draper D, Hadley WK: Etiology of acute salpingitis: influence of episode number and duration of symptoms. *Obstet Gynecol* 58:62, 1981.
37. Sweet RL, Mills J, Hadley WK, et al: Use of laparoscopy to determine the microbiologic etiology of acute salpingitis. *Am J Obstet Gynecol* 1334:68, 1979.
38. McCormack WM, Nowroozi K, Alpert S: Acute pelvic inflammatory disease: characteristics of patients with gonococcal infection and evaluation of their response to treatment with aqueous procaine penicillin G and spectinomycin hydrochloride. *Sex Transm Dis* 4:125, 1977.
39. Sweet RL, Schachter J, Robbie MO: Failure of beta-lactam antibiotics to eradicate *Chlamydia trachomatis* in the endometrium despite apparent clinical cure of acute salpingitis. *JAMA* 250:2641–2645, 1983.
40. Curtis AH: Bacteriology and pathology of fallopian tubes removed at operation. *Surg Gynecol Obstet* 33:621, 1921.
41. Studdiford WE, Casper WA, Scandron EN: The persistence of gonococcal infections in the adnexa. *Surg Gynecol Obstet* 67:176, 1938.
42. Tronca E, Handsfield HH, Wiesner PJ, Holmes

KK: Demonstration of *Neisseria gonorrhoeae* with fluorescent antibody in patients with disseminated gonococcal infection. *J Infect Dis* 129:583, 1974.

43. Lemcke R, Csonka GW: Antibodies against pleuropneumonia-like organisms in patients with salpingitis. *Br J Vener Dis* 38:212–217, 1962.

44. Mardh P-A, Westrom L: Tubal and cervical cultures in acute salpingitis with special reference to *Mycoplasma hominis* and T-strain mycoplasmas. *Br J Vener Dis* 46:169, 1970.

45. Møller BR: The role of mycoplasmas in the upper genital tract of women. *Sex Transm Dis* 10(S):281–284, 1983.

46. Taylor-Robinson D, Carney FE: Growth and effect of mycoplasmas in fallopian tube organ cultures. *Br J Vener Dis* 50:212, 1974.

47. Hare MJ, Barnes CFJ: Fallopian tube organ culture in the investigation of Bacteroides as a cause of pelvic inflammatory disease. In Philips I, Collier J (eds): *Metronidazole: Royal Society of Medicine International Congress and Symposium Series No. 18.* London, Academic Press, 1979.

48. Taylor-Robinson D, McCormack WM: The genital mycoplasmas. *N Engl J Med* 302:1003, 1980.

49. Møller BR, Freundt EA, Black FT, et al: Experimental infection of the genital tract of female grivet monkeys for *Mycoplasma hominis. Infect Immun* 20:248, 1978.

50. Mardh P-A, Westrom L, vanMecklenberg C, et al: Studies on ciliated epithelia of the human genital tract. I. Swelling of the cilia of fallopian tube epithelium in organ cultures infected with *Mycoplasma hominis. Br J Vener Dis* 52:52, 1976.

51. Schachter J: Chlamydial infections. *N Engl J Med* 298:428, 490, 540, 1978.

52. Eilard ET, Brorsson J-E, Hanmark B, Forssman L: Isolation of chlamydia in acute salpingitis. *Scand J Infect Dis* 9(S):82, 1976.

53. Mardh P-A, Ripa T, Svensson L, et al: *Chlamydia trachomatis* infection in patients with acute salpingitis. *N Engl J Med* 298:1377, 1977.

54. Treharne JD, Ripa KT, Mardh P-A, et al: Antibodies to *Chlamydia trachomatis* in acute salpingitis. *Br J Vener Dis* 5:26, 1979.

55. Paavonen J, Saikku P, Vesterinen E, Ako K: *Chlamydia trachomatis* in acute salpingitis. *Br J Vener Dis* 55:703, 1979.

56. Paavonen J: *Chlamydia trachomatis* in acute salpingitis. *Am J Obstet Gynecol* 138:957, 1980.

57. Mardh P-A, Lind I, Svensson L, et al: Antibodies to *Chlamydia trachomatis, Mycoplasma hominis* and *Neisseria gonorrhoeae* in serum from patients with acute salpingitis. *Br J Vener Dis* 57:125, 1981.

58. Ripa KT, Svensson L, Treharne JD, et al: *Chlamydia trachomatis* infection in patients with laparoscopically verified acute salpingitis: results of isolation and antibody determinations. *Am J Obstet Gynecol* 138:960, 1980.

59. Gjonnaess H, Dalaker K, Anestad G, et al: Pelvic inflammatory disease: etiological studies with emphasis on chlamydial infection. *Obstet Gynecol* 59:550–555, 1982.

60. Moller BR, Mardh P-A, Ahrons S, Nussler E: Infection with *Chlamydia trachomatis, Mycoplasma hominis,* and *Neisseria gonorrhoeae* in

patients with acute pelvic inflammatory disease. *Sex Transm Dis* 8:198–202, 1981.

61. Osser S, Poersson K: Epidemiology and serodiagnostic aspects of chlamydial salpingitis. *Obstet Gynecol* 59:206–209, 1982.

62. Svensson L, Westrom L, Ripa KT, et al: Differences in some clinical laboratory parameters in acute salpingitis related to culture and serologic findings. *Am J Obstet Gynecol* 138:1017, 1980.

63. Punnonen R, Terho P, Nikkanen V, et al: Chlamydial serology in infertile women by immunofluorescence. *Fertil Steril* 31:656, 1979.

64. Henry-Suchet J, Loffredo V, Sarfaty D: *Chlamydia trachomatis* and mycoplasma research by laparoscopy in cases of pelvic inflammatory disease and in cases of tubal obstruction. *Am J Obstet Gynecol* 138:1022, 1980.

65. Jones RB, Ardery BR, Hui SL, Cleary RE: Correlation between serum antichlamydial antibodies and tubal factor as a cause of infertility. *Fertil Steril* 38:553, 1982.

66. Moore DE, Foy HM, Dalin JR, et al: Increased frequency of serum antibodies to *Chlamydia trachomatis* in infertility due to tubal disease. *Lancet* 2:574, 1982.

67. Gump DW, Gibson M, Ashikaga T: Evidence of prior pelvic inflammatory disease and its relationship to *C. trachomatis* antibody and intrauterine contraceptive device use in infertile women. *Am J Obstet Gynecol* 146:153, 1983.

68. Cevanini R, Possati G, LaPlaca M: *Chlamydia trachomatis* infection in infertile women. In Mardh P-A, Holmes KK, Oriel JD, Piot P, Schachter J (eds): *Chlamydial Infections.* Amsterdam, Elsevier Biomedical Press, 1982, pp 182–192.

69. Gibson M, Gump D, Ashikaga T, Hall B: Patterns of adnexal inflammatory damage: chlamydia, the intrauterine device, and history of pelvic inflammatory disease. *Fertil Steril* 41:47–51, 1984.

70. Hutchinson GR, Taylor-Robinson D, Dourmashkin RR: Growth and effect of chlamydia in human and bovine oviduct cultures. *Br J Vener Dis* 55:194, 1979.

71. Ripa KR, Moller BR, Mardh P-A, et al: Experimental acute salpingitis in grivet monkeys provoked by *Chlamydia trachomatis. Acta Pathol Microbiol Scand* 87:65, 1979.

72. White HJ, Rank RG, Soloff BL, Barron AL: Experimental chlamydial salpingitis in immunosuppressed guinea pigs infected in the genital tract with agent of guinea pig inclusion conjunctivitis. *Infect Immun* 26:573, 1979.

73. Sweet RL, Banks J, Sung M, Donegan E, Schachter J: Experimental chlamydial salpingitis in the guinea pig. *Am J Obstet Gynecol* 138:952, 1980.

74. Swenson CE, Donegan E, Schachter J: *Chlamydia trachomatis*-induced salpingitis in mice. *J Infect Dis* 148:1101–1107, 1983.

75. Swenson CE, Schachter J: Infertility as a consequence of chlamydial infection of the upper genital tract in female mice. *Sex Transm Dis* 11:64–67, 1984.

76. Fitz-Hugh T: Acute gonococcal peritonitis of the right upper guadrant in women. *JAMA* 102:2084, 1934.

77. Stanley MM: Gonococcal peritonitis of the upper abdomen in young women. *Arch Intern Med* 78:1, 1946.
78. Wolner-Hanssen P, Westrom L, Mardh P-A: Perihepatitis and chlamydial salpingitis. *Lancet* 1:901, 1980.
79. Wang S, Eschenbach DA, Holmes KK, Wager G, Grayston JT: *Chlamydia trachomatis* infection in Fitz-Hugh-Curtis syndrome. *Am J Obstet Gynecol* 138:1034, 1980.
80. Dalaker K, Gjonnaess H, Kvile G, et al: *Chlamydia trachomatis* as a cause of acute perihepatitis associated with pelvic inflammatory disease. *Br J Vener Dis* 57:41–43, 1981.
81. Darougar S, Forsey T, Wood JJ, et al: Chlamydia and the Fitz-Hugh-Curtis syndrome. *Br J Vener Dis* 57:391–394, 1981.
82. Paavonen J, Valtonen VV: *Chlamydia trachomatis* as a possible cause of peritonitis and perihepatitis in a young woman *Br J Vener Dis* 56:341–343, 1980.
83. Paavonen J, Saikku P, vonKnorring J, et al: Association of infection with *Chlamydia trachomatis* with Fitz-Hugh-Curtis syndrome. *J Infect Dis* 144:176, 1981.
84. Bowie WR, Jones H: Acute inflammatory disease in outpatients: association with *Chlamydia trachomatis* and *Neisseria gonorrhoeae*. *Ann Intern Med* 95:686–688, 1981.
85. Eschenbach DA: Personal communication, 1984.
86. Nolan GJ, Osborne N: Gonococcal infection in the female. *Obstet Gynecol* 42:156, 1973.
87. Toth A, O'Leary WM, Ledger WJ: Evidence for microbial transfer by spermatozoa. *Obstet Gynecol* 59:556–559, 1982.
88. Carney FE, Taylor-Robinson D: Growth and effect of *Neisseria gonorrhoeae* in organ cultures. *Br J Vener Dis* 49:435, 1973.
89. Draper DL, James JF, Brooks GF, Sweet RL: Comparison of virulence markers of peritoneal-fallopian tube and endocervical *Neisseria gonorrhoeae* isolates from women with acute salpingitis. *Infect immun* 27:882, 1980.
90. Draper DL, James JF, Hadley WK, Sweet RL: Auxotypes and antibiotic susceptibilites of *Neisseria gonorrhoeae* from women with acute salpingitis. Comparison with gonococci causing uncomplicated genital tract infections in women. *Sex Transm Dis* 8:43, 1981.
91. Draper DL, Donegan EA, James JF, Sweet RL, Brooks GF: Scanning electron microscopy of attachment of *Neisseria gonorrhoeae* colony phenotypes to surfaces of human genital epithelia. *Am J Obstet Gynecol* 138:818, 1980.
92. Buchanan TM, Eschenbach DA, Knapp JS, Holmes KK: Gonococcal salpingitis is less likely to recur with *Neisseria gonorrhoeae* of the same principal outer membrane protein antigen type. *Am J Obstet Gynecol* 138:978–980, 1981.
93. Mardh P-A, Moller BR, Paavonen J: Chlamydial infection of the female genital tract with emphasis on pelvic inflammatory disease. A review of Scandinavian studies. *Sex Transm Dis* 8(S):140–155, 1981.
94. Bartlett JG, Onderdonk AB, Drude E, et al: Quantitative bacteriology of the vaginal flora. *J Infect Dis* 126:271, 1977.
95. Taylor ES, McMillan JH, Greer BE, Drogemueller W, Thompson HE: The intrauterine device and tubo-ovarian abscesses. *Am J Obstet Gynecol* 123:338, 1975.
96. Landers DV, Sweet RL: Tubo-ovarian abscess: contemporary approach to management. *Rev Infect Dis* 5:876–884, 1983.
97. Wolner-Hanssen P, Mardh P-A, Svensson L, Westrom L: Laparoscopy in women with chlamydial infection and pelvic pain: a comparison of patients with and without salpingitis. *Obstet Gynecol* 61:299–303, 1983.
98. Rees E, Annels EH: Gonococcal salpingitis. *Br J Vener Dis* 45:205, 1969.
99. Hager WD, Eschenbach DA, Spence MR, Sweet RL: Criteria for diagnosis and grading of salpingitis. *Obstet Gynecol* 61:113–114, 1983.
100. Westrom L, Skude G, Mardh P-A: Amylases of the genital tract. II. Peritoneal fluid isoamylases in acute salpingitis. *Am J Obstet Gynecol* 126:657, 1976.
101. Curtis AH: *Obstetrics and Gynecology.* Philadelphia, WB Saunders, 1933, vol, 2, p 497.
102. Hedberg E, Anberg A: Gonorrheal salpingitis: views on treatment and prognosis. *Fertil Steril* 16:125, 1965.
103. Falk V, Krook G: Do results of culture for gonococci vary with sampling phase of menstrual cycle? *Acta Derm Venereol (Stockh)* 47:190, 1967.
104. Viberg L: Acute inflammatory conditions of the uterine adnexa. *Acta Obstet Gynecol Scand* 43(S4):5, 1964.
105. Krook G, Juhlin I: Problems in diagnosis, treatment and control of gonorrheal infections. IV. The correlation between the dose of penicillin IC_{50} values of gonococci and results of treatment. *Acta Derm Venereol (Stockh)* 45:343, 1965.
106. Mardh P-A: An overview of infectious agents of salpingitis; their biology and recent advances in methods of detection. *Am J Obstet Gynecol* 138:933–951, 1980.
107. Weinstein WM, Onderdonk AB, Bartlett JG, et al: Experimental intra-abdominal abscesses in rats: development of an experimental model. *Infect Immun* 10:1250, 1974.
108. Weinstein WM, Onderdonk AB, Bartlett JG, et al: Antimicrobial therapy of experimental sepsis. *J Infect Dis* 132:282, 1975.
109. Centers for Disease Control: Sexually transmitted diseases treatment guidelines 1982. *MMWR*, August 20, 1982, Vol. 32, No. 25. US Department of Health and Human Services, Public Health Service, Atlanta, Georgia.
110. Westrom L, Iosif S, Svensson L, Mardh P-A: Infertility after acute salpingitis: results of treatment with different antibiotics. *Curr Ther*, pp 47–50, 1979.
111. Thompson SE, Holcomb G, Cheng S, et al: Antibiotic therapy of outpatient pelvic inflammatory disease. Abstract 671, presented at the Twentieth Interscience Conference on Antimicrobial Agents and Chemotherapy, New Orleans, Sept. 22–24, 1980.
112. Mourod A, Sweet RL, Sugg N, Schachter J: Relative resistance to erythromycin in *Chlamydia trachomatis. Antimicrob Agents Chemother*

18:696–698, 1980.

113. Lardaro HH: Spontaneous rupture of tubo-ovarian abscess within the free peritoneal cavity. *JAMA* 156:699, 1954.

114. Pedowitz P, Bloomfield RQ: Ruptured adnexal abscess with generalized peritonitis. *Am J Obstet Gynecol* 88:721, 1964.

115. Kaplan AL, Jacobs WL, Ehresman JB: Aggressive management of pelvic abscess. *Am J Obstet Gynecol* 98:982, 1967.

116. Franklin EW, Heuron JD, Thompson JD: Management of pelvic abscess. *Clin Obstet Gynecol* 16:66, 1973.

117. Ginsburg DS, Stern JL, Hammond KA, et al: Tubo-ovarian abscess: a retrospective review. *Am J Obstet Gynecol* 138:1055, 1980.

118. Joiner K, Lowe B, Dzink J, Bartlett JG: Comparative efficacy of 10 antimicrobial agents in experimental *Bacteroides fragilis* infections. *J Infect Dis* 145:561–568, 1982.

119. Collins CG, Nix FC, Cerrha HT: Ruptured tubo-ovarian abscess. *Am J Obstet Gynecol* 72:820, 1956.

120. Gerzof SG, Robbins AH, Johnson WC, et al: Percutaneous catheter drainage of abdominal abscesses. *N Engl J Med* 305:653–, 1981.

CHAPTER 5

Toxic Shock Syndrome

Toxic shock syndrome (TSS) is an acute and severe multisystem illness which has only recently been recognized (1–9). The disease is characterized by sudden onset of high fever, hypotension, vomiting, diarrhea, myalgias, and "sunburn-like" rash. Although first reported by Todd and colleagues in 1978 (10) in seven children (four girls and three boys), TSS occurs predominantly in women (2, 4, 9). Thus TSS is a disease which the obstetrician-gynecologist must be cognizant of in order to appropriately diagnose and treat this potentially life-threatening illness. Moreover, health care providers must recognize that while the overwhelming majority of TSS cases occur in association with menstruation, TSS not associated with menstruation may also occur (11).

EPIDEMIOLOGY

From 1970 through April 1982, 1654 cases of TSS were reported to the Centers for Disease Control (CDC). The peak number of reported TSS cases occurred from January to October, 1980. Between 90 and 95% of cases occurred in women (2, 4, 9) with the greatest risk being present for women less than 30 yr of age (2, 9). The overwhelming majority (>95%) of menstruation-associated TSS cases occur in white women. Approximately 95% of TSS cases in women occurred in association with menstruation (1, 2, 4, 8). Nearly 99% of women with menstruation-associated TSS wore tampons (2, 5, 13, 14). The estimated incidence of TSS has ranged from 3–15 cases per 100,000 menstruating women per year (2, 4, 5, 9, 15), with 6–7 cases per 100,000 menstruating women per year being the general consensus (4, 5, 9).

The sudden increase in TSS cases reported in 1980 may be the result of several factors: (a) the introduction of new tampon products; (b) changes in the constituent materials of tampons; or (c) a change in *Staphylococcus aureus.*

A dramatic decrease in the number of menstrually-associated TSS cases reported to the CDC has been noted since the removal of Rely tampons from the market in September, 1980 (16). However, Osterholm and Forfang reported that, using an active-passive surveillance system, they noted no decrease in the number of TSS cases in the state of Minnesota following the removal of Rely from the market (17). In addition, Davis and Vergeront have suggested that TSS reporting may have been influenced by news media publicity related to TSS in the late summer and fall of 1980 (18).

Whereas only 6% of TSS cases prior to 1981 were not associated with menstruation, the percentage of nonmenstrual cases of TSS has increased to 13.2% of reported cases in 1981 (11) and 15% in 1982 (12). As suggested by Duff, this increase is probably due to two factors: (a) a change in the patterns of tampon use, and (b) improved recognition of TSS in a variety of clinical settings (19). Nonmenstruation-associated TSS has been reported in a variety of conditions which are listed in Table 5.1. As reported by Reingold and co-workers, patients with TSS not associated with menstruation differ significantly in age and racial distribution from those with menstruation-associated TSS (11). Firstly, it can occur in males, and TSS associated with infections not involving the vagina occur equally in men and women. Of patients with nonmenstruation-associated TSS, 11% were nonwhite compared to only 2% among menstruation-associated TSS (11). The age range for nonmenstruation-associated TSS ranged from the newborn to the elderly rather than the reproductive age span seen with menstruation-associated TSS.

Based on observations made in investigations demonstrating TSS associated with surgical wound infections (20, 21), the incubation period for TSS ranged from 1 to 4 days, with a median of 2 days. These data clearly demonstrate the potential for rapid development of a fulminant disease in previously healthy individuals who have been exposed to the specific factor(s) responsible for TSS (11).

Table 5.1
Conditions Associated with Nonmenstrual Toxic Shock Syndrome

Surgical wound infections (11, 20, 21)
Soft tissue infections (10, 11, 22)

Cellulitis	Lung abscess
Subcutaneous abscess	Bursitis
Osteomyelitis	Purulent adenitis
Mastitis	Infected burns
Hydradenitis	Infected cuta-
Infected insect bite	neous ulcer

Postpartum cases (8, 9, 11, 12, 20, 21, 23, 24, 25)
Immediate neonatal period (23, 24)
   (concomitant maternal TNS)
Female genital tract cases (6, 7, 11, 21, 26, 27)
   Vaginal infections
   Acute salpingitis
   Diaphragm use
   Vaginal contraceptive sponge use (R. L. Sweet, unpublished data)

Initial reports suggested that the case-fatality rate for TSS was as high as 13% (1, 6). The three major causes of death in TSS are adult respiratory distress syndrome (ARDS), intractable hypotension, and hemorrhage due to disseminated intravascular coagulation (DIC). More recent data have noted that the case-fatality rate for the 1654 TSS cases reported to the CDC from 1970 to 1982 was 5.6% with a rate of 3.3% in 1981 (12). This improvement in survival is, most likely, a reflection of increased awareness of TSS by clinicians, with resultant early diagnosis and institution of appropriate therapeutic measures.

A recurrence rate of approximately 30% was noted by investigators at the CDC (1, 5). Multiple recurrences have been reported in the same patient (3, 5, 26). Interestingly, all reported recurrences have occurred in women in association with menstruation.

ETIOLOGY

A significant association between TSS and tampon usage was identified in a series of case-control epidemiologic studies (1, 2, 4, 5, 28, 29, 30). While nearly 70% of women in the United States used tampons during their menstrual period, a significantly greater proportion used tampons during the menstrual period in which TSS occurred than did matched controls.

Initial studies revealed no association between TSS and any specific brand of tampons (1, 2, 4, 5). However, more recent investigations demonstrated a significant association between TSS and use of Rely tampons (13, 15, 28–30). In September, 1980, the CDC reported that while

26% of controls used Rely, 71% of TSS cases were exclusive Rely users (13). Schlech and co-workers reported that the relative risk for the development of TSS among Rely users compared to users of other tampon brands was 7.7 (99% confidence intervals, 2.1 to 27.9) (30). These workers noted no significant influence of tampon absorbency that could be separated from the risk associated with use of Rely. Osterholm and associates demonstrated that the odds ratio for developing menstruation-associated TSS with any use of tampons compared to no use of tampons was 18 (p < 0.001) (29). When exclusive use of particular tampon brands were evaluated, Rely was the only brand with a significantly increased odds ratio (2.49; p = 0.005). This increased relative risk with Rely was beyond that predicted by absorbency alone. Osterholm's group (29), in contradistinction to the CDC findings (30), demonstrated that women who used high-absorbency tampons had a greater relative risk of developing TSS than women who used low-absorbency tampons.

TSS occurs in nonmenstruating females, menstruating females not using tampons, and in men. Thus, it is apparent that tampons by themselves are not the explanation for TSS. However, the composition of materials used in tampons may play an important role in the development of TSS (14). As noted by Shands et al (5), prior to 1977 all tampon products were made of rayon or a blend of rayon and cotton. Since 1977, 44% of tampon products with 65% of the market have contained more absorbent synthetic materials such as polyacrylate fibers, carboxymethylcellulose, high-absorbancy rayon-cellulose, and polyester foams. Tierno (31) and Hanna (32) have postulated that these synthetic components interact with the bacterial flora of the vagina to provide an environment that is appropriate for the growth of toxin-producing staphylococci.

The association of TSS with *S. aureus* was identified in the original case-control studies (4, 5). Davis et al reported that in 17 of 23 cervico-vaginal cultures obtained from TSS patients, *S. aureus* was recovered (4). Similarly, Shands and co-workers recovered *S. aureus* from 62 of 64 vaginal cultures from women with menstruation-associated TSS (5). Among TSS cases reported to the CDC as of October, 1982 *S. aureus* had been recovered from 210 of 215 patients (12). *S. aureus* may be present as part of the normal bacterial flora of the vagina and cervix in healthy women; it has been recovered in from 0–15% of vaginal specimens (5, 33–38), with 5–10% being the generally accepted prevalence. Interestingly, several studies have noted an increase in the incidence of *S. aureus* colonization of the female lower genital tract at the time of menses (39, 40). Noble et al (40) reported the recovery of *S. aureus* from 17% of their patients during menstruation, compared to 5.8% at midcycle in the same women. These investigators did not detect an association between tampon use and recovery of *S. aureus*. However, Guinan and co-workers noted that there was a significant association between the colonization rate of *S. aureus* and the use of Rely tampons (39). Patients using other types of tampons had an 8% colonization rate for *S. aureus* as compared to the 43% rate for users of Rely. Saunders and associates suggested that an imbalance among the normal microflora of the female genital tract may be crucial to the development of menstruation-associated TSS (41). They reported that lactobacilli, which play a major role in maintaining the normal vaginal environment, have an inverse relationship with staphylococci and postulated that lactobacilli served as a natural defense against *S. aureus*. Moreover, they suggested that an increase in *S. aureus* may occur because tampons (especially super absorbable types) remove substrates necessary for lactobacilli to exert this inhibitory effect.

As noted by Wager (14) the exact cause(s) of TSS has (have) not been completely elucidated. The abrupt onset of the clinical presentation, the multisystem involvement, rarity of bacteremia, and the similarity of TSS to other illnesses known to be caused by bacterial toxins led investigators to hypothesize that a toxin either alone or synergistically with other factor(s) was responsible for TSS. With the demonstration that *S. aureus* was recovered from nearly 100% of TSS cases, speculation focused on a staphylococcal toxin as the culprit.

Recent investigations have identified the presence of staphylococcal toxins associated with isolates of *S. aureus* recovered from patients with TSS (42–44). Schlievert identified a protein with an isoelectric point of 7.2 and a molecular weight of 22,000 daltons which he named pyrogenic extoxin C(PEC) (42). In this investigation PEC was present in 28 of 28 *S. aureus* recovered from TSS cases but in only 5 (16%) of 32 *S. aureus* recovered from controls (42). Altemeier et al found PEC was produced by 131 (91%) of 144 TSS isolates of *S. aureus* (44). Bergdoll and associates simultaneously identified a toxin with similar physical characteristics, which they called enterotoxin F (43). They reported that 61 (94%) of 65 *S. aureus* strains from TSS patients produced enterotoxin F, and only 4 (4.6%) of 87 non-TSS *S. aureus* strains produced enterotoxin F. Furthermore, in a prospective blinded study, Bergdole et al noted that all 34 *S. aureus* strains from TSS produced enterotoxin F as compared to 3 (11%) of 26 control strains (43). Recent opinion holds that PEC and staphylococcal enterotoxin F are identical (45, 46).

Although in experimental models neither of these toxins by itself produced the complete spectrum of disease seen in clinical cases of TSS, Schlievert has demonstrated that PEC significantly enhanced susceptibility to lethal endotoxin shock by 50,000 fold (47). Larsen and Schlievert suggested that this enhancement of endotoxin may explain the manifestations of gram-negative septic shock associated with TSS and that the combination of PEC and small amounts of circulating endogenous endotoxin from the normal bowel flora provides the best explanation for the pathogenesis of TSS (46).

Bergdoll and co-workers have also demonstrated that the immunologic status vis à vis enterotoxin F may also be important in the pathogenesis of TSS (43). They found that TSS patients had a greater serosusceptibility to enterotoxin F than did controls; anti-SEF antibody was present in titers ≥1:100 in 5 (17.2%) of 29 TSS patients, compared to 44 (78.6%) of 56 controls.

Duff noted that three conditions are required

for TSS to develop (19). First, the patient must be colonized or infected with *S. aureus*. Second, the staphylococci must be capable of producing the toxin(s) that are associated with the clinical manifestations of TSS. Lastly, there must be a portal of entry for the toxins(s) to enter the systemic circulation. In nonmenstrual TSS, *S. aureus* is present in a localized supportive infection, and as toxin is produced it is absorbed from the infected site into the bloodstream. Duff suggested several mechanisms by which staphylococcal toxin gains access to the systemic circulation in menstruation-associated TSS (19). Toxin could be absorbed through microulcerations in the vaginal mucosa secondary to trauma from tampons and/or inserters. The superabsorbable tampons may obstruct menstrual flow producing reflux of menstrual blood containing toxin through the fallopian tubes into the peritoneal cavity, resulting in absorption of toxin across the peritoneum. Alternately, toxin could be absorbed across the denuded endometrial surface.

CLINICAL PRESENTATION AND DIAGNOSIS

TSS is a multisystem disease with a wide range of symptoms, signs, and laboratory findings. Characteristically, TSS occurs abruptly with the sudden onset of high fever, chills, myalgias, vomiting, diarrhea, hypotension, and generalized "sunburn-like" rash: the updated case definition proposed by the CDC is described in Table 5.2. The major changes in this revised definition are that orthostatic syncope may replace demonstrated hypotension, and *S. aureus* bacteremia is no longer an exclusion (12).

The most commonly observed clinical signs and symptoms are presented in Table 5.3. Involvement of the skin and mucous membranes is one of the most characteristic findings in TSS. The rash which occurs early in the disease process presents as a "sunburn-like" macular erythema; it can evolve to where the patient appears like a "broiled lobster." From day 5–12 after onset of TSS a fine desquamation occurs on the face, trunk, and extremities. This is followed by the nearly pathognomonic full-thickness, peeling-like desquamation of the palms and/or soles. The staphylococcal toxin(s) has a predilection for mucous membranes, and their involvement is often a prominent feature of TSS (14). This manifests clinically as sore throat, oropharyngeal hyperemia, strawberry tongue, nonpurulent conjunctivitis, and/or vaginal hyperemia.

Gastrointestinal symptoms and signs are frequent and prominent in TSS. Vomiting and watery diarrhea have been noted in approximately 90% of cases. These symptoms occur early in the disease, are usually severe, and are associated with marked generalized abdominal tenderness. Hepatomegaly and pancreatitis have been reported on occasion.

Another early, characteristic finding is the presence of myalgias which have been reported in from 88–100% of TSS cases. (3, 6, 7, 8, 22). Exquisite muscle tenderness can be elicited by

Table 5.2
Case Definition of Toxic Shock Syndrome (12)

1. Fever (temperature $\geq 38.9°C$, 102°F)
2. Rash characterized by diffuse macular erythroderma
3. Desquamation occurring 1–2 weeks after onset of illness (in survivors)
4. Hypotension (systolic blood pressure ≤ 90 mm Hg in adults) or orthostatic syncope
5. Involvement of three or more of the following organ systems:
   a. Gastrointestinal (vomiting or diarrhea at onset of illness)
   b. Muscular (myalgia or creatine phosphokinase level twice normal)
   c. Mucous membrane (vaginal, oropharyngeal, or conjunctival hyperemia)
   d. Renal (BUN or creatinine level $\geq$twice normal or ≥ 5 WBC per HPF in absence of urinary tract infection)
   e. Hepatic (total bilirubin, SGOT or SGPT twice normal level)
   f. Hematologic (platelets $\leq 100,000/mm^3$)
   g. Central nervous system (disorientation or alterations in consciousness without focal neurological signs when fever and hypotension absent)
6. Negative throat and cerebrospinal fluid cultures (A positive blood culture for *S. aureus* does not exclude a case)
7. Negative serologic tests for Rocky Mountain spotted fever, leptospirosis, rubeola.

Table 5.3
Clinical Signs and Symptoms Commonly Seen in Patients with Toxic Shock Syndrome[a]

Symptom/sign	No. of patients	No. of patients with symptoms/sign	
		No.	%
Fever (≥38.9°C, 102°F)	140	140	100
Rash with desquamation	140	140	100
Myaligia	140	136	97
Vomiting	140	124	89
Diarrhea	140	123	88
Headache	133	102	77
Abdominal tenderness	64	48	75
Pharyngeal hyperemia	40	29	73
Sore throat	139	98	71
Conjunctivitis/conjunctival hyperemia	140	84	60
Photophobia	37	22	60
Decreased sensorium	140	82	59
Rigors/chills	114	63	55
"Strawberry" tongue	62	31	50
Vaginal hyperemia	87	35	40
Vaginal discharge	115	45	39
Arthralgia	54	15	28
Adnexal tenderness	38	10	26

[a] Based on references 3, 5, 6, 7, 8, 22, 26 and adapted from Wager GP: Toxic shock syndrome: a review. *Am J Obstet Gynecol* 146:93–102, 1983.

movement or touch. Additional musculoskeletal findings include arthralgias, synovitis of hand joints, and sterile joint effusions.

Neurologic involvement may be difficult to assess in face of the high fever and/or severe hypotension associated with TSS. In general, neurological symptoms and signs have included headache, confusion, loss of consciousness, disorientation, agitation, photophobia, seizures, meningeal irritation, and evidence of psychomotor retardation. Tofte and Williams (6) and Chesney et al (8) noted normal glucose and protein levels and very low counts of mononuclear or polymorphonuclear cells in the spinal fluid.

Hypotension and shock are prominent features of TSS. They occur early in the disease process and constitute one of the major criteria for the diagnosis of TSS. More recently the presence of orthostatic syncope has been accepted as an alternative criterion for documented shock. Multiple cardiac abnormalities have been reported in TSS cases. These include sinus or supraventricular tachycardia, first degree heart block, premature ventricular beats, nonspecific ST-T wave changes, and T-wave inversion in precordial leads (3, 6, 7, 8, 14, 22). In addition, Shands et al reported cases with

pericarditis and vasculitis (5). Chesney and co-workers noted low central venous pressure was present in their TSS cases (8) and McKenna and associates, using Swan-Ganz measurements, noted that TSS patients had high cardiac output, low peripheral resistance, normal pulmonary wedge pressure, and normal pulmonary resistance (3).

In more than 80% of patients with TSS renal involvement has been demonstrated (3, 5, 6, 7, 8, 22). This renal dysfunction has been manifested with sterile pyuria, mild proteinuria, hematuria, azotemia, hyponatremia, increased urinary sodium, hyperkalemia, and decreased creatinine clearance.

The prognosis for patients with TSS is often determined by the presence of pulmonary involvement, especially adult respiratory distress syndrome (ARDS) or "shock lung". Fisher and co-workers reported that tachypnea and hypoxemia ($PO_2 < 60$ mm Hg) were frequently present in TSS patients (7). Radiologic evidence of pulmonary edema and/or pleural effusions has also been reported (7, 8). Progression of these respiratory findings to ARDS in TSS patients is well documented (3, 5, 6, 7, 8, 22). Most likely ARDS occurs as a consequence of the enhanced activity of endotoxin caused by the staphylococcal toxin

PEC (47). Once ARDS develops the prognosis is poor, especially when extensive or prolonged ARDS is present (14).

The laboratory abnormalities reported in TSS cases reflect the multisystem involvement characteristic of the disease. A summary of the more frequent laboratory findings is presented in Table 5.4. Some of the more commonly reported metabolic and electrolyte abnormalities include metabolic acidosis, hypocalcemia, hypokalemia, hyponatremia, and hypophosphatemia. Among the frequent hematologic abnormalities are anemia, thrombocytopenia, leukocytosis, prolonged prothrombin time, prolonged partial thromboplastin time, and increased fibrin degradation products. Hepatic involvement is manifested by increased liver enzymes and hyperbilirubinemia. Renal involvement is signalled by the occurrence of azotemia, increased serum creatinine, pyuria, hematuria, and proteinuria. In addition, increase creatine phosphokinase connotes muscle involvement.

Despite the severe clinical manifestations of TSS, the vast majority of patients recover without residual effects. Chesney and colleagues (8) have arbitrarily divided the sequelae associated with TSS into two groups. The late onset findings occur between the 4th and 14th days of the acute illness. This group includes the desquamation of skin and peeling of palms and/or soles, impaired sensation of the fingers, swollen, denuded tongue, transient vocal cord paralysis, acute tubular necrosis with renal failure, ARDS, and most recently the carpal tunnel syndrome (48). The second group of late findings occurs on or after the 60th day from the onset of TSS episode. Included in this group are splitting of the nails, reversible loss of hair and nails, CNS sequelae, renal impairment, cardiac dysfunction, and, as suggested by Wager (14), recurrent episodes of TSS.

Of particular concern is the report by Rosene and co-workers demonstrating persistent neurologic sequelae in survivors of TSS (49). These investigators studied 12 women 2 to 12 months after recovery from episodes of TSS. They reported that 6 had demonstrable abnormalities in intellectual function, such as impaired memory, concentration, and ability to perform mathematical calculations. All 12 women were hyperreflexic at follow-up. In addition eight had abnormal electroencephalograms and five had disturbances in cerebellar function. Chesney et al, in a recent follow-up evaluation of 36 TSS pa-

Table 5.4
Laboratory Abnormalities Commonly Seen in Patients with Toxic Shock Syndrome[a]

Laboratory abnormality	No. of patients	No. of patients with abnormal laboratory test	
		No.	%
Metabolic acidosis	30	25	83
Pyuria	77	63	82
Decreased serum proteins	55	45	82
Hypokalemia	27	21	78
Increased SGOT	61	47	77
Hypocalcemia	122	85	70
Increased serum creatinine	128	83	65
Anemia	49	30	61
Leukocytosis	129	76	59
Proteinuria	66	39	59
Microhematuria	63	37	59
Decreased phosphorus	57	33	58
Increased LDH	23	13	57
Prolonged prothrombin time	51	28	55
Increased CPK	94	51	54
Thrombocytopenia	113	60	53
Azotemia	129	68	53
Increased SGPT	21	10	48
Hyponatremia	34	16	47
Prolonged partial thromboplastin time	48	22	46

[a] Based on references 3, 5, 6, 7, 8, 22 and 26; adapted from Wager GP: Toxic shock syndrome: a review. *Am J Obstet Gynecol* 146:93–102, 1983.

Table 5.5
Recurrence Categories for Toxic Shock Syndrome[a]

Major criteria	Definite recurrence	Probable recurrence	No recurrence
Temperature 38.9°C Rash Vomiting or diarrhea Myalgia	Desquamation and at least 3 of 4 major criteria	Desquamation and 2 of 4 major criteria, *or* 3 of 4 major criteria	Two major criteria or fewer; no desquamation

[a] Adapted from Davis JP, Chesney PJ, Wand PJ, LaVenture M, et al: Toxic shock syndrome: epidemiologic features, recurrence, risk factors, and prevention. *N Engl J Med* 303:1429–1435, 1980.

tients, noted a frequent incidence of late sequelae (50). Three patients were found to have prolonged neuromuscular dysfunction; one with vocal cord paralysis and two with diffuse myopathy. One patient with acute renal failure secondary to acute tubular necrosis during her acute episode of TSS had a markedly impaired creatinine clearance 9 yr later. In addition, they reported that one patient had persistent cyanosis of her feet and hands 9 months after the initial TSS episode.

It has been well documented that TSS can recur, especially in women with menstruation-associated disease. Recurrence rates of from 28 to 64% have been reported (3, 4, 5), with a recurrence rate of approximately one-third being the general consensus. Davis et al noted that recurrences were significantly less frequent in patients who received β-lactamase resistant, antistaphylococcal antibiotics during their initial episode of TSS (4).

As a result of confusion regarding what constitutes a recurrent episode of TSS, three categories based on the presence or absence of the major criteria for diagnosis of TSS have been proposed. These recurrence categories for TSS are presented in Table 5.5.

TSS associated with surgical wound infections generally presents as an early onset wound infection within 48 hr postoperatively. Unlike other early-onset wound infections which are caused by *Clostridia perfringens* or group A β-hemolytic streptococci, TSS-associated wound infections have minimal or absent local signs of infection such as erythema, fluctuence, or drainage (20, 21). However, *S. aureus* is nearly always recovered from these benign appearing wounds. As noted by Bartlett and co-workers (21), the key clinical point is the occurrence of watery diarrhea and diffuse erythroderma in association with high fever in the initial several days postoperatively. Such findings, especially if hypotension is coexistent, must result in prompt evaluation of the operative wound for evidence of *S. aureus* infection.

Table 5.6
Diagnostic Criteria of Probable Toxic Shock Syndrome (26)

≥3 criteria and desquamation
or
≥5 criteria without desquamation

Criteria
Temperature ≥38°C, 102°F
Rash
Hypotension, orthostatic dizziness or syncope
Myalgia
Vomiting, diarrhea or both
Mucous membrane inflammation (conjunctivitis, pharyngitis, vaginitis)
Clinical abnormalities of ≥2 organ systems
Reasonable evidence for absence of other etiologies

Tofte and Williams (26) have suggested that TSS is associated with a broad spectrum of clinical manifestations and that many cases do not fulfill the strict epidemiologic criteria defined by the CDC (12), are generally milder, and do not present with life-threatening hypotension. As a result these workers proposed a case definition of "probable TSS' (6). These criteria are presented in Table 5.6. It is important for clinicans to recognize these milder cases of TSS in order to institute early and appropriate therapy. These milder "probable TSS" cases may subsequently develop into the severe, life-threatening form of TSS. Over the past 2 yr, we have admitted two such patients with severe, classical TSS who had presented to the emergency room several days previous with, in retrospect, mild symptoms and signs of TSS. One case occurred with a vaginal contraceptive sponge, and the second was in association with a perirectal abscess.

DIAGNOSIS

As described above, TSS presents with a broad spectrum of clinical manifestations, and multiple organ systems are involved. No definitive diagnostic or confirmatory laboratory test has been developed for TSS. Nor are any of the variety of clinical and laboratory findings pathognomonic for the disease. Thus it is necessary to differentiate TSS from a multitude of other diseases which are listed in Table 5.7. An empiric diagnois must be based upon the typical constellation of clinical and laboratory findings which have been previously described. Clinicians should consider the possibility of TSS in any patient with an unexplained febrile, exanthematous, multisystem illness, especially if such an illness is associated with menstruation or a documented or suspected *S. aureus* infection. A high index of suspicion and early diagnosis are crucial to instituting appropriate therapy and gaining a favorable prognosis.

The majority of the differential diagnosis list are easily differentiated from TSS on clinical grounds and laboratory evaluation. However, several are very similar and may be difficult to differentiate. Streptococcal scarlet fever is unusual after 10 yr of age and generally occurs secondary to an upper respiratory tract illness from which the group A β-hemolytic streptococcus can be recovered. If seen early in the disease the rash of scarlet fever is described as a "sandpaper rash." Late in the disease the desquamation of scarlet fever and TSS are clinically similar, although microscopically they occur in different levels of the skin. Serum antibodies to streptococcal extracellular products such as antistreptolysin O are always present with scarlet fever.

Mucocutaneous lymph node syndrome (Kawasaki's disease) presents with a clinical picture very similar to TSS. In fact some investigators have suggested that this disease may be a variant form of TSS (3, 4, 6). However, mucocutaneous lymph node syndrome is primarily a pediatric disease, and the majority of cases have occurred at less than 5 yr of age. In addition, as noted by McKenna et al (3), myalgias, elevated CPK, abdominal pain, hypotension and shock, ARDS, thrombocytopenia, and renal failure are very rare or absent in mucocutaneous lymph node disease.

Diseases such as leptospirosis, rubeola, and Rocky Mountain spotted fever are clinically strikingly similar to TSS. However, serologic testing of acute and convalescent serum can establish or rule out the diagnosis of these diseases. In addition, *Leptospira* can be cultured from spinal fluid and/or blood.

TREATMENT AND PREVENTION

As stressed by Wager (14) and Duff (19) patients with suspected TSS require prompt and aggressive therapy. Initial evaluation of the patient commences simultaneously with aggressive fluid resuscitation aimed at maintaining adequate circulating volume, cardiac output, blood pressure, and perfusion of vital organs.

Table 5.7
Differential Diagnosis of Toxic Shock Syndrome[a]

Exanthematous diseases	
Mucocutaneous lymph node syndrome	Rubeola and rubella
Streptococcal scarlet fever	Meningococcemia
Staphylococcal scarlet fever	Staphylococcal scalded skin syndrome
Rocky Mountain spotted fever	Bullous impetigo
Leptospirosis	Erythema multiforme
Viral exanthematous disease	Toxic epidermal necrolysis
Drug eruptions	Acute rheumatic fever
Gastrointestinal diseases	
Staphylococcal food poisoning	Pancreatitis
Gastroenteritis	Dysentery
Appendicitis	
Miscellaneous diseases	
Septic shock	Systemic lupus erythematosus
Acute pyelonephritis	Reye's syndrome
Legionnaire's disease	Tick typhus
Pelvic inflammatory disease	Rhabdomyolysis
Hemolytic uremic syndrome	Tularemia
Stevens-Johnson syndrome	

[a]Adapted from Wager GP: Toxic shock syndrome: a review. *Am J Obstet Gynecol* 146:93–102, 1983.

This initial patient evaluation requires a thorough physical examination which includes a pelvic exam to look for and remove any tampon, diaphragm, cervical cap, or contraceptive sponge which may be present. If none of these is present a thorough search for a localized *S. aureus* infection must be undertaken. Cultures for *S. aureus* are obtained from the vagina, rectum, conjunctiva, oropharynx, anterior nares, and any localized sites of infection. Blood, urine, and spinal fluid are also obtained for culture.

Serum is obtained for serologic studies to rule out leptospirosis, rubeola, and Rocky Mountain spotted fever. Additional laboratory studies are obtained for a complete blood count with differential, platelet count, and coagulation screen; electrolytes, liver function tests, calcium, phosphorus, creatine phosphokinase, BUN, creatinine; and urinalysis, chest x-ray, and electrocardiogram.

Aggressive fluid replacement is the initial priority and is the cornerstone of therapy in patients with TSS. Massive amounts of fluid replacement are generally required with 8–12 liters per day not being uncommon (14). To facilitate and monitor administration of such massive volume replacement the placement of a Swans-Ganz catheter is necessary. In addition, this central line will allow for monitoring of cardiovascular status. An arterial line is established to allow for continuous blood pressure and arterial oxygenation assessment. A urinary catheter is inserted to monitor urine output. When no blood loss has occurred volume replacement is achieved with isotonic crystalloid solution such as normal saline or lactated Ringer's solution or colloids such as plasminate or salt-poor albumin, or combinations of crystalloid and colloid. In patients with blood loss secondary to DIC, packed red blood cells and coagulation factors should be included in the fluid replacement scheme.

The fluid replacement is guided by measurement of pulmonary artery wedge pressure (PAWP), which should be maintained at 10–12 mm Hg (19). Shubin et al have proposed a "7-3" rule for fluid replacement in shock patients (51). A fluid bolus of 5–20 ml/min for 10 min is given. If PAWP increases more than 7 mm Hg above baseline, the infusion is temporarily discontinued. On the other hand, if PAWP does not rise more than 3 mm Hg, a second similar fluid challenge is given and the "7-3" rule reapplied.

As fluid replacement is initiated, use of mili-tary antishock trousers (MAST unit) may be beneficial in producing immediate improvement in cardiac function. This unit mobilizes pooled blood from the lower extremities and lower abdomen/pelvis and returns it into the central circulation. McSwain has reported that the MAST unit results in an autotransfusion with 750–1000 cc of autologous blood (52). The MAST unit is a temporizing measure, and once fluid replacement has reestablished normal perfusion blood pressure, the unit should be gradually deflated (19).

If aggressive volume replacement does not promptly restore blood pressure and perfusion to vital organs, use of vasopressor therapy is indicated. The drug of choice is dopamine, which in low doses has a weak β-mimetic effect that results in an increased myocardial contractility and heart rate while simultaneously stimulating dopaminergic receptors that cause vasodilation of the renal, mesenteric, coronary, and cerebral vasculature (53). In addition, dopamine produces vasoconstriction in skeletal muscle which results in blood being diverted from peripheral beds to vital organs (i.e., heart, brain, kidney).

Dopamine is administered by continuous intravenous infusion. An initial dose of 2 to 5 μg/kg/min is instituted, and the infusion is increased in small increments until an appropriate perfusion pressure is obtained.

The use of glucocorticoids in the management of TSS remains controversial. Although Shumer noted significant improvement in survival of patients with septic shock treated early and aggressively with corticosteroids (54), their efficacy or necessity in TSS has not been demonstrated. Our policy is to administer corticosteroids to patients with septic shock who do not respond promptly to our initial efforts at volume replacement. Either methylprednisolone (30 mg/kg) or dexamethasone (3 mg/kg) as a single intravenous bolus is given. The dose is repeated in 4 hr if cardiovascular function has not improved (55).

Two additional therapeutic modalities have been suggested for management of TSS patients (as well as septic shock patients) with intractable hypotension. Several studies have demonstrated successful results with the use of naloxone (Narcon) (56, 57). This narcotic antagonist could block the action of endorphins which are present in elevated levels in stressed patients and which profoundly depress the cardiovascular system. While not of proven value in TSS this approach deserves further investigation.

Duff has suggested that hemodialysis might remove the toxin responsible for the hypotension (19). Such an approach has been used with success in clostridial septotoxemia secondary to the exotoxins of *C. perfringens* (58). This approach has also not been adequately evaluated in TSS.

While β-lactamase-resistant, antistaphylococcal antibiotics have not been demonstrated to shorten the acute episode of TSS or to be necessary for clinical response in the acute episode, they are recommended as part of the therapeutic approach. Firstly, they are advisable because of the risk of bacteremia with *S. aureus*. More importantly, patients who received β-lactamase resistant, antistaphylococcal antibiotics had a significantly lower rate of TSS recurrences (4, 6, 8). Available choices include methicillin, nafcillin, or oxacillin. For penicillin allergic patients vancomycin, clindamycin, or gentamicin are alternatives.

As emphasized by Duff (19), one of the major objectives in the management of TSS is preventing ARDS, which is one of the leading causes of death in TSS and is associated with very high mortality rates when it complicates septic shock. Oxygen is administered by mask or nasal cannula at the initiation of therapy. Arterial blood gases are monitored frequently to detect hypoxia and/or metabolic acidosis. Close monitoring of fluid replacement is mandatory to avoid excessive fluid replacement. There should be no hesitancy to intubate the patient and institute mechanical ventilation with the earliest signs of decreased pulmonary compliance. With such an aggresive approach, irreversible hypoxic damage to the pulmonary vasculature will, hopefully, be prevented (19).

Additional therapeutic measures may be necessary on an individual basis, depending on the clinical presentation of TSS. Coagulation abnormalities are treated with fresh frozen plasma, cryoprecipitate, fresh whole blood, and/or platelets. Calcium supplementation may be necessary if hypocalcemia and/or cardiac dysfunction is present. Electrolyte abnormalities must be corrected by administration of electrolyte solutions. Dialysis may be necessary in cases of acute renal failure. Finally, in nonmenstruation cases of TSS a thorough search for localized *S. aureus* infection(s) must be undertaken. Such infection sites must be appropriately managed as indicated by the particular type of infection (i.e., incision and drainage of abscesses, debridement of necrotic tissue).

Recommendations have been made to reduce the risk of TSS (5). Women can significantly decrease their risk of developing TSS by not using tampons. The risk may also be reduced by avoiding continuous tampon usage and alternating tampon use with napkins. Based on studies demonstrating a very significant increase risk to develop TSS among users of high-absorbancy tampons (29), it seems advisable for women to avoid the use of such tampons when possible. Women, especially young adolescents, must be educated about the signs and symptoms of TSS. They should be warned that if such signs and symptoms occur, the tampon must be removed and medical care sought promptly. Women with a previous history of TSS should, ideally, not use tampons.

In summary, good results in the management of TSS depend upon a high index of suspicion, prompt and aggressive fluid replacement, close monitoring of cardiovascular status, respiratory status and urine output, and prevention of ARDS (or early recognition of and treatment of ARDS).

References

1. Toxic-shock syndrome—United States. *MMWR* 29:229, 1980.
2. Follow-up on toxic-shock syndrome—United States. *MMWR* 29:297, 1980.
3. McKenna U, Meadows JA, Brewer NS, et al: Toxic-shock syndrome, a newly recognized disease entity: report of 11 cases. *Mayo Clin Proc* 55:663–672, 1980.
4. Davis JP, Chesney PJ, Wand PJ, LaVenture M, et al: Toxic shock syndrome: epidemiologic features, recurrence, risk factors, and prevention. *N Engl J Med* 303:1429–1435, 1980.
5. Shands KN, Schmid GP, Dan BB, et al: Toxic-shock syndrome in menstruating women: association with tampon use and *Staphylococcus aureus* and clinical features in 52 cases. *N Engl J Med* 303:1436–1442, 1980.
6. Tofte RW, Williams DN: Toxic-shock syndrome: clinical and laboratory features in 15 patients. *Ann Intern Med* 94:149–155, 1981.
7. Fisher RF, Goodpasture HC, Peterie JD, Voth DW: Toxic shock in menstruating women. *Ann Intern Med* 94:156–163, 1981.
8. Chesney PJ, David JP, Purdy WK, et al: Clinical manifestations of toxic-shock syndrome. *JAMA* 246:741–748, 1981.
9. Toxic-shock syndrome—United States, 1970–1980. *MMWR* 30:25, 1981.
10. Todd J, Fishaut M, Kapral F, Welch T: Toxic-shock syndrome associated with phage-group-1 staphylococci. *Lancet* 2:1116–1118, 1978.
11. Reingold AL, Shands KN, Dans BB, Broome CV: Toxic-shock syndrome not associated with menstruation. *Lancet* 1:1–4, 1982.
12. Toxic-shock syndrome—United States, 1970–1982. *MMWR* 31:201, 1982.
13. Follow-up on toxic-shock syndrome. *MMWR*

29:441, 1980.

14. Wager GP: Toxic-shock syndrome: a review. *Am J Obstet Gynecol* 146:93–102, 1983.

15. Toxic-shock syndrome—Utah. *MMWR* 29:495, 1980.

16. Reingold AL, Hargrett NT, Shands KN, et al: Toxic-shock surveillance in the United States, 1980–1981. *Ann Intern Med* 96:875–880, 1982.

17. Osterholm MT, Forfang JC: Toxic-shock syndrome in Minnesota: results of an active-passive surveillance system. *J Infect Dis* 145:458–464, 1982.

18. Davis JP, Vergeront JM: The effect of publicity on the reporting of toxic-shock syndrome in Wisconsin. *J Infect Dis* 145:449–457, 1982.

19. Duff P: Recognizing and treating toxic shock. *Contemp Obstet Gynecol* 22:43–60, 1983.

20. Dornan KJ, Thompson DM, Conn AR, et al: Toxic shock syndrome in the postoperative patient. *Surg Gynecol Obstet* 154:65–68, 1982.

21. Bartlett P, Reingold AL, Graham DR, et al: Toxic shock syndrome associated with surgical wound infections. *JAMA* 247:1448–1450, 1982.

22. Fisher CJ, Horowitz BZ, Nolan SM: The clinical spectum of toxic-shock syndrome. *West J Med* 135:175–182, 1981.

23. Green SL, LaPeter KS: Evidence for postpartum toxic-shock syndrome in a mother-infant pair. *Am J Med* 72:169–172, 1982.

24. Chow AW, Wittman BK, Bartlett BA, Scheifele DW: Variant postpartum toxic shock syndrome with probably intrapartum transmission to the neonate. *Am J Obstet Gynecol* 148:1074–1079, 1984.

25. Bracero L, Bowe E: Postpartum toxic-shock syndrome. *Am J Obstet Gynecol* 143:478–479, 1982.

26. Tofte RW, Williams DN: Toxic-shock syndrome: evidence of a broad clinical spectrum. *JAMA* 246:2163–2167, 1981.

27. Schlossberg D: A possible pathogenesis for recurrent toxic shock syndrome. *Am J Obstet Gynecol* 141:348–349, 1981.

28. Kehrberg MW, Latham RH, Haslam BT, et al: Risk factors for staphylococcal toxic shock syndrome. *Am J Epidemiol* 114:873–879, 1981.

29. Osterholm MT, Davis JP, Gibson RW, et al: Tristate toxic-shock syndrome study. I. Epidemiologic findings. *J Infect Dis* 145:431–440, 1982.

30. Schlech WF, Shands, KN Reingold AL, et al: Risk factors for development of toxic shock syndrome: association with a tampon brand. *JAMA* 248:835–839, 1982.

31. Tierno PM: Cellulase activity of microorganisms on carboxymethylcellulose from tampons. *Lancet* 2:746, 1981.

32. Hanna BA: Microbial degradation of carboxymethylcellulose from tampons. *Lancet* 1:279, 1982.

33. Gorbach SL, Menda KB, Thadepalli H, et al: Anaerobic microflora of the cervix in healthy women. *Am J Obstet Gynecol* 117:1053–1055, 1973.

34. Ohm MJ, Galask RP: Bacterial flora of the cervix from 100 prehysterectomy patients. *Am J Obstet Gynecol* 122:683–687, 1975.

35. Grossman JH III, Adams RL: Vaginal flora in women undergoing hysterectomy with antibiotic prophylaxis. *Obstet Gynecol* 53:23–26, 1979.

36. Bartlett JG, Onderdonk AB, Drude E, et al: Quantitative bacteriology of the vaginal flora. *J Infect Dis* 136:271–277, 1977.

37. Tasjian JH, Coulan CB, Washington JA III: Vaginal flora in asymptomatic women. *Mayo Clin Proc* 51:557–561, 1976.

38. Osborne NG, Wright RC: Effect of a preoperative scrub on the bacterial flora of the endocervix and vagina. *Obstet Gynecol* 50:148–151, 1977.

39. Guinan ME, Dan BB, Guidotti RJ, et al: Vaginal colonization with *Staphylococcus aureus* in healthy women. *Ann Intern Med* 96:944–947, 1982.

40. Noble VS, Jacobson JA, Smith CB: The effect of menses and use of catamenial products on cervical carriage of *Staphylococcus aureus*. *Am J Obstet Gynecol* 144:186–189, 1982.

41. Saunders CC, Saunders WE Jr, Fagnant JE: Toxic shock syndrome: an ecologic imbalance within the genital microflora of women? *Am J Obstet Gynecol* 142:977–982, 1982.

42. Schlievert PM, Shands KN, Dan BB, et al: Identification and characterization of an exotoxin from *S. aureus* associated with toxic-shock syndrome. *J Infect Dis* 143:509–516, 1981.

43. Bergdoll MS, Crass BA, Reiser RF, et al: A new staphylococcal enterotoxin, enterotoxin F, associated with toxic-shock syndrome *S. aureus* isolates. *Lancet* 1:1017–1021, 1981.

44. Altemeier WA, Lewis S, Schlievert PM, Bjornson HS: Studies of the staphylococcal causation of toxic shock syndrome. *Surg Gynecol Obstet* 153:481–485, 1981.

45. Bennett JV: Toxins and toxic-shock syndrome. *J Infect Dis* 143:631–632, 1981.

46. Larsen B, Schlievert PM: TSS: the mystery unfolds. *Contemp Ob/Gyn* 18:219–229, 1981.

47. Schlievert PM: Enhancement of host susceptibility to letal endotoxin shock by staphylococcal pyrogenic exotoxin type C. *Infect Immun* 36:123–128, 1982.

48. Sahs AL, Helms CM, DuBois C: Complication of toxic shock syndrome. *Arch Neurol* 40:414–415, 1983.

49. Rosene KA, Copass MK, Kastner LS, et al: Persistent neuropsychological sequelae of toxic shock syndrome. *Ann Intern Med* 96:865–870, 1982.

50. Chesney PJ, Crass BA, Polyak MB, et al: Toxic-shock syndrome: management and long-term sequelae. *Ann Intern Med* 96:847–851, 1982.

51. Shubin H, Weil MH, Carson RW: Bacterial shock. *Am Heart J* 94:112–114, 1977.

52. McSwain NE: Pneumonatic trousers and the management of shock. *J Trauma* 17:719–724, 1977.

53. Sweet RL: Septic abortion. In Sciarra J (ed): *Gynecology and Obstetrics.* Hagerstown, MD, Harper & Row, 1979.

54. Shumer W: Steroids in the treatment of clinical septic shock. *Ann Surg* 184:333–339, 1976.

55. Sheagren JN: Septic shock and corticosteroids. *N Engl J Med* 305:456–458, 1981.

56. Tiengo M: Naloxone in irreversible shock. *Lancet* 2:690, 1980.

57. Peters WP, Friedman PA, Johnson MW, et al: Pressor effect of naloxone in septic shock. *Lancet* 1:529–532, 1981.

58. Sweet RL: Anaerobic infections of the female genital tract. *Am J Obstet Gynecol* 122:891–901, 1975.

CHAPTER 6

Infectious Vulvovaginitis

Symptoms of vulvovaginitis, which include discharge, odor, itching or vaginal discomfort, account for a considerable proportion of outpatient gynecologic visits. In the past, patients with trichomonal or candidal vaginitis were properly treated. However, many patients with these infections experienced failed therapy or recurrence, and still others with less distinctive types of vaginitis often did not receive satisfactory therapy at all. In the last few years, with rising interest in all sexually transmitted diseases, vaginitis has been investigated more actively. As a consequence, there have been improvements in our understanding of pathophysiology, in diagnosis and in treatment.

PREVALENCE AND DISTRIBUTION OF VAGINITIS

In their classic paper, Gardner and Dukes analyzed 1181 private patients (602 obstetric, 579 gynecologic) in Houston (1). The vast majority were sexually active, premenopausal women. Microscopic examinations of wet mounts and stained smears were made of all patients with symptoms of vaginitis or with gross evidence of vaginitis on inspection. Also included were data from 78 clinically normal patients. These authors described normal vaginal secretions as usually white and curdy (i.e., not homogeneous), with a pH of 4.0–4.7. Their findings are summarized in Table 6.1. The most common type of vaginitis was nonspecific vaginitis, which they characterized clearly in that publication. Trichomoniasis and candidiasis each accounted for about one-quarter of cases.

Thirty years later, Osbourne and colleagues reported culture results (for eight selected organisms) from vaginal secretions of 253 college women with "genital symptoms suggestive of vulvovaginitis" and in 130 asymptomatic sexually active control women (2). Table 6.2 shows their findings. Although these authors did not provide the clinical diagnosis of cause of vaginitis in symptomatic patients, they noted *T.*

vaginalis and *G. vaginalis* each occurred in one-quarter of these students, while yeasts were found in 39%.

Thus, vaginal symptoms occur commonly. Trichomoniasis, moniliasis, and nonspecific vaginitis account for the vast majority of cases, but some cases (1–10%) cannot be accounted for by these three diagnoses. Further, the prevalence of vulvovaginal organisms varies from population to population, and commonly asymptomatic women will harbor yeasts, *T. vaginalis* or *G. vaginalis*.

TRICHOMONIASIS

This infection is caused by *Trichomonas vaginalis*, a protozoan first described in 1836. The organism is responsible for approximately a quarter of all cases of clinically evident vaginal infections (1, 2) and also occurs commonly among women without symptoms of vaginitis. McLellan and colleagues studied women attending a sexually transmitted disease clinic in Baltimore (3). Of 226 consecutive women, 44% had positive cultures for *T. vaginalis*, but only 50% of those with a positive culture complained of vaginal discharge and only 17% complained of pruritis.

In defining risk factors for *T. vaginalis*, McLellan and co-workers noted that a positive vaginal culture was significantly associated with multiple sexual partners (22/100 with versus 14/126 without *T. vaginalis*, p < 0.05), but a positive culture was not associated with age, day of cycle, type of contraceptive used, recent use of antibiotics, or frequency of coitus.

Among symptomatic women with trichomoniasis, the vaginal secretions are usually copious, homogeneous, malodorous, with a pH of >4.5. A frothy, yellow-green discharge is often cited as the typical finding, but in objective series frothiness was detected in only 12–34% (1, 3). Gardner and Dukes described the color of the discharge as grey in 46% of cases, yellow-green in 36%, and yellow-green in 10% (1). Punctate

Table 6.1
Etiology of Infectious Vaginitides in 1,181 Patients[a,b]

Clinical diagnosis	No. of cases	% of all patients	% of cases of vaginitis
Trichomoniasis[c]	71	6.0	24
Moniliasis[d]	79	6.7	27
Nonspecific vaginitis[e]	127	10.8	41
Gonorrhea	1	0.1	
Chancroid	1	0.1	
Granuloma inguinale	1	0.1	
Other bacterial vaginitis[f]	11	1.0	4

[a] Adapted from Gardner H, Dukes CD: Haemophilus vaginalis vaginitis: a newly defined specific infection previously classified "nonspecific" vaginitis. *Am J Obstet Gynecol* 69:962, 1955.
[b] Private patients of Dr. Herman Gardner, Houston, Texas.
[c] Trichomoniasis based upon typical symptoms and positive smear. In addition to these 71 cases, 9 other women had positive smears, but did not have typical symptoms.
[d] Moniliasis based upon typical signs, symptoms, and positive smear.
[e] Nonspecific vaginitis, which was called *Haemophilus vaginitis* vaginitis by these authors, was based upon typical findings and a positive culture of *H. Vaginalis*.
[f] In these cases, none of the other etiologies could be assigned. The authors found no uniform clinical or microbiologic pattern.

mucosal hemorrhages of the cervix, the so-called "strawberry" or "flea-bitten" cervix, are seen infrequently. Because of the variations in signs and symptoms, one cannot rely upon these findings. Under most circumstances, the clinical diagnosis can be confirmed by microscopic examination of a wet mount, made by mixing a drop of secretions with a few drops of saline on a slide. Because trichomoniasis may produce a heavy polymorphonuclear infiltrate, it is easy to miss the trichomonads. One must examine the preparation in an area with relatively few white cells. Usually, the trichomonads are evident by the extreme activity of these flagellates in freshly made preparations. There is not complete agreement regarding the reliability of wet mounts for diagnosis of trichomoniasis in symptomatic women. Some authors believe simple microscopy is as reliable as culture (4, 5), but most have found the sensitivity of culture to be greater than that of wet mounts (6–8).

The only effective treatment for trichomoniasis is metronidazole (Flagyl) or related 5-nitroimidazole derivatives (tinidazole, ornidazole). However, evidence developed in the early 1970s that metronidazole was carcinogenic in certain rodent species, but not in others. When tumors evolved, it was only after chronic, high-dose use, making the application of this data to use in humans difficult. The Food and Drug Administration interpreted the data as showing a very low risk of human carcinogenesis and denied a petition to remove metronidazole from the market (9). Recently, a study from the Mayo Clinic provided data of 771 women with metronidazole for trichomoniasis (10). With surveillance of 10–20 yr, these investigators found no appreciable carcinogenicity attributable to metronidazole.

In view of concerns about carcinogenicity, there was a reduction in standard dose of metronidazole (250 mg p.o. t.i.d. in women) from 10 to 7 days, and topical metronidazole preparations were removed from the market (9). Evaluation of a single dose of 2 g was undertaken and found to be effective (4, 5, 11). Recent direct comparisons of the 7 day versus single dose regimens have found them to be equivalent (12, 13). Cure rates with either regimen have varied from 86 to 97%. Aubert and Sesta reported that side effects were not significantly different between the two regimens (13). Nausea and vomiting occurred in 4% of 140 with the single dose and in 0 of 123 with the 7-day course; candidiasis was noted in 10.4% of the former and in 1.3% of the latter groups (p > 0.1). In 1982, the CDC recommended single dose treatment as the regimen of choice (14).

Possible causes of failure of metronidazole therapy include (1) pharmacokinetic problems in either absorption or delivery to the infected site, (2) inactivation of metronidazole by vaginal bacteria, (3) interference by other drugs, or (4) resistance to metronidazole. Until recently, resistance was usually discounted, but development of a suitable aerobic in vitro assay has permitted the demonstration of resistance in several strains from Europe and the United States. However, these strains have remained very infrequent, and failure of therapy is not likely to be the more frequent cause (15).

When sexual partners are symptomatic or when they harbor the organism, they should be treated also. Treatment is more problematic in an asymptomatic male partner who has a negative culture and smear or in whom no testing has been performed. Testing may be less reliable in asymptomatic males, and the female may become reinfected if the male is untreated. Thus,

Table 6.2
Prevalence of Selected Microorganisms in Genital Cultures in 383 Sexually Active College Students[a]

Organism	Symptomatic women (N = 253) (%)	p	Asymptomatic women (N = 130) (%)
T. vaginalis[b]	24.5	0.0002	6.9
Yeasts	39.1	0.0473	22.3
G. vaginalis	23.7	0.0001	5.4
Herpes simplex	12.6	0.0001	1.5
N. gonorrhoeae[c]	10.6	0.0001	2.3
C. trachomatis[c]	10.6	0.0001	6.9
M. hominis	25.7	0.0722	14.6
U. urealyticum	19.0	NS[d]	18.5
None of the above	9.1	0.0001	58.5

[a] Adapted from Osbourne NG, Grubin L, Pratson L: *Am J Obstet Gynecol* 142:962, 1982.
[b] Detected by wet mount and Papanicolaou smear.
[c] Cultures for *N. gonorrhoeae* and *C. trachomatis* were taken only from the endocervix.
[d] Authors did not provide a clinical diagnosis in symptomatic women.

there are concerns raised by prescribing metronidazole for the male partner who does not come to the office or clinic. It would seem advisable, however, to treat the consort in cases of reinfection. The CDC recently recommended concurrent treatment of male consorts of women with trichomoniasis (14).

Use of metronidazole is occasionally accompanied by headache, metallic or bitter aftertaste, or nausea and vomiting. Blood dyscrasias are rare consequences, but in the product information total and differential leukocyte counts are recommended before, during, and after treatment.

Metronidazole should be avoided in the first trimester of pregnancy. Use in later gestation is controversial. If used here, it should be restricted to cases in which *symptomatic relief* is not achieved by local measures such as administration of clotrimazole (Gyne-Lotrimin) (14).

YEAST INFECTION

Yeasts are commonly found in the vagina. Osbourne et al cultured yeasts in specimens from 22% of 130 asymptomatic college women and from 39% of 253 with vulvovaginal symptoms (2). Earlier, Oriel and colleagues cultured yeasts in vaginal specimens from 138 (26%) of 533 women attending a venereology clinic in London (16). In both studies, *Candida albicans* was the predominant yeast isolate (95 and 81%, respectively), with *Torulopsis glabrata* and other *Candida* species making up the remainder. Oriel and co-workers reported symptoms of vaginal

pruritis with or without discharge in 50%, symptoms of discharge alone in 30%, and no signs or symptoms in 20% of patients with a positive culture for *C. albicans*. In comparison, of these venereology patients with negative tests for both yeasts and *T. vaginalis*, 19% of 170 experienced pruritis with or without discharge, 38% noted discharge, and 43% were asymptomatic.

It is unclear why some women with vaginal yeasts develop symptoms. Commonly noted predisposing features to growth of yeast in vagina are: glycosuria, diabetes mellitus, pregnancy, obesity, and recent use of antibiotics, steroids, or immunosuppressants (17). The role of oral contraceptives (OC) is controversial, as noted by Oriel and colleagues (16). In Oriel's study, it was noted that users of oral contraceptives were more likely to have yeast isolates in vaginal cultures (32% of 241 women on O.C. versus 18% of women not taking O.C.), but symptoms or signs of vaginal yeast infection were not increased (23% on O.C. versus 26% not on O.C.). It is commonly suggested that wearing tight fitting undergarments predisposes to yeast infection by increasing local humidity and temperature.

Yeasts may be sexually transmitted. Oriel noted that 5 of 48 men seen after sexual contact with women harboring yeasts developed mycotic balanoposthitis (16).

The characteristic findings of vaginal candidiasis are reddened vulval or vaginal areas with vulval scaling, edema, or excoriation and raised, white or yellow adherent vaginal plaques. However, Oriel noted such findings in only 38% of women with positive cultures for *C. albicans* (16).

The diagnosis may be confirmed by observing mycelia and/or pseudohyphae upon direct microscopy in a 10% KOH preparation, but it is often impossible to detect yeast cells because of excess cellular debris. Oriel and colleagues found gram-stained specimens to be more satisfactory, but overall they found culture to be the most sensitive test (16). Only half of their patients with positive cultures showed organisms on direct microscopy, and they noted that often women with the most florid findings gave positive results only by culture. On the other hand, Van Slyke and colleagues found that among *symptomatic* patients the KOH wet mount was "usually sufficient for office use" (18). Compared to cultures, direct microscopy gave 2.3% false-positive and a 6.2% false-negative results.

Treatment of yeast infections results in acute relief of symptoms and eradication of yeasts in from 50 to 90%, and recurrence of infection is a common problem. In general, predisposing factors should be eliminated, when possible, and sexual partners should be treated if there is recurrence or clinical or mycologic evidence of infection. The traditional specific approach to vaginal candidiasis is local application of antifungal agents. For a number of years, nystatin suppositories, ointments, or cream (Mycostatin or Nilstat, b.i.d. for 15 days) had been the main therapy. Newer and effective commercial preparations are: miconazole cream (2%) (Monistat), one applicatorful daily 10–14 days and clotrimazole tablets, 100-mg suppository (Gyne-Lotrimin, Canesten) daily, 3 or 7 days.

In comparative studies, several investigations have reported significantly better cure rates with miconazole (19,20,21) than with mycostatin. Clotrimazole is as effective as nystatin (22) but offers the advantage of a shorter course. In a double-blind study, a 3-day course of 200 mg clotrimazole vaginally at bedtime has been found comparable to a 7-day course of 100 mg at bedtime (23). Robertson noted signs and symptoms were relieved in 19 (82%) of 23 patients treated for 3 days compared to 21 (91%) of 23 treated for 7 days (NS). There was no significant difference in recurrence 4 weeks after therapy, (three positive cultures of 20 women treated for 3 days versus one positive of 22 women treated for 7 days). There were no adverse reactions noted. Earlier, using 200 mg (two suppositories) nightly for 3 nights, Masterson and colleagues had noted a 99.1% cure rate

(negative cultures for *C. albicans*) at the end of 1 week and an 89.4% cure rate at 4 weeks (24).

Candidiasis may be more difficult to cure in pregnancy. There is more experience with nystatin than with the newer topical antifungal agents, and some favor its use in pregnancy for that reason. Yet, in a number of series studying pregnant women, no particular adverse effect in the mother or fetus was noted with miconazole or clotrimazole (19–21,25–26).

Because of better compliance with shorter courses and improved cure rates shown in a number of studies, the newer agents—miconazole and clotrimazole—have become increasingly popular.

Gentian violet (1% solution) may be used in cases of florid candidiasis to give acute symptomatic relief, but it is messy and results in marked drying and itching if used continuously.

Recently, Van Slyke and colleagues reported excellent results with boric acid powder (600 mg in a size 0 gelatin capsule) used daily for 14 days (18). In a double-blind study of boric acid versus capsules containing 100,000 units mystatin (in cornstarch), cure rates were significantly better with boric acid (92% at 7–10 days after treatment versus 64% with nystatin) (p = 0.001). There were no serious adverse effects from either preparation, but patients using boric acid capsulates often noted a slight watery discharge. Blood boron levels indicated little absorption from the vaginal preparation. However, because boric acid in large doses is toxic, the capsules or the powder must be kept out of reach of small children. Boric acid capsules should probably also be avoided in pregnancy. A major advantage of this treatment is its small cost. If 14 capsules and 600 mg of boric acid are prescribed, the total cost is approximately $3.00.

Availability of ketoconazole, a safe, effective oral preparation for the treatment of fungal infections, offers a new approach to therapy of vaginal yeast infections. This new agent has recently been reviewed (27). It is an imidazole antifungal drug, structurally related to miconazole, and is effective in a variety of superficial and systemic mycoses. The mechanism of action of ketoconazole may result from perturbations in sterol or fatty acid metabolism or to accumulation of toxic endoperoxides secondary to its effect on oxidative and peroxidative systems.

After oral ingestion of a 200-mg dose, ketoconazole is well absorbed resulting in peak serum levels of 1–3 μg/ml. These levels should be effective against many fungal infections. The drug is distributed widely and is detected in urine, saliva, and in cerebrospinal fluid in varying concentrations. Extensive metabolism of the drug occurs as only 2–4% is excreted in unchanged form in the urine. In healthy subjects, the elimination half-life is 8 hr after a usual 200-mg dose.

Overall, side effects are infrequent, but when present, gastrointestinal symptoms (in 5% of patients) and pruritis (in 2%) are the most common (27). Transient elevations of liver enzymes occur in about 10% of patients. In 281 patients undergoing treatment for vaginal candidiasis, Van Der Pas et al found side effects in 5% of patients (nausea 2%, headache, 1%, epigastric pain, somnolence, and weakness, less than 1% each) (28).

The dose for treating vaginal candidiasis is 200 mg b.i.d. for 5 days. Efficacy with this dose is approximately 90% (27,28). In two double-blind studies, ketoconazole (200 mg t.i.d. for 3 days) was as effective as miconazole (400 mg intravaginal capsule t.i.d. for 3 days) at the initial evaluation 4 days after therapy. Relapse tended to occur more frequently in the ketoconazole group (27). However, in this comparative study, the optimal duration of therapy with ketoconazole was not used.

The major advantages of ketoconazole in treating vaginal candidiasis appear to be (1) the convenience of its oral route of administration and (2) the potential benefit in eliminating a gastrointestinal reservoir of *C. albicans* in cases of recurrent vaginitis.

Although failure of therapy and recurrence of vaginal yeast infections are common, there is poor understanding of this problem. Miles and co-workers found 100% agreement between positive vaginal yeast cultures and positive stool cultures and suggested that therapy aimed at controlling the gastrointestinal "reservoir" of yeast might lead to improved results (29). Resistance of yeasts to antifungal drugs does not appear to be likely (17). In some cases, genital yeast infections are clearly transmitted sexually. One other practical consideration is poor patient compliance, especially with longer courses of vaginal preparations (30).

When a single course of therapy is unsuccessful, then a second course of treatment with vaginal preparations is often successful. Van Slyke et al noted that of ten patients who had not responded to nystatin, nine (90%) responded to boric acid (18). Also of four who had not responded to a first course of boric acid, three

(75%) responded to a second course. Similarly, in the study of McNellis et al, of 25 patients who did not respond to a first course of miconazole cream, 16 (64%) did respond to a second course (19). However, they noted a poor response to a second course of nystatin. Of 73 who did not respond to a first course, only 20 (27.4%) responded to a second course of vaginal nystatin. When there is still no response, treatment with oral ketoconazole may be more effective, but it has not been evaluated in such instances.

Finally, Oriel and colleagues raise the question of whether all patients with a positive yeast culture should be treated regardless of whether they have vaginal symptoms. They suggest treatment even in asymptomatic women to prevent subsequent development of symptomatic infection and transmission of yeast infection to sexual partners. However, there would seem to be few indications to perform cultures for yeast in asymptomatic women, and thus treatment of asymptomatic candidiasis is not a common dilemma.

"NONSPECIFIC VAGINITIS"

In 1955, Gardner and Dukes described a clinical syndrome of vaginitis with the following features: a grey (85% of cases), homogenous, odorous discharge with a pH of 5.0–5.5, without yeast forms or trichomonads (1). The volume of discharge was moderate, and upon examining a wet mount there were characteristic stippled or granulated epithelial cells called "clue cells." Leukocytes were not prominent. In a quarter of patients, the vaginal secretions were frothy. In the vaginal secretions of the cases, *Haemophilus vaginalis* (subsequently called *Corynebacterium vaginale* and now named *Gardnerella vaginalis*) was isolated, but they did not isolate it from any normal patients. Gardner and Dukes thus called this specific infection *H. vaginalis* vaginitis and suggested this term in preference to "nonspecific vaginitis," a designation which had been applied previously. During the next 20 yr, reports were largely confirmatory of the association between *G. vaginalis* and the characteristic syndrome, although some showed that this organism could be recovered from a considerable percentage of asymptomatic women (31,32).

However, recent reports have suggested that anaerobic bacteria play an important, if not predominant, role in pathophysiology of this condition. In Seattle (33,34), investigators have used basically the same features to diagnose "nonspecific vaginitis" (NSV). In addition, they noted that a "fishy" amine odor was liberated when 10% KOH was added to the discharge in preparing a wet mount. These authors have reported that *G. vaginalis* is recovered from over 90% of women with NSV, but it is also found in 30–40% of asymptomatic women when selective media are used. They noted, however, that patients with NSV had 4+ growth of *G. vaginalis* significantly more commonly. They point to evidence for a major anaerobic component in NSV as follows: (1) detection of organic acids produced by anaerobes when vaginal secretions are analyzed by gas-liquid chromatography; (2) isolation of anaerobes in high concentrations; and (3) the excellent clinical response to oral metronidazole (Flagyl) (33). This last point is impressive because of the extensive activity of metronidazole against anaerobes and its modest activity against *G. vaginalis* (35). In addition, with selective media, it has recently been shown that after successful treatment of NSV, up to 50% of patients still have *G. vaginalis* in vaginal secretions (34). In some patients with NSV, small curved rods, *Mobiluncus* species (39a), are seen. The role of these organisms is uncertain. Thus, within the last few years, there has been a greater interest in the etiology of this common condition. It would seem appropriate to conclude that, at present, certain anaerobes including *Bacteroides* species and anaerobic cocci act with *G. vaginalis* to cause NSV.

Despite the commonly used term of nonspecific vaginitis, this is a specific infection, and the diagnosis should *not* be based solely upon the absence of trichomonads and yeast forms.

The chief symptom is vaginal discharge, rather than pruritis. Some patients may note an offensive vaginal odor, which may be accentuated after coitus. Upon examination, the typical discharge is often evident at the introitus. Vulvovaginal irritation is less marked than with trichomoniasis or candidiasis.

Table 6.3 summarizes the characteristics of NSV and of normal vaginal secretions. Thus, the diagnosis of NSV should be based upon the general characteristics of volume, color, adherence, and viscosity and upon specific features of high pH, "amine" odor with KOH, homogeneous consistency, and presence of "clue" cells. True clue cells are epithelial cells which are so heavily stippled with bacteria that the borders are obscured; epithelial cells with few bacteria and clear borders should *not* be identified as clue cells. By limiting the clinical diagnosis of NSV to conditions with these features, there is little need for elaborate laboratory aids. Despite the likely role of anaerobes, there is no need to perform cultures for them, and there is no real diagnostic value in demonstrating the presence of *G. vaginalis* in vaginal secretions.

Treatment of NSV previously had been directed against *G. vaginalis*. In very few patients, Gardner and Dukes had reported good results with topical sulfa cream and tetracycline (1). Yet, *G. vaginalis* has been uniformly resistant to sulfonamide in vitro (31). Others had reported that ampicillin was highly effective. However, Pheifer reported poor responses with all of these agents, whereas, with metronidazole (500 mg, b.i.d., orally for 7 days) the cure rate was approximately 90% (33). In three later double-blind studies, metronidazole or tinadazole were confirmed to be highly effective. Balsdon and colleagues compared metronidazole (400 mg

Table 6.3
Characteristics of Nonspecific Vaginitis (NSV) and Normal Vaginal Secretion[a]

Feature	NSV	Normal secretions
Volume	++	+
Color	Gray (85%)	White (86%)
Consistency	Homogeneous	Nonhomogeneous, floccular
Viscosity	Low	High
Adherent	Yes	No
Clue cells	Positive	Negative
Amine odor when mixed with KOH	Yes	No
pH	>4.5	<4.5

[a] Adapted from Gardner H, Dukes CD: Haemophilus vaginalis vaginitis: a newly defined specific infection previously classified "nonspecific" vaginitis. *Am J Obstet Gynecol* 69:962, 1955 and Pheifer TA, Forsyth PS, Durfee MA, et al: Nonspecific vaginitis: role of *Haemophilus vaginalis* and treatment with metronidazole. *N Engl J Med* 298:1429, 1978.

b.i.d. for 7 days) oxytetracycline (500 mg b.i.d. for 7 days), and placebo (b.i.d. for 7 days) (35). Patients whose randomized therapy had failed were then treated with metronidazole. Altogether, 16 of 17 patients treated with metronidazole were clinically cured, and cultures of *G. vaginalis* became negative in 15, even though metronidazole has no in vitro activity. Oxytetracycline therapy led to clinical cure in 6 of 10 patients, and the placebo led to clinical cure in only 1 of 9 patients. In a larger double-blind study, Malouf and co-workers found that metronidazole was curative in 91% of 22 patients, while sulfa cream, doxycycline, and ampicillin were curative in 55% of 18, 64% of 33, and 48% of 23 patients, respectively (36). Recently, Piot and colleagues carried out a double-blind comparison of oral tinidazole (which has a longer half-life than metronidazole) to vaginal cream with or without sulfonamides (37). At 1 week, tinidazole had cured 29 (97%) of 30 patients, while the oral placebo plus vaginal creams had cured 16 (60%) of 27. It was suggested that cream containing sulfonamide was not more effective than the cream itself.

Use of metronidazole for NSV is currently not approved by the FDA. In view of potential side effects, some have advised treating this mild infection with ampicillin orally, at first (38). Alternatively, one may use metronidazole, but should advise the patient of its benefits, risks, and status for treating NSV. Good cure rates are achieved by treating the female, without treatment of her consorts (37). On the other hand, Gardner has pointed to the frequent isolation of *G. vaginalis* in sexual consorts and suggested treatment of the partner simultaneously (1). Further, Pheifer and colleagues noted the correlation of recurrent *G. vaginalis* infection with sexual reexposure and suggested that treatment of the partner may prove necessary to prevent reinfection (33). Malouf and colleagues in their comparative study treated the patients and partners with identical regimens (36).

Metronidazole should be avoided in the first trimester of pregnancy, and for NSV in later pregnancy, ampicillin would seem to be a wise choice. If marked symptoms persist, then metronidazole may be used.

References

1. Gardner H, Dukes CD: Haemophilus vaginalis vaginitis: a newly defined specific infection previously classified "nonspecific" vaginitis. *Am J Obstet Gynecol* 69:962, 1955.
2. Osbourne NG, Grubin L, Pratson L: Vaginitis in sexually active women: relationship to nine sexually transmitted organisms. *Am J Obstet Gynecol* 142:962, 1982.
3. McLellan R, Spence MR, Brockman M, et al: The clinical diagnosis of trichomoniasis. *Obstet Gynecol* 60:30, 1982.
4. Morton RS: Metronidazole in the single-dose treatment of trichomoniasis in men and women. *Br J Vener Dis* 48:525, 1972.
5. Woodcock KR: Treatment of trichomonal vaginitis with a single oral dose of metronidazole. *Br J Vener Dis* 48:65, 1972.
6. Hess J: Review of current methods for the detection of trichomonas in clinical material. *J Clin Pathol* 22:269, 1969.
7. McCann JS: Comparison of direct microscopy and culture in the diagnosis of trichomoniasis. *Br J Vener Dis* 50:450, 1974.
8. Spence MR, Hollander DH, Smith J, et al: The clinical and laboratory diagnosis of *Trichomonas vaginalis* infection. *Sex Transm Dis* 7:168, 1980.
9. Metronidazole (Flagyl) box warning. *FDA Drug Bull* 6:22, 1976.
10. Beard CM, Noller KL, O'Fallon WM, et al: Lack of evidence for cancer due to use of metronidazole. *N Engl J Med* 301:519, 1979.
11. Fugere P, Verschelden G, Caron M: Single oral dose of ornidazole in women with vaginal trichomoniasis. *Obstet Gynecol* 62:502, 1983.
12. Hager WD, Brown ST, Kraus SJ, et al: Metronidazole for vaginal trichomoniasis. *JAMA* 244:1219, 1980.
13. Aubert JM, Sesta HJ: Treatment of vaginal trichomoniasis, single 2-gram dose of metronidazole as compared with a seven-day course. *J Reprod Med* 27:743, 1982.
14. Sexually transmitted diseases treatment guidelines, 1982. *MMWR* 31:47(s), 1982.
15. Muller M, Meingassner JG, Miller WA, Ledger WJ: Three metronidazole-resistant strains of *Trichomonas vaginalis* from the United States. *Am J Obstet Gynecol* 138:808, 1980.
16. Oriel JD, Partridge BM, Denny MJ, Coleman JC: Genital yeast infections. *Br Med J* 4:761, 1972.
17. Vaginal candidosis. *Br Med J* 1:357, 1976.
18. Van Slyke KK, Michel VP, Rein MF: Treatment of vulvovaginal candidiasis with boric acid powder. *Am J Obstet Gynecol* 141:145, 1981.
19. McNellis D, McLeod M, Lawson J, Pasquale SA: Treatment of vulvovaginal candidiasis in pregnancy, a comparative study. *Obstet Gynecol* 50:674, 1977.
20. Wallenburg HCS, Wladimiroff JW: Recurrence of vulvovaginal candidosis during pregnancy, comparison of miconazole vs. nystatin treatment. *Obstet Gynecol* 48:491, 1976.
21. Davis JE, Frudenfeld JH, Goddard JL: Comparative evaluation of monistat myocstatin in the treatment of vulvovaginal candidiasis. *Obstet Gynecol* 44:403, 1974.
22. Gyne-Lotrimin for vaginal infections. *Med Lett Drugs Ther* 18:66, 1976.
23. Robertson WH: A concentrated therapeutic regimen for vulvovaginal candidiasis. *JAMA* 244:2549, 1980.
24. Masterson G, Napier IR, Henderson JN, et al: Three-day clotrimazole treatment in candidal vulvovaginitis. *Br J Vener Dis* 53:126, 1977.

25. Culbertson C: Monistat: a new fungicide for treatment of vulvovaginal candidiasis. *Am J Obstet Gynecol* 120:973, 1974.

26. Frerich W, Gad A: The frequency of candida infections in pregnancy and their treatment with clotrimazole. *Curr Med Res Opin* 4:640, 1977.

27. Heel RC, Brogden RN, Carmine A, et al: Ketoconazole: a review of its therapeutic efficacy in superficial and systemic fungal infections. *Drugs* 23:1, 1982.

28. Van Der Pas H, Peeters F, Janssens D, et al: Treatment of vaginal candidosis with oral ketoconazole. *Eur J Obstet Gynecol Reprod Biol* 14:399, 1983.

29. Miles MR, Olsen L, Rogers A: Recurrent vaginal candidiasis. Importance of an intestinal reservoir. *JAMA* 238:1836, 1977.

30. Masterson G, Henderson JN, Napier L, et al: Vaginal candidosis. *Br Med J* 1:712, 1976.

31. Dunkelberg WE: *Corynebacterium vaginale* (review). *Sex Transm Dis* 4:69, 1977.

32. Gardner HL: *Haemophilus vaginalis* vaginitis after twenty-five years. *Am J Obstet Gynecol* 137:385, 1980.

33. Pheifer TA, Forsyth PS, Durfee MA, et al: Nonspecific vaginitis: role of *Haemophilus vaginalis* and treatment with metronidazole. *N Engl J Med* 298:1429, 1978.

34. Spiegel CA, Amsel R, Eschenbach D, et al: Anaerobic bacteria in nonspecific vaginitis. *N Engl J Med* 303:601, 1980.

34a. Sprott MS, Ingham RS, Pottman RL, et al: Characteristics of motile curved rods in vaginal secretions. *J Med Microbiol* 16:175, 1983.

35. Balsdon MJ, Taylor GE, Pead L, et al: Corynebacterium vaginale and vaginitis: a controlled trial of treatment. *Lancet* 1:501, 1980.

36. Malouf M, Fortier M, Morin G, et al: Treatment of *Haemophilus vaginalis* vaginitis. *Obstet Gynecol* 57:711, 1981.

37. Piot P, Van Dyck E, Godts P, et al: A placebo-controlled, double-blind comparison of tinidazole and triple sulfonamide cream for the treatment of nonspecific vaginitis. *Am J Obstet Gynecol* 147:85, 1983.

38. Robbie MO, Sweet RL: Metronidazole use in obstetrics and gynecology: a review. *Am J Obstet Gynecol* 145:865, 1983.

CHAPTER 7

Genital Mycoplasmas

The mycoplasmas are a unique group of microorganisms that commonly inhabit the mucosa of the respiratory and genital tracts (1, 2). Many antigenically distinct species that are infectious in humans have been characterized. These include *Mycoplasma pneumoniae*, the agent responsible for atypical pneumonias and genital mycoplasmas. The latter consist of four species: *Mycoplasma fermentans*, *Mycoplasma primatum*, *Mycoplasma hominis*, and *Ureaplasma urealyticum* (formerly T-mycoplasmas or T strains). *M. fermentans* and *M. primatum* are uncommon, and there is no good evidence that these organisms produce clinical disease. *M. hominis* and *U. urealyticum* are common genital organisms which have been associated with a variety of clinical conditions, including low birth weight infants, spontaneous abortions, stillbirths, postpartum infections, chorioamnionitis, infertility, and pelvic inflammatory disease.

Phylogenetically, mycoplasmas fall between bacteria and viruses. All mycoplasmas have several characteristics in common: (1) absence of cell walls; (2) growth in cell-free media; (3) dependence on the availability of sterols for adequate growth; (4) inhibition of growth by specific antibody; and (5) susceptibility of antimicrobial agents that inhibit protein synthesis and resistance to agents that affect synthesis of cell walls. They differ from bacteria because they have no cell wall but rather a nonrigid triple-layered membrane encloses the cell. Mycoplasmas are the smallest known free-living organisms. They differ from viruses because they contain both DNA and RNA and because they can grow in cell-free media.

M. hominis is distinguished from *U. urealyticum* by differences in colonial morphology, metabolic characteristics, and susceptibility to antibiotics (Table 7.1). *M. hominis*, an aerobic organism, is recognizable as a "fried egg" colony. The organism converts arginine to ornithine with the liberation of ammonia. This reaction produces a color change when an appropriate pH indicator is incorporated into broth media containing arginine. *U. urealyticum* is a microaerophilic organism characterized by the small colony size and its ability to hydrolyze urea. Urea is an essential substrate for growth and is converted to ammonia. This reaction can be detected by a color change of a pH indicator in broth or agar containing urea.

EPIDEMIOLOGY

Infants become colonized with genital mycoplasmas during the birth process. Presumably the organisms are acquired from a contaminated cervix or vagina, because infants delivered by cesarean section are less frequently colonized with mycoplasmas than those delivered vaginally. Approximately one-third of newborn females have vaginal colonization with *U. urealyticum*, and a smaller percentage harbor *M. hominis*. Mycoplasmas are less frequently recovered from the genital tracts of infant males. Sequential studies have shown a progressive decrease in colonization during the first year of life.

Genital mycoplasmas are uncommon in prepubertal girls. After puberty, colonization with genital mycoplasmas occurs primarily through sexual contact. The recovery rate increases dramatically with the onset of sexual intercourse. A wide range in the recovery rate has been reported for *U. urealyticum* (40 to 95%) and for *M. hominis* (15 to 72%) among sexually active women. Differences in the number of sexual partners often is the sole determinant for the wide range of recovery rates for the genital mycoplasmas. McCormack et al have shown that the colonization rate of genital mycoplasmas is related to the number of sexual partners (3). Ureaplasma was recovered from only 6% of women who have no history of sexual contact, from 37.5% of women with single sexual partners, from 55% of women with two sexual partners, and rose to 75% of women with three or more sexual partners. *M. hominis* was less prevalent but followed a similar pattern.

Table 7.1
Characteristics of Genital Tract
Mycoplasmas

Characteristic		
Colony morphology	Small	Large fried egg
Colony size	20–30 μm	200–300 μm
Metabolic substrate	Urea	Arginine
Aerobic growth	−	+
Antibiotic suscepti- bility		
Tetracycline	+	+
Erythromycin	+	−
Lincomycin	−	+
Clindamycin	−	+
Penicillin	−	−
Cephalosporins	−	−

Genital mycoplasmas are commonly isolated from gravid women at approximately the same recovery rate as in nonpregnant women with the same degree of sexual activity. Braun et al reported that pregnant women at the Boston City Hospital had 79% and 48% isolation rates for *U. urealyticum* and *M. hominis*, respectively; both organisms were recovered in 41% of the study group (4). Genital mycoplasmas have been more frequently recovered from women of lower socioeconomic classes than from private patients and from black women than from white women. Investigations of the role of *M. hominis* and *U. urealyticum* in human disease must take into account this high background prevalence of the genital tract mycoplasmas.

CLINICAL MANIFESTATIONS OF GENITAL MYCOPLASMA INFECTION

Spontaneous Abortion and Stillbirth

Mycoplasmas, both ureaplasmas and *M. hominis*, have been associated with spontaneous abortion since the 1960s. Investigators reported the isolation of genital mycoplasmas from the chorion, amnion, and/or decidua of spontaneously aborted fetuses. However, a causal relationship has not been established. The major unresolved issue is the question of contamination when the products of conception pass through the cervix and vagina. In several studies mycoplasmas, especially ureaplasmas, were isolated more frequently from the fetal membranes of fetuses aborted spontaneously than from those therapeutically aborted. Stray-Pedersen and coworkers isolated ureaplasmas more often

from the endometrium in women who had repeated spontaneous abortions (28%) than from the endometrial cavity in a controlled group (7%) (5). In addition, Harwick and colleagues reported cases of mycoplasma septicemia in the mothers of spontaneous abortions (6). The results of these studies suggest that there is an association between spontaneous abortion and maternal infection or infection of the fetus, or both, because of genital mycoplasmas. However, it is not clear whether the association is valid because of the difficulty in evaluating the comparability of the study groups. Furthermore, the role of other microorganisms was not investigated.

Yet, even though *U. urealyticum* is isolated commonly in amniotic fluid of asymptomatic patients in labor (7), isolation of mycoplasmas from aborted fetuses and stillbirths cannot be explained completely by contamination, as these organisms have been isolated from the lungs, brain, heart, and viscera. Although their presence in the respiratory tract is most likely the result of aspiration of infected or contaminated amniotic fluid, their recovery from heart and viscera is probably indicative of hematogenous spread, either due to invasion of the fetus through the umbilical vessels or dissemination from infected lungs. However, as noted by Taylor-Robinson and McCormack, none of these observations provide an answer to the question of whether abortion occurs because mycoplasmas invade the fetus and cause its death or because the fetus dies from another cause, with subsequent invasion of necrotic tissue by the mycoplasmas (2).

Chromosomal damage and inhibition of mitosis have been observed in human tissue cultures infected with mycoplasmas, but these effects have been seen in vitro only. Mycoplasmas have not been associated with chromosomal abnormalities or congenital anomalies of the human fetus.

Because mycoplasmas are sensitive to antibiotics, it is possible that fetal loss, if caused by these organisms, could be prevented by appropriate antimicrobial therapy. Driscoll and coworkers have reported successful pregnancies after antibiotic therapy in women who were colonized by ureaplasmas and who had a history of frequent spontaneous abortions (8). More recently, Quinn and colleagues reported antibiotic treatment of 62 couples with histories of pregnancy wastage and with positive genital or urinary cultures for mycoplasmas (9). Doxycycline treatment before conception reduced the pregnancy loss rate to 48%, compared to a loss rate of 96% in the "no treatment" group. Erythromycin (250 mg qid from the 2nd or 3rd month until the end of pregnancy) further reduced the pregnancy loss rate to 16%, but this trial was small and poorly controlled. Stray-Pedersen and colleagues used doxycycline to treat women who had had repeated spontaneous abortions and reported that many of the women subsequently had normal pregnancies (5). These findings have led to the concept that subclinical mycoplasma infection is an important cause of spontaneous abortion, especially repeated abortions. However, these studies have not assessed other microorganisms (especially *C. trachomatis* and anaerobes) which are susceptible to the antibiotic regimens. Most significantly, the effectiveness of antibiotics in preventing spontaneous abortion remains controversial because all the antibiotic trials have been uncontrolled.

In summary, the evidence linking the genital mycoplasmas to spontaneous abortion is mainly anecdotal. Establishment of a causal relationship will require large scale investigations which assess other potential pathogens and include placebo-controlled trials of antibiotics in patients who have had repeat spontaneous abortions.

Chorioamnionitis and Neonatal Infection

Shurin and coworkers isolated *U. urealyticum* twice as frequently from neonates whose placentas showed a histologically severe chorioamnionitis than from newborns with less severe or no disease (10). Because inflammation is related to rupture of the membranes and ureaplasmas are more likely to gain access to the amniotic cavity and colonize the fetus when membranes have ruptured, any association between chorioamnionitis and neonatal colonization may be spurious. The chorioamnionitis could be due to any of the other microorganisms that could gain entry to the amniotic cavity at the same time. The data of Shurin and coworkers are impressive because they controlled for duration of membrane rupture and still noted a statistically significant association between chorioamnionitis and ureaplasmal infection.

The role of mycoplasmas in clinically evident amnionitis (also called intraamniotic infection or amniotic fluid infection) has been of interest also. A decade ago, case studies suggested that genital mycoplasmas were the cause of clinical amnionitis (11). In 1983, Blanco and colleagues

reported that *M. hominis* was isolated significantly more often in amniotic fluid of 52 patients with intraamniotic infection (35%) than in amniotic fluid of 52 matched controls (8%; p < 0.001) (7). Yet in the cases of intraamniotic infection (IAI) *M. hominis* was isolated more often (83% (15/18) of cases) in fluid also containing ≥10 (2) colony-forming units per ml of high virulence bacteria. *U. urealyticum*, on the other hand, was isolated in half of the fluids of both clinically infected and control patients. Further understanding of the pathogenic role of *M. hominis* in IAI may be delineated by quantitation of this organism in amniotic fluid, by attempts at isolation from the bloodstream, and by determination of antibody response.

The genital mycoplasmas acquired by the infant during labor have generally not been associated with serious neonatal infection.

Low Birth Weight

In the first systematic study of the effects of mycoplasma on infants, workers at Boston City Hospital reported that 22% of infants weighing less than 2500 g were colonized with *M. hominis* or *U. ureaplasma*, a rate significantly higher than the 12% colonization rate among infants weighing more than 2500 g (12). The colonized infants had a statistically lower mean birth weight (2605 g) than those who were not colonized (2952 g) (12). In a subsequent study at the same institution, it was reported that 28% of infants with a birth weight of 2500 g or less were colonized by ureaplasmas, whereas only 5% of those weighing more than 2500 g were colonized.

In a prospective study, Braun et al reported that women who were colonized with *U. urealyticum* gave birth to infants with a mean birth weight (3099 g) that was statistically lower than the mean birth weight of those not colonized (3297 g) (4). Colonization with mycoplasmas was not associated with other risk factors of low birth weight. Multiple regression analysis indicated that the relation of genital mycoplasmas to birth weight is independent of other variables such as age, race, parity, and maternal weight. Studies of other authors have corroborated the association of low birth weight and mycoplasmas colonization.

In double-blind controlled studies (conducted before the adverse effect of prenatal tetracycline exposure was recognized), tetracycline was administered to pregnant women (13). In these studies, women treated with tetracycline for 6 weeks gave birth to infants weighing less than

2500 g statistically less often than did women who were treated with placebo. These studies suggest an effect of the antibiotic therapy on the microbial flora, including mycoplasmas, which resulted in decreasing the incidence of low birth weight infants. More recently, Kass and colleagues showed an increase in birth weight when women with genital mycoplasmas in the genital tract were treated with erythromycin for the latter half of pregnancy, compared to women given placebo (14). However, microbiologic investigations were not conducted to isolate other microorganisms.

This observation has not been explained. It seems clear that in some populations the association between low birth weight and infection, particularly with ureaplasmas, is a real phenomenon. Despite this association it cannot be definitely concluded that genital mycoplasmas are directly responsible for low birth weight. Perhaps women who have a predisposition to smaller babies are selectively colonized with mycoplasmas. On the other hand, it is also possible that microorganisms present in the birth canal may cause placentitis, which could interfere with the nutrition of the developing fetus and result in lower birth weight.

Thus, an association between mycoplasma colonization of the newborn and/or mother and low birth weight exists, but a causal relation is unproved. In view of the important contribution of low birth weight to perinatal morbidity and mortality, future prospective large scale studies are warranted.

Postpartum Infection

Like other organisms present in the lower genital tract microflora, mycoplasmas can be recovered transiently in the bloodstream following vaginal delivery. McCormack and associates reported that mycoplasmas were recovered from blood cultures obtained a few minutes after delivery from 26 (8%) of 327 women. This bloodstream invasion did not persist and was not associated with postpartum fever (15).

M. hominis has also been isolated from the blood cultures in patients with postpartum fever, and an antibody response was noted in nearly all these cases. McCormack and colleagues and Wallace and co-workers recovered *M. hominis* from the bloodstream of a total of 10 febrile postpartum women (16, 17). In a larger series, Lamey and co-workers isolated bacteria and/or mycoplasmas in 20.8% (26/125) of blood cultures from febrile postpartum women (18). Gen-

ital mycoplasmas were isolated in 12.8% (16/125) of these cultures and from none of 60 afebrile postpartum patients (p < 0.005). *M. hominis* was isolated in nine blood cultures and *U. urealyticum* in eight. Finally, Platt and co-workers reported an association between a fourfold rise in mycoplasmacidal antibody and fever after vaginal delivery (19). Genital mycoplasmas are seldom recovered from the blood of postpartum women who are not febrile. Thus, it appears that *M. hominis* causes postpartum fever, most likely by causing endometritis. In general, the patients have a low-grade fever for 1–2 days, minimal clinical findings, including a mildly tender uterus, and recovery uneventfully even without specific antibiotic therapy.

The frequency with which endometritis due to *M. hominis* occurs without bloodstream invasion and the percentage of endometritis caused by *M. hominis* is not clear. Recent work suggests that *M. hominis* is a common cause of postpartum infection. However, further studies are needed to elucidate the role of mycoplasmas in postpartum infections, especially in relation to that of other microorganisms common to the vaginal flora.

Pelvic Inflammatory Disease

The role of genital mycoplasmas in pelvic inflammatory disease is discussed in Chapter 4. It is probable that mycoplasmas, especially *M. hominis*, have a primary pathogenic role in a proportion of cases of pelvic inflammatory disease (20). Based solely in serologic data, one would estimate that in 25% of patients with PID, *M. hominis* plays a role.

DIAGNOSIS

The diagnosis of mycoplasma infection may be based on isolation of the organism from a site of infection and on demonstration of a rise in antibody. In women, vaginal specimens are more likely to contain mycoplasmas than are specimens obtained from other sites in the lower genital tract. For optimal isolation of mycoplasmas, specimens should be inoculated immediately into medium, kept at 4°C, and transported to the laboratory as soon as possible.

The basic medium is a beef-heart infusion broth, available commercially as pleuropneumonia-like organism (PPLO) broth, supplemented with fresh yeast extract and horse serum. Antibacterials are added to inhibit bacterial growth. The metabolic activity of mycoplasmas can be used to detect their growth in broth medium. Clinical specimens are added to vials of broth containing phenol red and arginine or urea. *M. hominis* metabolizes arginine to ammonia, thus raising the pH of the medium. Ureaplasmas break down urea to form ammonia, resulting in a similar elevation of the pH. Aliquots of the medium from urea broth cultures are subcultured onto agar medium containing urea and manganese sulfate (to detect ammonia); ureaplasma colonies are dark brown and are inhibited by erythromycin discs. If *M. hominis* is present, an alkaline change occurs in the arginine broth. This broth medium is subcultured on basic PPLO agar containing erythromycin; colonies of *M. hominis* appear in 1-4 days which are visualized at ×100 magnification. Positive identification *M. hominis* can be performed by showing inhibition of growth on agar by a paper disc containing anti-*M. hominis* antibodies.

Various serologic procedures, including agglutination, complement fixation, indirect hemagglutination, metabolic inhibition test, and ELISA have been used to detect serologic response to the genital mycoplasmas. In the metabolic inhibition test, specific metabolites (arginine for *M. hominis* and urea for ureaplasmas) are incorporated into broth containing phenol red, organisms, and antibody. The antibody inhibits multiplication and metabolism of homologous organisms, thus preventing a change in color of the pH indicators. With ELISA, specific antibody classes (IgG, M, or A) can be detected. It should be noted that a significant antibody rise indicates a recent infection, but does not demonstrate the site of infection.

TREATMENT

Since the mycoplasmas lack cell walls, they are resistant to cell wall active antimicrobial agents. Thus, the penicillins, cephalosporins, and vancomycin are ineffective. The antimicrobial agents that inhibit protein synthesis are active against most mycoplasmas. Tetracyclines are effective against both *M. hominis* and *U. ureaplasma*. *M. hominis* is sensitive to lincomycin but resistant to erythromycin. Ureaplasmas, on the other hand, are sensitive to erythromycin but not to lincomycin. In addition, *M. hominis* is highly sensitive to clindamycin; ureaplasmas are moderately sensitive to clindamycin. The aminoglycosides have some activity against mycoplasmas.

Because of the still unproved causal relationship between genital mycoplasmas and genital disease, treatment should be restricted to clinical situations where mycoplasmas have either been isolated, or are likely to be isolated, from a body fluid of a focus of infection and appear to be significantly related to the disease process. Thus, treatment of patients with repeated abortions or unexplained infertility should be considered experimental. Furthermore, in clinical conditions involving *M. hominis*, such as intraamniotic infection or puerperal fever, good responses are usually seen even with antibiotics having poor activity against *M. hominis*.

References

1. McCormack WM, Braun P, Lee Y-H, et al: The genital mycoplasmas. *N Engl J Med* 288:78, 1973.
2. Taylor-Robinson D, McCormack WM: The genital mycoplasmas. *N Engl J Med* 302:1003-1010, 1063, 1980.
3. McCormack EM, Almeida PC, Bailey PE: Sexual activity and vaginal colonization with genital mycoplasmas. *JAMA* 221:1375, 1972.
4. Braun P, Lee Y-H, Klein JO, et al: Birth weight and genital mycoplasmas in pregnancy. *N Engl J Med* 284:167, 1971.
5. Stray-Pedersen B, Eng J, Reikvam TM: Uterine T-mycoplasma colonization in reproductive failure. *Am J Obstet Gynecol* 130:307, 1978.
6. Harwick HJ, Purcell RH, Iuppa J, et al: Mycoplasma hominis and abortion. *J Infect Dis* 121:260, 1970.
7. Blanco JD, Gibbs RS, Malherbe H, et al: A controlled study of genital mycoplasmas in amniotic fluid from patients with intra-amniotic infection. *J Infect Dis* 147:650, 1983.
8. Driscoll SG, Kundsin RB, Horne HW, et al: Infections and first trimester losses: possible role of mycoplasmas. *Fertil Steril* 20:1017, 1969.
9. Quinn PA, Shewchuk AB, Shiber J, et al: Efficacy of antibiotic therapy in preventing spontaneous pregnancy loss among couples with genital mycoplasmas. *Am J Obstet Gynecol* 145:239, 1983.
10. Shurin PA, Alpert S, Rosner B, et al: Chorioamnionitis and colonization of the newborn infant with genital mycoplasmas. *N Engl J Med* 293:5, 1975.
11. Brunell PA, Dische RM, Walker MB: Mycoplasma, amnionitis and respiratory distress syndrome. *JAMA* 207:2097, 1969.
12. Klein JO, Buckland D, Finland M: Colonization of newborn infants by mycoplasmas. *N Engl J Med* 280:1025, 1969.
13. Elder HA, Santamaria BAG, Smith S: The natural history of asymptomatic bacteriuria during pregnancy: the effect of tetracycline in clinical course and the outcome of pregnancy. *Am J Obstet Gynecol* 111:441, 1971.
14. Kass EH, McCormack WM, Lin J-S, et al: Genital mycoplasmas as a cause of excess premature delivery. *Trans Assoc Am Phys* 94:261, 1981.
15. McCormack WM, Rosner B, Lee Y-H, et al: Isolation of genital mycoplasmas from blood obtained shortly after vaginal delivery. *Lancet* 1:596, 1975.

16. McCormack WM, Lee Y-H, Lin J-S, et al: Genital mycoplasmas in postpartum fever. *J Infect Dis* 127:193, 1973.

17. Wallace RJ, Alpert S, Browne K, et al: Isolation of *Mycoplasma hominis* from blood cultures of patients with postpartum fever. *Obstet Gynecol* 51:181, 1978.

18. Lamey JR, Eschenbach DA, Mitchell SM, et al: Isolation of mycoplasmas and bacteria from the blood of postpartum women. *Am J Obstet Gynecol* 143:104, 1982.

19. Platt R, Lin-J-L, Warren JW, et al: Infection with *Mycoplasma hominis* in postpartum fever. *Lancet* 2:1217, 1980.

20. Moller B: The role of mycoplasmas in upper genital tract of women. *Sex Transm Dis* 10:281, 1983.

CHAPTER 8

Chlamydial Infections

The United States is currently in the midst of an epidemic of sexually transmitted diseases (STD). Parallel with concern over this major public health problem has been the recognition that a much broader spectrum of STD exists. Included in this expanded scope of STD are over 20 diseases, syndromes, and complications in addition to the classic venereal diseases of gonorrhea, syphilis, chancroid, lymphogranuloma venereum, and granuloma inguinale. The most prevalent of these STD in the United States is *Chlamydia trachomatis*. During the past decade, an increasing number of sexually transmitted infections have been attributed to *C. trachomatis* (1, 2) (Table 8.1). Chlamydial infections are more common than gonococcal infections, and it is currently estimated that there are upwards of 3 million chlamydial infections annually in the United States (3–5). Economically it is estimated that more than $1 billion in direct and indirect costs are expended annually on chlamydial infections (6).

C. trachomatis has long been known as the causative agent of trachoma, a disease which is hyperendemic in many developing countries and considered to be the leading preventable cause of blindness in the world (7). In addition, chlamydia is the pathogen long known to cause inclusion conjunctivitis in the newborn and lymphogranuloma venereum (LGV). More recently, chlamydial infections of the genital tract and the consequences of perinatal exposure, both maternal and neonatal, have received considerable attention (8).

Although *C. trachomatis* affects and causes important diseases in men, women, and infants, this review will primarily focus on the genital tract disease associated with chlamydial infections in women and in the newborn. Indeed, it is women that bear the brunt of the chlamydia burden because of their increased risk for adverse reproductive consequences. With the increasing awareness for the role of *C. trachomatis* as a sexual pathogen has come an increased awareness by clinicians of the chlamydia prob-

lem. *C. trachomatis* is a high prevalence agent and is associated with a wide variety of complications. In addition, an unknown percent of chlamydial infection progresses to complications such as acute salpingitis. Other long-term consequences of chlamydial infection include infertility, ectopic pregnancies, neonatal conjunctivitis, and chlamydial pneumonia of the newborn; an association of chlamydial infection with fetal wastage, premature ruptured membranes, preterm labor and/or delivery, and postpartum endometritis has been suggested.

THE ORGANISM

The characteristics of the two species which make up the genus *Chlamydia* are characterized in Table 8.2. *Chlamydia psittaci* is the causative agent of psittacosis, a common pathogen in avian species and lower mammals. *C. trachomatis* seems to be a specifically human pathogen (except for a few strains of rodent origin). *C. psittaci* is differentiated from *C. trachomatis* on the basis of sulfonamide resistance and failure of inclusions to stain with iodine. *C. trachomatis* is sensitive to sulfonamides and has iodine-staining inclusions.

Although all chlamydiae share a common genus-specific antigen, *C. trachomatis* may be further differentiated on serologic basis. There are currently 15 serotypes recognized (2) (Table 8.2). The *C. trachomatis* serotypes are responsible for three major groups of infections. Three of these serotypes (L1, L2, L3) represent the agents causing lymphogranuloma venereum. LGV appear to have different receptor sites and a much broader tissue spectrum in vivo and host spectrum in vitro than the other *C. trachomatis* strains. In addition, the LGV serotypes are more invasive than the remaining chlamydial serotypes. Serotypes A, B, Ba, and C are the agents responsible for endemic blinding trachoma. The remaining serotypes of *C. trachomatis* (D, E, F, G, H, I, J, K) are the sexually transmitted agents which cause inclusion conjunctivitis, newborn pneumonia, urethritis, cervicitis, epididymitis,

Table 8.1.
Clinical Spectrum of Sexually Transmitted *C. Trachomatis* Infections

Men	Women	Infants
Urethritis	Cervicitis	Conjunctivitis
Postgonococcal urethritis	Bartholinitis	Pneumonia
Epididymitis	Endometritis	Asymptomatic pharyngeal carriage
Prostatitis	Salpingitis	Asymptomatic gastrointestinal tract carriage
Proctitis	Perihepatitis	Otitis media[a]
Conjunctivitis	Urethritis	
Pharyngitis	Lymphogranuloma venereum	
Lymphogranuloma venereum	Conjunctivitis	
Reiter's syndrome	Pharyngitis	
Sterility	Sterility	
	Dysplasia[a]	
	Postpartum endometritis[a]	
	Prematurity[a]	
	Stillbirth[a]	

[a] Indicates relationship not firmly established.

Table 8.2.
Chlamydiae: Taxonomy and Association with Human Disease

Chlamydia psittaci		*C. trachomatis*	
Resistant to sulfonamides		Sensitive to sulfonamides	
Inclusions do not stain with iodine		Inclusions stain with iodine	
Common pathogen in birds and lower mammals		Mostly of human origin	
Serotypes	Disease	Serotypes	Disease
Many	Psittacosis	A, B, Ba, C	Hyperendemic blinding trachoma
		D, E, F, G, H, I, J, K	Inclusion conjunctivitis, nongonococcal urethritis, cervicitis, salpingitis, proctitis, epididymitis, pneumonia of newborn
		L1, L2, L3	Lymphogranuloma venereum

salpingitis, acute urethral syndrome, and perinatal infections.

The chlamydiae are separated into their own order, Chlamydiales, on the basis of a unique growth cycle (Fig. 8.1), which distinguishes them from all other microorganisms (9). The chlamydial organism exists in two forms: (1) the elementary body which is the infectious particle and capable of entering uninfected cells, and (2) the initial body which multiplies by binary fission to produce the inclusions that are identified in properly stained cells.

The initiation of infection depends on what appears to be specific attachment sites on susceptible host cells (10). After the chlamydial particle (the elementary body is the infectious particle) attaches to the host cell, it is ingested by a phagocytic process which is similar to ordinary bacterial phagocytosis (11). This process is an enhanced phagocytosis, which is directed by the chlamydiae; chlamydial particles are selectively taken up by the susceptible host cell. Intracellularly, chlamydiae exist within a cytoplasmic vacuole. Chlamydiae remain within this phagosome throughout their entire growth cycle. It has been suggested that in this state chlamydiae may be protected from host defense mechanisms, and such protection perhaps is responsible for the chronicity of certain chlamydial infections (13). This cycle takes approximately 48 hr to complete, and while in the cell, the infecting elementary body undergoes reorganization into what is called a reticulate or initial body, which represents the metabolically active and dividing form of the organism. These forms are not infectious and will not survive outside the cell. They divide for approximately 8–24 or 36 hr and then condense and reorganize to form new elementary bodies which are released when the infected cell bursts. For their entire intracellular life, the chlamydiae reside within the phagosome, but they successfully prevent phagolysosomal fusion (10). Recognition of the characteristic cytoplasmic inclusion is the means by which chlamydiae are detected. Infectivity increases as the number of elementary bodies increases, and by 48–72 hr, the host cell bursts and liberates these infectious particles. The cycle then starts anew. The complete infectious cycle takes 2–3 days.

C. trachomatis is an obligatory intracellular bacterium (9). It is an extremely well-adapted human parasite which depends on the host cell for nutrients and energy (12). Although chla-

mydiae are capable of limited metabolic activities, they do not possess an enzyme system capable of generating ATP and have been considered energy parasites. Primarily they inhabit columnar and pseudostratified columnar epithelial surfaces. Although chlamydiae do not stain with the gram stain, in many respects they are bacteria-like. They contain DNA and RNA, are susceptible to certain antibiotics, have a rigid cell wall, similar in structure and content to that of a gram-negative bacteria, and multiply by binary fission. However, they differ from bacteria but are similar to viruses in that they are obligate intracellular parasites and may be regarded as bacteria that have adapted to an intracellular environment. Thus, they need viable cells for their multiplication and survival.

EPIDEMIOLOGY AND TRANSMISSION

C. trachomatis (serotypes A, B, Ba, C) has long been recognized as the causative agent of

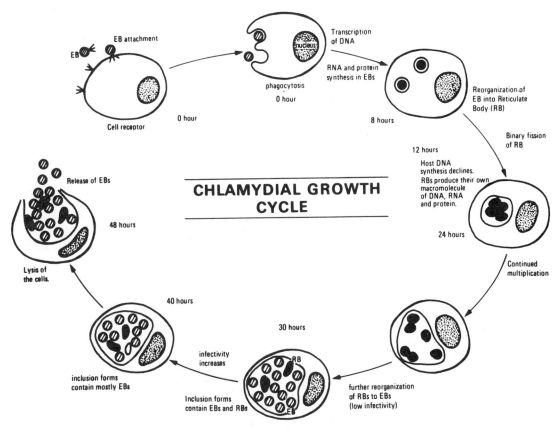

Figure 8.1. Chlamydial growth cycle. *EB*, elementary body. *RB*, reticulate body. (From Thompson SE, Washington AE: Epidemiology of sexually transmitted *Chlamydia trachomatis* infections. *Epidemiol Rev* 5:96–123, 1983.)

trachoma, a chronic conjunctivitis affecting hundreds of millions of people in developing countries and resulting in millions of cases of blindness. However, the child to child and intra-familial patterns of infection in trachoma endemic areas are not applicable to the clinical manifestation of infections associated with the oculogenital *C. trachomatis* strains (serotypes D, E, F, G, H, I, J, and K).

For these oculogenital serotypes, which are the major focus in this chapter, the primary method of transmission is sexual. Schachter (1) has stated that *C. trachomatis* is probably the most common sexually transmitted pathogen in Western industrialized society (1). Chlamydiae cause between one-third and one-half of nongonococcal urethritis in men (14, 15). Double infections with gonococci are common in both men and women, and between 20 and 40% of men and between 40 and 60% of women with lower genital gonorrheal infection have concomitant chlamydial infection (14–16). Men having gonorrhea and being treated with penicillins often develop postgonococcal urethritis due to this concomitant chlamydial infection. Epididymitis is an important complication of chlamydial infection of the male urethra (17), and *C. trachomatis* is the major cause of epididymitis in men under the age of 35. Rectal and pharyngeal infections also occur in both sexes (18–20).

A number of clinical conditions in the female have been attributed to *C. trachomatis* (21). These include cervicitis, endometritis, salpingitis, urethral syndrome, urethritis, and perinatal infections. The anatomic site within the female genital tract which is most commonly infected with *C. trachomatis* is the cervix. Unfortunately, there are no specific symptoms associated with the cervical infections, and thus many of the chlamydial infections of the cervix are clinically inapparent. This is unfortunate because mucopurulent cervicitis (the female equivalent of nongonococcal urethritis) caused by *C. trachomatis* predisposes to acute pelvic inflammatory disease in nonpregnant women and to maternal and infant infections during pregnancy. In addition, asymptomatic chlamydial cervicitis is a major reservoir for sexual transmission of *C. trachomatis*. Many sexually active women have been exposed to chlamydiae; from 20% to 40% have microimmunofluorescent chlamydial antibody titers. Most of the women with antibody titers against chlamydia do not have a current infection. In general, between 3 and 5% of unselected nonpregnant women have *C. trachomatis* isolated from their cervices. In selected populations *C. trachomatis* is more prevalent. *C. trachomatis* has been recovered from 15–33% of patients examined in venereal disease clinics (22–26), from 29–68% of female consorts of men with nongonococcal urethritis (14, 24, 27–30), in 67–74% of female consorts of men with culture positive *C. trachomatis* urethritis (14, 27, 30), and from 34–63% of women with mucopurulent endocervicitis (25, 31). In a recent screening program in family planning clinics in Northern and Central California, Schachter et al demonstrated that from 5.5 to 22.5% of asymptomatic women were positive for *C. trachomatis* (32). Overall, there were 265 (9%) of 2935 cultures positive for chlamydia. Among pregnant women, the prevalence of chlamydial cervical infection has ranged from 2 to 30% (33–40).

A general consensus is that in the United States 4–5% of sexually active women carry chlamydia in their cervix. However, high risk populations can be readily identified. A number of studies have shown that the same populations that are at risk for other sexually transmitted infections are at highest risk for chlamydial infections. Thus, young unwed mothers are often found to have high rates of chlamydial infections of the cervix (37, 39). Additional high risk groups include women on oral contraceptives (24, 27), women with cervical ectopy (3, 23, 27, 30), and women who are partners of men with nongonococcal urethritis (14, 24, 27–30). In both sexually active asymptomatic and symptomatic women, there is a higher incidence of *C. trachomatis* than of *Neisseria gonorrhoeae* or herpesvirus hominis. Schachter previously reported that the carriage rate for asymptomatic women in San Francisco was 3.5% for chlamydia, as compared to 0.5% for herpesviruses and 0.4% for gonococci. In symptomatic women, although the herpesvirus and gonococci increased significantly, the chlamydiae still were more common, with an isolation rate of 15% versus 5.3% of herpesviruses and 4.7% for gonococci (3). This pattern of chlamydia being recovered from the cervices of sexually active asymptomatic women 5–7 times more frequently than gonorrhea has recently been confirmed by Schachter's review (32) of the family planning clinic experience in California, where the overall GC recovery rate is less than 1% compared to the *C. trachomatis* rate of 9%. The majority of women with chlamydial disease remain untreated because their infection is either asymptomatic or relatively inapparent. If not treated, the infection can persist for several years (1).

Over 1 million women acquire pelvic inflammatory disease (PID) each year in the United States. Recent studies in the U.S. suggest that 20–30% of these cases are associated with *C. trachomatis* (41). Thus, 200,000–300,000 cases of chlamydia-associated PID occur annually in the U.S. and are estimated to require over 400,000 physician office visits and 40,000 hospitalizations each year. The implications of these data are discussed in greater detail in Chapter 4. Washington has estimated that 50,000 women/year are involuntarily rendered infertile due to chlamydial infections in the U.S. (6). In addition, these women are exposed to a significantly increased risk for ectopic pregnancies.

The infant born to a woman with a chlamydial infection of the cervix is at 60–70% risk of acquiring the infection during passage through the birth canal (33–36). Approximately 25–50% of exposed infants will develop chlamydial conjunctivitis in the first 2 weeks of life, and 10–20% of the infants will develop chlamydial pneumonia within 3–4 months of birth. In utero transmission is not known to occur. Those infants delivered by cesarean section are not at risk of acquiring chlamydial infection via vertical transmission from maternal cervical infection. Prolonged ruptured membranes prior to cesarean section might be an exception to this statement.

Attack rates for inclusion conjunctivitis of the newborn in prospective studies have ranged from 7 to 63/1000 live births, and attack rates of chlamydial pneumonia have ranged from 3 to 10/1000 live births (1, 33–40). Studies of serial admissions for pneumonia in infants of less than 6 months have implicated *C. trachomatis* in 10–50% of these cases. Thus, chlamydial infection is responsible for a major portion of pneumonias in this age group.

CLINICAL SPECTRUM OF CHLAMYDIAL INFECTION

C. trachomatis has been recovered from multiple sites in the male anogenital tract. These include the urethra (1, 14–16), epididymis (17, 42), prostate (42, 43), and rectum (44). There has been considerable data presented over the past decade demonstrating that *C. trachomatis* is a primary pathogen in infections involving these sites.

C. trachomatis is a major cause of nongonococcal urethritis (NGU) (1, 14) and postgonococcal urethritis (PGU). Nongonococcal urethritis is an extremely common sexually transmitted disease. In Great Britain, where NGU is a reportable disease, it is now three times as common as gonorrhea in men. In the United States, where national statistics are not available, it is estimated that NGU is at least twice as common as gonorrhea and that 2.5 million cases of NGU occur each year in the U.S. Investigations have shown that *C. trachomatis* can be isolated from 26 to 72% of men with NGU; most investigators report isolation of *C. trachomatis* in 25–50% of NGU (16). In contradistinction, chlamydiae have been recovered from less than 7% of asymptomatic men without disease. In addition to the high isolation rates for *C. trachomatis* from men with NGU, other data support the etiologic role of *C. trachomatis* in NGU. Sexual partners of men with chlamydial NGU have positive endocervical cultures for *C. trachomatis* in 45–68% of cases while only 4–18% of sexual partners of controls or men with chlamydia-negative nongonococcal urethritis have recovery of *C. trachomatis* (12, 14, 17, 45). Seroconversion with rising titers of immunoglobulin G antibody or presence of immunoglobulin M antibody occurs more frequently among men with chlamydia-positive NGU than in those with chlamydia-negative NGU (14, 45). Chlamydia-positive NGU responds better clinically to antimicrobial agents with demonstrated in vitro activity against *C. trachomatis* than to agents without such activity (15). Several investigators have fulfilled Koch's postulates by establishing *C. trachomatis* urethral infections in experimental primates (46, 47).

Between 20 and 40% of men with urethral gonorrhea have concomitant *C. trachomatis* isolated from the urethra. While postgonococcal urethritis will develop in 5–38% of patients with chlamydia-negative gonococcal urethritis, this complication will develop in approximately 80–100% of men with chlamydia-positive gonococcal urethritis (48–51). Because chlamydial infections do not respond to the short course of penicillins used to treat gonorrhea, these men have a persistent urethritis despite eradication of *N. gonorrhoeae*. Diagnosis of NGU is made in men who either complain of dysuria, frequency, or discharge, or have urethral discharge on examination; who are found to have an abnormal number of polymorphonuclear cells in the urethral discharge or first-voided urine specimen; and who do not have the typical gram-negative intracellular diplococci suggestive of gonorrhea or a culture positive for gonorrhea. Establishing that NGU is due to *C. trachomatis* requires chlamydial isolation or use of monoclonal antibody-staining of direct smears (Tam et al (127)).

Patients with NGU should be treated with tetracycline hydrochloride (500 mg four times/day for at least 7 days or doxycycline 100 mg b.i.d. for 7 days). Because of the high incidence of concomitance between *N. gonorrhoeae* and *C. trachomatis*, it has been recommended by the Center for Disease Control that tetracycline (2 g/day for 7 days) be considered as a first treatment choice for gonorrhea. Thus, it seems that a tetracycline regimen is a reasonable treatment of choice for all male urethritis. If tetracycline is contraindicated, erythromycin or sulfisoxazole for 14 days can be given. Because of concern over compliance with a 7-day tetracycline regimen, a combined approach for treatment of uncomplicated gonorrhea has been suggested. An initial single-dose regimen effective against *N. gonorrhoeae* (i.e., ampicillin 3.5 g with 1.0 g probenecid) is followed by a 7-day course of tetracycline. Routine treatment of female sex partners of men with NGU is indicated. One-third of women whose male partners have NGU will have a chlamydial infection of the cervix; more than two-thirds of those whose male partners with NGU are chlamydia-positive will have such infections.

Epididymitis

A major role for *C. trachomatis* causing epididymitis in young men under the age of 35 has recently been suggested by the investigation of Berger et al, with the isolation of *C. trachomatis* from epididymal aspirates in five of six men (17). Epididymitis thus appears to be a major complication of chlamydial urethritis in men, and *C. trachomatis* appears to be the cause of "idiopathic" epididymitis. Recently it has been suggested that 50% of the estimated 500,000 cases of acute epididymitis that occur in the U.S. annually are due to *C. trachomatis* (4). In men over the age of 35, coliform organisms were the major cause of epididymitis.

Prostatitis

A link between chlamydial infection and prostatitis has not been definitely established. Paavonen estimated that prostatitis accompanies NGU in up to 20% of cases (45). Mardh and co-workers suggested that *C. trachomatis* is associated with acute rather than chronic prostatitis (43). However, Bruce et al recovered *C. trachomatis* from early morning urine specimens and/or prostatic fluid or semen in 56% of 70 patients with chronic prostatitis (42).

Proctitis

Chlamydiae have been associated with proctitis in both men and women (18, 20). Quinn et al have recently demonstrated that non-LGV immunotypes of *C. trachomatis* are associated with a mild proctitis, with or without symptoms in male homosexual populations (52). In 96 homosexual men with symptoms suggestive of proctitis, 8 isolates of *C. trachomatis* (non-LGV type) were obtained.

Reiter's Syndrome

Reiter's syndrome develops in some men following bouts of nongonococcal urethritis. Kousa and co-workers isolated *C. trachomatis* from 60% of men with Reiter's syndrome and signs of urethritis (53). Schachter has suggested that *C. trachomatis* infection may be a trigger mechanism for Reiter's syndrome. For instance, modification by chlamydiae of the membrane of the cytoplasmic vacuole in which chlamydiae exist intracellularly could trigger an autoimmune reaction. However, because Reiter's syndrome seems to occur in a genetically predisposed population (approximately 95% of patients are HLA B-27 positive) and the agent is rarely recovered from extragenital sites, the exact relationship of chlamydia to this disease still remains obscure (54).

LOWER GENITAL DISEASE OF WOMEN

As described by Thompson and Washington, the clinical spectrum and epidemiology of *C. trachomatis* infection in women are similar to those associated with gonococcal infection (13). However, there are also major differences. Chlamydial infection may be asymptomatic, may be associated with nonspecific symptoms, or may exist in the absence of any visible signs of infection. The diagnosis can only be proven by culture or use of monoclonal antibody technology.

Despite the absence of clinically apparent disease, women infected with *C. trachomatis* may harbor the organism for long periods of time. The incubation period for *C. trachomatis* is probably 6–14 days, which is considerably longer than that for *N. gonorrhoeae*.

As a result of the longer incubation period, the high rate of asymptomatic infection, and the persistent carrier state, there exists a large reservoir of *C. trachomatis* infection in the population.

Bartholinitis

Davies and co-workers recovered *C. trachomatis* from Bartholin duct exudates in 9 of 30 patients (55). Concurrent infections with gonococci were present in seven of these patients. The two without gonococcal concomitant infection were sexual partners of men with NGU. Although it is possible that the chlamydial isolation reflected contamination of the vulval epithelium by *C. trachomatis* from the cervical or urethral infection, it seems reasonable that *C. trachomatis* can cause a true infection of the Bartholin gland duct. At the present time, the proportion of cases of bartholinitis that may be regarded as chlamydial is not known.

Endocervicitis

The anatomic site within the female genital tract which is most commonly infected with *C. trachomatis* is the cervix. The organism can be shown to cause endocervicitis. However, it is clear that asymptomatic infections also occur. *C. trachomatis*, however, will not cause vaginitis, as it does not appear to grow in vaginal squamous cells. The organism seems to be a specific parasite of squamocolumnar cells, and thus grows only within the transitional zone and the endocervix. It is not associated with ectocervicitis. The infected cervix may range from a clinically normal examination to a severely eroded cervix with a hypertrophic cervical erosion and a mucopurulent endocervical discharge. Dunlap and co-workers were the first to describe follicle-like lesions (similar to those seen in the conjunctivae) that occur in the cervix in association with chlamydial infection (18). They describe this finding of follicular cervicitis in 90% of mothers whose babies had chlamydial inclusion conjunctivitis of the newborn. Rees and co-workers employed colposcopy to evaluate the sexual partners of men with NGU (48). Of the women with positive endocervical cultures for *C. trachomatis*, more than 80% had hypertrophic cervicitis with mucopurulent endocervical discharge. Paavonen et al have recently confirmed this association between mucopurulent endocervicitis and isolation of *C. trachomatis* from the endocervix (56). These workers used the term "positive swab test" to connote the presence of a yellow or green discoloration to an endocervical swab secondary to the presence of a mucopurulent endocervical discharge.

The complex microflora of the lower genital tract makes it difficult to delineate a single pathogen as the putative agent in cervicitis. However, recent data indicate that *C. trachomatis* is a major etiologic agent in mucopurulent endocervicitis. Paavonen reported that *C. trachomatis* is recovered from the cervix with greater frequency in women with signs of cervicitis than in those without such signs (56). More recently, Paavonen has noted that severe inflammatory atypia and/or dyskaryotic changes in Pap smears occurred significantly more frequently in chlamydia-positive than in chlamydia-negative women (57). Mardh and co-workers have suggested that this chlamydia-associated atypia represents a reparative atypia related to an infectious process (58). Paavonen et al obtained cervical biopsy specimens during colposcopy in patients with *C. trachomatis* isolation from the cervix. Severe inflammatory changes were noted in 45% of cases; the inflammation was characterized by heavy leukocytic and lymphocytic infiltration and intraepithelial microabscesses and by epithelial necrosis and ulceration (59). In addition, cervical dysplasia occurred significantly more often in *C. trachomatis* culture-positive patients than in age-matched controls with signs of cervicitis on clinical examination but without the presence of sexually transmissible organisms (59). Schachter and co-workers demonstrated that patients with cervical neoplasia had a significant excess of anti-chlamydia antibodies, as compared to that of controls (60). Ectopy is often associated with *C. trachomatis*, but it can be induced by a number of other stimuli. In addition to ectopy, other frequently associated findings with *C. trachomatis* cervical infection include use of oral contraceptives, partners of men with NGU, and age under 20 years. The suggested clinical criteria for a diagnosis of mucopurulent endocervicitis includes the presence of ectopy, edema, erythema, and friability, and demonstration of 10 white blood cells per high power field and a positive swab test.

Rees and colleagues noted that only two organisms are found to be associated with chronic cervicitis and purulent endocervical discharge; these are *C. trachomatis* and *N. gonorrhoeae* (48). It seems justified for the clinician lacking availability of chlamydial isolation facilities to consider managing cervicitis in the same manner that nongonococcal urethritis in the male is managed; thus, he would test for other pathogens, such as *N. gonorrhoeae* and, if they are not found, treat with tetracyclines for the chlamydial infection. Chlamydial infections of the cervix respond to antichlamydial therapy. The recommended regimens are 2 g/day for 7 days or 1 g/day for 14 days of tetracycline orally. Alternately, doxycyline 100 mg b.i.d. for 7 days could be used. Erythromycin in similar dosages would be indicated for pregnant women or those unable to tolerate tetracycline. Bowie has recently demonstrated that sulfisoxazole (2 g daily for 10 days) is also an effective alternative (61).

It seems apparent that cervical infection with *C. trachomatis* is a major reservoir for the male and neonatal infections associated with this agent. In addition, the cervix is the source for major complications involving the upper genital tract, such as acute salpingitis. Thus, it is imperative that efforts be made to identify those women who are symptomatic and asymptomatic carriers of *C. trachomatis* in their cervix.

Acute Urethral Syndrome

The acute urethral syndrome, which is defined as acute dysuria and frequent urination in women with pyuria but whose voided urine is sterile or contains less than 10^5 microorganisms/ml, is a common and perplexing problem for the clinician. Paavonen noted that 25% of women whose male partners had chlamydial urethritis had chlamydial infection in their urethra (62). Recently, Stamm and co-workers have identified a causative role for *C. trachomatis* in up to 25% of women presenting with the acute urethral syndrome (63). These workers were able to show that *C. trachomatis* infection was present in 10 of the 16 patients with the urethral syndrome, sterile bladder urine, and pyuria. Among the 32 patients with the urethral syndrome and sterile bladder urine, evidence of recent infection with *C. trachomatis* was demonstrated in 10 of 16 with pyuria, while only 1 of 16 without pyuria had such evidence. On the other hand, *C. trachomatis* was unlikely to be recovered from women with acute cystitis or those women with the urethral syndrome and bladder bacteriuria.

It should be recognized, however, that the majority of the *C. trachomatis* isolates were obtained from the cervix of women with the acute urethral syndrome in these studies. In only 4 of the 10 women with acute urethral syndrome and sterile pyuria was *C. trachomatis* isolated from the urethral cultures. The remaining patients either had cervical isolates or four-fold rises in antibodies to *C. trachomatis*. The clinician must be aware that *C. trachomatis* will not be recovered from the urine, but that culture attempts must be performed via urethral swabs.

Several findings on history are suggestive of *C. trachomatis* being the causative agent in women presenting with symptoms of acute urethral syndrome (63). These include a recent change in sexual partner, the use of oral contraceptives, and a longer duration of presenting symptoms (approximately 14 days), as compared to women with acute cystitis or bacteriuria who present within 4 days. In addition, women with chlamydia associated as the cause of their acute urethral syndrome are less likely to give a history of recurrent urinary tract infections, which is in contradistinction to those women with acute cystitis or bladder bacteriuria.

More recently, Stamm and colleagues have shown that antimicrobial therapy of the acute urethral syndrome which utilized an agent effective against *C. trachomatis* was significantly more effective than placebo in eradicating urinary symptoms, pyuria, and the infecting microorganism among women with the urethral syndrome due to coliforms, staphylococci, or *C. trachomatis* (64). In contradistinction, those women with acute urethral syndrome and no pyuria did not benefit from antibiotic therapy.

Nonpuerperal Endometritis

Recent investigations have suggested that endometritis in nonpregnant women is another manifestation of genital chlamydial infection (65, 66). Mardh and co-workers (65) recovered *C. trachomatis* from the endometrium of three women with concomitant signs of salpingitis. These workers suggested that chlamydia ascends from the cervix and affects the uterine mucosa and then spreads intracanalicularly from the endometrium to the fallopian tubes. Interestingly, these workers noted that the endometrial cultures could be positive despite negative cervical cultures. More recently, Mardh et al reported that in 9 of 18 patients with laparoscopically confirmed PID, *C. trachomatis* was recovered from endometrial aspirates (58). Endometrial biopsy specimens in women in whom *C. trachomatis* was isolated demonstrated heavy infiltration of monocytes. Similarly, Paavonen has confirmed the presence histologically of endometritis (based on presence of 5 plasma cells per high power field) in 47% of women with chlamydial endocervicitis (67). Recently, Sweet et al also recovered *C. trachomatis* from the endometrial cavity of women with signs and symptoms of acute salpingitis (41). In this report *C. trachomatis* was recovered from the endometrial cavity in 17 of 71 (24%) patients with acute salpingitis. Despite prompt clinical response to antibiotic therapy, 13 women treated with β-lactam antibiotics still had positive endometrial cultures for *C. trachomatis* at posttherapy evaluation. This suggests the presence of a subclinical, persistent chlamydial endometritis among patients with resolving acute PID.

Acute Salpingitis

The most serious systemic complication of chlamydial infection in women is acute salpingitis. The role of *C. trachomatis* as a pathogen in this disease has received considerable recent attention. Interestingly, the association of chlamydial infection of the female genital tract (as determined by giving birth to an infant that developed inclusion conjunctivitis of the newborn) and pelvic inflammatory disease in the postpartum patient was initially recognized by ophthalmologists in the 1930s (68).

There is considerable evidence from European investigations (predominantly Scandinavian) that *C. trachomatis* is an important etiologic agent in acute salpingitis (69–75). However, the rate at which this disease occurs is not known, and there is controversy as to the importance of this agent in various geographic locales. Scandinavian investigations suggest that approximately half of acute salpingitis occurring in that area is due to *C. trachomatis* (69–75), whereas in North America, results have not been as clear cut (67–78). The first direct evidence of an association with *C. trachomatis* in acute salpingitis was documented by Eilard and colleagues, who isolated *C. trachomatis* from tubal specimens in 2 of 22 women with acute salpingitis undergoing laparoscopy (69). Of major importance was the report of Mardh et al of a 30% isolation of *C. trachomatis* from the fallopian tubes of women with acute salpingitis in whom isolation attempts were performed on material aspirated from the involved fallopian tubes visualized by laparoscopy (70).

In addition to the isolation studies previously noted, a number of investigations have indirectly associated acute salpingitis with chlamydial infection. Paavonen et al recovered *C. trachomatis* from the cervix in 51 (33%) of 156 women with acute salpingitis (73). In Scandinavia, serologic studies have indicated that *C. trachomatis* is a frequent causative agent in acute salpingitis. Treharne and colleagues suggested that *C. trachomatis* is the probable etiologic agent in 67% of 143 women with pelvic inflammatory disease in their investigation (72).

They reported high levels of chlamydial antibody, both in sera and fluids aspirated from the cul-de-sac. These antibody titers were correlated with the severity of clinically graded tubal inflammation seen at the time of laparoscopy. Paavonen in Finland provided additional indirect support for the concept that acute salpingitis may in many cases be due to infection with *C. trachomatis*. This group of investigators reported that 26% of salpingitis patients showed serial conversion in a single agent immunofluorescent test (71). In paired sera, 10 (46%) of 22 chlamydia-positive patients and 9 (18%) of 50 chlamydia-negative patients showed significant (greater than four-fold) change in immunofluorescent antibody titer; the positive cultures were obtained from the cervix in this patient group. This difference was statistically significant. In a subsequent report, 32 of 167 (19%) of salpingitis patients demonstrated a four-fold rise in chlamydial antibody (74). Mardh and colleagues recently reported that antibodies to *C. trachomatis*, either IgM or IgG or both were present in the sera from 80% of patients with acute salpingitis (75). By comparison, in the control group of 50 women, antibodies to *C. trachomatis* were noted in only 8%. This group of Swedish investigators also demonstrated that the results of the chlamydial antibody test correlated with the severity of the tubal inflammation as shown by laparoscopy. Taken together, these studies from Scandinavia suggest that the major etiologic agent for acute salpingitis in that geographic area is *C. trachomatis*. This is a dramatic change in the etiologic pattern from that of the previous decades. In the middle 1960s almost 50% of acute salpingitis cases in this area had gonorrhea, whereas at the present time, less than 10% of all salpingitis cases are infected with gonococci. Based on culture data (30%) and based on serologic data, somewhere between 30 and 67% of acute salpingitis is now associated with chlamydia as the etiologic agent in Scandinavia.

Until recently, in the United States, evidence suggested that chlamydia-associated acute salpingitis was much less frequent than what has been reported from Scandinavia (76–78). In the United States, initial studies noted the recovery of *C. trachomatis* from the fallopian tube or cul-de-sac aspirate in 0–10% of patients with acute salpingitis (76–78). Sweet and co-workers did not isolate a single *C. trachomatis* from the fallopian tube exudate of 37 women undergoing laparoscopic evaluation with a confirmed diagnosis of acute salpingitis (78). Eschenbach and colleagues recovered chlamydia on one occasion from 102 patients (76), and Thompson and co-workers were able to recover chlamydia from intraperitoneal sites from 3 of 30 patients with acute salpingitis; however, 2 of their 3 isolates were from the cul-de-sac fluid, and it is uncertain whether this reflected vaginal contamination or true intraperitoneal infection (77). Indirect evidence for *C. trachomatis* as a causative agent for acute salpingitis in the United States did, however, exist. Cervical isolation rates in patients diagnosed to have acute salpingitis ranged from 5 to 20% (76–78). More recently, Bowie et al have presented evidence that supports a major etiologic role for *C. trachomatis* in acute salpingitis in North America. In a venereal disease clinic in Vancouver, they reported that *C. trachomatis* was recovered from the cervix of 50% of women diagnosed as having pelvic inflammatory disease, compared to 20% of women attending the venereal disease clinic who did not have acute salpingitis (79). In summary, studies emanating from Scandinavia demonstrated a 2-fold increased cervical isolation rate of *C. trachomatis* and a 20-fold increased fallopian tube isolation rate, as compared to the initial U.S. studies. Despite apparent differences in these recovery rates, the serologic evidence for an association between chlamydia and PID were quite similar.

These documented differences in the initial studies between isolation rates in Sweden and the United States lead to controversy relative to the role of *C. trachomatis* as an etiologic agent in acute salpingitis in North America. Several factors were postulated to explain these differences between Swedish isolation rates and those in the United States. Firstly, there were significant differences in the methods of collecting specimens. Swedish investigations utilized needle aspiration and/or needle biopsy of the fimbria at the time of laparoscopy. In the U.S., culture attempts had been made on purulent exudates. Because *C. trachomatis* is an intracellular organism, successful isolation may require the presence of fresh infected cells in the innoculum. Recently, in an animal model, Schachter et al noted that *C. trachomatis* can be recovered from the tissue of the fallopian tube for a much greater period than it can be recovered from the tubal exudate (80). A second explanation for these differences may be that the high rate of GC in the United States (30–80%) in salpingitis patients may submerge the role of *C. trachomatis* in this country, while in Sweden, with a 10% prevalence rate of GC in salpingitis patients,

chlamydia has assumed a prominent role in the etiology of this disease. A third possible explanation is that the patient groups which have been studied in the United States and Sweden are not comparable. Investigations utilizing intraperitoneal cultures in the United States have been based on hospitalized patients who in general have presented to emergency rooms with acute disease. Swedish investigators, on the other hand, admit all patients with acute salpingitis. Svensson et al noted that patients presenting with acute salpingitis and *C. trachomatis* tend to have a milder clinical disease, are less often febrile, and have had mild symptoms for longer periods of time than women admitted with gonococcal or nongonococcal-nonchlamydial salpingitis; paradoxically, though, those women documented to have chlamydial salpingitis in Svensson's group had the highest erythrocyte sedimentation rates and the more severe inflammatory changes noted at the time of laparoscopy (81).

Recently, Sweet and co-workers, employing methodology similar to that used by the Scandinavian investigators, reported the recovery of *C. trachomatis* from the upper genital tract in 17 (24%) of 71 patients with acute salpingitis (41). Similarly, Eschenbach and colleagues are isolating *C. trachomatis* from the upper genital tract in acute salpingitis and have confirmed these findings (82). Thus, current investigations have documented that *C. trachomatis* is also a major etiologic agent for acute PID in the U.S., and it is estimated that this organism is associated with 20–30% of acute PID.

Further support for a role in salpingitis for *C. trachomatis* arises from studies performed on infertility patients. Punnonen and co-workers noted in infertility patients with abnormal hysterosalpingograms that 21 of 23 (91%) had antibody titers against *C. trachomatis* (83). This compared to 52 of 105 (50%) patients who were infertile but had normal hysterosalpingograms, and 20 of 68 (29%) pregnant women who were used as controls. In addition, they noted that the mean geometric titer of antibody against *C. trachomatis* was significantly higher in those infertility patients with abnormal hysterosalpingograms, as compared to the infertility patients with normal hysterosalpingograms or to the pregnant women. More recently, Henry-Souchet et al reported that in patients undergoing tubal corrective surgery for infertility with tubal obstruction but no active inflammation, antibody was present against *C. trachomatis* in

12 of 24 patients (50%), as compared to 5 of 28 controls (18%). In addition, she was able to recover *C. trachomatis* from the peritoneal cavity or fallopian tube cultures in 6 of 29 (20.7%) patients with no inflammation, as compared to 0 of 36 controls (84). These two studies suggest a possible role for *C. trachomatis* in both salpingitis and subsequent infertility in women with tubal sterility and chronic inflammation.

Several recent studies have confirmed an association between infertility due solely or in part to tubal factors and the presence of antibodies to *C. trachomatis* (85–90) (Table 8.3). These studies have demonstrated that infertility patients with serologic evidence of previous infection with *C. trachomatis* were two to three times more likely to have tubal abnormalities than infertile women without evidence of antibody to *C. trachomatis*. Those women with tubal factor infertility had two to four times the prevalence rate of antichlamydial antibodies than the infertile patients with normal fallopian tubes or pregnant women had. Surprisingly, in the studies by Punnonen et al (83), Jones et al (86), and Gump et al (88), less than half of these women with antichlamydial antibodies had a history of having had PID. This led Rosenfeld to suggest that chlamydial infection of the upper genital tract in women may in many instances be subclinical and thus may be an insidious cause of tubal factor infertility (91).

Despite the impressive seroepidemiologic data documenting an association between antibodies against *C. trachomatis* and tubal factor infertility, attempts to recover *C. trachomatis* from the fallopian tubes and/or cul-de-sac in such infertility patients has yielded inconsistent results. Henry-Souchet isolated *C. trachomatis* from the tubes and/or peritoneum in 35% of infertile women with chronic tubal inflammation, in 21% with no evidence of inflammation, and in none of her controls (84). Sayed and co-workers recently reported the recovery of *C. trachomatis* from fallopian tube biopsies of five infertile women with cornual obstruction (92). On the other hand, Cevenini et al (89) and Moore et al (87) were unable to isolate *C. trachomatis*. Moreover, the remaining studies did not attempt to recover chlamydia from the fallopian tubes and/or peritoneum in their infertility patients.

Taylor-Robinson and Carney have developed an in vitro model for the study of infection of the human fallopian tube (93). Gonococci introduced into this model based on organ cultures of fallopian tubes cause extensive damage to the fallopian tube within a 7-day period of time. When this model was applied to infection with *C. trachomatis* Hutchinson and co-workers found the agent to replicate but cause no discernible damage (94). However, because the host response might be important in causing chlamydial salpingitis, further focus has recently centered on experimental animal model infections. Ripa et al have demonstrated that *C. trachomatis* can cause an acute salpingitis when it reaches the fallopian tubes of grivet monkeys (95). They inoculated *C. trachomatis* directly into the fallopian tubes of two experimental animals through the cervical canal and into the uterine cavity of a third. A self-limited acute

Table 8.3.
Studies Demonstrating an Association between *C. trachomatis* Infection and Infertility

Study	Findings
Punnonen et al (83)	Infertile women with abnormal HSG had an increased prevalence of and higher titers of antichlamydial antibodies than infertile women with normal HSG or pregnant women.
Henry-Souchet et al (84, 85)	Infertile women with tubal obstruction were significantly more likely to have antichlamydial antibodies and were nearly twice as likely to have positive cultures for *C. trachomatis*.
Jones et al (86)	Infertile women with tubal factor as the sole or contributing factor had 3.5 times the prevalence of antichlamydial antibodies.
Moore et al (87)	75% of infertile women with tubal occlusion had antibodies to chlamydia, while none of the women with normal tubes had such antibodies.
Gump et al (88)	Infertile women with antichlamydial antibodies were nearly 3 times more likely to have an abnormal HSG than infertile women without chlamydial antibodies.
Cevenini et al (89)	Infertile women with salpingitis were 3.2 times more likely to have elevated antichlamydial antibodies.

salpingitis occurred in the three animals, and chlamydiae were recovered up to 3 weeks following inoculation. At laparotomy, they documented the finding of acute salpingitis in these animals and a lymphocytic infiltrate in the mucosal muscular and serosal-subserosal layers. Additional animal work has been performed utilizing the guinea pig inclusion conjunctivitis (GPIC) agent which is an infection in guinea pigs with a pathogenesis similar to that of sexually transmitted human chlamydial infections. When the GPIC agent is inoculated into the vagina, it results in an acute self-limited infection which can be modified by immunosuppression to become chronic and progressive. Thus, Rank et al (96) and White et al (97) have produced ascending infections with salpingitis and peritonitis. Sweet et al (98) have reported the use of a nonimmunosuppressed guinea pig model for acute salpingitis. These workers inoculated GPIC agent directly into the uterine horn. This resulted in the development of an acute self-limited salpingitis. The disease is largely a luminal one and results in severe inflammatory reaction, with purulent discharge at the end of the fimbriated tube. Moller et al have reported on the histologic findings in the fallopian tube in two patients with acute salpingitis due to *C. trachomatis* (99). The light microscopy findings of the histological changes in the tubes from these patients were similar to those described for gonococcal salpingitis. In addition, they reported that the inflammatory changes were similar to those seen in the grivet monkeys experimentally infected with *C. trachomatis*.

Swenson et al recently reported that the inoculation of the mouse pneumonia biovar of *C. trachomatis* into the ovarian bursa of mice resulted in acute salpingitis (100). Inclusions were seen in histologic sections, and the organism could be recovered from infected tissues for up to 21 days postinoculation. The inflammatory response decreased after 20 days. In 5 of 11 mice examined between 23 and 48 days postinoculation, gross hydrosalpinges were found. Such a finding has been described by Gibson and co-workers in humans; they reported that women with tubal factor infertility and antichlamydial antibodies were significantly more likely to have hydrosalpinx than infertility patients without chlamydial antibodies (90). In a subsequent investigation, Swenson and Schachter demonstrated that chlamydial infection of the upper reproductive tract of mice prior to mating can result in infertility (101). Most significant was

their finding that chlamydial infection of the upper reproductive tract in mice has an adverse effect on fertility long after apparent resolution of the infection.

Although the final answer to the role of *C. trachomatis* in acute salpingitis in the United States and the contribution this agent makes to the total number of cases of acute salpingitis and its sequelae must await further investigations, the current consensus is that *C. trachomatis* is a major pathogen in acute salpingitis in the U.S. and is associated with 20–30% of acute salpingitis cases. Recommendations for the treatment of acute salpingitis now include agents effective against chlamydia. Based on estimates that 20% of women will be infertile postacute salpingitis, approximately 20,000–30,000 women become sterile each year secondary to chlamydial salpingitis.

Fitz-Hugh-Curtis Syndrome

Acute perihepatitis is a localized fibrinous inflammation affecting the anterior surface of the liver and the adjacent parietal peritoneum. The sequelae are fibrous adhesions between the liver and the diaphragm (Fig. 8.2). When this condition occurs in association with acute salpingitis, it has been known as the Fitz-Hugh-Curtis (FHC) syndrome. It is important to recognize, though, that the symptoms of salpingitis are often moderate or even absent in this syndrome. The clinical picture is often characterized by an acute onset of severe right upper quadrant abdominal pain resembling that of acute cholecystitis. This syndrome was first described in 1919 by Stajano (102). In 1930 Curtis (103) and in 1934 Fitz-Hugh (104) related the syndrome to gonococcal infection. In fact until recently the Fitz-Hugh-Curtis syndrome was believed to be a complication of gonococcal infection.

C. trachomatis as a possible cause of Fitz-Hugh-Curtis syndrome was first suggested by Muller-Schoop et al (105). These investigators found serologic evidence of recent chlamydial infection in 9 of 11 patients with both perihepatitis and peritonitis. Subsequently, additional investigations have confirmed an association between *C. trachomatis* and Fitz-Hugh-Curtis syndrome (106–111). In 1980 Paavonen and Valtonen reported a case of a 20-year-old woman who developed pelvic peritonitis and perihepatitis (107). *C. trachomatis* had been isolated from the cervix and a significant rise in

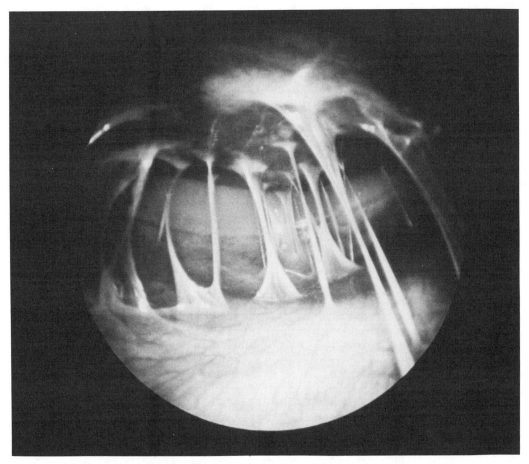

Figure 8.2. Laparoscopic view of Fitz-Hugh-Curtis syndrome.

antibody titer against *C. trachomatis* was noted. Subsequently, Paavonen and co-workers reported that *C. trachomatis* was isolated from the cervix and/or urethra in 6 of 11 patients tested among 15 hospitalized with the Fitz-Hugh-Curtis syndrome in Finland (108). Results of the microimmunofluorescent test indicated that 10 of 15 patients were infected with *C. trachomatis*. In the United States, Wang and colleagues have similarly identified a relationship between *C. trachomatis* and FHC syndrome (109). In 19 women with the Fitz-Hugh-Curtis syndrome, chlamydial antibodies against *C. trachomatis* were present in 17 of 19, and the geometric mean titer of the microimmunofluorescent antibody was 1:724. In comparison, in women with uncomplicated acute salpingitis, antibody against *C. trachomatis* was noted in 9 of 19, and the titer of antibody was only 1:138. Darougar reported that a diagnosis of FHC syndrome was confirmed laparoscopically in 5 of 10 women with

acute right upper quadrant abdominal pain, but negative results were reported for biliary tract disease. *C. trachomatis* was isolated from the endocervical canal in one of six patients examined. Of the sera from 9 patients tested by the microimmunofluorescent antibody test, 9 and 6 samples, respectively, showed type specific IgG and IgM antibodies against *C. trachomatis* serotypes D through K (110). Dalaker and associates confirmed four cases of FHC syndrome by laparoscopy. *C. trachomatis* was cultured from the cervix in two and from both the cervix and Fallopian tubes in two of these patients (111). Neither gonococci nor aerobic nor anaerobic bacteria were isolated from the Fallopian tubes in this report. Moller and Mardh have described the presence of perihepatitis in a grivet monkey whose tubes had been ligated and who had had experimental inoculation of *C. trachomatis*. Thus, an etiologic relationship between *C. trachomatis* and the FHC syndrome seems evident.

However, other organisms involved in acute salpingitis also probably are associated with the FHC syndrome.

PERINATAL INFECTION WITH C. TRACHOMATIS

Infections of the Neonate

The infant delivered vaginally to a woman with chlamydial infection of the cervix has a 60–70% risk of acquiring the infection during passage through the birth canal (33–36). Approximately 25–50% of exposed infants will develop conjunctivitis in the first 2 weeks of life, and 10–20% of the infants will develop pneumonia within 3–4 months. In utero transmission is not known to occur, and infants delivered by cesarean section are not at risk of acquiring chlamydial infection, unless there has been a premature rupture of the membranes.

The determinant of whether or not chlamydial infections of the newborn represent a major medical problem in a specific population group will be the prevalence rate of chlamydial infections of the cervix in that population. This carriage rate can vary broadly, and the reported incidence has ranged from 2 to 24% (1, 33–37, 40, 112–114) (Table 8.4), with most studies in the 7 to 12% range. The higher prevalence rates occur in inner city and lower socioeconomic patient groups. In addition, young unmarried women, a history of greater past sexual activity, black ethnicity, and oral contraceptive usage are associated with an increased risk for cervical chlamydia during pregnancy.

CONJUNCTIVITIS

Acute conjunctivitis of the newborn (inclusion conjunctivitis of the newborn or inclusion blennorrhea) was initially described in 1910. It was recognized that the agent which caused inclusion conjunctivitis of the newborn was also present in the genital tract of the mother; intracytoplasmic inclusions similar to those produced by trachoma were seen in scrapings of the conjunctiva of infants with conjunctivitis and in those from the cervix of their mothers. This mucopurulent conjunctivitis generally develops 5–14 days after birth. It is now recognized as the most common conjunctivitis in the first month of life (115).

The organism replicates extensively in superficial epithelial cells of the conjunctiva and causes considerable cell damage. There is an exuberant inflammatory reaction, and pseudomembranes may form (which may result in scar formations). Follicles such as are seen in adults or older children with chlamydial infection of the conjunctiva are not usually observed unless the disease has been active for 1 or 2 months. The majority of untreated infants will resolve spontaneously during the first few months of

Table 8.4.
Prospective Studies of Perinatal Chlamydial Infection

Study	Prevalence of maternal infection (%)	Prevalence of maternal antibody (%)	Attack rate of infant infection		Cases per 1000 live births	
			Conjunctivitis	Pneumonia	Conjunctivitis	Pneumonia
Chandler et al (36)	12.7	44	50	Not studied	63	Not studied
Schachter (1)	5.0		40	Not studied	20	Not studied
Frommel et al (35)	8.8	Not studied	44	11	40	10
Schachter et al (34)	4.0	?63	35	20	14	8
Hammerschlag et al (33)	2.0	73	33	16	7	3
Mardh (112)	9.0		23	Not studied	20	Not studied
Heggie (37)[a]	18.0	Not studied	21	3	32	5.4
Grossman et al (40)		53	18	18	7	7
Thompson et al (113)	16	Not studied				
Harrison et al (114)	24	81				

[a] Only 95 of 210 infants born to chlamydia-positive mothers were available for follow-up evaluation.

life. Occasional infants maintain persistent conjunctivitis; pannus formation and scarring typical of trachoma have been reported. Visual loss is rare. Micropannus and some scarring will most likely occur in infants if they are not treated within the first 2 weeks of the disease. If they are treated early, no sequelae will develop.

The disease often starts with a watery eye discharge which rapidly and progressively becomes very purulent. The eyelids are usually markedly swollen. The conjunctivae become very reddened and somewhat thickened throughout. The follicular nature of the infection, so characteristic of trachoma, is missing, since the conjunctivae of the neonate lacks lymphoid tissue.

In severe cases, diagnosis is readily made by demonstrating the typical inclusion bodies by means of Giesma stain of conjunctival scrapings. The chlamydial organisms are also readily cultured from the eye. Serologic diagnosis is not helpful because of the presence of maternally transmitted antichlamydial IgG antibody and the uncertain appearance of IgM in this disease. Since chlamydial infections appear to be unaffected by silver nitrate prophylaxis, it seems reasonable to recommend a prophylactic regimen, which would be active against both chlamydia and gonococci. A preliminary trial of prophylactic erythromycin ointment has been shown to prevent development of inclusion conjunctivitis of the newborn (116). However, the regimen does not affect chlamydial infection in extraocular sites in infants (117–118).

PNEUMONIA

Until 1975, it was assumed that chlamydial infection in the infant was restricted to the conjunctiva. During a prospective study on the development of inclusion conjunctivitis of the newborn, an infant who had been successfully treated for conjunctivitis developed pneumonia and yielded chlamydia from the respiratory tract (88). In 1977, Beem and Saxon published a series of retrospective and prospective cases of chlamydial pneumonia in young infants (119). This report was followed by studies from other centers (34, 120), and the clinical entity of chlamydial pneumonia became well defined. During the ensuing years it has become clear that this disease is very common, probably one of the three most common pneumonias seen in infancy. The many reported series have helped to delineate the clinical features of this infection (119–121).

Of the vast majority of chlamydial pneumonia cases present between the 4th and 11th weeks of life, virtually all will be symptomatic before the 8th week. Initially, they present with upper respiratory symptoms. The infants are usually afebrile or have only a minimal amount of fever. The upper respiratory tract symptoms are those of congestion and obstruction of the nasal passages without significant discharge. The finding of abnormal bulging eardrums is common, occurring in more than one-half the cases described. The history or presence of conjunctivitis can be elucidated in half the cases. Lower respiratory tract symptoms consist of tachypnea and a very prominent stacatto-type cough. Some infants have apneic periods. Crepitant inspiratory rales are commonly heard; on the other hand, expiratory wheezes are uncommon. The radiographic findings are those of hyperexpansion of the lungs, with bilateral symmetrical interstitial infiltrates.

Laboratory findings include a normal white blood count and an increased number of eosinophils. Blood gas analysis usually shows that many of the infants have a mild or moderate degree of hypoxia. Serum immunoglobulins, both the IgG and IgM variety, are generally elevated.

Initially, it was speculated that chlamydia pneumonia of infants resulted from *C. trachomatis* draining into the respiratory tract from involved conjunctivae and that the eye was the portal of entry. Prospective studies have shown that conjunctivitis is not a prerequisite and, indeed, prevention of conjunctivitis by appropriate ocular prophylaxis does not prevent respiratory tract infection and pneumonia (116–118). While it seems likely that some respiratory tract infections may result from conjunctivae seeding at birth, it is apparent that the respiratory tract can be directly infected during the birth process. Hammerschlag et al have shown that neonatal prophylaxis with erythromycin ointment could prevent the development of ICN, but had no apparent effect on nasopharyngeal infection or pneumonia (116).

The long incubation period for chlamydial pneumonia in infants seen in most cases is perplexing. There have been some suggestions in the literature that the pneumonia in infants is likely to reflect a hypersensitivity response to the organism in the lung. While it is clear that the host inflammatory reaction is a major contributing factor in any disease process, there is scant evidence to support chlamydia pneumonia of infants as a hypersensitivity reaction. In large part, the speculation is based upon the relative eosinophilia seen in some cases and the difficulties in obtaining appropriate lung specimens for either isolation attempts or sequential pathologic analysis of the development of the disease. Schachter and colleagues have recovered *C. trachomatis* from 3 of the 4 lung specimens that have been tested from infants with chlamydial pneumonia (122). These data support the assertion that *C. trachomatis* may be a causative agent for pneumonia in human infants. The isolation of chlamydia from a defined clinical syndrome, such as described by Beem and Saxon, and the findings of high antibodies in the sera of patients with this syndrome suggests that this organism is one of the major causes of infant pneumonia.

OTHER CLINICAL MANIFESTATIONS IN THE NEONATE

Serologic evidence of infection with chlamydia is present in 60 to 70% of infants passing through an infected cervix (33–36). Although conjunctivitis and pneumonia are the only two firmly established and clearly delineated clinical entities, there is suggestive evidence that chlamydia plays a role in otitis media, obstruction of nasal passages, and lower airway disease (bronchiolitis) in young infants. Because chlamydial infection may result in nasopharyngeal obstruction and apnea, it is likely that some infants with sudden infant death syndrome have chlamydial infection. Unpublished studies by Schachter and Grossman suggest that the chlamydial contribution to this syndrome is sparse (less than 5% of cases). All these entities in infants need further study and delineation. Furthermore, it is clear that many infants, as well as older children, acquire antibodies to *C. trachomatis* without having experienced a discrete and recognized infection, suggesting that there may be other, not yet described, clinical entities caused by this organism.

Infections in Pregnant Women

POSTPARTUM ENDOMETRITIS

Preliminary investigation by Wager and coworkers from Seattle suggested that pregnant women in whom *C. trachomatis* was recovered at their initial prenatal visit have a significant increased risk for developing late onset endometritis following a vaginal delivery (123). Late endometritis developed in 7 (22%) of 32 women with *C. trachomatis* isolated during prenatal care, as compared to 18 (5%) of 359 chlamydia-negative women. However, attempts to recover chlamydia from the patients during their acute infection were not performed. Cytryn et al have reported the occurrence of a severe pelvic infection from *C. trachomatis* after cesarean section (124). Recently, Harrison and co-workers and Thompson and colleagues failed to demonstrate an association between postpartum endometritis and *C. trachomatis* infection alone (113, 114). Thus, the elucidation of the role this organism has as a causative agent in postpartum endometritis must await further prospective studies utilizing chlamydia culture techniques during the acute infection.

SPONTANEOUS ABORTION AND FETAL DEATH

Martin and colleagues in Seattle have reported a significant increase in the occurrence of spontaneous abortions and fetal deaths among women who had *C. trachomatis* recovered from the cervix at their initial prenatal visit (38). Proof of causation for these events is not available and requires additional large scale prospective investigations. In our prospective studies in San Francisco of vertical transmission from mothers to neonates of *C. trachomatis*, we have been unable to corroborate these findings (unpublished data). Similarly, Harrison et al noted no increased risk for spontaneous abortion or fetal deaths among women with chlamydial infections (114).

PREMATURITY, LOW BIRTH WEIGHT, PREMATURE RUPTURED MEMBRANES

A great deal of interest and controversy has revolved around what role, if any, *C. trachomatis* infection of the cervix plays in the etiology of preterm labor and delivery, low birth weight, or premature rupture of the membranes. Once again, conflicting studies exist. Martin and coworkers in Seattle noted a significant increase in the occurrence of preterm delivery among chlamydia-positive women (38). In addition, they reported an increased incidence of low birth weight babies and of perinatal mortality in the chlamydia-positive group; the major cause of mortality was intrauterine death. In this study only women seen prior to 18 weeks of gestation were included. Of the 18 women with chlamydia isolated, stillbirth occurred in three and preterm delivery and perinatal death in another three. Thus there was a 33% incidence of perinatal mortality in the Seattle study; this is in significant contrast with results in the 238 uninfected mothers in which only 8 (3%) had similar complications. Subsequent studies performed in New Orleans by Martin et al failed to confirm these findings (125). Our prospective studies in San Francisco also have failed to confirm an association between chlamydial infection and preterm delivery, premature ruptured membranes, perinatal mortality, or low birth weight. Similarly, Harrison et al (114) and Thompson et al (113) have reported no association between *C. trachomatis* cervical infection and prematurity, low birth weight, stillbirths, or premature rupture of the membranes.

Of considerable interest was the finding by Harrison and colleagues that there was a subset of chlamydia-positive mothers who showed evidence of active invasive infection by the presence of significant titers of IgM antibody against *C. trachomatis* (114). In this subgroup there was significantly increased incidence of low birth weight, shorter gestational length, and more premature ruptured membranes. Only large scale prospective investigations will resolve the dilemma of *C. trachomatis* as a cause of preterm labor and delivery, low birth weight, and/or perinatal loss.

DIAGNOSIS OF CHLAMYDIAL INFECTIONS

Schachter and Dawson have suggested that the principles for diagnosing chlamydial infections are essentially the same as those for diagnosing any other microbial infection (126). The agent may be demonstrated by cytology on clinical specimens; serologic means may be used to demonstrate rising antibody titers to chlamydial antigens; or the agent may be isolated from the patient's tissues. Recently, fluorescein-labeled monoclonal antibody has been used to perform direct immunofluorescence tests for chlamydia on specimens of genital secretions (127).

Cytology

Both the intracellular nature of chlamydia and their unique growth cycle provide specific markers for cytologic diagnosis. Demonstration of inclusions in scrapings from genital tract specimens was the method used to elucidate the epidemiology and clinical spectrum of chlamydial infections prior to the availability of cultures. However, these procedures cannot be recommended because of poor sensitivity. Schachter and Dawson reported that cervical infection with chlamydia can only be recognized by cytologic means in approximately 20% of cases (128). Cytology (usually using the Giemsa stain) is still useful in areas where more sophisticated laboratory technology is not available, or in some instances where rapid diagnosis can be achieved. It is a useful and sensitive means for diagnosing inclusion conjunctivitis of the newborn. However, it is not successful in diagnosing cervical infections because of limited sensitivity. Failure to demonstrate inclusions will not rule out chlamydial infection.

Serology

Despite an abundant immune response to chlamydial infections (2), serology is not particularly useful in diagnosing *C. trachomatis* infections of the genital tract (129). Virtually all individuals who are not treated very early in the course of their infection will develop a measurable antibody response, and cell-mediated immune response is also stimulated (130). The high background rates of antichlamydial antibodies in sexually active populations renders serodiagnosis inconclusive. Because many chlamydial infections are chronic, the patients may not be seen at an appropriate time for collection of acute and convalescent sera to document increasing titers. It is important to recognize that a single antibody titer as a screening procedure will suggest previous chlamydial infection but not active infection. The exception would be extremely high IgG levels or IgM levels.

The two serologic tests that have been used for chlamydial infections are the complement fixation (CF test) and the microimmunofluorescent (Micro-IF) test. The CF test is most useful in diagnosing LGV. The Micro-IF test is a much more sensitive test for diagnosing *C. trachomatis* and allows determination of the immunoglobulin class of antibody. It is possible that in some specific clinical instances, serologic tests may be helpful to the clinician in diagnosing chlamydial infection. For example, in an adult's first acquisition of chlamydia, paired sera will show rising titers. In some disease involving systemic complications of superficial chlamydial infections, an exceptionally high titer may possibly provide some corroboration for clinical diagnosis (34, 72, 119). For example, women who develop acute salpingitis from a chlamydial infection will have much higher antibody levels than women with uncomplicated cervicitis. Men with chlamydial epididymitis will have much higher antibody titers than men with chlamydial urethritis. A similar pattern is seen in infants with perinatally acquired infection. An infant with pneumonia will have much higher antibody titers than a child with uncomplicated conjunctivitis (34, 119). Schachter and Grossman have suggested the rule of thumb that systemic complications result in higher antibody titers quite similar to the high titers observed in individuals with proven LGV infections (5). The serologic test of choice is the Micro-IF test of Wang and Grayston (129).

Cultural Methods

The optimum laboratory test on a routine basis for the diagnosis of chlamydial infections of the female genital tract is isolation of the organism from the involved site. Because chlamydiae are obligatory intracellular parasites, isolation attempts cannot be performed on ar-

tificial media but require a susceptible tissue culture cell line. The methods of choice involve treating a susceptible cell monolayer with an antimetabolite that interferes with the replication or metabolism of the host cell, while allowing chlamydial functions. Treatment of McCoy cells with either 5-iodo-2-deoxyuridine or cyclohexamide are the two most commonly used methods (131, 132). The most important step in the isolation procedure involves centrifuging the organisms onto the cell monolayers; this method has increased the sensitivity of the cell culture method 100-fold. Cyclohexamide treatment appears to be simple and inexpensive and, above all, provides the most sensitive system. After an appropriate incubation period, which varies from 24 to 72 hours, depending on staining procedures used, the monolayers are stained and examined microscopically for the presence of inclusions. This can be done with either iodine and/or Giemsa stain (Fig. 8.3). Although isolation procedures for *C. trachomatis* are useful in diagnosis on a routine basis, the isolation procedures are not without drawbacks. The involved anatomic site must be appropriately sam-

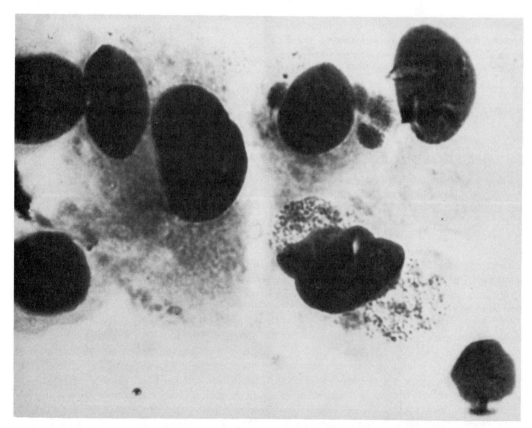

Figure 8.3.   Giemsa stain demonstrating *C. trachomatis* inclusions.

pled. Culture of discharges is inadequate, and an adequate sample of involved epithelial cells must be obtained. The sensitivity of chlamydial culture techniques is unknown. Schachter and Grossman estimated that in nongonococcal urethritis or cervicitis the sensitivity of culture techniques is 70–80% (5).

Monoclonal Antibodies

In an attempt to simplify the diagnosis of genital tract infection with chlamydia, fluorescein-labeled monoclonal antibody has been used to perform direct immunofluorescence tests for chlamydia on clinical specimens. Tam and coworkers have recently demonstrated that this direct method is an effective, culture-independent means of detecting chlamydial infection in specimens from patients attending a sexually transmitted diseases clinic (127). The direct test was used in 926 patients who presented with overt urethritis (men) or mucopurulent endocervicitis (women) and demonstrated a sensitivity of 93% and a specificity of 96% when compared with cultures. Uyeda and colleagues reported that the direct immunofluorescence test in 401 asymptomatic female patients had a sensitivity of 96% and a specificity of more than 99% (133).

Tam et al estimated that the direct immunofluorescence monoclonal antibody test will detect 90% or more of chlamydial infections that would be culture positive (127). They suggested that the use of the direct immunofluorescence test will permit laboratories that are not versed in cell culture techniques to perform rapid diagnostic testing for chlamydial infection.

THERAPY OF CHLAMYDIAL INFECTIONS

Given the morbidity associated with chlamydial infections, some efforts at control measures are indicated. In the past, such measures required the introduction of chlamydial isolation procedures on a much broader scale than was feasible. The introduction of monoclonal diagnostic methodology should facilitate establishing large scale screening efforts for chlamydia. A first step would be that chlamydial diagnostic techniques be introduced in the management of genital tract complaints in women. They are at the greatest risk for developing serious complications of the infection and are epidemiologically crucial in both vertical and horizontal transmission. It seems appropriate that pregnant women should be the first focus of chlamydial control measures. Each year in the

United States, 155,000 infants are exposed to chlamydial infections and more than 100,000 will acquire these infections, with approximately 75,000 cases of conjunctivitis and 30,000 cases of pneumonia each year (4). In addition, these women may be at risk for developing complications of pregnancy (i.e., PROM, preterm delivery) or postpartum endometritis.

There are three general approaches which can be employed as control measures. The first deals with the effort to reduce the reservoir. The routine use of tetracycline (as recommended by the Center for Disease Control) for the treatment of gonorrhea would remove the approximately 20–30% of men and 30–50% of women with gonorrhea who have coexistent chlamydial infection from the infective pool. Effective treatment of men with nongonococcal urethritis with tetracyclines or erythromycins and routine treatment of their sexual contacts would also be appropriate. Management of mucopurulent endocervicitis in women in the same manner as one deals with NGU in men would also help to reduce the pool.

There are specific approaches to preventing perinatal infection with *C. trachomatis* that could be initiated. One can substitute erythromycin ointment for silver nitrate in ocular prophylaxis for neonates. Silver nitrate is clearly ineffective in preventing chlamydial infections. Topical erythromycin is active against *C. trachomatis*, and pilot studies have shown that it prevents the development of chlamydial conjunctivitis, although it does not prevent respiratory tract infection or pneumonia. Since erythromycin is also effective in preventing gonococcal ophthalmia neonatorum and is less irritating to the eye than the silver nitrate which has been in common use, it would seem appropriate to recommend that a routine shift be made to ocular prophylaxis with erythromycin ointment.

The third method is aimed at preventing the exposure of infants to chlamydia during the birth process. It involves routine testing of pregnant women for chlamydial infection and treating those found to carry the organism. While this can be an expensive undertaking (less so with monoclonal direct smears), Schachter and Grossman have shown that it can be justified, not only as a public health measure but also as cost-effective in selected populations (5). The consistency of attack rates observed in prospective studies allow reasonable certainty in predicting the outcomes of exposure to chlamydia during vaginal deliveries. It is the prevalence of chlamydial infection in the maternal cervix that is the crucial determinant in the incidence of disease in infants. The cost-benefit analysis developed by Schachter and Grossman noted that when the prevalence of chlamydial cervical infection is 5% or less, it costs more to detect and treat infections than it would to treat the resulting diseases in newborns. This analysis may be an underestimate. It was made on the basis of disease in infants, and possible complications of the pregnant woman have not been included, since their frequency of occurrence is not known. In addition, monoclonal diagnostic technology should lower the cost of screening. At above the 6% cervical infection rate, the costs of treating disease in the infants would exceed the costs for identifying and treating pregnant women with cervical chlamydia to prevent the perinatal exposure. Since infection rates of 15–30% are commonly reported in selected populations, it seems obvious that routine screening for chlamydial infections should be initiated for these expectant mothers, as an adjunct to perinatal care. The treatment of choice in managing chlamydial infection during pregnancy has not been defined. Macrolide antibiotics are the likeliest candidates. Preliminary studies have documented the efficacy of erythromycin treatment in eradicating chlamydial infection in pregnant women and preventing vertical transmission of chlamydia to neonates (134). However, these results must be expanded and confirmed, and optimal regimens must be determined.

The recommended treatment for NGU is tetracycline HCl (250 to 500 mg four times/day for 7–14 days). The exact length of time has not been definitively established. Seven days of therapy is adequate (61) and, indeed, 2 g/day for 5 days may be sufficient (although this has not been tested). Alternately, doxycycline (100 mg b.i.d. for 7 days) may be used. If tetracycline is contraindicated, erythromycin in similar dosage schedules may be utilized. Sulfisoxazole (2 g/day for 10–14 days) is also effective. Additional drugs which have demonstrated in vitro activity against *C. trachomatis* include sulfamethoxazole-trimethoprim, rifampin, and clindamycin (135, 136). Single dose regimens of penicillin-G or ampicillin are ineffective, but prolonged treatment with ampicillin (2 g/day for 10 days) may be effective (61).

Women with chlamydial cervicitis may be treated with the regimens recommended for men with NGU. Bowie has reported equal efficacy with tetracycline, erythromycin, and sulfisoxazole regimens (61). Tetracycline HCl is the antibiotic of choice for chlamydial salpingitis in a dosage schedule of 500 mg four times/day for 7–10 days; alternately doxycycline (100 mg b.i.d. for 7 days) can be used. As discussed in Chapter 4, an antichlamydial agent is part of a combination therapy approach to the treatment of acute PID. Clindamycin may be a viable alternative in doses of 450 mg q6h.

Chlamydial inclusion conjunctivitis is usually treated with tetracycline or erythromycin eyedrops. For chlamydial pneumonia, systemic erythromycin therapy is advocated. General consensus suggests that chlamydial conjunctivitis of the newborn should also be treated with systemic erythromycin, because of high failure rates observed with topical treatment. A 2-week course of erythromycin in a dose of 40 mg/kg per day is recommended. Systemic therapy will also eradicate nasopharyngeal colonization and prevent pneumonia secondary to chlamydia.

References

1. Schachter J: Chlamydial infections. *N Engl J Med* 298:428–435, 490–495, 540–549, 1978.
2. Grayston JT, Wang S-P: New knowledge of chlamydiae and the diseases they cause. *J Infect Dis* 132:87–105, 1975.
3. Schachter J, Hanna L, Hill EC, Massad S, Sheppard CW, Conte JE, Meyer KF: Are chlamydial infections the most prevalent venereal disease? *J Am Med Assoc* 231:1252–1255, 1975.
4. National Institute of Allergy and Infectious Diseases: Summary and Recommendations of the National Institute Allergy and Infectious Diseases Study Group on Sexually Transmitted Diseases, 1980.
5. Schachter J, Grossman M: Chlamydial infections. *Annu Rev Med* 32:45–61, 1981.
6. Washington AE: Chlamydia: a major threat to reproductive health. Research Highlights Institute for Health Policy Studies. University of California, San Francisco 2:1–3, 1984.
7. Jones BR: Laboratory tests for chlamydial infection: their role in epidemiological studies of trachoma and its control. *Br J Ophthalmol* 58:438–454, 1974.
8. Sweet RS, Schachter J, Landers DV: Chlamydial infections in obstetrics and gynecology. *Clin Obstet Gynecol* 26:143–164, 1983.
9. Page LA: The rickettsias. In Buchanan RE, Gibbons NE (eds): *Bergey's Manual of Determinative Bacteriology*, ed 8. Baltimore,Williams & Wilkins, 1974, pp 914–918.
10. Kuo C-C, Wang S-P, Grayston JT: Effect of polycations, polyanions and neuroaminidase on the infectivity of trachoma-inclusion conjunctivitis and lymphogranuloma venereum organisms in HeLa cells: sialic acid residues as possible receptors for trachoma-inclusion conjunctivitis. *Infect Immun* 8:74–79, 1973.

11. Friis RR: Interaction of L cells and *Chlamydia psittaci*: entry of the parasite and host responses to its development. *J Bacteriol* 110:706–721, 1972.

12. Moulder JW: The relation of the psittacosis group (chlamydiae) to bacteria and viruses. *Ann Rev Microbiol* 20:107–130, 1966.

13. Thompson SE, Washington AE: Epidemiology of sexually transmitted *Chlamydia trachomatis* infections. *Epidemiol Rev* 5:96–123, 1983.

14. Holmes KK, Handsfield HH, Wang S-P, Wentworth BB, Turck M, Anderson JB, Alexander ER: Etiology of nongonococcal urethritis. *N Engl J Med* 292:1199–1206, 1975.

15. Richmond SJ, Oriel JD: Recognition and management of genital chlamydial infection. *Br Med J* 2:480–482, 1978.

16. Oriel JD, Reeve P, Thomas BJ, Nicol CS: Infection with Chlamydia group A in men with urethritis due to *Neisseria gonorrhoeae*. *J Infect Dis* 131:376–382, 1975.

17. Berger RE, Alexander ER, Monda GD, Ansell J, McCormick G, Holmes KK: *Chlamydia trachomatis* as a cause of acute "idiopathic" epididymitis. *N Engl J Med* 298:301–304, 1978.

18. Dunlop EMC, Harper IA, Al-Hussaini MK, et al: Relation of TRIC agent to "non-specific" genital infection. *Br J Vener Dis* 42:33–42, 1966.

19. Schachter J, Atwood G: Chlamydial pharyngitis? *J Am Vener Dis Assoc* 2:12, 1975.

20. Goldmeier D, Darougar S: Isolation of *Chlamydia trachomatis* from throat and rectum of homosexual men. *Br J Vener Dis* 55:184–185, 1977.

21. Schachter J, Grossman M: Chlamydia. In Remington J, Klien JO (eds): *Infections of the Fetus and Newborn*, ed 2. Philadelphia, WB Saunders, 1983, pp 450–463.

22. Wentworth BB, Bonon P, Holmes KK, et al: Isolation of viruses, bacteria and other organisms from venereal disease clinic patients: methodology and problems associated with multiple isolations. *Health Lab Sci* 10:75–81, 1973.

23. Oriel JD, Powis PA, Reeve P, et al: Chlamydial infection of the cervix. *Br J Vener Dis* 50:11–16, 1974.

24. Hilton AL, Richmond SJ, Milne JD, et al: *Chlamydia* A in the female genital tract. *Br J Vener Dis* 50:1–10, 1974.

25. Hobson D, Johnson FWA, Rees E, et al: Simplified method for diagnosis of genital and ocular infections with Chlamydia. *Lancet* 2:555–556, 1974.

26. Burns DCM, Darougar S, Thin RN, et al: Isolation of *Chlamydia* from women attending a clinic for sexually transmitted disease. *Br J Vener Dis* 51:314–318, 1975.

27. Arya OP, Mallinson H, Goddard AD: Epidemiological and clinical correlates of chlamydial infection of the cervix. *Br J Vener Dis* 57:118–124, 1981.

28. Tait IA, Rees E, Hobson D, et al: Chlamydial infection of the cervix in contacts of men with nongonococcal urethritis. *Br J Vener Dis* 56:37–45, 1980.

29. Dunlap EMC, Jones BR, Darougar S: Chlamydia and non-specific urethritis. *Br Med J* 2:575–577, 1972.

30. Oriel JD, Reeve P, Powis P, et al: Chlamydial infection: isolation of *Chlamydia* from patients with non-specific genital infection. *Br J Vener Dis* 48:419–436, 1972.

31. Kuo C-C, Wang S-P, Wentworth BB, et al: Primary isolation of TRIC organisms in HeLa 229 cells treated with DEAE-dextran. *J Infect Dis* 125:665–668, 1972.

32. Schachter J, Stoner E, Moncoda J: Screening for chlamydial infections in women attending Family Planning Clinics: evaluations of presumptive indicators for therapy. *West J Med* 138:375–379, 1983.

33. Hammerschlag MR, Anderka M, Semine DZ, McComb D, McCormack WM: Prospective study of maternal and infantile infection with *Chlamydia trachomatis*. *Pediatrics* 64:142–148, 1979.

34. Schachter J, Holt J, Goodner E, Grossman M, Sweet R, Mills J: Prospective study of chlamydial infection in neonates. *Lancet* 2:377–380, 1979.

35. Frommel GT, Rothenberg R, Wang S-P, McIntosh K, Wintersgill C, Allaman J, Orr I: Chlamydial infection of mothers and their infants. *J Pediatr* 95:28–32, 1979.

36. Chandler JW, Alexander ER, Pheiffer TA, Wang S-P, Holmes KK, English M: Ophthalmia neonatorum associated with maternal chlamydial infections. *Trans Am Acad Ophthalmol Otolaryngol* 83:302–308, 1977.

37. Heggie AD, Lumicao CG, Stuart LA, Gyues MT: *Chlamydia trachomatis* infection in mothers and infants. A prospective study. *Am J Dis Child* 135:507–511m, 1981.

38. Martin DH, Koutsky L, Eschenbach DA, et al: Prematurity and perinatal mortality in pregnancies complicated by maternal *Chlamydia trachomatis* infections. *JAMA* 247:1585–1588, 1982.

39. Thompson S, Lopez B, Wong KH, et al: The relationship of low birthweight and infant mortality to vaginal microorganisms. Presented at the 3rd International Meeting on Sexually Transmitted Diseases. Antwerp, Belgium, October 2–3, 1980.

40. Grossman M, Schachter J, Sweet R, Bishop E, Jordan C: Prospective studies of Chlamydia in newborns. In Mardh P-A, Holmes KK, Oriel JD, Piot P, Schachter J (eds): *Chlamydial Infections*. Fernstrom Foundations Series, Amsterdam, Elsevier, 1982, vol 2, pp 213–216.

41. Sweet RL, Schachter J, Robbie MO: Failure of B-lactam antibiotics to eradicate *Chlamydia trachomatis* in the endometrium despite apparent clinical cure of acute salpingitis. *JAMA* 250:2641–2645, 1983.

42. Bruce AW, Chadwick D, Willett WS, et al: The role of chlamydiae in genitourinary disease. *J Urol* 126:625–629, 1981.

43. Mardh P-A, Ripa K-T, Colleen S, et al: Role of *Chlamydia trachomatis* in non-acute prostatitis. *Br J Vener Dis* 54:330–334, 1978.

44. Quinn TC, Goodell SE, Mkrtichian SE, et al: *Chlamydia trachomatis* proctitis. *N Engl J Med* 305:195–200, 1981.

45. Paavonen J, Kousa M, Saikku P, et al: Examination of men with nongonococcal urethritis and their sexual partners for *Chlamydia trachomatis* and *Ureaplasma urealyticum*. *Sex Transm Dis*

5:93–96, 1978.

46. Digiacomo RF, Gale JL, Wang S-P, et al: Chlamydial infection of the male baboon urethra. *Br J Vener Dis* 51:310–313, 1975.

47. Jacobs NJ, Arum ES, Kraus SJ: Experimental infection of the chimpanzee urethra and pharynx with *C. trachomatis. Sex Transm Dis* 5:132–136, 1978.

48. Rees E, Tart AA, Hobson D, et al: Chlamydia in relation to cervical infection and pelvic inflammatory disease. In Holmes KK, Hobson D (eds): *Nongonococcal Urethritis and Related Infections.* Washington, D.C., American Society for Microbiology, 1977, pp 67–76.

49. Richmond SJ, Hilton AL, Clarke SKR: Chlamydial infection: Role of Chlamydia subgroup A in nongonococcal and post gonococcal urethritis. *Br J Vener Dis* 48:437–444, 1972.

50. Oriel JD, Reeve P, Thomas BJ, Nocl CS: Infection with Chlamydia group A in man with urethritis due to *Neisseria gonorrhoeae. J Infect Dis* 131:376–382, 1975.

51. Oriel JD, Ridgway GL, Reeve P, et al: The lack of effect of ampicillin plus probenecid given for genital infections with *Neisseria gonorrhoeae* on associated infections with *Chlamydia trachomatis. J Infect Dis* 133:568–571, 1976.

52. Quinn TC, Goddell SE, Mkrtichian E, et al: *Chlamydia trachomatis* proctitis. *N Engl J Med* 305:195–200, 1981.

53. Kousa M, Saikku P, Richmond SJ, Lassus A: Frequent association of chlamydial infection with Reiter's syndrome. *Sex Transm Dis* 5:57–61, 1978.

54. Schachter J: Can chlamydial infections cause rheumatic disease? In Dumonde DE (ed): *Infection and Immunology in the Rheumatic Diseases.* Oxford, Blackwell Scientific, 1976, pp 151–157.

55. Davies JA, Rees E, Hobson D, Karayiannis P: Isolation of *Chlamydia trachomatis* from Bartholin's ducts. *Br J Vener Dis* 54:409–413, 1978.

56. Paavonen J, Brunham R, Kiviat N, et al: Cervicitis: etiologic, clinical and histopathologic findings. In Mardh P-A, Holmes KK, Oriel JD, Piot P, Schachter J (eds): *Chlamydial Infections.* Amsterdam, Elsevier Biomedical Press, 1982, pp 141–145.

57. Paavonen J: Chlamydial infections: microbiological, clinical and diagnostic aspects. *Med Microbiol* 57:135, 1979.

58. Mardh P-A, Moller BR, Paavonen J: Chlamydia infection of the female genital tract with emphasis on pelvic inflammatory disease. A review of Scandinavian studies. *Sex Transm Dis* 8:140–155, 1981.

59. Paavonen J, Meyer B, Vesterinen E, Saksela E: Colposcopic and histologic findings in cervical chlamydial infection. *Lancet* 2:320, 1980.

60. Schachter J, Hill EC, King E, et al: Chlamydia trachomatis and cervical neoplasia. *JAMA* 248:2134–2138, 1982.

61. Bowie WR, Manzon LM, Barrie-Hume CJ, et al: Efficacy of treatment regimens for lower urogenital *Chlamydia trachomatis* infection in women. *Am J Obstet Gynecol* 142:125–129, 1982.

62. Paavonen J: *Chlamydia trachomatis*-induced urethritis in female partners of men with nongonococcal urethritis. *Sex Transm Dis* 6:69-71, 1979.

63. Stamm WE, Wagner KF, Ansel R, et al: Causes of the acute urethral syndrome in women. *New Engl J Med* 303:409–415, 1980.

64. Stamm WE, Running K, McKevitt M, et al: Treatment of the acute urethral syndrome. *N Engl J Med* 304:956–958, 1981.

65. Mardh P-A, Moller BR, Ingerselv HJ, et al: Endometritis caused by *Chlamydia trachomatis. Br J Vener Dis* 57:191–195, 1981.

66. Gump DW, Dickstein S, Gibson M: Endometritis related to *Chlamydia trachomatis* infection. *Ann Int Med* 95:61–63, 1981.

67. Paavonen J: Endometritis. In Murdh P-A, Holmes K, Oriel JD, Piot P, Schachter J (eds): *Chlamydial Infections.* Amsterdam, Elsevier Biomedical Press, 1982.

68. Thygeson P, Mengert WF: The virus of inclusion conjunctiitis: further observations. *Arch Ophthalmol* 15:377–410, 1936.

69. Eilard T, Brorsson J-E, Hamark B, Forssman L: Isolation of chlamydia in acute salpingitis. *Scand J Infect Dis Suppl* 9:82–84, 1976.

70. Mardh P-A, Ripa KT, Svensson L, Westrom L: *Chlamydia trachomatis* in patients with acute salpingitis. *N Engl J Med* 296:1377–1379, 1977.

71. Paavonen J, Saikku P, Vesterinen E, Aho K: *Chlamydia trachomatis* in acute salpingitis. *Br J Vener Dis* 55:203–206, 1979.

72. Treharne JD, Ripa KT, Mardh P-A, Svensson L, Westrom L, Darougar S: Antibodies to *Chlamydia trachomatis* in acute salpingitis. *Br J Vener Dis* 55:26–29, 1979.

73. Ripa KT, Svensson L, Treharne JD, Westrom L, Mardh P-A: *Chlamydia trachomatis* infection in patients with laparoscopically verified salpingitis: results of isolation and antibody determinations. *Am J Obstet Gynecol* 138:960–964, 1980.

74. Paavonen J: *Chlamydia trachomatis* in acute salpingitis. *Am J Obstet Gynecol* 138:957–959, 1980.

75. Mardh P-A, Lind I, Svensson L, Westrom L, Moller BR; Antibodies to *Chlamydia trachomatis, Mycoplasma hominis* and *Neisseria gonorrhoeae* in sera from patients with acute salpingitis. *Br J Vener Dis* 57:125–129, 1981.

76. Eschenbach DA, Buchanan TM, Pollock HM, Forsyth PS, Alexander ER, Lin J-S, Wang S-P, Wentworth BB, McCormack WM, Holmes KK: Polymicrobial etiology of acute pelvic inflammatory disease. *N Engl J Med* 293:166–171, 1975.

77. Thompson SE, Hager WD, Wong K-H, Lopez B, Ramsey C, Allen SD, Stargel MD, Thornsberry C, Benigno BB, Thompson JD, Shulman JA: The microbiology and therapy of acute pelvic inflammatory disease in hospitalized patients. *Am J Obstet Gynecol* 126:179–186, 1980.

78. Sweet RL, Draper DL, Schachter J, James J, Hadley WK, Brooks GF: Microbiology and pathogenesis of acute salpingitis as determined by laparoscopy: What is the appropriate site to sample? *Am J Obstet Gynecol* 138:985–989, 1980.

79. Bowie WR, Jones H: Acute pelvic inflammatory disease in outpatients: association with *Chlamydia trachomatis* and *Neisseria gonorrhoeae. Ann Int Med* 95:685–688, 1981.

80. Schachter J, Banks J, Sung M, Sweet R: Hydrosalpinx as a consequence of Chlamydial salpingitis in the guinea pig. In Mardh P-A, Holmes KK, Oriel JD, Piot P, Schachter J (eds): *Chlamydial Infections.* Amsterdam, Elsevier Biomedical Press, 1982.

81. Svensson L, Westrom L, Ripa KT, Mardh P-A: Differences in some clinical and laboratory parameters in acute salpingitis related to culture and serologic findings. *Am J Obstet Gynecol* 138:1017–1021, 1980.

82. Eschenbach DA: Personal communication, 1984.

83. Punnonen R, Terho P, Nikkanen V, Meurman O: Chlamydial serology in infertile women by immunofluorescence. *Fertil Steril* 31:656–659, 1979.

84. Henry-Souchet J, Catalan F, Loffredo V, et al: Microbiology of specimens obtained by laparoscopy from controls and from patients with pelvic inflammatory disease or infertility with tubal obstructions: *Chlamydia trachomatis* and *Ureaplasma urealyticum. Am J Obstet Gynecol* 138:1022–1025, 1980.

85. Henry-Souchet J, Catalan F, Loffredo V, et al: *Chlamydia trachomatis* associated with chronic inflammation in abdominal specimens from women selected for tuboplasty. *Fertil Steril* 36:599–605, 1981.

86. Jones RB, Ardery BR, Hui SL, et al: Correlation between serum antichlamydial antibodies and tubal factors as a cause of infertility. *Fertil Steril* 38:553–555, 1982.

87. Moore DE, Spadoni LR, Roy HM, et al: Increased frequency of serum antibodies to *Chlamydia trachomatis* in infertility due to distal tube disease. *Lancet* 2:574–577, 1982.

88. Gump DW, Gibson M, Ashikaga T: Evidence of prior pelvic inflammatory disease and its relationship to *Chlamydia trachomatis* antibody and intrauterine contraceptive device use in infertile women. *Am J Obstet Gynecol* 146:153–159, 1983.

89. Cevenini R, Possati G, LaPlaca M: *Chlamydia trachomatis* infection in infertile women. In Mardh P-A, Holmes KK, Oriel JD, Piot P, Schachter J (eds): *Chlamydial Infections.* Amsterdam, Elsevier Biomedical Press, 1982, pp 189–192.

90. Gibson M, Gump D, Ashsikaga T, Hall B: Patterns of adnexal inflammatory damage: chlamydia, the intrauterine device, and history of pelvic inflammatory disease. *Fertil Steril* 41:47–51, 1984.

91. Rosenfeld DL, Seidman SM, Bronson RA, et al: Unsuspected chronic pelvic inflammatory disease in the infertile patient. *Fertil Steril* 39:44–48, 1983.

92. Sayed H, Allen H, Kirk M: Chlamydia trachomatis in tubal infertility. Abstract from the 81st Annual Meeting of the American Society for Microbiology, Dallas, TX, March 14, 1981. Washington, D.C., American Society for Microbiology, 1981, p 291.

93. Taylor-Robinson D, Carney FE: Growth and effect of mycoplasmas in Fallopian tube organ cultures. *Br J Vener Dis* 50:212, 1974.

94. Hutchinson GR, Taylor-Robinson D, Dourmashkin RR: Growth and effect of *Chlamydia* in human and bovine oviduct organ cultures. *Br J Vener Dis* 55:194, 1979.

95. Ripa KT, Moller BR, Mardh P-A, Freundt EA, Melson F: Experimental acute salpingitis in grivet monkeys provoked by *Chlamydia trachomatis. Acta Pathol Microbiol Scand* 87:65, 1979.

96. Rank RG, White HJ, Barron AL: Humoral immunity in the resolution of genital infection in female guinea pigs infected with the agent of guinea pig inclusion conjunctivitis. *Infect Immun* 26:573, 1979.

97. White HJ, Rank RG, Soloff BL, Barron AL: Experimental chlamydial salpingitis in immunosuppressed guinea pigs infected in the genital tract with agent of guinea pig inclusion conjunctivitis. *Infect Immun* 26:728, 1979.

98. Sweet RL, Schachter J, Banks J, Sung M: Experimental chlamydial salpingitis in the guinea pig. *Am J Obstet Gynecol* 138:952–956, 1980.

99. Moller BR, Westrom L, Ahrons S, et al: *Chlamydia trachomatis* infection of the Fallopian tubes: Histologic findings in two patients. *Br J Vener Dis* 55:422–428, 1979.

100. Swenson CE, Donegan E, Schachter J: *Chlamydia trachomatis*: induced salpingitis in mice. *J Infect Dis* 148:1101–1107, 1983.

101. Swenson CE, Schachter J: Infertility as a consequence of chlamydial infection of the upper genital tract in female mice. *Sex Transm Dis* 11:64–67, 1984.

102. Stajano C: La Reaccion frenica on ginecologica. *Semana Med Buenos Aires* 27:243–428, 1920.

103. Curtis AH: A cause of adhesions in the right upper quadrant. *JAMA* 94:1221–1222, 1930.

104. Fitz-Hugh T: Acute gonococcie peritonitis of the right upper quadrant. *JAMA* 102:2094–2096, 1934.

105. Muller-Schoop JW, Wang SP, Munzinger J, et al: *Chlamydia trachomatis* as a possible cause of peritonitis and perihepatitis in young women. *Br Med J* 1:1022–1024, 1978.

106. Wolner-Hanssen P, Westrom L, Mardh P-A: Perihepatitis in chlamydial salpingitis. *Lancet* 1:901–904, 1980.

107. Paavonen J, Valtonen VV: *Chlamydia trachomatis* as a possible cause of peritonitis and perihepatitis in a young woman. *Br J Vener Dis* 56:341–343, 1980.

108. Paavonen J, Saikku P, von Knorring J, Aho K, Wang SP: Association of infection with *Chlamydia trachomatis* with Fitz-Hugh-Curtis syndrome. *J Infect Dis* 144:176, 1981.

109. Wang SP, Eschenbach DA, Holmes KK, Wager G, Grayston JT: *Chlamydia trachomatis* infection in Fitz-Hugh-Curtis syndrome. *Am J Obstet Gynecol* 138:1034–1038, 1980.

110. Darougar S, Forsey T, Wood JJ, Bolton JP, Allan A: Chlamydia and the Curtis-Fitz-Hugh syndrome. *Br J Vener Dis* 57:391–394, 1981.

111. Dalaker K, Gjonnaess H, Kuile G, et al: *Chlamydia trachomatis* as a cause of acute perihepatitis associated with pelvic inflammatory disease. *Br J Vener Dis* 57:41–43, 1981.

112. Mardh P-A, Helin I, Bobeck S, et al: Colonization of pregnant and puerperal women and neonates with *Chlamydia trachomatis. Br J Vener Dis* 56:96–100, 1980.

113. Thompson S, Lopez B, Wang KG, et al: A prospective study of chlamydia and mycoplasmal infections during pregnancy. In Mardh P-A, Holmes KK, Oriel JD, Piot P, Schachter J (eds): *Chlamydial Infections*, Fernstrom Foundation Series. Amsterdam, Elsevier, 1982, pp 155–158, vol 2.

114. Harrison HR, Alexander ER, Weinstein L, et al: Cervical *Chlamydia trachomatis* and mycoplasmal infections in pregnancy. Epidemiology and

outcomes. *JAMA* 250:1721–1727, 1983.

115. Schachter J, Lum L, Gooding CA, Ostler B: Pneumonitis following inclusion blennorrhea. *J Pediatr* 87:779–780, 1975.

116. Hammerschlag MR, Chiang WT, Chandler JW, English M, Alexander ER: Effectiveness of erythromycin neonatal ocular prophylaxis in prevention of infant *Chlamydia trachomatis* infection. In Programs and Abstracts of the 11th International Congress of Chemotherapy and 19th Interscience Conference on Antimicrobial Agents and Chemotherapy. Washington, D.C., American Society for Microbiology, 1979, abstract 524.

117. Rowe S, Aicardi E, Dawson CR, Schachter J: Purulent ocular discharge in neonates: significance of *Chlamydia trachomatis*. *Pediat Pediau* 63:628–632, 1979.

118. Beem MO, Saxon EM, Tipple M: Treatment of chlamydial pneumonia in infancy. *Pediatrics* 63:198–203, 1979.

119. Beem MO, Saxon EM: Respiratory-tract colonization and a distinctive pneumonia syndrome in infants infected with *Chlamydia trachomatis*. *N Engl J Med* 296:301–310, 1977.

120. Harrison HR, English MG, Lee CK, Alexander ER: *Chlamydia trachomatis* infant pneumonitis: comparison with matched controls and other infant pneumonitis. *N Engl J Med* 298:702–708, 1978.

121. Tipple M, Beem MO, Saxon E: Clinical characteristics of the afebrile pneumonia associated with *Chlamydia trachomatis* infection in infants less than 6 months of age. *Pediatrics* 63:192–197, 1979.

122. Arth C, VonSchmidt B, Grossman M, Schachter J: Chlamydial pneumonitis. *J Pediatr* 93:447–449, 1978.

123. Wager GP, Martin DH, Koutsky L, et al: Puerperal infectious morbidity: relationship to route of delivery and to antepartum *Chlamydia trachomatis* infection. *Am J Obstet Gynecol* 138:1028–1033, 1980.

124. Cytryn A, Sen P, Haingsub R, et al: Severe pelvic infection from *Chlamydia trachomatis* after cesarean section. *JAMA* 247:1732–1734, 1982.

125. Martin DH, Faro S, Pastorek G: High prevalence of chlamydial infections in an inner city obstetrical population. Program and Abstracts of the 21st Interscience Conference on Antimicrobial Agents and Chemotherapy. American Society for Microbiology. November 4–6, 1981. Chicago, IL, 1981, abstr 515.

126. Schachter J, Dawson CR: Psittacosis-lymphogranuloma venereum agents/TRIC agents. In Lennette EH, Schmidt N (eds): *Diagnostic Procedures for Viral and Rickettsial Infections*, ed 5. Washington, D.C., Am Publ Health Assoc, 1982, pp 1021–1059.

127. Tam MR, Stamm WE, Handsfield HH, et al: Culture-dependent diagnosis of *Chlamydia trachomatis* using monoclonal antibodies. *N Engl J Med* 310:1146–1150, 1984.

128. Schachter J, Dawson CR: Comparative efficiency of various diagnostic methods for chlamydial infection. In Hobson D, Holmes KK (eds): *Nongonococcal Urethritis and Related Infections*. Washington, D.C., American Society for Microbiology, 1977, pp 337–341.

129. Wang SP, Grayston JT: Immunologic relationship between genital TRIC, lymphogranuloma venereum and related organisms in a new microtiter indirect immunofluorescence test. *Am J Ophthalmol* 70:367–374, 1970.

130. Hanna L, Schmidt L, Sharp M, Sittes D, Jawetz E: Human cell-mediated immune response to chlamydial antigens. *Infect Immun* 23:412–417, 1979.

131. Wentworth BB, Alexander ER: Isolation of *Chlamydia trachomatis* by use of 5-iodo-2-deoxyuridine treated cells. *Appl Microbiol* 27:912–916, 1974.

132. Ripa KT, Mardh P-A: Cultivation of *Chlamydia trachomatis* in cycloheximide-treated McCoy cells. *J Clin Microbiol* 6:328–331, 1977.

133. Uyeda CT, Welborn PP, Ellison-Birang N, et al: Evaluation of Micro Frak direct specimen test for identification of *Chlamydia trachomatis* in clinical specimens. Presented at the Annual Meeting of the American Society for Microbiology, St. Louis, March 4–9, 1984, abstract, p 254.

134. Podgore JK, Belts R, Alden E, Alexander ER: Effectiveness of maternal third trimester erythromycin in prevention of infant *Chlamydia trachomatis* infection. In Programs and Abstracts of the 20th Interscience Conference on Antimicrobial Agents and Chemotherapy. Washington, D.C., American Society for Microbiology, 1980, abstr 524.

135. Mourad A, Sweet RL, Sugg N, Schachter J: Relative resistance to erythromycin in *Chlamydia trachomatis*. *Antimicrob Agents Chemother* 18:696–698, 1980.

136. Bowie WR: In vitro activity of clindamycin against *Chlamydia trachomatis*. *J Sex Transm Dis* 8:220–221, 1981.

CHAPTER 9

Mixed Anaerobic-Aerobic Pelvic Infection

Despite the introduction of potent antimicrobial agents, infection remains a major source of morbidity and mortality on obstetrical and gynecological services. However, the focus of concern has shifted dramatically over the past several decades. Initially, obstetrician-gynecologists focused on the group A β-hemolytic streptococcus, which was the primary cause in the preantibiotic era of maternal mortality. In the 1950s the emphasis was on gram-negative enterobacteriaceae, especially *Escherichia coli*. Beginning in the 1960s the importance of anaerobic bacteria became apparent, and now current investigations have demonstrated the importance of mixed anaerobic and facultative bacteria in the pathogenesis of pelvic infections (1–6).

ETIOLOGY

In order to prevent significant morbidity or potential mortality, the obstetrician-gynecologist must develop appropriate management plans for the treatment of pelvic infections. These plans must be based on several factors, including a knowledge of the microorganisms involved, the microbiologic techniques capable of isolating the mixed anaerobic and facultative bacteria present, knowledge of the available antibiotics and their spectrum of activity, an awareness of the potential side effects of these antibiotics and, lastly, a realization that surgical intervention may be necessary to eradicate the infection.

There are two basic underlying principles which are crucial to an understanding of the pathogenesis of female genital tract infections. The first of these is that except for the group A β-hemolytic streptococcus, *N. gonorrheae*, and *C. trachomatis*, the pathogens which cause upper genital tract infections in the pelvis arise from the normal microflora of the vagina and cervix. The lower genital tract of healthy women is a complex ecosystem that harbors multiple bacterial species, both anaerobic and facultative bacteria. An average of 6–7 organisms reside in the vagina and cervix and are present in concentrations of 10^8–10^9 bacteria per ml (7). In this milieu, anaerobes are the most prevalent organisms and outnumber the facultative bacteria by a factor of 10 to 1. The anaerobic bacteria commonly indentified in the normal microflora of the vagina and cervix include: lactobacilli; anaerobic gram-positive cocci (peptococci, peptostreptococci, and gaffkya); and *Bacteroides* species (*B. bivius*, *B. disiens*, *B. fragilis*). Recently, *B. bivius* and *B. disiens* have been identified as the major components of the anaerobic vaginal flora. In recent investigations *B. fragilis* was recovered from the vagina and cervix of less than 5% of healthy, normal women. Thus, *B. bivius* and *B. disiens* appear to be the unique anaerobes for the female genital tract, analogous to the role of *B. fragilis* as the predominant anaerobe in the colon and rectum. The most common facultative bacteria of the normal vagina and cervix appear to be lactobacilli, streptococci, *Staphylococcus epidermidis* and *Gardnerella vaginalis*. *E. coli* is recovered in 5–30% of healthy female lower genital tracts; other enterobacteriaceae are generally found in less than 10% of the population.

The second guiding principle is the recognition that Pasteur and Koch's theorem that a single pathogen is responsible for a single infection no longer holds (8). No longer can soft tissue infections of the female pelvis be explained by this single pathogen theory of etiology. Rather, identification of the presence in pelvic infections of a complex microflora which includes multiple aerobic and anaerobic bacteria has led to the so-called polymicrobic etiology of infection. In general, anaerobic bacteria are recovered from nearly two-thirds of pelvic infections and are the only isolates in approximately one-third of such infections (Table 9.1).

Table 9.1
Prevalence of Anaerobic Organisms in Pelvic Infections

Study	Infection	No. of cases	Anaerobes recovered (%)
Altemeier, 1940 (9)	TOA	25	22 (88)
Rotheram and Shick, 1969 (10)	Septic abortion	76	48 (63)
Swenson et al, 1973 (11)	Various	24	21 (87)
Thadepalli et al, 1973 (12)	Abscess	16	16 (100)
Chow et al, 1975 (13)	PID	21	10 (48)
Golde et al 1977 (14)	TOA	37	32 (87)
Sweet, 1979 (4)	Various	125	75 (60)
Gall et al, 1981 (15)	Various	43	37 (86)
Cunningham et al, 1981 (16)	Various	100	71 (71)
Cunningham et al, 1982 (17)	Post c-section	136	98 (72)
Gibbs et al, 1983 (18)	Post c-section	113	79 (70)
Sweet et al, 1983 (19)	PID	74	68 (92)
Sweet et al, 1984 (20)	Various	60	54 (90)

Whereas the older literature emphasized anaerobic gram-positive cocci and clostridia, more recent investigations have documented the important role of anaerobic gram-negative bacteria in pelvic infections. It has become apparent that anaerobic bacteria are probable pathogens in virtually all types of bacterial infections of the female pelvis (Table 9.2). The recovery rate for *B. fragilis* in pelvic infections has ranged from 0 to 79% (Table 9.3). More recent studies have shown the importance of *B. bivius* and *B. disiens* which have been recovered from pelvic infections in 19–44% and 2–16% of patients, respectively (6, 15, 18, 19, 24).

While it is true that anaerobic bacteria are recovered in a high percentage of genital tract infections and only anaerobic bacteria may often be isolated, the majority of these infections are mixed with facultative and/or aerobic organisms. Thus, the term mixed anaerobic and aerobic infections is often applied to soft tissue infections of the upper female genital tract.

Alterations in the normal environment as a result of medical therapy or operative intervention can produce conditions appropriate for selective anaerobic survival and proliferation (1). These conditions are provided by a lowering of the oxidation-reduction potential of tissue. A variety of factors facilitate the access of this normal microflora of the cervix and vagina to the upper genital tract and allow the appropriate environmental conditions for the organisms to act as pathogens producing clinical infection in the pelvis. These factors contributing to an environment conducive to anaerobic growth include impairment of local vascular supply, presence of traumatized or necrotic tissue, the presence of foreign bodies, and the growth of exogenous organisms which produce tissue destruction. The blood supply to the distal ends of surgical pedicles is interrupted, and when such pedicles have been exposed to the bacteria of the lower genital tract during a surgical procedure (i.e., vaginal hysterectomy), a nidus for infection may be established. Such avascular necrotic tissue is an ideal environment for the growth and multiplication of anaerobic bacteria. Foreign bodies have long been recognized as a nidus for infections, such as septic abortions. More recently, it has been appreciated that suture material in the skin and subcutaneous tissue of abdominal wounds may serve as a nidus for infection. Intrauterine contraceptive devices (IUDs) have been proposed as foreign bodies that predispose to the development of pelvic infections involving the uterus, fallopian tubes, and ovaries. Traumatized necrotic tissue may be present following a long, neglected labor and/or surgical procedure. A prime example of the importance of tissue destruction in the pathogenesis of infection is cesarean section. In this procedure, necrotic uterine musculature results from the surgical incision and closure of this incision with a running locked suture. The necrotic tissue is exposed to the vaginal and cervical bacteria that have gained access to the amniotic fluid as a result of labor, ruptured membranes, and multiple vaginal examinations during labor. It should not be surprising, therefore, that women undergoing cesarean section have a significantly greater risk of endomyometritis than do those delivered vaginally (1). The initial growth of exogenous microorganisms such as *N. gonorrhoeae* or *C. trachomatis* in acute salpingitis cause tissue destruction and alteration of the local environment that may

Table 9.2
Pelvic Infections in Which Anaerobic Bacteria Are Commonly Recovered

Endomyometritis	Skene's abscess
Parametritis	Acute salpingitis
Pelvic cellulitis	Pyosalpinx
Pelvic abscess	Tuboovarian abscess
Septic pelvic thrombophlebitis	Intra amniotic infection
Pelvic peritonitis	Abscess of adjacent tissue
Bacteremia	Groin, perirectal, abdominal wall
Wound infection	Nonspecific vaginitis
Necrotizing fasciitis	Septic abortion
Bartholin gland abscess	

Table 9.3
Prevalence of B. fragilis in Pelvic Infections

Study	Type of pelvic infection	No. of patients	No. of patients with B. fragilis
Rotheram and Shick, 1969 (10)	Septic abortion	34	9 (26%)
Swenson et al, 1973 (11)	Various types	91	15 (16%)
Thadepalli et al, 1973 (12)	Various types	33	26 (79%)
Chow et al, 1975 (13)	PID	30	0
Eschenbach et al, 1975 (2)	PID	54	14 (26%)
Golde et al, 1977 (14)	Tuboovarian abscess	37	19 (51%)
Gibbs et al, 1978 (21)	Post c-section endomyometritis	127	35 (28%)
Sweet and Ledger, 1979 (4)	Various types	109	20 (18%)
Harding et al, 1980 (22)	Various types	25	18 (72%)
Cunningham et al, 1981 (16)	Various types	100	10 (10%)
Gall et al, 1981 (15)	Various types	43	4 (9%)
Sweet, 1981 (6)	Various types	125	24 (19%)
Sweet, 1983 (19)	Various types	53	4 (7.5%)
Hemsell, 1984 (23)	Post c-section endomyometritis	102	24 (23%)

pave the way for lower genital tract flora, especially anaerobes, to gain access to the upper genital tract.

Thus, it should not be surprising that the majority of female genital tract infections are polymicrobic and are mixtures of anaerobic and facultative bacteria. Table 9.4 is a schematic depiction of the common pathogenic organisms involved in female genital tract infections. Of the facultative or aerobic organisms, the most common gram-positives are streptococci, including hemolytic and nonhemolytic species and *S. epidermidis*. The major clinical streptococci based on Lancefield grouping are groups A, B, and D. This identification is important in selecting antimicrobial therapy. Although many streptococci are exquisitely susceptible to penicillin G, the group D, and especially the enterococci, are notable exceptions. Of the staphylococci, *S. epidermidis* is most commonly recovered from sites of pelvic infection; the pathogenicity of this organism in pelvic sepsis is controversial. *Staphylococcus aureus*, although not as common, is a recognized pathogen in occasional pelvic infections. Recently, *S. aureus* strains capable of producing a pyrogenic exotoxin have been implicated in the etiology of toxic shock syndrome. Of the gram-negative facultative organisms, *E. coli* is by far the most common. *Klebsiella*, *Proteus*, and *Enterobacter* are much less frequent; *Pseudomonas* is extremely rare in nonimmunosuppressed obstetric and gynecologic patients as a source of soft tissue infection. *G. vaginalis* is a major component of the normal vaginal flora, being isolated in 50–60% of healthy women. It is recognized as a putative agent in synergy with anaerobic bacteria in nonspecific vaginitis. More recently, *G. vaginalis* has been recovered from the upper genital tract (uterus and/or fallopian tube) of patients with pelvic inflammatory disease or endomyometritis. *N. gonorrhoeae* is a gram-negative diplococcus which is an exogenous, sexually transmitted organism which is a frequent

Table 9.4
Schematic Depiction of the Major Pathogens in the Etiology of Acute Salpingitis

Potential pathogens			
Facultative (aerobes)		Anaerobes	
Gram +	Gram −	Gram +	Gram −
Streptococci	*E. coli*	Peptostreptococcus	*Bacteroides* species
Staphylococci	*Klebsiella*	Peptococcus	*B. fragilis*
	Proteus	Gafkya	*B. bivius*
	Enterobacter	Clostridia	*B. disiens*
	Pseudomonas		*B. melaninogenicus*
			Fusobacterium

pathogen in PID. *C. trachomatis*, an obligatory intracellular bacterium, is now recognized with increasing frequency as a major pathogen in PID. At San Francisco General Hospital, *C. trachomatis* has been recovered from 24% of patients with PID (19). The role of *C. trachomatis* as a putative agent in postpartum endomyometritis is not definitely established.

Of the gram-positive anaerobic organisms, the cocci, peptostreptococci, and peptococci are most common. At the present time, clostridia is infrequently recovered from obstetric and gynecologic infections. Of the gram-negative anaerobes, *B. bivius* and *B. disiens* are the most common. *B. fragilis*, although less frequent, is still a major cause of morbidity and serious infection on obstetric and gynecologic services. The virulence of *B. fragilis*, despite its lower incidence of occurrence, probably accounts for the attention this organism has received. *Fusobacterium* species are also very common.

MICROBIOLOGIC TECHNIQUES FOR ISOLATION OF PATHOGENS FROM PELVIC INFECTIONS

Because soft tissue upper genital tract infections are caused by pathogens which are derived from the normal endogenous flora of the vagina and cervix and because these infections often include anaerobic bacteria, special culture methodology must be employed to both prevent contamination by the normal microflora and to ensure isolation and recovery of anaerobic bacteria. In Table 9.5 the common obstetric and gynecologic infections are listed, and the appropriate site from which to obtain cultures in these particular infections is also noted. In addition, the microorganisms that are cultured from the site of infection are also listed. The specifics as to the anaerobic technology and methods of recovery for *N. gonorrheae*, *C. tra-*

chomatis, and mycoplasma are described in detail in Chapter 2. In patients with endomyometritis following either cesarean section, vaginal delivery, or abortions, the appropriate site for obtaining specimens is the endometrial cavity, not the cervix or lochia. We utilized a telescoping double-lumen plastic cannula with a wire brush as described by Knuppel et al (25). This provides an ideal uncontaminated specimen from the endometrial cavity. The wire brush is promptly placed in an anaerobic tube and transported to the laboratory for processing. In addition, the wire brush can be used to obtain cultures for the gonococcus and chlamydia. As described in detail in Chapter 4, microbiologic specimens for pelvic inflammatory disease may be obtained from several sites. From the cervix it is appropriate to only culture for *N. gonorrheae* and *C. trachomatis*. The ideal specimen site is the fallopian tube, obtained via laparoscopy, but this is not universally applicable. Therefore, either an endometrial aspirate, which is our preference, or a culdocentesis may be utilized. In patients with pelvic abscesses it is relatively useless to culture the lower genital tract, but rather the appropriate specimen is from the abscess itself. The role of percutaneous aspiration of abscesses is described in Chapter 4. At the time of surgical management of abscesses, both an aspirate from the purulent material and, most importantly, a piece of the abscess wall should be sent to the laboratory for processing. Lastly, it is crucial to recognize that posthysterectomy pelvic infections do not occur in the vagina. Thus, vaginal cultures are an inappropriate method to obtain isolates. If it is pelvic cellulitis that has developed postoperatively, the infection is in the peritoneal cavity, and the appropriate specimen is peritoneal fluid, obtained via culdocentesis. For a postoperative cuff abscess, aspiration of the purulent material from the apex of the vagina is accepteble. These

Table 9.5
Female Pelvic Adhesions

Type of infection	Sites for cultures	Microorganisms
Endomyometritis	Endometrial aspiration	Anaerobes-facultatives
		N. gonorrhoeae
		C. trachomatis
Pelvic inflammatory disease	Endocervical	N. gonorrhoeae
		C. trachomatis
	Culdocentesis	N. gonorrhoeae
	Endometrial aspirate	Anaerobes-facultatives
	Laparoscopy	C. trachomatis
		M. hominis
Pelvic abscess	Aspiration of abscess	Anaerobes-facultatives
	Abscess wall	
Posthysterectomy		
Pelvic cellulitis	Culdocentesis	Anaerobes-facultatives
Cuff abscess	Aspiration	Anaerobes-facultatives

specimens should be processed for anaerobic and facultative bacteria.

MANAGEMENT OF PELVIC INFECTIONS

Selection of antimicrobial agents for the treatment of pelvic infections should be based on knowledge of the microorganisms involved. Whereas the older literature documented the role of anaerobic gram-positive cocci and clostridia, recent studies have emphasized the importance of anaerobic gram-negative rods. Attention in the late 1960s and 1970s focused on *B. fragilis* as a major cause of morbidity due to infection in obstetrics and gynecology. More recently, studies have reported the emergence of *B. bivius* and *B. disiens* as frequent pathogens in female genital tract infections (6, 24). Not only are the latter two organisms frequently recovered from the site of pelvic infections, but they also have unique antimicrobial susceptibility patterns very similar to those of *B. fragilis*, and thus are often resistant to penicillins and first generation cephalosporins (26). It is currently recognized that infections of the female pelvis are characteristically due to mixtures of anaerobic bacteria, especially peptococcus species, peptostreptococcus species, *B. fragilis, B. bivius, B. disiens*, and *Bacteroides melaninogenicus*; facultative gram-negative enterobacteriaceae such as *E. coli* ; and facultative streptococci.

Although there have been tremendous strides made in utilization of anaerobic microbiologic technology for isolating, identifying, and testing the antimicrobial susceptibility of organisms, the initial choice of antimicrobial therapy must often be empiric. In addition to recognizing the

susceptibility patterns of the potential pathogens, several other factors are also beneficial in determining the initial selection of antimicrobial therapy for these mixed pelvic infections. It is crucial that the antimicrobial agent be capable of penetrating into the infected space, such as an abscess or soft tissue spaces of the pelvis. The efficacy of new antimicrobial agents can be compared in experimental animal models and, finally, the efficacy of antibiotics can be compared in prospective randomized clinical trials.

The intraabdominal sepsis model of Weinstein et al is an excellent description of the pathogenesis of mixed aerobic-anaerobic infections of the abdomen and pelvis (27). The initial stage of peritonitis, sepsis, and an associated high mortality rate of approximately 40% appears to be due to gram-negative facultative bacteria, especially *E. coli*. The surviving animals over the next several days develop a secondary phase characterized by the development of intraabdominal abscesses. The microorganisms associated with these abscesses are anaerobes, in particular *B. fragilis*. A similar biphasic disease process occurs in many clinical entities that are encountered in obstetrics and gynecology. While pelvic inflammatory disease, pelvic cellulitis, and endomyometritis are analogous to the initial phase of peritonitis in this model, these infections, if untreated or inadequately treated, will progress to an abscess stage characterized by the presence of entities such as pyosalpinx, tuboovarian abscess, or pelvic abscess. In this model, while *E. coli* by itself produced a high rate of mortality and *B. fragilis* (the encapsulated strain) by itself produced abscesses almost universally, the enterococcus, neither by itself nor in synergy with *E. coli* or *B. fragilis*, appeared to be a pathogen. Whether the enterococcus plays a major etiological role in mixed anaerobic-aerobic infections of the pelvis is controversial. At least in the animal model, it appears not to.

This animal model was also utilized in an attempt to identify the appropriate management for mixed infections (28). Classically, physicians have been trained to apply a single antimicrobial agent to treat a monoetiologic agent in infection. With the recognition that we were dealing with multiple organisms, both aerobes and anaerobes, it became crucial to determine whether or not the majority of organisms recovered from the site of infections must be treated, or whether only identifiable important agents require therapy. In this animal model it became apparent that treatment of only the peritonitis stage with agents effective against only the gram-negative facultative bacteria such as *E. coli* would prevent only the initial stage of peritonitis and sepsis with almost no effect on the subsequent development of abscesses (Table 9.6). On the other hand, with agents only effective against anaerobic bacteria such as clindamycin or metronidazole, while the abscess stage was prevented, the animals universally developed peritonitis with a high mortality rate. In this animal model it became apparent that either combination therapy with agents effective against both anaerobic bacteria and gram-negative facultative bacteria, or single agents effective against both components, was necessary in order to prevent peritonitis, sepsis and its associated high mortality, and the development of intraabdominal abscesses (28, 29). This basic tenet of utilizing combination or single agent therapy which is effective against the resistant gram-negative an-

aerobes such as *B. fragilis* early in the disease process has been demonstrated to be appropriate and applicable to the clinical situation as well. The investigation by diZerega et al clearly identified the benefits of this early aggressive approach in the therapy against resistant anaerobes (30). In a study involving postcesarean section endometritis, these investigators were able to demonstrate that those patients who received an agent effective against *B. fragilis* (clindamycin) had significantly less morbidity, required less additional antibiotics or surgical intervention, had less serious infection complications such as abscesses or septic pelvic thrombophlebitis, and spent a mean of 1.6 less days in the hospital than those women receiving an agent that did not cover *B. fragilis* (penicillin).

Table 9.7 is an attempt to simplify the approach to managing pelvic infections by organizing the pathogenic organisms into five major groups according to antimicrobial susceptibility patterns. The anaerobes, other than *B. fragilis*, *B. bivius*, or *B. disiens* but especially peptococci and peptostreptococci, are extremely common in pelvic infections. They are sensitive to multiple antibiotics, including penicillin, ampicillin, first, second, and third generation cephalosporins, chloramphenicol, clindamycin, and extended spectrum penicillins such as carbenicillin, ticarcillin, piperacillin, and mezlocillin. Gram-negative enterobacteriaceae, especially *E. coli*, are also very common in pelvic infections. Increasingly, these organisms are resistant to ampicillin and the first generation cephalosporins. They generally required aminoglycosides for excellent coverage. The second and third generation cephalosporins are also very active against the enterobacteriaceae. Somewhat less effective are the extended spectrum penicillins,

Table 9.6
Effect of Antimicrobial Treatment on the Mortality Rates and Incidence of Abscess Formation in an Animal Model of Intraabdominal Sepsis[a]

Treatment regimen	Mortality rate (%)	Abscess formation (%)
Untreated controls	58/157 (37)	99/99 (100)
Cefazolin	2/30 (7)	14/28 (50)
Gentamicin	2/57 (4)	54/55 (98)
Clindamycin	21/60 (35)	2/39 (5)
Clindamycin plus gentamicin	5/58 (7)	3/53 (6)
Cefoxitin	0/30	2/30 (7)

[a] Based on ref. 28.

Table 9.7
Frequency of Bacterial Pathogens Recovered from Pelvic Infections

1. Anaerobes other than *B. fragilis*, *B. bivius*, or *B. disiens*. (especially peptococci and peptostreptococci)	Common
2. Gram-negative enterobacteriaceae (especially *E. coli*, *Klebsiella*, *Proteus*)	Common
3. Enterococci (? primary pathogen)	10%
4. Facultative streptococci (nonenterococcal)	Common
5. *B. fragilis*, *B. bivius*, *B. disiens*	Common

such as carbenicillin, ticarcillin, piperacillin, and mezlocillin.

The enterococcus is isolated from the site of pelvic infections in 5–10% of patients. The role of this organism in pelvic infections remains controversial. Most investigators hold that the enterococcus is not (as a general rule) a primary pathogen (6, 31). On occasion the enterococcus has been recovered as the sole pathogen from an infection site of the upper genital tract. In most instances, this occurs in patients who have recently received broad spectrum antibiotics. The enterococcus has a unique antimicrobial susceptibility pattern; ampicillin or a combination of penicillin plus aminoglycoside are most effective. Vancomycin is the drug of choice for penicillin-allergic patients. The new extended spectrum penicillins such as piperacillin and mezlocillin are also effective against the enterococcus.

The aerobic streptococci are also common in pelvic infections. These organisms are sensitive to a variety of penicillins, ampicillins, first and second generation cephalosporins, extended spectrum penicillins, and clindamycin. However, the coverage against these organisms by third generation cephalosporins is not equal to that of the first and second generation cephalosporins. The remaining fifth group is comprised of the resistant gram-negative anaerobes, which includes *B. fragilis, B. bivius,* and *B. disiens.* These are very common organisms in pelvic infections and have patterns of susceptibility demonstrating resistance to penicillin, ampicillin, and first generation cephalosporins (24, 26).

The in vitro activity of available antimicrobial agents against the gram-negative facultative and aerobic bacteria commonly recovered from the site of pelvic infections is depicted in Table 9.8. It is important for the clinician to recognize that a pattern has evolved across the United States of increasing resistance of *E. coli* to both ampicillin and first generation cephalosporins such as cefazolin and cephalothin. Prior to the introduction to clinical medicine of the second and third generation cephalosporins, the clinician had to rely on aminoglycosides such as gentamicin and tobramycin to provide excellent coverage against these gram-negative facultative organisms. The second generation cephalosporins cefamandole and cefoxitin are very effective against these organisms. The newer penicillins, such as carbenicillin, ticarcillin, piperacillin, and mezlocillin, are more effective than ampicillin but not quite as effective as the second and third generation cephalosporins. The third generation

**Table 9.8
In Vitro Activity of Antimicrobial Agents against Gram-negative Facultative Bacteria Commonly Recovered from Pelvic Infections**

	E. coli	Klebsiella	Proteus
Ampicillin	++	+	++++
First generation cephalosporins	++	+++	+++
Gentamicin/ tobramycin	++++	++++	++++
Cefamandole	++++	+++	++++
Cefoxitin	++++	+++	++++
Carbenicillin-ticarcillin	+++	+	++++
Piperacillin	+++	+++	++++
Third generation cephalosoporins	++++	++++	++++
Monobactams	++++	++++	++++

cephalosporins have exquisite activity against this group of organisms. Recent clinical trials have evaluated monobactam type antibiotics; these are described in Chapter 19 in more depth. Although not available to the clinician at the present time, with their introduction into clinical medicine in the near future, they will provide a very good alternative to the use of the aminoglycosides in the treatment of gram-negative facultative organisms.

As can be seen in Table 9.9, penicillin G and ampicillin remain extremely effective antimicrobial agents against gram-positive anaerobic cocci such as peptococcus, peptostreptococci, and many of the *Bacteroides* species. However, these penicillins have little if any activity against resistant gram-negative anaerobes such as *B. fragilis, B. bivius,* and *B. disiens.* In addition, 10–20% of *Bacteroides melaninogenicus* is now resistant to penicillin G and ampicillin. The extended spectrum penicillins such as ticarcillin, piperacillin, and mezlocillin, when used in large doses, do provide fairly good activity against the gram-negative-resistant anaerobes. These extended spectrum penicillins are described in detail in Chapter 19. They, in a simplistic manner, are an ampicillin-like drug which provides extended activity against *B. fragilis, B. bivius,* and the *Pseudomonas* organism. While more effective than ampicillin or penicillin against these anaerobic organisms, they are not as effective as chloramphenicol, clindamycin, cefoxitin, or metronidazole. Preliminary studies with these newer penicillin drugs have shown them to be

Table 9.9
In Vitro Activity of Penicillins against Anaerobic Bacteria Commonly Recovered from Pelvic Infections

	Penicillin G	Ampicillin	Ticarcillin, piperacillin, and mezlocillin
Peptococcus	++++	++++	++++
Peptostreptococcus	++++	++++	++++
Clostridia	++++	++++	++++
Bacteroides species	++++	++++	++++
B. fragilis	+	+	+++
B. bivius	++	++	+++
B. disiens	++	++	+++
B. melaninogenicus	+++	+++	+++

fairly effective in the management of mixed aerobic and anaerobic infections in the pelvis. Mezlocillin has been studied in comparison with ampicillin in the treatment of endomyometritis (32). However, it is important to recognize that ampicillin is by no means the gold standard against which we should be comparing antimicrobial agents. Sweet et al, in a comparative study, demonstrated that piperacillin, in a dose of 4.5 g every 6 hr, was equally efficacious to a cefoxitin treatment regimen of 2 g every 6 hr in the management of a variety of mixed aerobic and anaerobic infections of the female pelvis (33). Although Sweet and co-workers had good results with the piperacillin therapy, *E. coli* became resistant to piperacillin during therapy. There were no clinical infections or problems with this developed resistance, but because of this there is concern about the use of piperacillin as a single agent in severe mixed aerobic and anaerobic infections where *E. coli* is a potential pathogen.

The use of cephalosporins in the management of pelvic infections is described in detail in Chapter 19. As can be seen in Table 9.10, the first and second generation cephalosporins, much like the penicillins, are very effective against all anaerobic organisms other than the resistant gram-negative group of *B. fragilis, B. bivius,* and *B. disiens.* Of the second generation cephalosporins, cefamandole still lacks adequate coverage against *B. fragilis, B. bivius,* and *B. disiens.* Cefoxitin, on the other hand, was demonstrated to be an efficacious antimicrobial agent in in vitro studies against these resistant anaerobes. Eighty-five to ninety-five percent of *B. fragilis* organisms are sensitive to cefoxitin, and upwards of 95% of *B. bivius* and *B. disiens* are susceptible to easily obtained levels of cefoxitin.

Over the past several years there has been a plethora of third generation cephalosporins which have been developed, tested, and introduced into clinical medicine; Table 9.11 is a partial list of these newer cephalosporins. These third generation cephalosporins are discussed in detail in Chapter 19. Experience with all these agents is relatively limited at the present time, but preliminary studies will be discussed. Cefotaxime has been evaluated in both open and comparative studies. These studies by Hemsell et al have demonstrated that a dose of 2 g three times/day is effective in the treatment of both endomyometritis following cesarean section, and pelvic inflammatory disease including tuboovarian abscesses (23). When compared in a prospective comparative matter to clindamycin-gentamicin, the use of cefataxime was reported to have a 97% cure rate, 79 of 81 patients, compared to 37 of 39, or 95%, in the clindamycin-gentamicin group. While cefataxime is a very active agent against gram-negative facultative bacteria, it is lacking in its coverage against *B. fragilis,* and because of this it may have a limited role as a single agent in the management of mixed pelvic infections. In addition, as with the other third generation cephalosporins, the improvement in the gram-negative susceptibility coverage has resulted in a loss of coverage against gram-positive organisms. Of special note in the pelvis is the decreased activity against *S. aureus* and the group B streptococcus.

Moxalactam has been investigated in several open studies (5, 16, 17). These studies have revealed moxalactam to be effective in from 86 to 95% of cases in the management of mixed pelvic infections. More recently, Gibbs et al (18) demonstrated that moxalactam was equally efficacious to a clindamycin-gentamicin regimen

Table 9.10
In Vitro Activity of First and Second Generation Cephalosporins against Anaerobic Bacteria Recovered from Pelvic Infections

	Cephalothin and cefazolin	Cefamandole	Cefoxitin
Peptococcus	++++	++++	++++
Peptostreptococcus	++++	++++	++++
Clostridia	++++	++++	++++
Bacteroides species	++++	++++	++++
B. fragilis	+	+	++++
B. bivius	+	++	++++
B. disiens	+	++	++++
B. melaninogenicus	+++	+++	++++

Table 9.11
Third Generation Cephalosporins

Cefotaxime[a]	Cefmenoxime
Moxalactam[a]	Cefsulodin
Cefoperazone[a]	Cefotetan
Ceftizoxime[a]	Cefodizime
Ceftazidime[a]	Cefotian
Ceftriaxone[a]	Imipenem

[a] Available in the U.S.

in the treatment of postcesarean section endometritis, with cure rates of 96% and 98%, respectively. Sweet et al (20) have demonstrated that moxalactam was equally efficacious to a clindamycin-gentamicin regimen in the treatment of gynecologic infections, including tuboovarian abscesses, with cure rates of 97% for the moxalactam group and 97% for the clindamycin-gentamicin group. However, these studies of good efficacy with moxalactam usage were based on a dosing regimen of 2 g three times/day, or a total of 6 g. With the recent admonition not to use more than 4 g of moxalactam per day because of concern with bleeding problems secondary to hypoprothrombinemia, the final evaluation of the use of moxalactam as a single agent in mixed pelvic infections must await future clinical trials comparing this 4-g dose to the more standard clindamycin-aminoglycoside type regimens.

Cefoperazone has been used in a limited fashion in the treatment of mixed aerobic-anaerobic infections of the pelvis, and these preliminary studies (34, 35) have revealed cefoperazone to be an efficacious agent in these limited trials. However, cefoperazone has poor activity against *B. fragilis* and, consequently, its role as a single agent in the pelvis is limited. More recently Blanco and coworkers (36), in a comparative trial of mixed pelvic infections, noted that cef-

tazidime was equally effective when compared to a clindamycin-tobramycin regimen, with cure rates of 89.5% and 87.2%, respectively. It is important to recognize that in this trial, clindamycin was dosed in 600 mg 3 times/day rather than the standard 4 times/day dosing of clindamycin. Thus it is possible that the clindamycin regimen, when used in an appropriate dosage, might have been more effective. Recently, imipenem (Thienamycin) has been demonstrated to be an extremely broad spectrum effective third generation cephalosporin (37, 38). In vitro studies revealed this third generation cephalosporin to be as effective, if not more effective, than aminoglycosides against gram-negative facultative enterobacteriaceae such as *E. coli*, *Klebsiella*, and *Serratia*. In addition, Thienamycin was demonstrated to be as effective as aminoglycosides against *Pseudomonas aeruginosa*. Its coverage against the enterococcus was equal to that of ampicillin and against *S. aureus* was as effective as nafcillin or methicillin. Thus it is the only third generation cephalosporin which has maintained exquisite activity against gram-positive facultative or aerobic organisms and is the only cephalosporin effective against the enterococcus. Against anaerobic organisms, imipenem demonstrated greater efficacy against *B. fragilis, B. bivius*, anaerobic gram-positive cocci, and clostridia than did penicillins, cefoxitin, clindamycin, or metronidazole. Preliminary trials with imipenem, both open and comparative studies, have confirmed the excellent in vitro activity of this agent. These studies have resulted in an overall 97% cure rate of a variety of mixed aerobic-anaerobic infections (39). The final evaluation of this agent must await greater numbers of patients treated with the agent, especially to ensure that the enterococcal coverage maintains its in vitro anticipated good results.

In Table 9.12 it is demonstrated that clinda-

Table 9.12
In Vitro Activity of Clindamycin, Chloramphenicol and Metronidazole against Anaerobic Bacteria Recovered from Pelvic Infections

	Clindamycin	Chloramphenicol	Metronidazole
Peptococcus	+++	++++	+++
Peptostreptococcus	++++	++++	+++
Clostridia	++++	++++	++++
Bacteroides species	++++	++++	++++
B. fragilis	++++	++++	++++
B. bivius	++++	++++	++++
B. disiens	++++	++++	++++
B. melaninogenicus	++++	++++	++++

mycin, cloramphenicol, and metronidazole have excellent activity against anaerobic bacteria, including the gram-positive cocci, clostridia, *Bacteroides* species, *B. fragilis, B. bivius, B. disiens,* and *B. melaninogenicus*. All three of these agents are described in detail in Chapter 19. While all three are very effective against anaerobic bacteria, each has a drawback which the clinician must be cognizant of. Clindamycin is associated with pseudomembranous colitis, as described in Chapter 19. Fortunately, this is a rare occurrence. Chloramphenicol has been reported to result in aplastic anemia in approximately 1 in 100,000 patients receiving the drug. Again, this is a rare occurrence, but is often fatal when it does occur. With metronidazole short-term side effects are relatively rare, but the unanswered question as to its carcinogenic potential is a drawback to its widespread use. In in vitro studies all three of these agents have been demonstrated to be very effective against anaerobic bacteria, and prospective clinical studies have confirmed their clinical efficacy.

The importance of providing antimicrobial coverage against the gram-negative-resistant anaerobes such as *B. fragilis, B. bivius,* and *B. disiens* is well demonstrated in Table 9.13. In these studies 81–86% of patients had anaerobic bacteria recovered. Most importantly, 35–69% of these patients had resistant anaerobes such as *B. fragilis, B. bivius,* and *B. disiens* recovered from the site of their pelvic infections. Tally and coworkers have recently reported a large series evaluation of the resistance rates of the *B. fragilis* group. In over 700 isolates of *B. fragilis* from 12 medical institutions across the United States they noted no resistance to chloramphenicol or metronidazole. Clindamycin resistance by *B. fragilis* was noted in 6%, while there was 8% resistance to cefoxitin, 12% to piperacillin, and 22% to moxalactam. Fifty-four percent of the isolates of *B. fragilis* group were resistant to

cefotaxime, and 57% were resistant to cefoperazone.

In evaluating the therapeutic response of obstetric and gynecologic infections, several factors must be taken into account. Not only is the patient's initial response to antimicrobial therapy crucial, but we must evaluate the need for alternative antibiotic agents, the need for use of anticoagulants for the treatment of septic pelvic thrombophlebitis and, most importantly, the need for surgical intervention for either drainage or surgical extirpation of abscesses.

In addition to elucidation of the common pathogens involved in pelvic infection and the important role played by resistant gram-negative anaerobes such as *B. fragilis, B. bivius,* and *B. disiens*, a major advance in our knowledge has been the recognition of the importance that early treatment, especially against these gram-negative-resistant anaerobic bacilli, plays in resolving pelvic infections and preventing severe morbidity and mortality due to infection in obstetric and gynecologic patients (4, 6, 31). Both animal model work (29, 41) and clinical studies (30) have demonstrated the need for early aggressive antimicrobial therapy in the management of mixed aerobic-anaerobic infections that includes antibiotics effective against the gram-negative anaerobic bacilli, especially *B. fragilis, B. bivius,* and *B. disiens*.

A schematic approach to the therapy of mixed aerobic-anaerobic pelvic infections is depicted in Figure 9.1. The traditional approach to the management of these infections has been the utilization of a penicillin-aminoglycoside regimen, ampicillin by itself, or a first generation cephalosporin by itself. With such antimicrobial regimens, cure rates were obtained in 70–90% of patients. Those patients not responding within an appropriate period of time were then treated with clindamycin or chloramphenicol for supposed *B. fragilis* infection. Once again the vast

Table 9.13
The Recovery of Anaerobic Bacteria from the Site of Infection in Obstetric and Gynecologic Patients

	Gall and Hill (%)	Sweet	Gibbs
Patients with anaerobes recovered	37/43 (86)	34/42 (81)	52/62 (84)
Anaerobic bacteria isolates	207/313 (66)	128/251 (51)	82/201 (41)
B. fragilis	4 (9)	6 (14)	2 (3)
B. bivius	19 (44)	13 (31)	12 (19)
B. disiens	7 (16)	1 (2)	8 (13)

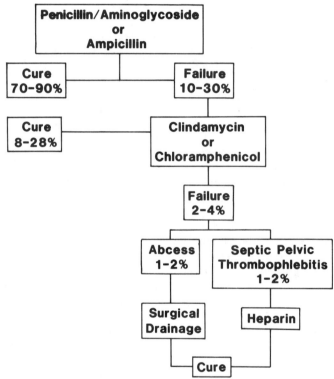

Figure 9.1.   Traditional approach to the treatment of mixed anaerobic-aerobic soft tissue pelvic infections.

majority of patients would respond, but there consistently remained a small number of failures, of which 1–2% had pelvic abscesses requiring surgical drainage and 1–2% developed septic pelvic thrombophlebitis requiring anticoagulation therapy with heparin. More recently, a more aggressive approach has been utilized in which therapy is commenced at the level of agents effective against *B. fragilis* and *B. bivius*, rather than waiting for the patient to fail to respond. It is inappropriate to expose 10–30% of patients with pelvic infections to potential life-threatening complications such as abscess formation and septic pelvic thrombophlebitis.

A major turning point in the approach to management of pelvic infections was the classic study by diZerega et al (30) in which the benefits of this early aggressive approach in the therapy against resistant anaerobes was demonstrated to yield significant improvement in medical outcome and decreased hospital costs. In this study of postcesarean section endomyometritis, patients were randomized into either a penicillin-gentamicin or a clindamycin-gentamicin treatment regimen. Those patients who received clindamycin (an agent effective against *B. fragilis*) had significantly less morbidity, required less additional antibiotics or surgical intervention, had less serious infection complications, such as abscesses or septic pelvic thrombophlebitis, and spent a mean of 1.6 less days in the hospital than those women receiving penicillin (an agent that does not cover *B. fragilis*), with a resultant significant savings in health care costs.

More recently Ledger (31) has noted that whereas the traditional approach with ampicillin or an aminoglycoside-penicillin regimen resulted in clinical cures for 316 of 416 patients (76%), 8% of these patients required additional antimicrobial agents, 2% required heparin, and 14% required surgical intervention. With the use of a clindamycin-aminoglycoside or clindamycin-aminoglycoside-ampicillin regimen in 204 patients, the cure rate overall was 87%; 8% of these patients required additional antibiotics, but none required heparin for septic pelvic thrombophlebitis, and only 4.4% required surgical intervention. Similarly, in this review the use of cefoxitin or third generation cephalosporins effective against *B. fragilis* in 285 patients was associated with an overall cure rate of 85%; 8% of patients required additional antibiotics, 0.4% required heparin, and 4.9% required surgical intervention. Thus in this large review it was demonstrated that treatment effective against resistant anaerobic organisms resulted in a significant decrease in the need for anticoagulation for septic pelvic thrombophlebitis and surgical intervention for the management of abscesses.

Prior to these studies, the traditional approach to therapy for obstetrical and gynecological infections commonly employed regimens that included ampicillin, a first generation cephalosporin, a penicillin-aminoglycoside combination, a first generation cephalosporin-aminoglycoside combination, or a penicillin/tetracycline. Only when the patient did not respond to these intial regimens were agents such as clindamycin or chloramphenicol added to provide coverage for *B. fragilis*. However, the introduction of newer and safer β-lactam antimicrobial agents which are effective against organisms such as *B. fragilis* and *B. bivius* and a demonstration in clinical practice that early treatment with combinations of agents or single agents which are effective against both components of mixed anaerobic and facultative pelvic infections reduced the incidence of serious complications of pelvic sepsis (i.e., pelvic abscess and septic pelvic thrombophlebitis), has led to a reevaluation of this approach. It is our present feeling that the traditional approach to the

treatment of pelvic infections is inappropriate. Studies of pelvic infection which utilized antimicrobials that did not provide coverage for *B. fragilis* or other resistant anaerobes have reported cure rates ranging from 70 to 90% but noted that these regimens result in a 5–29% occurrence rate of severe infections (i.e., pelvic abscess, wound abscess, and/or septic pelvic thrombophlebitis). On the other hand, studies that included antimicrobial regimens effective against resistant anaerobes such as *B. fragilis* and *B. bivius* reported cure rates in the 87–100% range and, most significantly, a lower incidence of severe infections ranging from 0 to 15% (6). An additional impetus to this more aggressive approach in the management of pelvic infections due to mixtures of anaerobic and facultative bacteria has been the realization that many anaerobic bacteria other than *B. fragilis* are now resistant to penicillin and first generation cephalosporins; among these are more than 20% of *B. melaninogenicus* strains and the newly recognized anaerobic species of *B. bivius* and *B. disiens*. Because these resistant anaerobes occur in upwards of 30% of women with pelvic infections, it seems inappropriate to not provide coverage against these organisms as part of the initial empiric antimicrobial therapy for mixed anaerobic-aerobic pelvic infections.

There are a variety of antimicrobial combinations and single antimicrobial agents which provide effective therapy against the anaerobic bacteria, including *B. fragilis* and *B. bivius*, and many of the facultative bacteria associated with the infections of the female genital tract (Table 9.14). These include an aminoglycoside in combination with either clindamycin, metronidazole, ticarcillin, piperacillin, mezlocillin, or chloramphenicol. Potential single agent therapy would be cefoxitin or, possibly, moxalactam. For obstetric and gynecologic infections it would generally be unnecessary to add an aminoglycoside to either of these agents because of the paucity of *P. aeruginosa* as a pathogen in nonimmunosuppressed obstetric and gynecologic patients. The very high incidence of *B. fragilis* resistance to cefoperazone and cefotaxime (upwards of 50%) demonstrated in a recent collaborative study by Tally and colleagues limits their use as single agent therapy for serious mixed anaerobic-aerobic infections of the pelvis (40). The use of piperacillin or mezlocillin as single agent therapy in mixed pelvic infections seems appropriate but must await further investigative efforts. Sweet et al noticed the development of

Table 9.14
Possible Antimicrobial Regimens for the Treatment of Mixed Anaerobic-Aerobic Soft Tissue Pelvic Infections

Combination therapy

Clindamycin		
or		Aminoglycoside
Metronidazole		or
or	*plus*	Third generation cephalosporin
Chloramphenicol		
or		or
Mezlocillin/pipera-cillin		Monobactam[a]

Single agent therapy
  Cefoxitin
    or
  Mezlocillin/piperacillin
    or
  Moxalactam
    or
  Imipenem[a]

[a] Investigational drug as of August 1984.

resistance by *E. coli* to piperacillin while patients were undergoing therapy (33); thus, we recommend the addition of an aminoglycoside to piperacillin in treating moderate to severe mixed anaerobic-aerobic infections of the pelvis. Other potential combination regimens, which require clinical trials, include combining a third generation cephalosporin with either clindamycin or metronidazole and the combination of a monobactam antimicrobial with clindamycin or metronidazole.

In approximately 1% of pelvic infections, patients fail to respond to appropriate antimicrobial therapy and do not have an abscess or hematoma requiring surgical intervention. In these patients, a diagnosis of septic pelvic thrombophlebitis should be considered. Heparin therapy is commenced (antimicrobial therapy is continued) as both a diagnostic and therapeutic tool. The goal is to achieve a partial thromboplastin time (PTT) that is 2.5 times control. If the diagnosis is correct, the patient should rapidly respond and become afebrile within 24–36 hr. Heparin therapy is continued for 10 days, unless septic pulmonary emboli occur. In this circumstance long-term anticoagulation is necessary.

At times the best antimicrobial agent for the management of pelvic infections is the good surgeon who applies prophylactic antibiotics properly, utilizes good surgical technique, and utilizes surgical drainage and excision of ne-crotic tissue where appropriate. It is of crucial importance that the clinician caring for women with pelvic infections recognize that often surgical intervention is the critical factor for resolution of pelvic soft tissue infection associated with mixed anaerobic-facultative bacteria. Investigators at the Tufts New England Medical Center have demonstrated a significant improvement in mortality rates in patients with intraabdominal abscesses over the last decade (42). These investigators have identified that the improved survival among patients with intraabdominal abscesses was due to earlier diagnoses being made, the employment of aggressive broad spectrum antimicrobial treatment which included agents effective against *B. fragilis* and other resistant gram-negative anaerobes, and the utilization of early surgical intervention when the patient did not respond to antimicrobial therapy. Anaerobic bacteria are recognized as pathogens in the pathogenesis of pelvic and intraabdominal abscesses. These abscesses are unique anaerobic environments in which there is an extremely low oxidation reduction potential and low pH. As a result, white blood cells cannot phagocytose and cannot kill bacteria. In addition, an abscess contains high numbers of microorganisms in the range of 10^7–10^9 organisms/ml. This results in an inoculum effect in which, although in vitro testing with 10^5 organisms shows susceptibility, the in vivo situation is very different. Finally, this abscess environment provides sufficient opportunity for the microorganisms to produce a multitude of inactivating enzymes which preclude activity of various antimicrobial agents. This is the mechanism by which chloramphenicol is rendered inactive inside an abscess environment. In addition, many of the penicillins and first generation cephalosporins are inactivated by the β-lactamase enzymes produced by this multitude of bacteria. Of the antimicrobial agents available, animal model studies have demonstrated that only clindamycin, cefoxitin, moxalactam, and metronidazole penetrated into the abscess environment in sufficient quantities to be effective (41).

In the past, the general consensus held that pelvic abscesses required surgical intervention. However, our recent studies have demonstrated that such a dictum is not necessarily true, especially for tuboovarian abscesses (TOA) (43). Among 232 tuboovarian abscesses managed at the San Francisco General Hospital over the past 10 years, in the group of women receiving antibiotics effective against *B. fragilis* (i.e., clindamycin in the majority of cases) nearly 70% of these abscesses responded to antimicrobial therapy alone without surgical drainage. It is our feeling that antimicrobial therapy as the first step is appropriate in the management of these abscesses and that either clindamycin, metronidazole, cefoxitin, or moxalactam should be the antimicrobial agent used because of their demonstrated penetration into and stability within the abscess environment. The detailed approach to management of pelvic abscesses is described in detail in Chapter 12.

SUMMARY

The selection of antimicrobial agents for gynecological and obstetrical patients with mixed aerobic-anaerobic pelvic infections must be based on a knowledge of the microorganisms involved. It is now recognized that infections of the female upper genital tract are due to multiple bacterial organisms. In general these infections are associated with mixtures of anaerobic bacteria, especially *Peptococcus* species, *Peptostreptococcus* species, *B. fragilis*, *B. bivius*, *B. disiens*, and *B. melaninogenicus*; the facultative gram-negative enterobacteriaceae, especially *E. coli*; and facultative streptococci.

In clinical situations the choice of antimicrobial agent(s) must often be empiric and must be based on known susceptibility patterns of the microorganisms generally recognized to be involved in gynecological and obstetrical infections. A major advance in the approach to the treatment of mixed aerobic-anaerobic pelvic infections has been the recognition that early treatment which effectively eradicates gram-negative anaerobic bacilli (*B. fragilis, B. bivius, B. disiens*) results in higher cure rates and lower incidences of severe infection, such as pelvic abscesses, bacteremia, and septic pelvic thrombophlebitis, than does the traditional approach to treatment with regimens such as ampicillin, a first generation cephalosporin, or a penicillin plus aminoglycoside combination. This more aggressive approach will result in prevention of significant morbidity and, hopefully, the occasional mortality that still occurs on obstetric and gynecologic services due to infection.

References

1. Sweet RL: Anaerobic infections of the female genital tract. *Am J Obstet Gynecol* 122:891–901, 1975.
2. Eschenbach DA, Buchanan TM, Pollack HM, et al: Polymicrobial etiology of acute pelvic inflammatory disease. *N Engl J Med* 293:166–171, 1975.
3. Ledger WJ, Norman M, Gee C, Lewis W: Bacteremia on an obstetric/gynecologic service. *Am J Obstet Gynecol* 121:205–212, 1975.
4. Sweet RL, Ledger WJ: Cefoxitin: Single agent treatment of mixed aerobic-anaerobic pelvic infections. *Obstet Gynecol* 54:193–198, 1979.
5. Gibbs RS, Blanco JC, Casteneda YS, St. Clair PJ: Therapy of obstetrical infections with moxalactam. *Antimicrob Agents Chemother* 17:1004–1007, 1980.
6. Sweet RL: Treatment of mixed aerobic-anaerobic infections of the female genital tract. *J Antimicrob Chemother* 8(Suppl D):105–114, 1981.
7. Bartlett JG, Onderdonk AB, Drude E: Quantitative microbiology of the vaginal flora. *J Infect Dis* 136:271–277, 1977.
8. Gorbach SL, Bartlett JG: Anaerobic infections: old myths and new realities. *J Infect Dis* 130:307–310, 1974.
9. Altemeier WA: The anaerobic streptococci in tubo-ovarian abscess. *Am J Obstet Gynecol* 3:1038–1042, 1940.
10. Rotheram EB, Schick SF: Nonclostridial anaerobic bacteria in septic abortion. *Am J Med* 46:80–89, 1969.
11. Swenson RM, Michaelson TC, Daly MJ, et al: Anaerobic bacterial infections of the female genital tract. *Obstet Gynecol* 42:538–541, 1973.
12. Thadepalli H, Gorbach SL, Keith L: Anaerobic infections of the female genital tract: bacteriologic and therapeutic aspects. *Am J Obstet Gynecol* 117:1034–1040, 1973.
13. Chow AW, Marshall JR, Guze LB: Anaerobic infections of the female genital tract: prospects and prospectives. *Obstet Gynecol Surv* 30:477–487, 1975.
14. Golde SH, Isreal R, Ledger WJ: Unilateral tuboovarian abscess: a distinct entity. *Am J Obstet Gynecol* 127:807–810, 1977.
15. Gall SA, Kohan AP, Ayers OM, et al: Intravenous metronidazole or clindamycin with tobramycin for therapy of pelvic infections. *Obstet Gynecol* 57:51–58, 1981.
16. Cunningham FG, Hemsell DL, DePalma RT, et al: Moxalactam for obstetric and gynecologic infections. *Am J Obstet Gynecol* 139:915–921, 1981.
17. Cunningham FG, Gibbs RS, Hemsell DL: Moxalactam for treatment of pelvic infections after cesarean delivery. *Rev Infect Dis* 4(Suppl):696–700, 1982.
18. Gibbs RS, Blanco JD, Duff P, et al: A double-blind randomized comparison of moxalactam versus clindamycin-gentamicin in treatment of endomyometritis of cesarean section delivery. *Am J Obstet Gynecol* 146:769, 1983.
19. Sweet RL, Schachter J, Robbie MO: Failure of β-lactam antibiotics to eradicate *Chlamydia trachomatis* in the endometrium despite apparent clinical cure of acute salpingitis. *JAMA* 250:2641–2645, 1983.
20. Sweet RL, Ohm-Smith M, Landers DV, Robbie MO: Moxalactam versus clindamycin plus tobramycin in the treatment of obstetric and gynecologic infections. *Am J Obstet Gynecol*, in press, 1984.
21. Gibbs RS, Jones PM, Wilder CJ: Antibiotic therapy of endometritis following cesarean section:

treatment success and failures. *Obstet Gynecol* 52:31–37, 1978.

22. Harding GKM, Buckwold FJ, Ronald AR, et al: Prospective randomized comparative study of clindamycin, chloramphenicol, and ticarcillin, each in combination with gentamicin, in therapy for intra-abdominal and female genital tract infections. *J Infect Dis* 142:384–393, 1980.

23. Hemsell DL, Cunningham FG, DePalma RT, et al: Cefotaxime sodium therapy for endomyometritis following cesarean section: dose finding and comparative studies. *Obstet Gynecol* 62:489–497, 1983.

24. Snydman DR, Tally FP, Knuppel R, et al: *Bacteroides bivius* and *Bacteroides disiens* in obstetrical patients: clinical findings and antimicrobial susceptibilities. *J Antimicrob Chemother* 6:519–525, 1980.

25. Knuppel RS, Scerbo JC, Mitchell GW, et al: Quantitative transcervical uterine cultures with a new device. *Obstet Gynecol* 57:243–248, 1981.

26. Kirby BD, George WL, Sutter VL, et al: Gram negative anaerobic bacilli: their role in infection and patterns of susceptibility to antimicrobial agents. I. Little known *Bacteroides* species. *Rev Infect Dis* 2:914–951, 1980.

27. Weinstein WM, Onderdonk AB, Bartlett JG, Gorbach SL: Experimental intraabdominal abscesses in rats: development of an experimental model. *Infect Immun* 10:1250–1255, 1974.

28. Weinstein WM, Onderdonk AB, Bartlett JG, Louie TJ, Gorbach SL: Antimicrobial therapy of experimental intra-abdominal sepsis. *J Infect Dis* 132:282–286, 1975.

29. Bartlett JG, Louie TJ, Gorbach SL, Onderdonk AB: Therapeutic efficacy of 29 antimicrobial regimens in experimental intra-abdominal sepsis. *Rev Infect Dis* 3:535–542, 1981.

30. diZerega G, Yonekura L, Roy S, Nakamura RM, Ledger WJ: A comparison of clindamycin-gentamicin and penicillin-gentamicin in the treatment of postcesarean section endomyometritis. *Am J Obstet Gynecol* 134:238–242, 1979.

31. Ledger WJ: Selection of antimicrobial agents for treatment of infections of the female genital tract. *Rev Infect Dis* 5(Suppl):98–104, 1983.

32. Sorrell TC, Marshall JR, Yoshimori R, Chow AW: Antimicrobial therapy of postpartum endomyometritis. II. Prospective, randomized trial of mezlocillin versus ampicillin. *Am J Obstet Gynecol* 141:246–251, 1981.

33. Sweet RL, Robbie MO, Ohm-Smith M, Hadley WK: Comparative study of piperacillin versus cefoxitin in the treatment of obstetric and gynecologic infections. *Am J Obstet Gynecol* 145:342–349, 1983.

34. Strausbaugh LJ, Llorens AS: Cefoperazone therapy for obstetric and gynecologic infections. *Rev Infect Dis* 5(Suppl):P154–160, 1983.

35. Sarver DK, Christensen GD, Hester MG, et al: Clinical and laboratory evaluation of cefoperazone. *Clin Ther* 4:164–174, 1981.

36. Blanco JD, Gibbs RS, Duff P: Randomized comparison of ceftazidime versus clindamycin-tobramycin in the treatment of obstetrical and gynecological infections. *Antimicrob Agents Chemother* 24:500, 1983.

37. Sweet RL, Ohm-Smith M, Hadley WK: In vitro activity of n-formimidoyl Thienamycin (MK 0787) and other antimicrobials against isolates from obstetric and gynecologic infections. *Antimicrob Agents Chemother* 22:711–714, 1982.

38. Sweet RL, Ohm-Smith M, Hadley WK: In vitro activity of N-formimidoyl Thienamycin (MK 07787). *Antimicrob Agents Chemother* 18:642–644, 1980.

39. Sweet RL: Imipenem cilastatin in the treatment of obstetric and gynecologic infections. *Rev Infect Dis*, in press, 1984.

40. Tally FP, Cuchural GJ, Jacobus NV, et al: Susceptibility of the *Bacteroides fragilis* group in the United States in 1981. *Antimicrob Agents Chemother* 23:536–540, 1983.

41. Joiner K, Lowe B, Dzink J, Bartlett JG: Comparative efficacy of ten antimicrobial agents in experimental *Bacteroides fragilis* infections. *J Infect Dis* 145:561–568, 1982.

42. Sani S, Kellum JM, O'Leary MP, et al: Improved localization and survival in patients with intraabdominal abscesses. *Am J Surg* 154:136, 1983.

43. Landers DV, Sweet RL: Contemporary management of tubo-ovarian abscesses. *Rev Infect Dis* 5:876–884, 1983.

CHAPTER 10

Postabortal Infection and Septic Shock

POSTABORTAL INFECTION

In the last decade, medical and legal decisions have changed the practice and outcome of pregnancy termination. Death from abortion has decreased across the country, but complications have doggedly persisted (1). Data from the Centers for Disease Control indicate that death from abortion is still a problem, and infection is the leading cause (2). Fever and infection also were among the leading causes of nonlethal complications after legal abortion (3). Among 42,548 women undergoing abortion, 4303 (10%) experience some complication. Pelvic infection was diagnosed in 436 (1%), infection and hemorrhage in 307 (0.7%), and fever only in 865 (2%) (2).

Risk factors for complications after abortion are: greater duration of pregnancy and technical difficulties. For suction curettage in the first trimester, major complications were least frequent (<0.5%), as was risk of death (1.3/100,000 abortions) (4, 5). For intrauterine injections, the major complication rate was higher (2%), and the relative risk of death was 9 times greater (12.5/100,000) (4, 5). For either hysterotomy or hysterectomy, the risk of death (41.3/100,000) was 32 times greater than for curettage (3, 4). Because of the increased risk of complications with injection techniques for second trimester termination, interest has developed in suction curettage for midtrimester procedures. In the hands of experienced operators (using laminaria and special instruments), curettage of these pregnancies has been found to have significantly fewer complications (6).

Pathophysiology and Diagnosis

Infection after abortion is an ascending process, and it occurs more commonly in the presence of retained products of conception or operative trauma. Perforation of the uterus may be followed by severe infection whether or not there is bowel trauma (7, 8). Infection frequently follows hysterotomy because there is necrosis, foreign body (suture material), and blood clot in the thick uterine incision, contamination from the lower genital flora and, often, poor drainage of the uterine cavity.

For patients who have had an abortion, the diagnosis of postabortal infection is often made readily. Symptoms may include fever, chills, malaise, abdominal pain, and vaginal bleeding, perhaps with the passage of placental tissue. Postoperative infection may be more difficult to diagnose in patients who have illegal abortions because of patient denial of the procedure. Septic abortion should still be considered in every woman with lower abdominal pain, especially in the presence of fever and vaginal bleeding.

Physical findings include an elevated temperature, tachycardia, and tachypnea. Because bacteremia occurs more commonly with infected abortion than with other pelvic infections, shock may arise from sepsis as well as from blood loss. In the presence of sepsis, the patient may appear agitated, toxic, or disoriented. There is usually lower abdominal tenderness. On the pelvic examination, there is often blood and perhaps a foul odor in the vagina. It is important to look for cervical and vaginal lacerations, especially in a suspected illegal abortion. The cervix is most often open and will readily admit a sponge forceps. If a catheter from an illegal abortion is still in the cervix, it should *not* be removed immediately, since radioopaque dye may be injected through it to rule out perforation.

On the bimanual examination, uterine tenderness is often noted, and parametrial cellulitis or abscess may also be detected. Rarely, gas gangrene of the uterus may be detected by crepitation in the pelvis.

Laboratory diagnostic evaluation should include: complete blood count; urinalysis; a culture and gram stain of cervical material; two sets of blood cultures; an anterior-posterior roentgenogram of the abdomen and pelvis; and an upright chest x-ray film. Free hemoglobin may be noted in the serum or in the urine. Gram stain of cervical exudate may reveal the predominant organism immediately. The results of blood cultures are positive commonly in septic abortion (9). This yield is much greater than with other pelvic infections. Roentgenograms in patients with suspected illegal abortions help rule out a foreign body or free air under the diaphragm from perforation. Gas in the uterus is a late sign of uterine gangrene and commonly does not develop at all. Blood should be obtained for typing and crossmatching.

Prevention

Prevention of infected abortion consists mainly of avoiding unwanted pregnancies by proper use of contraceptives. Technical complications such as retained products of conception and perforation are commonly followed by infection. Hysterotomy is accompanied by such a relative increase in risk that it is rarely, if ever, indicated, and hysterectomy for abortion and sterilization is best reserved for women with additional uterine conditions.

Treatment

The essentials of treatment of infected abortion are replacement of blood and fluids, surgical removal of the infected tissue, and appropriate antibiotic therapy. After proper diagnostic studies have been carried out, vigorous parenteral antibiotic therapy should be administered. Because of the likelihood of multiple organisms and of bacteremia in septic abortion, broad spectrum antibiotic therapy such as clindamycin plus gentamicin is appropriate for initial therapy. In the patient who is in septic shock, addition of penicillin G would be advisable.

Whatever antibiotic therapy is selected, surgical drainage is essential. In most cases, the infection can be controlled by prompt curettage of the retained products of conception, shortly after admission.

When the uterus is too large for an operator to undertake suction curettage, then high dose oxytocin administration is often successful. Rather than increasing the dose of oxytocin stepwise, we start with 300 mU/min of oxytocin in normal saline (0.9%) or in Ringer's solution. At this dose, oxytocin exerts an antidiuretic effect. To avoid water intoxication, it is necessary to:

1. Administer the oxytocin in an electrolyte solution (not in 5% dextrose)
2. Avoid administration of electrolyte free solution via other intravenous catheters
3. Observe closely for decrease in urine output
4. Determine serum sodium concentration, if symptoms arise.

If these precautions are undertaken, very few adverse effects occur. After the products of conception are passed, a gentle curettage is advisable to be certain the uterine cavity is empty.

Use of prostaglandin E_2 suppositories is contraindicated in the presence of acute pelvic inflammatory disease. Furthermore because of fairly common side effects, fever, chills, and hypertension, they can not be recommended in patients with septic abortion. In a few situations, however, laparotomy may be indicated to control infection. Indications for laparotomy and hysterectomy include:

1. Failure to respond to curettage and appropriate medical therapy
2. Perforation and infection with suspected bowel injury
3. Pelvic or adnexal abscess
4. Poor response to vigorous medical therapy and debridement techniques
5. Gas gangrene (clostridial necrotizing myometritis).

It must be emphasized that the mere isolation of *Clostridium* species from the pelvis does not signify life-threatening infection nor the need for laparotomy. Instead, the initial treatment for the patient with presumed clostridial infection is penicillin in large doses, curettage, and supportive therapy. A pelvic roentgenogram should be obtained since it may reveal myometrial gas, but this occurs late, if at all. Then, if there is no response or deterioration, laparotomy is indicated.

Prognosis

The overall outlook for the patient with infected abortion is good, but this condition must still be considered a life-threatening infection. In the United States from 1972 to 1978, 320 women died of abortion complications, many from infection; this is startling testimony to the need for vigorous therapy.

Reproductive potential after an infected abortion may also be compromised by Asherman's syndrome, pelvic adhesions, or incompetent cervix.

BACTEREMIA

A potentially serious complication of genital infection is the development of bacteremia. The principal pathogens responsible for bacteremia in obstetric-gynecologic patients are coliform organisms, particularly *Escherichia coli*; group B streptococci; anaerobic streptococci; and *Bacteroides* species (10, 11). Other significant causative organisms include clostridia species, enterococci and, rarely, *Staphylococcus aureus* and *Streptococcus pneumoniae*. In certain patients, multiple aerobic and anaerobic organisms may be responsible for bacteremia (12). Blanco and colleagues reported an overall incidence of 7.5/1000 obstetric admissions (10) and Ledger and colleagues noted a very similar rate of 7.0/1000 admissions.

Most obstetric-gynecologic patients with bacteremia respond promptly to intravenous antibiotic therapy, and their prognosis is better than that of medical patients with bacteremia. Indeed, Blanco and colleagues were unable to discern any difference in outcome when they compared bacteremic obstetrical patients and non-bacteremia obstetrical patients with similar infections (10). However, on occasion, septic shock, the life-threatening complication of bacteremia, develops. Septic shock is an acute medical and surgical emergency with an appreciable mortality rate.

SEPTIC SHOCK (Tables 10.1 and 10.2)

Predisposing Factors

All patients in shock suffer from decreased tissue perfusion. Sepsis is the third most common cause of shock in the general hospital population and is exceeded by acute hemorrhage and myocardial infarction.

Although any organism may cause septic shock, the principal offenders are the endotoxin-producing aerobic gram-negative bacilli. In most clinical series, *E. coli* is implicated in approximately 50% of cases of septic shock. Infection due to species of *Klebsiella*, *Enterobacter*, *Serratia*, *Proteus*, and *Pseudomonas aeruginosa* account for an additional 30% of cases. The remaining cases result from infections with atypical organisms such as gram-positive aerobic bacteria, anaerobic bacteria, viruses, and rickettsiae (3).

The microorganisms responsible for sepsis may be endogenous or acquired during hospitalization. Risk factors for septic shock include advanced age, chronic debilitating diseases, disseminated malignancies, and immune deficiency disorders. Patients receiving immunosuppressive drugs, cytotoxic agents, and parenteral hyperalimentation are also at increased risk. Surgical procedures in the biliary, urinary, intestinal, and genital tracts clearly predispose the patient to increased risk of septicemia.

The prognosis for survival is affected by the patient's underlying medical illness. In selected series, the mortality associated with bacteremia alone is 40%. If clinical shock develops, the proportion of fatalities increases to 50–80%. In a study of 270 patients with gram-negative bacteremia, Freid and Vosti emphasized the importance of underlying disease as having "rapidly fatal," and "nonfatal" diseases and observed fatality ratios of 86%, 46%, and 16%, respectively (14). The vast majority of obstetric patients with septic shock would be included in the latter category of "no underlying fatal disease." In such patients, Freid and Vosti have shown that prognosis is adversely affected by imprecise initial medical and surgical therapy. Successful management of septic shock requires an understanding of its pathophysiology and appropriate therapy.

Pathophysiology of Septic Shock

Endotoxin is a complex lipopolysaccharide which is present in the cell wall of gram-negative bacteria. The critical component of endotoxin is a substituent termed lipid A, which has a β-1-6-diglucosamine backbone joined in an ester and amide linkage to long-chain fatty acids (15). Endotoxin is released into the host's circulation upon bacterial cell disruption and initiates an intricate series of derangements.

One of the first effects of endotoxin is direct activation of Hageman factor (XII) which, in turn, initiates the intrinsic clotting cascade. Hageman factor also directly activates factor VII, which stimulates the extrinsic coagulation pathway. Activation of the coagulation system leads to concurrent activation of the fibrinolytic system. Plasmin, the active component of the latter system, then acts upon Hageman factor to produce fragments termed prekallikrein activators. These substances activate prekallikrein to form kallikrein, which causes conversion of plasminogen to plasmin and also directly activates Hageman factor. These reactions enhance

Table 10.1
Laboratory Studies in Septic Shock

Laboratory test	Purpose/result
For all patients with septic shock	
1. White blood cell count	Initially decreased, then increased
2. Hematocrit	Variable—depending on blood loss and plasma volume
3. Platelet count	Decreased with DIC
4. Fibrinogen and fibrin degradation products (FDP)	Decreased with DIC
5. Prothrombin time (PT), activated partial thromboplastin time (aPTT), thrombin time (TT)	Increased with DIC
6. pH	Initially increased due to respiratory alkalosis, then decreased due to metabolic and respiratory acidosis
7. Arterial pO_2	Decreased
8. Arterial pCO_2	Decreased initially due to respiratory alkalosis, then variable
9. Bicarbonate	Decreased
10. Potassium	May be increased because of acidosis
11. Glucose	Increased, but utilization is impaired
12. Blood urea nitrogen (BUN)	Increased if renal function is impaired
13. Creatinine	Increased if renal function is impaired
14. Urine culture	Determine source of infection
15. Sputum culture	Determine source of infection
16. Operative-site culture (endometrium), wound culture, culture of abscess cavity	Determine source of infection
17. Aerobic and anaerobic blood culture	Determine organism responsible for septicemia
18. Chest x-ray	Evaluate for pneumonia, ARDS
19. Abdominal films	Evaluate for intestinal obstruction, perforated viscus, abscess
20. Electocardiogram	Detect arrhythmia or ischemia
For selected cases	
21. CT scan or ultrasound	Delineate abscess
22. Intravenous pyelogram	Rule out perinephric abscess, ureteral fistula, ureteral injury
23. Lactic acid	Increased, may predict outcome

coagulation, accelerate fibrinolysis, and precipitate disseminated intravascular coagulation. Kallikrein activation also leads to production of inflammatory mediators such as hydrogen peroxide, free radicals, and bradykinin. These substances cause intense inflammatory injury to vital organs (16).

Inflammatory injury also occurs as a result of endotoxin-induced activation of the complement cascade. Activation of the complement sequence may occur through the classic pathway, the alternate (properdin) pathway, and direct activation of the first component of complement (17, 18). In the classic activation sequence, bacteria-antibody complexes combine to activate C_1. C_1 activates a sequence of components, ultimately leading to activation of C_3 and then C_5-C_9 (17). In the alternate pathway, endotoxin interacts with properdin, a proesterase. C_3 is activated in the absence of the early complement components (C_1, C_4, or C_2) and without immunoglobulins.

Table 10.2
Treatment of Septic Shock in Obstetrics and Gynecology

Correct hemodynamic abnormalities
1. Restore intravascular volume through large bore IV catheter
2. Establish reliable methods for monitoring
3. Administer pharmacologic doses of glucocorticoids
   a. Methylprednisolone (30 mg/kg) or dexamethasone (3 mg/kg)
   b. Administer as an intravenous bolus at the time fluid resuscitation is initiated. Repeat in 4 hr, if necessary
4. If necessary, improve perfusion of vital organs by administering dopamine
   a. Dilute 4 ampules (800 mg) in 500 ml of sterile saline or 5% dextrose to give a concentration of 1600 μ/ml
   b. Begin infusion at the rate of 2–5 μg/kg/min; 0.1–0.2 ml/min for 50-kg patient
   c. Titrate dosage to achieve adequate tissue perfusion
5. Consider use of shock trousers as an adjunct to fluid resuscitation
6. Digitalize patient if overt congestive heart failure develops

Treat the underlying infection
1. Initially, administer antibiotics covering all potential pathogens in source of infection
2. Surgery, as indicated

Support the respiratory system
1. Administer oxygen
2. Monitor arterial blood gases frequently to detect onset of respiratory failure
3. Early use of mechanical ventilation with volume-cycled respirator

Correct coagulation abnormalities
Keep records of medication and fluid given

There are three major effects of complement activation. First, a chemotactic effect is exerted, resulting in migration of leukocytes into injured tissue with accelerated inflammation, bacterial lysis, and enhanced release of endotoxin. Second, release of inflammatory mediators by leukocytes causes injury to vascular endothelium with resultant platelet aggregation, release of platelet factor 3, and intensification of the coagulation cascade. Third, some complement components (C_{3a} and C_{5a}) interact to cause degranulation of mast cells and release of histamine.

Histamine release has several pathophysiologic effects, including disruption of endothelial integrity, increase in capillary permeability, decrease in plasma volume, vasodilation, and hypotension. In response to this initial state of hypotension, there is an increase in the host's heart rate and cardiac output. Accordingly, in this early stage of sepsis, the patient appears to be warm, flushed and maximally vasodilated; this stage of septic shock is referred to as "warm shock" (14, 17, 18).

This early stage of vasodilation, decreased peripheral resistance, and increased cardiac output usually is short lived. As sepsis progresses, the sympathetic nervous system responds by increased catecholamine release. This sympathetic discharge leads to generalized vasoconstriction, which is intensified by the release of prostaglandins from injured endothelial tissue (19, 20).

As a consequence of generalized vasoconstriction, there is profound decrease in perfusion of vital organs, localized tissue hypoxia, and lactic acidosis. This metabolic acidosis results in relaxation of smooth muscle in arterioles and constriction of smooth muscle in venules. Extensive pooling, increased hydrostatic pressure, and transudation of intravascular fluid into the extravascular space are the consequences (13). Because of generalized capillary pooling, circulating blood volume decreases, with a resultant decrease in venous return to the heart, progressive decrease in cardiac output, and falling systemic blood pressure (19).

Although decreased venous return is the single most important cause of decreased cardiac output, two other factors play a contributing role. In shock, levels of endogenous β-endorphins are increased significantly. These peptides are released from the pituitary gland along with adrenocorticotropin hormone in response to stress; their principal hemodynamic effect is to lower blood pressure (21–23). In addition, several studies in both laboratory animals and humans have suggested that there is a myocardial depressant factor (MDF) arising from the ischemic pancreas during evolution of the shock state (24, 25). As cardiac output initially begins to fall, local regulatory changes occur in an attempt to preserve perfusion of the coronary and cerebral vascular beds. If the cardiac output is not maintained, the prognosis worsens (24).

At the end point in evolution of the shock state, there is development of irreversible circulatory failure characterized by intractable hypotension, severe metabolic acidosis, and extensive cellular autolysis. Clinically, this end state is manifested by complete vasomotor collapse, coma, renal failure, and cardiopulmonary failure.

Although the major effects of endotoxin are on the cardiovascular system, this substance also has other pathophysiologic effects. Endotoxin adheres to the cell membrane of circulating leukocytes, causing margination or sequestration of these cells. Thus, in the early shock state, there is neutropenia. As cell-mediated immunologic defenses are mobilized, however, leukocytosis usually ensues (13).

Endotoxin also exerts a prominent effect on the temperature-regulating center of the hypothalamus. Because the hypothalamic center may be depressed in the early phase of sepsis, hypothermia may be present. Later, endotoxin activates the hypothalamic center and causes elevation of body temperature, an effect mediated by endogenous pyrogen released from host leukocytes (15).

Finally, endotoxin frequently causes severe damage to the host's pulmonary system. Endotoxin directly damages the endothelium of the pulmonary vasculature. As disruption of capillaries occurs, fragmented collagen is exposed; platelets then adhere to the area of injury. Release of platelet factor 3 activates the intrinsic coagulation cascade, resulting in microembolization and stasis of blood flow in the pulmonary microcirculation (13). Prostaglandins are released from platelets and injured endothelium, and these substances cause pulmonary vasoconstriction, with subsequent increase in pulmonary vascular resistance. The net effect of these processes is impairment of pulmonary perfusion, ischemia, and progressive injury to the vascular endothelium (26). Endotoxin-mediated endothelial injury also leads to activation of the complement cascade. Complement activation causes further damage to the lung by enhancing leukocyte aggregation into the pulmonary bed, with resultant release of additional inflammatory mediators and intrapulmonary leukostasis (27). Continued inflammation leads to increased capillary permeability, transudation of fluid into the interstitium and alveolus, and destruction of surfactant. In a baboon model, Moss and DasGupta have presented excellent histochemical and electromicroscopic evidence of disruption of the surfactant lining of the alveolus (28). Sibbald and associates, in a clinical study of patients with septic shock and acute respiratory distress syndrome (ARDS), have documented marked changes in capillary permeability (29).

The functional consequence is extensive atelectasis, perfusion-ventilation imbalance, decreased compliance, interstitial and intraalveolar edema, severe hypoxemia and, ultimately, respiratory failure.

Clinical Manifestations

One of the earliest manifestations of septic shock is an alteration in the patient's sensorium, including combativeness, anxiety, confusion, disorientation, and impaired intellect and judgment. Other early signs of evolving septicemia include temperature instability, flushing, and peripheral vasodilation. As noted, the early findings of increased cardiac output and peripheral vasodilation are usually followed by a state of intense vasoconstriction, leading to progressive decrease in cardiac output and blood pressure and decrease in perfusion of vital organs (13, 19, 30, 31). Diminished blood flow leads to myocardial impairment, manifested by tachycardia, arrhythmia, and myocardial ischemia, perhaps with infarction and biventricular failure.

Approximately 50% of patients with septic shock will develop evidence of the adult respiratory distress syndrome, the most frequent manifestations of which are tachypnea, dyspnea, stridor, cyanosis, lobar consolidation, and pulmonary edema (32).

In the obstetric-gynecologic patient with septic shock, the abdominopelvic examination is critically important. There may be evidence of intestinal obstruction, wound infection, evisceration, peritonitis, or pelvic abscess.

Other pertinent clinical manifestations include oliguria or anuria, hematuria or pyuria, jaundice, nausea, and vomiting. Development of a coagulopathy may be heralded by spontaneous hemorrhage from the gastrointestinal or genitourinary tract and by bleeding form venipuncture sites.

Diagnosis

In the differential diagnosis of septic shock, the most important element is hypovolemic shock. Much less common causes in obstetric-gynecologic patients are acute pulmonary embolus, amniotic fluid embolus, cardiogenic shock, cardiac tamponade, dissection of the aorta, hemorrhagic pancreatitis, and diabetic ketoacidosis.

In the early stage of septic shock, the white blood cell count may be low, but almost invariably rises with a marked shift to the left. Because acute blood loss may commonly accompany sepsis, the hematocrit may be low. Alternatively, the hematocrit may be elevated as a result of the decreased effective circulating plasma volume resulting from pooling in the capillary bed. A diminished platelet count, a decreased fibrinogen level, and an elevated level of fibrin degradation products are the earliest and most sensitive indicators of disseminated intravascular coagulation (13, 19, 30).

In the early stage of septic shock, the patient may have a transient respiratory alkalosis due to endotoxin-induced hyperventilation, but this is quickly superceded by a severe metabolic acidosis. Lactic acid is the major organic acid responsible for the metabolic acidosis. Lactate levels correspond to the severity of circulatory failure in shock. Patients with the highest levels of lactate have the worse prognosis for ultimate survival. In a clinical study of 56 patients with shock of various types, Broder and Weil found that no individual survived when the excess lactate level exceeded 4 millimoles/liter (33).

In patients with concurrent ARDS, respiratory failure leads to a superimposed respiratory acidosis, and this *acute* state will be manifested by decreased arterial pH, decreased serum bicarbonate, diminished arterial pO_2 and increased arterial pCO_2 (32). Serum potassium concentrations may increase as intracellular potassium flows from the cell in exchange for hydrogen ion.

With marked decrease in renal blood flow, urine output will first diminish and then cease. Creatinine clearance will decrease, and serum concentrations of substances normally handled by the kidney, such as urea, creatinine, and uric acid, then will increase (13).

Plasma glucose levels in septic shock usually are normal or high (34). In the early stage of septic shock, when cardiac output is high and peripheral resistance is low, both plasma glucose and plasma insulin levels are elevated. Despite the presence of high concentrations of insulin, however, glucose uptake by peripheral cells is impaired, reflecting a state of at least partial insulin antagonism.

Microbiologic studies are essential in confirming the diagnosis of septic shock and determining the origin of infection. A sample of urine should be obtained aseptically through the urethral catheter for microscopic examination and bacteriologic culture. Sputum culture and gram stain should be performed in patients with pulmonary findings or symptoms. At least two sets of blood cultures should be obtained to determine the pathogenic organism responsible for septicemia. Blood specimens also should be evaluated for fungi, especially in patients receiving parenteral hyperalimentation and those receiving immunosuppressive drugs. Finally, cultures of the operative site wound or abscess cavity should be obtained when appropriate.

Selected radiographic procedures may be helpful in the evaluation of the patient with septic shock. Posteroanterior and lateral films of the chest may indicate whether a primary respiratory infection is present and may also permit early detection of septic pulmonary emboli, cardiomegaly, pulmonary edema, or ARDS (32). Immediate recognition of the pulmonary changes associated with ARDS is essential in view of the fact that the disorder so adversely affects the prognosis in septic shock. These radiographic changes may develop after clinical changes of ARDS already have become apparent.

Abdominal films should be obtained if there is suspicion of intestinal obstruction, perforated viscus, foreign body, or abdomino-pelvic abscess. In some instances, computerized axial tomography and ultrasonography may be helpful in delineating the presence of an abscess, particularly in obese patients in whom pelvic examination alone is difficult. In addition, excretory urography may be indicated in certain patients when there is a need to establish the presence or absence of perinephric abscess, ruptured renal pelvis, ureteral fistula, or operative ureteral injury.

Accurate monitoring of cardiovascular performance is of paramount importance in the patient with septic shock (31). Standard electrocardiography should be utilized to detect myocardial ischemia or arrhythmias. Finally, central pressure monitoring provides invaluable data in assessing adequacy of venous return and determining pulmonary artery systolic and diastolic pressures, pulmonary vascular resistance, pulmonary capillary wedge pressure, and cardiac output.

Management

CORRECTION OF HEMODYNAMIC ABNORMALITIES

The first priority in treating septic shock is correction of hemodynamic abnormalities. The immediate goal of therapy is to restore the patient's effective circulating blood volume. A large-bore intravenous catheter should be inserted. If the patient has experienced acute blood loss, this objective should be accomplished by administering either packed red cells or whole blood. In the absence of blood loss, plasma volume loss may initially be corrected by infusion of isotonic crystalloids, such as normal saline or lactated Ringer's solution, or colloid solutions, such as plasmanate or albumin. Fluid resuscitation should be started, even before the central monitoring catheters have been inserted. In women without cardiac or respiratory signs, initial fluid replacement should be administered at 200 cc over 10 min. Later, adjustments may be made on the basis of blood pressure, pulse, jugular venous pulse, urine output, and Swan-Ganz or central venous pressure readings.

To monitor the septic patient (31), a Swan-Ganz catheter should be used to evaluate cardiac function. If this is not possible, a central venous pressure catheter should be inserted. An arterial line may be inserted to provide continuous assessment of both blood pressure and arterial oxygenation, and a urethral catheter should be placed to monitor urine output.

Continued restoration of intravascular volume should be guided by measurements of the patient's pulmonary artery wedge pressure (PAWP). PAWP should be maintained at a level of 10–12 mmHg. Lower levels do not provide adequate filling pressures for the left atrium and left ventricle, and higher levels may overload the cardiovascular system (13). Shubin and associates have proposed the "7-3" rule for fluid replacement in patients with septic shock (19). They recommend administration of a bolus of 50–200 ml in 10 min with continuous monitoring of PAWP. If PAWP increases more than 7

mmHg above the patient's base line, then the infusion should be discontinued temporarily. If the PAWP does not rise more than 3 mmHg above base line, then a second fluid challenge with the same volume should be given, and the "7-3" rule reapplied. If central venous pressure, rather than PAWP, is used as a guideline, the upper and lower decision points are 5 cm H_2O and 2 cm H_2O, respectively (see Table 10.3).

Intravenous fluid administration should include glucose solutions. To avoid low oncotic pressure, approximately one-third of the fluid volume should be given as protein solution. Serum potassium levels should be checked regularly.

While fluid resuscitation is being initiated, some authors advise use of shock trousers to improve cardiac function (35, 36). The principal effect of the pneumatic trousers is to mobilize blood that has pooled in the lower extremities and lower abdomen. McSwain estimates that 750–1000 cc of autologous blood is returned to the circulation by this maneuver (36). This autotransfusion effect occurs without compromising the arterial supply to the lower abdomen and lower extremities. Early use of the shock trousers may decrease the amount of fluid needed for resuscitation, thereby reducing the risk of extensive fluid replacement leading to pulmonary edema. Use of the pneumatic trousers is a temporary measure only, however, and the garment should be gradually deflated as normal perfusion pressure is reestablished by intravenous fluid therapy. The only absolute contraindications to use of the shock trousers are congestive heart failure and cerebral edema resulting from head trauma.

Table 10.3
Fluid Administration in Patients with Septic Shock[a]

	Volume administered
Initial reading:	
PAWP <12 mm Hg or CVP <10 cm water	200 ml in 10 min
PAWP 12–20 or CVP 10–15 cm water	100 ml in 10 min
PAWP >20 or CVP >15 cm water	50 ml in 10 min
During infusion:	
PAWP ↑ more than 7	Stop and reevaluate
CVP ↑ more than 5	
Postinfusion:	
PAWP ↑ less than 3	Repeat infusion
PAWP ↑ more than 7	Wait 10 min and reevaluate
CVP ↑ less than 2	Repeat infusion
CVP ↑ more than 5	Wait 10 min and reevaluate

[a] From Shubin H, Weil MH: *JAMA* 235:421, 1976.

TREATMENT OF INFECTION

As hemodynamic parameters are being corrected, attention also must be directed toward elimination of the underlying source of infection. Treatment of life-threatening septicemia requires administration of broad-spectrum antibiotics. Although it is not the only acceptable regimen, the antibiotic combination of penicillin (5 million units every 6 hr), tobramycin or gentamicin (initially, 1.5 mg/kg every 8 hr), and clindamycin (600 mg every 6 hr) will provide effective coverage against pelvic pathogens. Aminoglycoside dose may need adjustment based upon serum levels (37). Therapy with this or another appropriate antibiotic combination should be initiated promptly after cultures have been obtained.

The most common side effect related to use of clindamycin is diarrhea, but the most worrisome complication is the development of pseudomembranous enterocolitis. In patients who have diarrhea initially or who develop this symptom, metronidazole or chloramphenicol could be used.

There are certain unique situations in which the obstetrician may need to utilize different antibiotic combinations. For example, immunosuppressed patients with neutropenia may require use of carbenicillin or ticarcillin in conjunction with amikacin in treating infections due to resistant *Pseudomonas* organisms (13). Antifungal agents such as amphotericin or miconazole may be necessary to eliminate fungal septicemia in a patient receiving parenteral hyperalimentation or in an immunosuppressed patient. A semisynthetic penicillin should be substituted for aqueous penicillin G when *S. aureus* is suspected or actually isolated (13).

Elimination of the source of infection may require surgery. Definitive surgical therapy should not be delayed simply because the patient's blood pressure and tissue perfusion respond initially to fluid resuscitation.

The management of the gravid patient with septic shock due to chorioamnionitis presents a particularly difficult problem for the obstetrician. Several investigators have demonstrated that the maternal and fetal prognosis in chorioamnionitis has improved remarkably in recent years, presumably due to early diagnosis and aggressive use of potent broad-spectrum antibiotics (38-40). In these studies, chorioamnionitis alone was not considered an indication for cesarean section, which was performed for standard obstetric complications. Septic shock-complicated chorioamnionitis developed in only 2 of 378 patients. The maternal and fetal prognosis may not be so favorable when both chorioamnionitis and septic shock coexist. In a study of pregnant baboons, Morishima and associates noted that several ominous pathophysiologic changes occurred after administration of endotoxin to the mother (41). Uterine activity increased significantly, and uterine blood flow decreased. Maternal and fetal temperature increased. The base line fetal heart rate decreased in all subjects, and all fetuses developed persistent late decelerations. All of the mothers and fetuses developed metabolic acidosis, and all of the fetuses died in utero 2-6 hr after injection of endotoxin.

Given these experimental observations, we would recommend prompt delivery of the fetus, by cesarean section if necessary, if the parturient's cardiovascular dysfunction does not improve with the measures outlined above. If maternal blood pressure, cardiac output, and tissue perfusion do improve, continuation of labor is acceptable, provided that the fetus is continuously monitored. Immediate delivery by the most expeditious route is indicated if there is any evidence of deterioration in the condition of the fetus or worsening of maternal cardiovascular performance.

Surgery in the presence of deteriorating maternal cardiovascular function clearly is hazardous. It may be necessary, however, to remove the focus of infection. Most investigators recommend endotracheal intubation and general anesthesia for emergency abdominal delivery, particularly in a patient with hemodynamic abnormalities (2). Regional anesthetics, which often require more time to administer, may aggravate maternal hypotension which, in turn, may result in further decrease in uterine blood flow and progressive fetal hypoxia and acidosis.

The preferred agents for general anesthesia are those that produce the least depressive effect on the cardiovascular system of the mother and fetus. Inhalation gases that result in marked uterine relaxation, such as halothane, should be avoided in patients with chorioamnionitis and septic shock since such patients already are particularly susceptible to uterine atony and postoperative hemorrhage. One anesthetic regimen that has been widely advocated for emergency cesarean section is the combination of thiopental, nitrous oxide, and oxygen. In addition, succinylcholine is given concurrently to facilitate intubation. In selected instances, cyclopropane and ketamine also may be used for anesthesia in unstable hypotensive patients because they tend to minimize cardiovascular depression (42).

ADMINISTRATION OF CORTICOSTEROIDS

Many investigators also advocate the use of glucocorticoids in the treatment of septic shock (43–45). Several recent laboratory and clinical studies have demonstrated improvement in both circulatory hemodynamics and survival in subjects treated with these agents. Other investigators have failed to document improved survival in patients receiving corticosteroids (46, 47).

There are several reasons for the apparent discordant conclusions reached by different study groups (48). First, it is very difficult to separate the effect of corticosteroid administration from the effect of other treatment modalities such as fluid resuscitation, ventilatory support, and timing of surgical intervention. Second, the dosages of steroids used in different studies often are not comparable. Finally, the timing of corticosteroid administration also appears to be critically important in determining a beneficial effect. In most of the investigations reporting lack of success with steroid administration, the medication was not given until the shock state was already fully developed.

As proposed by Shumer, corticosteroids should be given in pharmacologic doses very early in the shock state (43). If there is not an immediate response to fluid resuscitation, we follow the regimen of Shumer: methylprednisolone (Solumedrol, 30 mg/kg) or dexamethasone (3 mg/kg) as a single intravenous bolus. The infusion may be repeated in 4 hr if necessary. The drugs may be discontinued abruptly without precipitating adrenal crisis.

When given early in the disease state and in proper dosage, corticosteroids appear to have several beneficial effects in improving the pathophysiologic derangements precipitated by sepsis. They exert a positive inotropic effect on the heart (48). They dilate the peripheral vasculature and cerebral vasculature and improve tissue perfusion. They promote gluconeogenesis, and may thus enhance the availability of glucose to the central nervous system. Most importantly, glucocorticoids inhibit the intense inflammatory reaction mediated by initiation of the complement cascade and leukocyte aggregation (27, 49). Accordingly, they stabilize lysosomal membranes and preserve the integrity of capillary endothelium, thus preventing cellular autolysis and transudation of intravascular fluid into the interstitial spaces. This latter effect of glucocorticoids is important in preventing serious inflammation of the pulmonary vasculature (29, 49, 50).

Shumer noted that serious side effects occur in approximately 6% of patient receiving pharmacologic doses of corticosteroids for the treatment of septic shock. Complications of steroid therapy include gastrointestinal bleeding, hyperosmolar diabetes, and acute psychosis (43).

USE OF VASOACTIVE AGENTS

If fluid resuscitation and corticosteroids do not restore adequate tissue perfusion, administration of dopamine may be valuable. Dopamine is an agent with unique pharmacologic properties (51). In low doses, dopamine has a weak beta-mimetic effect on the heart that increases myocardial contractility and heart rate without causing a disproportionate increase in myocardial oxygen consumption. The drug also stimulates special dopaminergic receptors in the renal, mesenteric, coronary, and cerebral vasculature to cause vasodilation. Unlike pure β-stimulants, dopamine causes vasoconstriction in skeletal muscle. Its net effect is to preserve renal, splanchnic, coronary, and cerebral blood flow.

These actions of dopamine are dose dependent. In doses exceeding 15–20 μg/kg/min, the principal effect of dopamine is stimulation of α-receptors with resultant vasoconstriction, an effect also noted with use of older vasopressors such as metaraminol and ephedrine. The ultimate results of this vasoconstriction is a transient increase in cardiac output followed by a sustained decrease in tissue perfusion, clearly an undesirable effect in shock.

Dopamine should be administered by continuous intravenous infusion. The solution for infusion may be prepared by mixing 4 5-ml ampules (200 mg/ampule) in 500 ml of sodium chloride, 5% dextrose, 5% dextrose and 0.9% sodium chloride, lactated Ringer's solution, or 5% dextrose and lactated Ringer's solution. Dopamine should not be mixed with bicarbonate solution since it is inactivated in an alkaline medium. The concentration of dopamine will be 1600 μg/ml. The recommended starting dose for intravenous infusion is 2–5 μg/kg/min. For a 50-kg woman, the initial dose would be approximately 0.1–0.2 ml/min. The infusion should be titrated upward to obtain the desired blood pressure and organ perfusion.

In patients with overt congestive heart failure complicating septic shock, digitalization is indicated. This may be accomplished by administering a loading dose of 0.75 mg of digoxin in three divided doses, 4–6 hr apart, followed by a daily maintenance dose calculated to provide a serum digoxin level of 0.5–2.5 ng/ml. Dosage of digoxin must be adjusted in the presence of impaired renal function; usual maintenance doses will be in the range of 0.125–0.375 mg/day.

SUPPORT THE RESPIRATORY SYSTEM

The most common cause of death in septic shock is respiratory failure due to ARDS. Kaplan and associates have demonstrated that the mortality rate in septic shock complicated by respiratory failure may be as high as 90%, almost twice that in septic shock without ARDS (32). Clowes and co-workers also have confirmed the poor prognosis in patients with septic shock who develop ARDS (50).

A major objective in the management of the critically ill patient is *prevention* of respiratory failure. Because patients with septicemia and shock are hypoxic and acidotic, oxygen by nasal cannula or face mask should be instituted immediately. Arterial blood gases should be monitored frequently to detect early onset of respiratory failure. Excessive fluid replacement should be avoided. Most importantly, the patient should be managed with mechanical ventilation at the earliest manifestation of decreased pulmonary compliance, thereby preventing irreversible hypoxic damage to the pulmonary vasculature. Clowes and associates have provided valuable clinical confirmation of the importance of effective ventilatory support in the treatment of the septic patient and have emphasized the unique application of volume-cycled respirators and positive-end expiratory pressure in this clinical setting (50).

ADDITIONAL SUPPORTIVE MEASURES

Coagulation abnormalities should be identified promptly and corrected by administration of cryoprecipitate, fresh frozen plasma, fresh whole blood, or platelets in patients with disrupted circulation (13). Only in rare circumstances should it be necessary to consider use of heparin for management of a consumption coagulopathy.

FUTURE TREATMENT MODALITIES

Several experimental modalities may have more widespread clinical application in management of septic shock. McCabe and associates have demonstrated that mortality in gram-negative bacteremia is reduced significantly in patients who develop antibodies directed against certain common antigens shared by the Enterobacteriaceae (52). In 175 patients with bacteremia due to gram-negative bacilli, these investigators noted that both shock and death were one-third as frequent in patients with high titers of antibody directed against an antigen present in the cell wall of rough mutant strains of bacteria. This discovery raises the intriguing possibility of passively immunizing debilitated hospitalized patients prior to the development of septicemia.

Several investigators have documented elevated plasma levels of prostaglandin in experimental animals receiving injections of endotoxin. Fletcher and Ramwell have demonstrated that increases in prostaglandin levels correlate with disturbances in hemodynamic parameters such as cardiac output, mean arterial pressure, heart rate, and pulmonary artery pressure (20). They also have shown that pretreatment with indomethacin, a nonsteroidal anti-inflammatory agent, prevents these hemodynamic derangements in the dog subjected to endotoxic shock.

Similarly, Cefalo and co-workers have suggested that increased prostaglandin levels are specifically responsible for vasoconstriction of the pulmonary vasculature with resultant development of pulmonary hypertension, pulmonary edema, and respiratory failure (26). Using a sheep model, these authors have confirmed that the increase in prostaglandins E and F_2 can be blocked by pretreatment of the animals with indomethacin or ibuprofen. Rao and associates, utilizing a primate model, have demonstrated that pretreatment of experimental subjects with aspirin reduces platelet aggregation in the small vessels of the kidney, and presumably also of the lung, thereby minimizing stasis, microembolization, and release of inflammatory mediators such as prostaglandins and complement (53).

Finally, there now is experimental evidence implicating endogenous β-endorphin in the pathophysiology of septic shock. In laboratory animals, endorphin exerts a profound depressant effect on the cardiovascular system. Holaday and Fader have shown that this hypotensive effect of endorphin can be reversed by administration of the narcotic antagonist naloxone (Narcan) (23). Two reports have described the use of endorphin antagonists in patients with seemingly irreversible septic shock (54, 55). Despite the apparent efficacy of these experimental modalities of treatment, however, additional clinical research is needed to establish their value in the management of septic shock.

References

1. Centers for Disease Control, Abortion Surveillance. Annual Summary 1978, U.S. Department of Health and Human Services, November 1980, p. 61.
2. Centers for Disease Control, Abortion Surveillance. Annual Summary 1978, U.S. Department of Health and Human Services, November 1980, p. 50.
3. Tietze C, Lewit S: Legal abortions: early medical complications: an interim report of the Joint Program for the Study of Abortion. *J Reprod Med* 8:193, 1972.
4. Tietze C, Lewit S: Legal abortions: early medical complications: an interim report of the Joint Program for the Study of Abortion. *J Reprod Med* 8:193, 1972.
5. Tietze C, Lewit S: Legal abortions: early medical complications: an interim report of the Joint Program for the Study of Abortion. *J Reprod Med* 8:193, 1972.
6. Grimes DA, Schulz KF, Cates W, et al: Midtrimester abortion by dilatation and evacuation. A safe and practical alternative. *N Engl J Med* 296:1141, 1977.
7. Grimes DA, Cates W, Selik RM: Fatal septic abortion in the United States, 1975–1977. *Obstet Gynecol* 57:739, 1981.
8. Cates W, Grimes DA: Deaths from second trimester abortion by dilatation and evacuation: causes, prevention, facilities. *Obstet Gynecol* 58:401, 1981.
9. Rotheram EB, Schick SF: Nonclostridial anaerobic bacteria in septic abortion. *Am J Med* 46:80, 1969.
10. Blanco JD, Gibbs RS, Castaneda YS: Bacteremia in obstetrics: clinical course. *Obstet Gynecol* 58:621, 1981.
11. Ledger WJ, Norman M, Gee C, et al: Bacteremia on an obstetric-gynecologic service. *Am J Obstet Gynecol* 121:205, 1975.
12. Monif GRG, Baer H: Polymicrobial bacteremia in obstetric patients. *Obstet Gynecol* 48:167, 1976.
13. Eskridge RA: Septic shock. *Crit Care Q* 2:55, 1980.
14. Freid MA, Vosti KL: The importance of underlying disease in patients with gram-negative bacteremia. *Arch Intern Med* 121:418, 1968.
15. Bernheim HA, Block LH, Atkins E: Fever: pathogenesis, pathophysiology, and purpose. *Ann Intern Med* 91:261, 1979.
16. Mason JW, Kleeberg U, Dolan P, Colman RW: Plasma kallikrein and Hageman factor in gram-negative bacteremia due to gram-negative organisms. *Ann Intern Med* 73:545, 1970.
17. McCabe WR: Serum complement levels in bacteremia due to gram-negative organisms. *N Engl J Med* 288:21, 1973.
18. Fearon DT, Ruddy S, Schur PH, McCabe WR: Activation of the properdin pathway of complement in patients with gram-negative bacteremia. *N Engl J Med* 292:937, 1975.
19. Shubin H, Weil MH, Carlson RW: Bacterial shock. *Am Heart J* 94:112, 1977.
20. Fletcher JR, Ramwell PW, Herman CM: Prostaglandins and the hemodynamic course of endotoxin shock. *J Surg Res* 20:589, 1976.
21. Guillemin R, Vargo T, Rossier J, Minick S, Ling N, Rivier C, Vale W, Bloom F: β-endorphin and adrenocorticotropin are secreted concomitantly by the pituitary gland. *Science* 197:1367, 1977.
22. Moberg GP: Site of action of endotoxins on hypothalamic-pituitary-adrenal axis. *Am J Physiol* 220:397, 1971.
23. Holaday JW, Faden AI: Naloxone reversal of endotoxin hypotension suggests role of endorphins in shock. *Nature* 275:450, 1978.
24. Weisel RD, Vito L, Dennis RC, Valeri CR, Hechtman HB: Myocardial depression during sepsis. *Am J Surg* 133:512, 1977.
25. Raffa J, Trunkey DD: Myocardial depression in sepsis. *J Trauma* 118:617, 1978.
26. Cefalo RC, Lewis PE, O'Brien WF, Fletcher JR, Ramwell PW: The role of prostaglandins in endotoxemia. *Am J Obstet Gynecol* 137:53, 1980.
27. Hammerschmidt DE, White JG, Craddock PR, Jacob HS: Corticosteroids inhibit complement-induced granulocyte aggregation. *J Clin Invest* 63:798, 1979.
28. Moss GS, DasGupta TK: The normal electron histochemistry and the effect of hemorrhagic shock on the pulmonary surfactant system. *Surg Gynecol Obstet* 140:53, 1975.
29. Sibbald WJ, Anderson RR, Reid B, Holliday RL, Driedger AA: Alveolar-capillary permeability in human septic ARDSK. *Chest* 79:133, 1981.
30. Tramont EC: The diagnosis and treatment of septic shock. *Milit Med* 144:153, 1979.
31. Weil MH, Nishijima H: Cardiac output in bacterial shock. *Am J Med* 64:920, 1978.
32. Kaplan RL, Sahn SA, Petty TL: Incidence and outcome of the respiratory distress syndrome in gram-negative sepsis. *Arch Intern Med* 139:867, 1979.
33. Broder G, Wil MH: Excess lactate: an index of reversibility of shock in human patients. *Science* 143:1457, 1964.
34. Clowes GHA, O'Donnell TF, Ryan NT, Blackburn GL: Energy metabolism in sepsis. *Am Surg* 179:684, 1974.
35. Paris PM: Antishock garments. *N Engl J Med* 305:960, 1981.
36. McSwain NE: Pneumatic trousers and the management of shock. *J Trauma* 17:719, 1977.
37. Zaske DE, Cipolle RJ, Strate RG, Malo JW, Koszalka MF: Rapid gentamicin elimination in obstetric patients. *Obstet Gynecol* 56:559, 1980.
38. Koh KS, Chan FH, Monfared AH, Ledger WJ, Paul RH: The changing perinatal and maternal outcome in chorioamnionitis. *Obstet Gynecol* 53:730, 1979.
39. Gibbs RS, Castillo MS, Rodgers RJ: Management of acute chorioamnionitis. *Am J Obstet Gynecol* 136:709, 1980.
40. Yoder PR, Gibbs RS, Blanco JP, et al: A prospec-

tive, controlled study of maternal and perinatal outcome after intra-amniotic infection at term. *Am J Obstet Gynecol* 145:695, 1983.

41. Morishima HO, Niemann WH, James LS: Effects of endotoxin on the pregnant baboon and fetus. *Am J Obstet Gynecol* 131:899, 1978.

42. Shnider SM: Choice of anesthesia for labor and delivery. *Obstet Gynecol* 58:24S, 1981.

43. Shumer W: Steroids in the treatment of clinical septic shock. *Ann Surg* 184:333, 1976.

44. Sladen A: Methylprednisolone—pharmacologic doses in shock lung syndrome. *J Thorac Cardiovasc Surg* 71:800, 1976.

45. Kusajima K, Wax S, Webb WR: Effects of methylprednisone on pulmonary microcirculation. *Surg Gynecol Obstet* 139:1, 1974.

46. Klastersky J, Cappel R, Debusscher L: Effectiveness of betamethasone in management of severe infections. *N Engl J Med* 284:1248, 1971.

47. Kreger BE, Craven DE, McCabe WR: Gram-negative bacteremia. *Am J Med* 68:344, 1980.

48. Sheagren JN: Septic shock and corticosteroids. *N Engl J Med* 305:456, 1981.

49. Jacob HS: Role of complement and granulocytes in septic shock (monograph). Kalamazoo, MI, Upjohn, 1978.

50. Clowes GHA, Hirsch E, Williams L, Kwasnik E, O'Donnel TF, Craven P, Saini VK, Morade I, Farizan M, Saravis C, Stone M, Kuffler J: Septic shock and shock lung in man. *Ann Surg* 181:681, 1975.

51. Goldberg LI: Dopamine—clinical uses of an endogenous catecholamine. *N Engl J Med* 291:707, 1974.

52. McCabe WR, Kreger BE, Johns M: Type-specific and cross-reactive antibodies in gram-negative bacteremia. *N Engl J Med* 287:261, 1972.

53. Rao PS, Cavanagh D, Lamont WG: Endotoxic shock in the primate: effects of aspirin and dipyridamole administration. *Am J Obstet Gynecol* 140:914, 1981.

54. Tiengo M: Naloxone in irreversible shock. *Lancet* 2:690, 1980.

55. Peters WP, Friedman PA, Johnson MW, Mitch WE: Pressor effect of naloxone in septic shock. *Lancet* 1:529, 1981.

CHAPTER 11

Wound and Episiotomy Infections

WOUND INFECTIONS

Abdominal wound infection following cesarean section or gynecologic surgery is a common complication, accounting for significant extension of hospital stay and adding considerable cost to hospital bills. Surveys of abdominal surgery (1, 2), in general, have revealed wound infection in 4.8–7.5% of cases. For abdominal hysterectomy, the wound infection rate was 6.1%, and for oophorectomy, it was 3.1% (1). After cesarean section, wound infection has been reported in an average of 10% (range 0–15%) of patients in control groups in prophylaxis studies (3). In San Antonio, a prospective study of infection after cesarean section revealed that 4.6% of 413 consecutive cases were complicated by wound infection (4). Sweet and Ledger reported that abdominal wound infection complicated 6% of cesarean sections (5). Prospective studies have suggested an increased incidence of wound infection if membranes have been ruptured greater than 6 hr.

According to the definition of wound infection adopted by the National Research Council in 1964, a wound is defined as "infected" if pus discharges and "possibly infected" if it develops the signs of inflammation or serous discharge. Possibly infected wounds are inspected daily until pus discharge (infected) or they resolve (not infected) (1).

In 1964, the Ad Hoc Committee of the Committee on Trauma of the National Research Council formulated a standard classification of surgical wound into four categories (1): *Clean wound*—the gastrointestinal, respiratory, or genitourinary tract is not entered. No inflammation is encountered, and no break in aseptic technique occurs. Cruse, in a large prospective study noted that of 36,383 clean wounds, only 624 (1.7%) became infected (6). *Clean-contaminated*—the gastrointestinal or respiratory tract is entered without significant spillage. Included in this category are procedures involving entry into the vagina or the uninfected biliary tract.

Cesarean section in the presence of ruptured membranes falls into this category. Cruse's study observed that of 7,335 clean-contaminated wounds, wound infection was diagnosed in 646 (8.8%). An expected rate of 10% is the generally quoted estimate of infection in these cases. *Contaminated*—acute inflammation (without pus formation) is encountered. There is a major break in aseptic technique, or gross spillage from the gastrointestinal tract occurs. Incisions into infected biliary or urinary tracts are also included in this category. A cesarean section performed in the presence of chorioamnionitis belongs in the contaminated group. The expected infection rate in contaminated cases is about 20%. Cruse reported that 458 of 2,613 contaminated wounds (17.5%) became infected in his prospective surveillance study. *Dirty*—presence of pus, a perforated viscus, and traumatic wounds are included here. The definition implies the presence of organisms in ordinarily sterile tissue prior to the operation. A 30% infection rate is considered a reasonable estimate. Cruse documented that in 1,586 dirty wounds, infection occurred in 660 (41.6%).

Cost

The cost of wound abscess results primarily from extension of hospital stay, but other costs, including antibiotics, supplies, and additional treatments, such as operations, may be incurred. Haley and colleagues (7) estimated the direct costs of surgical wounds of all types to be $884 in 1980. Based upon just five wound infections after cesarean section, Green and Wenzel (8) reported the additional cost to be $527 in 1977.

Pathogenesis

The two major factors which determine whether a wound will become infected are the amount of bacterial contamination and the resistance of the patient. Bacterial contamination is either of endogenous origin, from the patient's own microbial flora, or exogenous, from the environment. The influence of endogenous contamination is readily documented by the progressive increase from a clean infection rate through a 30% rate in dirty operative cases. In general, the source of endogenous bacteria in obstetric or gynecologic abdominal wound infections is either the abdominal skin or the flora of the vagina and cervix.

The condition of the wound is important in determining local resistance and is to a large extent a reflection of surgical technique. Gentle tissue handling, complete hemostasis, debridement of devitalized tissue, adequate blood supply, obliteration of dead space and closing the wound without tension are commonly recognized principles of good surgical technique. The presence of hematomas or foreign bodies in the wound predispose to the development of infection. Hemoglobin interferes with leukocyte migration and phagocytosis. An inadequate blood supply leads to a lower oxygen tension and acidosis in the wound, with the resultant inability of macrophages to kill bacteria.

In general surgery, risk factors for wound abscess have been reported in excellent studies (1, 2). Factors identified (1, 2) are: bacterial contamination of the wound, age, obesity, operating time, use of drains, and duration of preoperative hospitalization. Although both studies reported increases with diabetes and malnutrition, Howard et al (1) concluded that these were indirect factors, and, if corrected for age, length of operation, etc., the differences were no longer apparent. Use of steroids was associated with an increase in wound infections in the study by Howard et al (1), but not in that by Cruse and Foord (2). Cruse and Foord (2) reported an increase in wound infection in operations performed between midnight and 8 a.m., while Howard et al (1) concluded that time of day had no substantial direct effect. In addition, Howard et al (1) found an increase in wound infections when there was an infection which was remote from the operative incision. Finally, Cruse and Foord (2) also noted increases in infection rates with puncture of the surgeon's gloves and shaving or clipping of hair at the operative site (as compared to the use of depilatory cream or no hair removal at all).

However, risk factors for wound abscess after cesarean delivery may be different from those for abscess after other surgical procedures. Patients undergoing cesarean delivery have a limited age range, usually experience only a brief preoperative hospital stay, and rarely have debilitating diseases; furthermore, the operation itself is relatively short. On the other hand, many cesarean sections are performed as emergency procedures, often in a field contaminated with large numbers of bacteria (9, 10). It is likely that this fluid leads to contamination of the wound and, in some patients, results in wound abscess.

Studies of wound abscess after cesarean section have been limited. In 1977, Stage and coworkers (11) performed a discriminant analysis on data from 25 patients having cesarean delivery to determine risk factors for wound infection. The highest correlations were found with temperature on admission, total number of vaginal examinations, and number of vaginal examinations after membrane rupture. A moderate degree of correlation was found with length of surgical procedure and hours in labor prior to surgery, but only a poor correlation was found with presence of ruptured membranes or hours that membranes had been ruptured. Recently, Dommisse and Kilpert (12) reported on wound sepsis after 232 cesarean deliveries in Cape Town, South Africa. Wounds became septic in 22 patients (9.5%). Although none of the associations studied achieved statistical significance, these authors did note that wound sepsis was more frequent in nonelective compared with elective cases (10.4% versus 7.7%), in cases with labor for more than 12 hr compared with labor for less than 12 hr compared with no labor (14.6% versus 8.7% versus 6.7%), and in cases with membrane rupture for more than 12 hr compared with rupture for less than 12 hr compared with no rupture (16.2% versus 12% versus 5.8%).

Using a retrospective case-control design, Gibbs and colleagues found that selected features of labor were strongly associated with wound abscess after cesarean section. These features were duration of labor, interval from rupture of membranes to delivery, number of vaginal examinations, and duration of internal fetal monitoring. These features were also the ones associated with intrauterine infection on the authors' service (13).

In addition, other risk factors were operating time and estimated blood loss, but age, parity, weight, preoperative stay, preoperative hematocrit, surgeon's year of training, time of day, type of anesthesia, and presence of other maternal disease (hypertension, diabetes, etc.) were not significantly associated with wound abscess. In patients with abscess, 31% had transverse skin incision, while 17% of controls had this type of incision (p = 0.08).

Microbiology

The most prevalent bacteria in the lower genital tract include facultative (aerobic) organisms such as: *Staphylococcus epidermidis, Escherichia coli, Proteus, Peptostreptococcus,* and *Bacteroides* species (*Bacteroides fragilis* and *Bacteroides bivius*). Clostridial organisms have also been noted as part of the normal lower genital tract flora. Because the normal flora is comprised of aerobic and anaerobic bacteria, endogenous wound infections are often of the mixed aerobic and anaerobic (polymicrobic) type. It requires a relatively large number of bacteria to produce an infection; 10^5 bacteria/ml or g is the crucial inoculum. The presence of a foreign body such as suture material reduces the required inoculum by a factor of 10,000. *Staphylococcus aureus* may find its way into the abdominal wound from the skin, the genital tract (where it is found in 5–10% of women), or the environment (including surgical personnel). Yet, detailed study of wound infections after obstetric-gynecologic surgery has not been done.

Clinical Presentation and Treatment

EARLY ONSET WOUND INFECTION

This type of infection occurs within the first 48 hr postoperatively, often in the initial 12–24 hr. Patients present with an elevated temperature and an alteration in appearance of the abdominal wound. This may be a spreading cellulitis or discoloration of the skin in association with an advancing margin of active infection. Early wound infection is usually caused by a single bacterial pathogen, most commonly group A streptococcus or *Clostridium perfringens*. A gram stain of material aspirated from the active margin of infection is diagnostic. Gram-positive rods are strongly suggestive of clostridia; and gram-positive cocci indicate the probable presence of group A streptococci. Infection due to group A streptococci should be suspected if the patient develops a diffuse cellulitis or systemic illness or both. Group B streptococci may present a similar picture. In clostridial infection, cellulitis of the skin and subcutaneous tissue is associated with a watery discharge. This is followed by the characteristic bronze appearance

of the skin and crepitation in the vicinity of the wound.

The treatment of early wound infection consists of antibiotics and excision of necrotic tissue. Penicillin is the antibiotic of choice for both clostridia and group A streptococcus; alternatives include ampicillin, cephalosporins, erythromycin, or chloramphenicol. Extensive debridement and excision of necrotic tissue may be required. It is crucial to remove all nonviable tissue. Failure to treat aggressively these early onset wound infections exposes patients to the risks of necrotizing fasciitis, bacteremia, and disseminated intravascular coagulation.

LATE ONSET WOUND INFECTION

Late onset wound infections occur at about 4–8 days postoperatively. They present with fever and a swollen, erythematous, draining wound. The basic treatment modality for late wound infection is incision and drainage. Antibiotics are not generally required, unless there is extensive coexistent cellulitis present. Once the wound has been opened and drained and nonviable tissue excised, the patient should rapidly become afebrile, usually within 12 hr. If a response does not occur within this time, broad spectrum antibiotic therapy aimed at mixed aerobic-anaerobic bacteria should be instituted, and the possibility of a more extensive infectious process such as *necrotizing fasciitis* must be entertained.

The diagnosis of fasciitis is based on the presence of edema and necrosis, with partial liquefaction of the fascia adjacent to the wound site. Necrotizing fasciitis is a polymicrobic infection; the bacterial isolates include such anaerobes as peptostreptococci, peptococci, and *B. fragilis*, as well as such facultatives as *E. coli, Klebsiella* species, *Proteus* species, and *S. aureus*. Although necrotizing fasciitis is a rare clinical entity after cesarean section, the necessity for early recognition, extensive surgical debridement, aerobic and anaerobic cultures, and antimicrobial therapy are well documented. Treatment must be aggressive and must include extensive drainage and debridement and administration of appropriate antibiotics, as indicated by gram stain and cultures, in high dosage as adjunctive therapy. In view of the mixed aerobic-anaerobic nature of these infections, appropriate antimicrobial regimens would be a broad spectrum combination such as clindamycin-aminoglycoside.

Another form of severe wound infection is *progressive synergistic bacterial gangrene*. Classically described by Meleney and co-workers, this process appears to have a central ulcer, surrounded by a characteristic deep red or purple zone (Fig. 11.1). In turn, this is surrounded by an outer zone of erythema (14–16). At times, the ulcerated area is dark grey or even black. The process is slowly progressive, and there is often severe pain. A mixture of organisms may be responsible, and appropriate therapy consists of broad spectrum antibiotics and sharp debridement. Often serial debriding procedures are necessary to contain this process.

More fulminant in nature is *clostridial gas gangrene* (clostridial *anaerobic myonecrosis*) (14). *C. perfringens* is responsible in 60–80% of cases, with other clostridial species responsible in the rest. The clinical signs are sudden onset of severe pain in the wound with mild local edema, and thin watery exudate issuing from the wound. Systemic signs are usually present and vary from fever and tachycardia to septic shock. In advanced states, the wound has a bronzed appearance, with bullae, cutaneous gangrene, and crepitus. A radiograph may show gas,

but this is a late sign. The main stay of treatment is adequate surgical debridement. Because of systemic findings, antibiotic therapy is necessary; penicillin G (20 million IV in divided doses) would be preferred. Hyperbaric chambers and polyvalent antitoxin are of unproved value.

Prevention

Several simple suggestions will help decrease the risk for development of postcesarean section abdominal wound infection. These include: (a) limiting duration of preoperative hospitalization; (b) when possible, correcting malnutrition or anemia; (c) stabilizing diabetes; (d) decreasing steroids or immunosuppressive agents, if possible; (e) eradicating all infection such as urinary tract infection; (f) shaving at the operative site just prior to the surgery; (g) preparing the skin with an iodine-containing disinfectant; (h) surgeons scrubbing for greater than 5 min; (i) limiting operating room traffic; (j) using appropriate operating room ventilation and airflow; and (k) using proper surgical technique. Prophylactic antibiotics are of value in some operations, as discussed in Chapter 20.

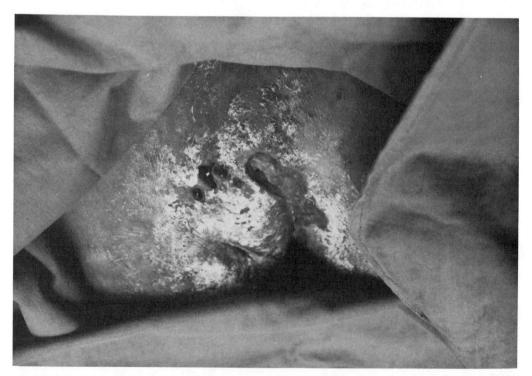

Figure 11.1. Progressive synergistic bacterial gangrene in a patient with stage IV carcinoma of the cervix. A central ulcerated area is seen in the crural region. This is surrounded by an irregular, darker zone (which is purple in color).

Where there is a good likelihood of wound infection, such as pelvic abscess, a delayed primary wound closure may be indicated (17). This approach will significantly reduce the risk of wound infection. On the 4th postoperative day, if the wound appears clean, it is closed. There is no increase in hospital stay required by the approach, and the wound heals very much like a primary closure.

EPISIOTOMY INFECTIONS

Although episiotomy with repair is performed in most vaginal deliveries, infection is an infrequent complication of this operation. However, recent papers have drawn attention to occasional, severe consequences (18–21). Shy and Eschenbach have recently classified episiotomy infections in a helpful way, according to the structures involved (18).

Simple Episiotomy Infection

This form is a localized infection involving only the skin and subcutaneous tissue (including Scarpa's fascia of the perineum) adjacent to the episiotomy. Signs are local edema and erythema with exudate; more extensive findings should raise the suspicion of a deeper infection. Treatment consists of opening, exploring, and debriding the perineal wound. Drainage alone is usually adequate, but appropriate antibiotics would be indicated if there is marked, superficial cellulitis or isolation of group A streptococci. The episiotomy incision should not be resutured at this time. Most will heal by granulation. Those involving the sphincter muscle or rectal mucosa may be repaired when the field is free of infection.

Superficial Fascial Necrosis

This type of episiotomy infection is a variant of "necrotizing fasciitis" (19–21). Both layers of the superficial perineal (i.e., Camper's and Colles' fascia) become necrotic, and infection spreads along the fascial planes to the abdominal wall, thigh, or buttock. Typically, the deep perineal fascia (i.e., inferior fascia of the urogen-

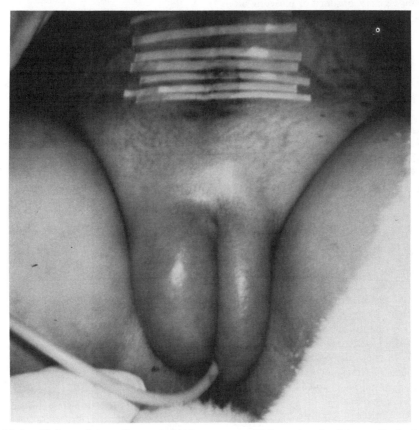

Figure 11.2. Vulvar edema of a noninfectious source. This patient had generalized edema from nephrotic syndrome with superimposed preeclampsia. Edema is bilateral and does not extent to buttocks or abdominal wall.

ital diaphragm) is not involved. Skin findings are variable, but initially include edema and erythema without clear borders. Later, there is progressive, brawny edema of the skin. The skin becomes blue or brown, and bullae or frank gangrene may occur. As the infection progresses, there may be loss of sensation or hyperesthesia.

Associated findings upon admission include marked hemoconcentration, although after fluid replacement the patient often is anemic. Hypocalcemia may also develop due to saponification of fatty acids. Traditionally, this infection has been associated with group A streptococci, but from more recent papers, anaerobic bacteria also play important roles.

In order for therapy to be effective, appropriate antibiotics must be complemented with adequate debridement. Indications for surgical exploration are (a) extension beyond the labia; (b) unilateral edema; (c) signs of toxicity or deterioration; and (d) failure of the infection to resolve within 24–48 hr. At surgery, necrotizing fasciitis may be recognized by separation of the skin from the deep fascia, absence of bleeding along incision lines, and a serosanguinous discharge. Dissection should be carried out until all necrotic tissue is debrided.

Myonecrosis

This infection involves the muscles beneath the deep fascia (14). Often this form is caused by myotoxin from *C. perfringens*, but may occasionally result from an extension of necrotizing fasciitis. Onset may be early and is typically accompanied by severe pain. Treatment for this form is also extensive debridement and high dose antibiotics including penicillin when clostridia species are suspected.

Differential Diagnosis

Not all puerperal vulvar edema signifies perineal infection (Fig. 11.2). Indeed, in most cases, vulvar edema results from less serious cause, such as vulvar hematoma, prolonged bearing down in labor, generalized edema from toxemia, allergic reactions, and trauma without serious infection. With these disorders, though, edema is usually bilateral, does not extend to the buttock and abdominal wall, and is not accompanied by signs of toxicity.

References

1. Howard JM, Barker WF, Culbertson WR, et al: Postoperative wound infections: the influence of ultraviolet irradiation of the operating room and various other factors. *Ann Surg* 160(S):1, 1964.
2. Cruse PJE, Foord R: A five-year prospective study of 23,649 surgical wounds. *Arch Surg* 107:206, 1973.
3. Swarz WH, Grolle K: Use of prophylactic antibiotics in Cesarean section, a review of the literature. *J Reprod Med* 26:595, 1981.
4. Gibbs RJ, Jones PM, Wilder CJ: Antibiotic therapy of endometritis following Cesarean section. Treatment successes and failures. *Obstet Gynecol* 52:31, 1978.
5. Sweet RL, Ledger WJ: Puerperal infections: a two year review. *Am J Obstet Gynecol* 117:1093, 1973.
6. Cruse PE, Foord R: Epidemiology of wound infection. A 10-year prospective study of 62,930 wounds. *Surg Clin North Am* 60:27, 1980.
7. Haley RW, Schaberg DR, Von Allmen, SD, et al: Estimating the extra charges and prolongation of hospitalization due to nosocomial infections: a comparison of methods. *J Infect Dis* 141:248, 1980.
8. Green JW, Wenzel RP: Postoperative wound infection: a controlled study of the increased duration of hospital stay and direct cost of hospitalization. *Ann Surg* 185:264, 1977.
9. Gilstrap LC, Cunningham, FG: The bacterial pathogenesis of infection following Cesarean section. *Obstet Gynecol* 53:545, 1979.
10. Blanco JD, Gibbs RS, Castandea YS, et al: Correlation of quantitative amniotic fluid cultures with endometritis after Cesarean section. *Am J Obstet Gynecol* 143:897, 1982.
11. Stage AH, Long H, Silberman R, et al: Wound infection following Cesarean section. *Surg Gynecol Obstet* 145:882, 1977.
12. Dommisse J, Kilpert B: Factors influencing Cesarean section wound sepsis. *S African Med J* 59:585, 1981.
13. Gibbs RS, Listwa HM, Read JA: The effect of internal fetal monitoring on maternal infection following Cesarean section. *Obstet Gynecol* 48:653, 1976.
14. Dellinger EP: Severe necrotizing soft-tissue infections. *JAMA* 246:1717, 1981.
15. Daly JW, Lukowski MJ, Monif GRG: The spontaneous occurrence of progressive synergistic bacterial gangrene on the abdominal wall. *Am J Obstet Gynecol* 131:624, 1978.
16. Brewer GE, Meleny FL: Progressive gangrenous infection of the skin and subcutaneous tissues, following operation for acute perforative appendicitis. *Ann Surg* 84:438, 1926.
17. Brown SE, Allen HH, Robins RN: The use of delayed primary wound closure in preventing wound infections. *Am J Obstet Gynecol* 127:713, 1977.
18. Shy KK, Eschenbach DA: Fatal perineal cellulitis from an episiotomy site. *Obstet Gynecol* 54:292, 1979.
19. Golde S, Ledger WJ: Necrotizing fasciitis in postpartum patients: a report of four cases. *Obstet Gynecol* 50:670, 1977.
20. Meltzer RM: Necrotizing fasciitis and progressive bacterial synergistic gangrene of the vulva. *Obstet Gynecol* 61:757, 1983.
21. Ewing TL, Smale LE, Elliott FA: Maternal deaths associated with postpartum vulvar edema. *Am J Obstet Gynecol* 134:173, 1979.

CHAPTER 12

Pelvic Abscess

Despite the clinical availability of many new and potent broad spectrum antimicrobial agents for treatment of pelvic infections and the widespread use of prophylactic antibiotics in surgical procedures, pelvic abscesses remain a diagnostic and therapeutic challenge for obstetrician-gynecologists (1–3). Mead has suggested that a pelvic abscess can be categorized on the basis of its etiologic origin (3). The major types of pelvic abscess include those which: (a) occur secondary to ascending intracanalicular spread of microorganisms from the cervix via the endometrial cavity to the adnexa (i.e., tuboovarian abscess); (b) arise after puerperal infections via lymphatic or hematogenous spread from the endometrium and/or myometrium to the adnexa; (c) are an infectious complication of pelvic surgery; or (d) may be secondary to infection in nongynecologic pelvic organs (i.e., appendicitis or diverticulitis).

Although pelvic abscesses constitute a small proportion of gynecologic inpatient admissions or hospital acquired infections on obstetric and gynecologic services, they are among the most serious complications seen by practicing obstetrician-gynecologists and are associated with prolonged hospitalization and significant morbidity. Tuboovarian abscesses have been reported to constitute 1.6–2.2% of gynecologic admissions at urban public hospitals (4, 5). In the case of hospital acquired infection following pelvic surgery, the reported incidence of pelvic abscess formation has ranged from 0.7 to 2.0% (6–8).

The major emphasis in this chapter will be on the pathogenesis, diagnosis, and management of tuboovarian abscesses. Infection occurring during the puerperium or following abortion are discussed thoroughly in Chapters 17 and 10, respectively. Soft tissue pelvic infections occurring postpelvic surgery are discussed in Chapter 9 and will only briefly be covered in this discussion.

POSTOPERATIVE ABSCESS

Although the frequency of postoperative soft tissue pelvic infections has been reduced by the use of prophylactic antibiotics (see Chapter 20), they remain a significant problem for the clinician. Ledger et al, in a prospective surveillance study, reported that 14% of gynecologic admissions were treated with antibiotics for hospital acquired infection (9). In a retrospective analysis of 12,000 hospital discharges, Ledger and Child demonstrated that nearly 50% of patients undergoing abdominal or vaginal hysterectomy were treated with antibiotics (10).

Such common occurrence of posthysterectomy infection is not unexpected (11). The surgical procedure is performed in the vagina, which is a microbiologically contaminated field. The presence of traumatized, devitalized tissue secondary to crush clamp technique and suture ligatures results in an ideal nidus for infection with the vaginal microorganisms. Moreover, hemoglobin, which accumulates at the operative site, interferes with natural host defense mechanisms by inhibiting the ability of leukocytes to phagocytose bacteria.

Posthysterectomy abscesses are divided into two major categories. The vaginal apex cuff abscess or infected hematoma usually presents with fever and a sensation of fullness or vague discomfort in the lower abdomen. Examination typically discloses an infected, foul smelling hematoma which can be easily drained per vagina with resultant prompt response. Cuff abscesses characteristically occur after 48 hr postoperatively but during the initial hospitalization. Hevron and Llorens reported the occurrence of 36 cuff abscesses among 1600 major pelvic operations (2%) and noted that cuff abscess drainage occurred on an average of 8 days after surgery (6). The second group are the true pelvic abscesses which tend to present at a later time, often after initial discharge from the hospital (6, 7). In fact, as noted by Ledger et al (7), posthysterectomy adnexal abscess may occur from postoperative day 6 to 133 days following surgery. Postoperative pelvic abscess has been reported to occur in 13 (0.7%) of 1600 major pelvic operations by Hevron and Llorens (6) and in 1% of patients undergoing hysterectomy by Ledger et al (7). In Ledger's series, nearly 3% of vaginal hysterectomies (preprophylactic antibiotic use) developed adnexal abscesses requiring surgical intervention. In both of these series the vast majority of postoperative abscesses occurred following vaginal hysterectomy. These abscesses present with abdominal pain, fever, and a tender, palpable pelvic mass. Characteristically, posthysterectomy adnexal masses are high in the pelvis. Although they may, on occasion, respond to antimicrobial therapy, our recommendation for the management of posthysterectomy adnexal abscess(es) is to initiate antimicrobial therapy that includes coverage for resistant anaerobes such as *Bacteroides fragilis* and to promptly proceed to exploratory laparotomy for extirpation and/or drainage of infected tissues. That vaginal drainage is not the optimal approach for management of posthysterectomy abscesses is confirmed by the findings of Hevron and Llorens, who noted that of the nine cases of pelvic abscess with primary treatment via vaginal drainage, five (55%) required subsequent laparotomy for eradication of infection.

TUBOOVARIAN ABSCESS

As discussed in Chapter 4, acute salpingitis or pelvic inflammatory disease (PID) is the most significant economic and medical consequence of the sexually transmitted disease epidemic in women (12). One of the major complications and/or sequelae of acute PID is the tuboovarian abscess (TOA).

Tuboovarian abscess has been reported to occur in as many as 34% of patients hospitalized with salpingitis (13–19). Although the TOA has been referred to as an end stage in the progression of upper genital tract infections (18, 19), a number of studies have shown that a prior history of PID is obtained in only one-third to one-half of patients presenting with TOAs (15, 19–21). This may indicate that subclinical infections are more prevalent than suspected or that upper genital tract infections may progress to abscess stage during the initial presentation, possibly dependent on the organisms involved.

Diagnosis

CLINICAL FINDINGS

TOAs occur most commonly in the third and fourth decades of life (13, 19, 22–24). The parity of these patients is variable, with approximately 25–50% being nulliparous (13, 15, 19–21).

Abdominal or pelvic pain is the most frequent presenting complaint and was the major complaint in more than 90% of TOA patients reported in the literature (14, 15, 19, 22, 23). Very few investigations have commented on other presenting symptoms; Landers and Sweet reported that of 232 patients with TOAs, a complaint of fever and chills was elicited in 50%, vaginal discharge in 28%, nausea in 26% and abnormal vaginal bleeding in 21% (15). A number of investigators have reported on the incidence of fever and leukocytosis, but definitions were variable. Temperature of at least 100.1°F, and usually higher, has been reported in from 60–80% of patients; and leukocytosis, although often undefined, was reported in from 66–80% of patients (13–15, 20, 22, 23). The clinical significance of this lies in the fact that many patients harboring TOAs may present with normal temperatures and white blood counts. In the series reported by Landers and Sweet, 35% of patients with surgically confirmed TOAs were afebrile, and 23% had WBC in the normal range (15). Thus, the absence of fever and/or leukocytosis should not, by itself, exclude a diagnosis of TOA and preclude initiation of appropriate management for TOAs.

In general, the presenting clinical findings for patients with uncomplicated salpingitis (i.e., no inflammatory mass) and those with tuboovarian abscesses are similar. Differentiation requires determination of the presence of an inflammatory adnexal mass. This illustrates the importance of recognizing the presence or abscence of a pelvic mass in patients presenting with the signs and symptoms of acute salpingitis. Physical exam alone may often be insufficient because pain and tenderness may preclude an adequate pelvic examination. Several relatively noninvasive imaging techniques may be utilized to aid in the diagnosis of pelvic abscesses and should be used whenever suspicion of an abscess arises. Differentiation of a TOA from inflammatory masses with adherent bowel or omentum is appreciably improved with such techniques. Laparoscopy may also be helpful as a diagnostic clinical tool, especially when the diagnosis is in question.

IMAGING TECHNIQUES

Several noninvasive imaging techniques are available and currently being used in the diagnosis and management of patients suspected to have abdominal or pelvic abscesses (25–34). These include radionucleotide scanning, ultrasound (sonography), and computed tomography (CT). The commonly employed radionucleotide scans are gallium-67- and indium-111 labeled WBC scanning, which have been highly accurate in the localization of intraabdominal abscesses (27–30). Their advantage is ease of performance. The disadvantages include expense, 24–48 hrs' delay before interpretation (gallium-67), and false-positive scans due to the high affinity of these radionucleotides to inflammatory tissue, such as infected or neoplastic tissue, rather than just discrete abscesses. The most promising technique seems to be indium-111-labeled WBC scans with reported accuracy of 87% (29). Bicknell and associates reported nearly 100% accuracy with indium-111-labeled autologous leukocytes in differentiating pancreatic abscesses from pseudocysts (30). None of the radionucleotide scanning techniques have been well studied for diagnostic accuracy in patients with TOAs. In general, the radionucleotide techniques are utilized in cases of suspected intraabdominal infection to rule in or out the presence of an abscess rather than to confirm that a palpable mass is an abscess.

Ultrasonography has become a frequently used confirmatory test when the diagnosis of a TOA is suspected; this relatively inexpensive scan can be useful in both confirming the clinical impression and measuring response to therapy. A number of retrospective studies have looked at the accuracy of ultrasound in the diagnosis of pelvic abscesses (25, 31–33). The largest of these, by Taylor et al, included 220 patients with surgically proven abdominal or pelvic abscesses (31). In this series, 36 of 40 abdominal and 32 of 33 pelvic abscesses were correctly identified, while 112 of 113 suspected abdominal and 33 of 34 suspected pelvic abscesses were correctly ruled out. Landers and Sweet reported a series of 98 patients who were evaluated with ultrasound, of which 31 had surgically confirmed TOAs. Twenty-nine of thirty-one surgically confirmed TOAs had been reported as complex adnexal masses or cystic type masses with multiple internal echoes and were felt to be consistent with an abscess. The remaining two were simple cystic masses. A mass was correctly identified in all surgically confirmed TOAs and in

90% of the 67 patients with clinically diagnosed TOAs (15). One would expect a typical sonogram of a TOA to reveal a discreet mass, with internal echoes indicating its complex nature. A sonogram of a surgically documented TOA is shown in Figure 12.1. Sonograms may also be useful in assessing response to therapy by detecting changes in the size and architecture of these masses. As technology continues to improve the quality of ultrasound, and ultrasonographers gain experience with techniques that combine the use of real-time and static imaging, the accuracy of this technique in the diagnosis and management of TOAs may be further enhanced. In addition to a high degree of accuracy, the availability of ultrasound to the physician and the ease of performing the exam are also attractive features of this procedure.

CT scans have been used extensively, both in the diagnosis and the treatment of abdominal abscesses. There is, however, very little information available on the accuracy of these scans, specifically, for the diagnosis of tuboovarian or other pelvic abscesses. In a recent study, Moir and Robins compared the accuracy of ultrasound, gallium, and CT scanning in the diagnosis of abdominal abscesses (34). They reported sensitivity of ultrasound, gallium, and CT as 82, 96, and 100%, respectively. Specificity was reported as 91, 65, and 100%, respectively, for the techniques. Thus, CT scans appear to be very accurate, at least in the abdomen, in detecting the presence of an abscess. It is unclear as to whether the sensitivity and specificity in the pelvis are similar and whether the increased accuracy of CT will justify the expense. Our current approach is to obtain ultrasound as the initial diagnostic aid and reserve CT scans for those patients in whom ultrasound fails to provide adequate information. A large pelvic abscess is seen on a CT scan in Figure 12.2. In the near future, nuclear magnetic resonance (NMR) may become the imaging technique of choice. To date there is very limited experience with NMR in the evaluation of pelvic masses. Only clinical experience can determine if the theoretic advantages in accuracy with NMR are applicable to clinical use in differentiating pelvic masses.

Etiology and Pathogenesis

MICROBIOLOGY OF TOAs

The microbiology of TOAs is predominantly a mixed flora of anaerobes and facultative or

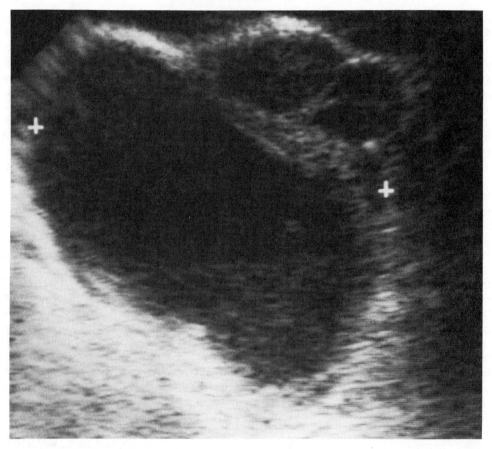

Figure 12.1. Ultrasound scan demonstrating a large left tuboovarian abscess which subsequently required surgical extirpation.

aerobic organisms (15, 35). Anaerobic organisms are particularly prevalent in these abscesses, having been isolated from 63–100% of adnexal abscesses in which appropriate anaerobic microbiological technology was used (36, 40). We obtained cultures directly from the abscess at surgery in 53 patients, of whom all but three had received antibiotics preoperatively. Anaerobic bacteria were isolated in 85% of 27 positive cultures; however, 26 (49%) of those cultured grew no organisms. The vast majority of these "no growth" cultures were performed prior to the institution of our anaerobic research laboratory. Most likely, the concept of a sterile abscess may well be a misnomer, and the lack of success in recovering organisms is more likely related to a lack of proper anaerobic collection, transport, and culturing techniques. The major role played by anaerobes in TOAs was initially demonstrated by Altemeier in the early 1940s, when he isolated anaerobic organisms from 92% of the TOA specimens that had been previously

reported by the clinical laboratory as "no growth" (38). We are now evaluating the microbiology of abscesses by aspirating the pus and sampling the abscess wall for anaerobic bacteria, facultative (aerobic) bacteria, *Neisseria gonorrhoeae*, *Mycoplasma hominis*, and *Chlamydia trachomatis*. The predominant organisms isolated from TOA aspirates were *Escherichia coli*, *B. fragilis*, other *Bacteroides* species, aerobic streptococci, *Peptococcus*, and *Peptostreptococcus* (15). These are many of the same organisms noted to be involved in a biphasic aerobic-anaerobic animal model of intraabdominal sepsis and abscess formation (41). In this model the investigators implanted colonic organisms into the peritoneal cavity of Wistar rats. These colonic bacteria are very similar to those found in the normal microflora of the vagina and cervix. The investigators noted the development of a biphasic disease process in which there is an initial stage of peritonitis and sepsis with an approximately 40% mortality rate. All the sur-

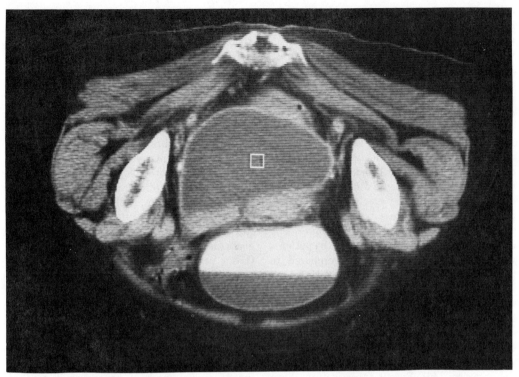

Figure 12.2.   CT scan demonstrating a large pelvic abscess.

viving animals went on to develop intraabdominal abscesses. While the bacteria associated with the peritonitis-sepsis stage were facultative, especially *E. coli*, the organisms recovered from these abscesses were predominantly anaerobes, especially *B. fragilis* and *Bacteroides* species. Hammill and co-workers were able to produce similar abscess formation with uterotuboovarian abscesses in rats by injecting *B. fragilis* into ligated uterine horns (42). Thus, anaerobic organisms, in particular *B. fragilis*, seem to be strongly associated with abscess formation. In animal (mice) experiments, it has been shown that abscess formation may be prevented by treatment with drugs active against *B. fragilis* in vitro, with the exception of chloramphenicol, which may be inactivated by anaerobic bacterial enzymes acting on the nitro group (43, 44).

One of the virulence factors associated with *B. fragilis* seems to be related to its capsular polysaccharide. A number of *Bacteroides* species failed to produce significant numbers of abscesses in experimental rats; however, when encapsulated *B. fragilis* was used alone, 95% of the rats developed abscesses (45). In one experiment, unencapsulated *Bacteroides distasonis* caused abscesses in only 17%, but when 200 μg of *B. fragilis*-purified capsular polysaccharide

alone were implanted, 100% of the rats developed abscesses (45). It has further been shown that encapsulated strains of *B. fragilis* are more resistant to opsonophagocytosis than other *Bacteroides* species (46). Thus, not only are *B. fragilis* strains by themselves capable of causing abscesses, but even the capsular polysaccharide of *B. fragilis* potentiates abscess formation. It has also been shown that active immunization of rats with the capsular polysaccharide of *B. fragilis* results in protection against abscess development when challenged with *B. fragilis* (47). This protection was specific for *B. fragilis* or related species but did not protect against abscess formation when a mixture of fecal microflora was used. *B. fragilis*, however, was eliminated from the infecting microflora. More recent investigation has shown that a T-cell-dependent immune response is involved in protection against abscess development after immunization with *B. fragilis* capsular antigen. Serum antibodies only afford protection against *B. fragilis* bacteremia, whereas the protection against abscess formation appears to be T-cell mediated and does not require the presence of serum antibody (48). In addition, the virulence of anaerobes may be due to the variety of enzymes they produce (49). Among these enzymes are collagenase and hyaluronidase, which may inhibit walling-off of infection, and heparinase, which may promote clotting in small vessels which may further decrease blood supply to infected tissue and consequently decrease oxygenation of the infected area. Superoxide dismutase, which is also produced by some anaerobes, may assist these anaerobes in surviving under aerobic conditions.

It has been observed that antibody levels to B. fragilis rise following infections in which the organism is a likely pathogen. Polk and coworkers studied 53 patients undergoing elective hysterectomy who were evaluated for rise in antibody titer to B. fragilis polysaccharide. A significant rise ($p < 0.05$) in titer from a mean of 5.6 to a mean of 13.0 was seen in the patients with postop abscess formation compared to those without complications, those with wound infections, those with pelvic cellulitis, and those with febrile morbidity (50). The importance of humoral factors is still unclear, but there is some suggestive evidence that B. fragilis immunoglobulin activates the alternative complement pathway leading to opsonization and phagocytosis of the organism (46). Recent investigations have emphasized the emergence of and recognition of B. bivius and B. disiens as major pathogens in infections of the upper female genital tract (15, 44). B. bivius, and to a lesser degree B. disiens, are major components of the normal vaginal-cervical flora and, thus, are not unexpectedly present as frequent pathogens on obstetric and gynecologic services. Whether these organisms contain unique characteristics, such as B. fragilis, which facilitate their ability to produce abscesses has not been studied yet.

Until recently N. gonorrhoeae (GC) was considered to be "the" major pathogen in the etiology of salpingitis. The arbitrary division into gonococcal and nongonococcal salpingitis, as determined by the presence or absence of endocervical GC, has given way to newer concepts of etiology which are based on Fallopian tube and peritoneal fluid culture data. The recovery of GC from TOAs is very uncommon. Landers and Sweet recovered GC from only 3.8% of 53 TOA aspirates, while the overall recovery rate of GC from the endocervix was 31% in these 53 patients with TOA (15). Some investigators have proposed that the gonococci may antecede and predispose for anaerobic invasion of the Fallopian tubes (51, 52). There may be an initial penetration of the endocervical barrier by the gonococci, while the other facultative and anaerobic organisms may gain access to the upper genital tract at the same time as, or soon after, the gonococci. Certain of these organisms might even suppress the growth of N. gonorrhoeae, preventing its recovery (53).

As described more fully in Chapter 4, it seems clear that other mechanisms for the etiology of salpingitis also exist. As newer techniques are utilized to obtain microbiologic specimens from the Fallopian tubes, we are identifying a larger number of patients with polymicrobial salpingitis in whom microbiologic, serologic, or epidemiologic evidence of current or recent gonococcal infection is absent. Eschenbach has proposed an interesting concept. In an attempt to explain the etiology of salpingitis in women without gonorrhea, chlamydia, or an intrauterine device (IUD), he suggested a relationship to anaerobic vaginitis (nonspecific vaginitis) (54). He pointed out the high concentrations of anaerobic bacteria in patients with this vaginitis. Perhaps an altered physiologic immunologic host defense system in the genital tract promotes bacterial attachment and invasion of the upper genital tract. Another possible explanation could be that a crucial mass of anaerobes is reached which simply overwhelms local defenses, leading to upper genital tract colonization and infection with these organisms. Possibly, a yet to be identified agent may inhibit local immune mechanisms in the endocervix. The resultant suppression could lead to ascending infection through the cervical canal.

C. trachomatis is now recognized as a major etiologic agent in acute salpingitis (55–61). The role of this organism in TOAs has not been determined. We have recently consulted on a patient with a surgically excised TOA cultured for anaerobic and aerobic organisms, as well as C. trachomatis, and only the chlamydia cultures were positive (Wilcox DF and Hohe PT, personal communication). Although C. trachomatis was the sole organism cultured from this abscess, it is not clear as to whether it was the causal organism or a secondary invader. The fact that the patient had been treated with antibiotics prior to surgery adds further confusion. We must, therefore, await additional reports to confirm the possibility of chlamydial abscesses.

The role of mycoplasma in salpingitis is still unclear. It has been supported by the isolation of M. hominis from tuboperitoneal cultures (62) and the recovery of Ureaplasma urealyticum from the Fallopian tubes (63) in a small number of cases. In addition, M. hominis has been shown to produce a parametritis, as well as tubal inflammation in the grivet monkey (64). It is, however, rarely the sole isolate in salpingitis. There is very little in the literature relating mycoplasms to TOAs, with the exception of one case report of *Mycoplasma pneumoniae* being the only organism isolated from a TOA after 2 weeks of antibiotic therapy (65).

Actinomycetes, most commonly *Actinomyces israelii*, a gram-positive anaerobe, has occasionally been recovered from patients with PID, especially in association with TOAs. A relationship between this organism and IUD use has been suggested by several investigators (66–68). It is felt by some that the presence of actinomycetes on Papanicolaou smears is associated with a higher risk of hospitalization with PID. Burkman et al noted that PID associated with the presence of actinomycetes was more likely to be of increased clinical severity (16). Seven of eight (87.5%) of their PID patients with actinomycetes present had a TOA, as compared to 11 of 38 (28.9%) PID patients without actinomycetes. However, this organism was not recovered from the microbiological specimens in several TOA series (15, 22, 35). However, it is a very difficult organism to culture, often requiring maintenance of anaerobic conditions for as long as 2 weeks. Most actinomycetes are actually identified by histology in pathology specimens or by cytology on Papanicolaou smears. Although actinomycotic infections have been stereotypically characterized by fistula formation with chronic draining sinuses, in fact, as Schmidt et al pointed out, the clinical diagnosis of actinomycetes in genital tract infections is seldom made prior to surgery (69). The exact role of actinomycetes in abscess formation remains unclear, as does the mechanism of its apparent relationship to the IUD. Whether *A. israelii* is a sole pathogen or a marker for mixed anaerobic-facultative infection is unclear. If actinomyces is demonstrated in association with a tuboovarian abscess, long-term antibiotic therapy for up to 6 weeks to 3 months must follow surgical extirpation of the infected tissue. Penicillin is the drug of choice; cephalosporins, clindamycin, cefoxitin, or chloramphenicol are alternative agents.

Pathogenesis of TOAs

The mechanism by which TOA formation occurs is difficult to establish because of the variety of presentations and degrees of tubal damage present when the infection is noted. Studies done with the gonococcus have demonstrated that once it ascends to the Fallopian tube, it attaches to the mucosal epithelial cells, penetrates the epithelial cells via phagocytosis, and causes the destruction of the epithelial cells. Within 2–7 days, ciliary motility is lost in Fallopian tube organ cultures inoculated with gonococci (70, 71). Recently, Gregg and co-workers have demonstrated that the gonococcus produces an exotoxin, which is a lipopolysaccharide, that destroys the cilia of the tubal epithelium (72). The destruction of the endosalpinx results in the production of a purulent exudate. In the early stages of disease, the tubal lumen is open, and the purulent exudate exudes from the fimbriated end, resulting in peritonitis. In addition, the gonococci may extend from the mucosa through the subepithelial tissue to involve the muscularis and the serosa of the Fallopian tube in the inflammatory process (71). During this initial inflammatory phase or during a recurrent infection, the ovary (as well as other pelvic structures) may become involved in the inflammatory process. Presumedly, an ovulation site in the ovary serves as the portal of entry for organisms into the ovary, with subsequent tissue invasion. Eventually, tissue planes become lost, and the separation of tube and ovary is obscured as the abscess forms. The abscess may remain localized, with involvement of tube and ovary alone. It may involve other contiguous pelvic structure, such as bowel, bladder, or the opposite adnexa, which may be undergoing similar inflammatory changes. At any point in the progression, rupture may occur, usually at the site of an adhesion to a nearby organ (11). Hare and Barnes and co-workers have demonstrated that *B. fragilis* is more virulent than the gonococcus in Fallopian tube explant systems. Within 4 days of inoculation into the explant system, *B. fragilis* destroyed the tubal epithelium (73).

IUD Use and TOAs

The frequency of IUD usage in patients presenting with TOAs has been reported in several studies to range from 20–54% (15, 20, 21, 35, 74–76). In the mid-1970s it was believed that there was a strong correlation between IUD use and the development of unilateral TOAs. Taylor et al reported on 16 patients who developed unilateral TOAs while wearing or soon after the removal of an IUD (77). Dawood and Birnbaum, in the same year, reported four additional cases and stressed the IUD association with unilateral TOAs as a distinct clinical entity (78). Subsequent investigation by Golde et al suggested that unilateral TOAs were a distinct entity, with or without an IUD (35). They did, however, report that 62.5% of IUD users with TOAs had unilateral disease, compared with 32.1% in nonusers. Several investigators have since compared the incidence of unilateral abscesses in IUD users and nonusers (15, 20, 21, 75, 76). These results and those of Golde et al are summarized in Table 12.1. In these studies, the incidence of unilateral TOAs ranged from 20 to 71%. The incidence of unilateral TOAs in IUD users was 25–89%. Thus, there was little difference in the incidence of unilateral TOAs with or without IUD use in the majority of these studies.

The pathogenesis of IUD-related salpingitis and adnexal abscess formation has yet to be clearly demonstrated. Several investigators have put forth tenable hypotheses; however, none of these alone can account for the diversity of clinical manifestations associated with IUD-related infections. Burnhill suggested in 1973 that a syndrome of progressive endometritis was associated with IUDs in which menorrhagia, metrorrhagia, and leukorrhea were noted and were followed by progressive endometritis, parametritis, peritonitis, and pelvic abscess formation (79). It has become clear that bacterial colonization of the endometrium is not merely a result of contamination at the time of insertion (80). The currently accepted hypothesis is that the IUD tail, projecting through the cervical canal, allows easy access of vaginal bacteria to the upper genital tract. In 1981, Sparks et al published a series of 22 IUD users undergoing hysterectomy that were evaluated by a multiple biopsy technique (81). They found bacteria in the uterus in 15 of 17 women with tailed IUDs. They also noted that all five uteri with a tailless IUD were sterile. They found no difference in

bacteria counts between monofilamentous and multifilamentous devices. In another study published in 1982 in which a group of 33 baboons with IUDs were studied, the multifilament tail and, especially, cracked multifilament tails were associated with considerably greater intrusion of bacteria into the uterine cavity than the monofilament tail (82). This difference was not related to the type of IUD (Lippes Loop, Dalkon shield). Another interesting feature of this study, which was carried out for 16 months, is that no animal that had bacteria present in the uterus showed any evidence of local disease by clinical signs, endoscopy, or histological examination of the endometrium. Persistence of bacterial flora, combined with a breakdown of the host defense mechanisms, may be enough to cause a chronic endometritis with progressive spread either via lymphatics in the parametrium and broad ligament to involve the adnexa or by intracanilicular spread from the endometrium to the Fallopian tube(s) and/or ovary.

Treatment Approach

MEDICAL THERAPY OF TOAs

The controversy over the management of TOAs revolves around the traditional dictum that abscesses cannot be adequately eradicated by antibiotics alone and require surgical drainage or extirpation. Saini and co-workers at the Tufts New England Medical Center attribute the improved survival of patients at their institution with intraabdominal abscesses to the combination of earlier diagnosis and improved localization of abscesses (with the use of newer imaging techniques), earlier drainage, and the use of broad spectrum antimicrobial regimens effective against anaerobes, especially *B. fragilis* (83). However, the issue is whether or not a TOA can be treated conservatively, without significant risk to the patients, in the hope of

Table 12.1
Incidence of Unilateral TOAs in IUD Users and Nonusers

Study (reference)	No. of TOAs	No. of unilateral TOAs (%)	No. of TOAs in IUD users (% unilateral)	No. of TOAs in nonusers (% unilateral)
Landers and Sweet (15)	232	164 (71)	76 (71)	156 (70.5)
Ginsberg et al (20)	160	90 (56)	75 (61)	85 (52)
Edelman and Berger (21)	318	65 (20)	67 (25)	251 (19)
Golde et al (35)	85	35 (43.5)	32 (62.5)	53 (32)
Scott (75)	66	28 (42)	19 (42)	47 (43)
Manara (76)	41	29 (71)	9 (89)	32 (66)
Total	902	411 (46)	278 (55)	624 (42)

preserving fertility and/or ovarian function. There is general acceptance that rupture of a TOA is an indication for immediate surgical intervention; however, there remains controversy in the management of the unruptured TOA. Opinions range from prompt surgical intervention, with complete removal of the uterus and adnexa (14, 84), to treatment with intravenous antibiotics, where surgery is reserved for patients who fail to respond or in whom there is suspicion of rupture (15, 19, 20). More recently, it has also been suggested that in those patients with unilateral TOAs requiring surgical intervention, unilateral adnexectomy may be an appropriate alternative in terms of preserving future fertility and hormonal production (4). Landers and Sweet have also raised the question as to whether unilateral adnexectomy is indicated in hopes of preventing future flare-ups and improving future fertility on the contralateral uninvolved side (15).

Kaplan et al treated 71 patients with total abdominal hysterectomy and bilateral salpingo-oophorectomy within 24–72 hr of instituting antibiotics. With this aggressive approach, bowel injury (serosal tears) occurred in 8.4% of patients (84). Such an approach, although often curative, eliminates future reproductive and/or hormonal function. It would seem prudent to question whether such an aggressive approach is necessary in all patients with TOAs. Several investigators have since reported favorable results, with a more conservative approach aimed at preservation of future reproductive potential (15, 19, 20). Franklin et al reported the results in 120 patients treated with an initial conservative approach. Eighty-five patients were treated with antibiotics alone, and 35 patients were treated with antibiotics plus colpotomy drainage. The overall failure rate was 26.5%, of which 10% were early failures. Ninety-seven patients were followed for from 2½–8 years after discharge with a subsequent intrauterine pregnancy rate of 10.3% (19). In 1980, Ginsberg and co-workers reported a series of 160 patients initially treated with antibiotics alone, of which 31% were early failures and 35% late failures. Long-term follow-up, ranging from 1 month to 10 years, was obtained in 95 patients; the subsequent intrauterine pregnancy rate was 9.5% (20). More recently, in a group of 232 patients with TOAs, Landers and Sweet reported that 217 were treated initially with antibiotics alone (15). Early failure was seen in 19.4% and late failure in 31%. Long-term follow-up greater than 2 years was available in 58 patients, and the subsequent intrauterine pregnancy rate was 13.8%. These studies demonstrate that response to medical therapy is successful in 33–74% of patients. The rate of subsequent intrauterine pregnancy ranged from 9.5 to 13.8%. This is a minimum and overly pessimistic estimate of fertility chances because those women using contraception are not excluded.

It may be difficult, clinically, to distinguish a TOA from a pyosalpinx, ovarian abscess, or some other inflammatory complex. This becomes less crucial when patients are treated with a conservative approach, as the initial therapy would be appropriate if any of these pelvic masses were present in association with pelvic infection. Future reproductive capability is a significant concern to most patients with TOAs and plays a major role in the desire for a more conservative approach to therapy.

A variety of antibiotic regimens were employed in the major reviews of TOAs in which the therapeutic regimens were stated. In the series by Franklin et al (19), patients were treated primarily with penicillin and streptomycin (1963–1968). Ginsberg et al (20) did not specifically state antibiotic regimens, except to say patients were treated with "broad spectrum antibiotics, with multiple agents being employed frequently" (1969–1979). Manara and co-workers evaluated patients treated with IV penicillin plus an aminoglycoside (1965–1979). Of their 41 patients, 25 were treated initially with antibiotics alone, of which 15 (60%) failed to respond (76). Hager recently reported the results of 32 TOA patients treated in the early 1970s (1970–1974) initially with parenteral penicillin or a first generation cephalosporin in combination with an aminoglycoside (17). Anaerobe coverage (unspecified, but presumably clindamycin or chloramphenicol) was added in most patients with an abscess. They reported clinical improvement, defined as afebrile, with a decrease in size of abscess in only 15.6%. Table 12.2 is a summary of conservative antibiotic therapy of TOAs. There appears from these data to be a tremendous variation in response rates to antimicrobial therapy alone. This confusion relates in part to the variety of definitions for response and also the degree of aggressiveness in using surgical intervention. A major disadvantage in most of these studies was the lack of detailed analysis comparing responses to particular antibiotic regimens. If one accepts that these abscesses contain high concentrations of the resistant gram-negative anaerobes, such as *B. fragilis*, *B. bivius*, and *Bacteroides disiens*, then improved results should be noted in patients treated aggressively with antibiotics effective against these resistant gram-negative anaerobes, such as clindamycin, metronidazole, cefoxitin, or moxalactam. There is, however, insufficient data available to confirm this suspicion.

In Landers' and Sweet's series of 232 TOAs (1970–1980), treatment regimens varied. Patients treated in the earlier years received high dose penicillin (15). In later years, an aminoglycoside was added, and the dose of penicillin was reduced. In more recent years, patients were treated primarily with combination therapy which included clindamycin. The regimens most commonly used were "triple therapy" with penicillin, an aminoglycoside, and clindamycin, or an aminoglycoside and clindamycin in combination. A small number of patients were treated with a second generation cephalosporin (cefoxitin). Response to therapy was determined on the basis of improvement in symptoms, absence of fever, reduction of pelvic tenderness, and decrease in size of the mass. Since all patients not requiring surgery during the initial hospitalization became afebrile with symptomatic improvement, evaluation of the mass was used to assess differences in therapeutic response.

The result of this evaluation is summarized in Table 12.3. Of the patients treated with antibiotics alone, a total of 167 were examined prior to discharge. Reduction in mass size was seen in 25% of patients treated with penicillin alone, 49% of patients treated with penicillin and an aminoglycoside, and 68% of patients treated with regimens that included clindamycin (p < 0.01). A total of 104 patients who were available for follow-up had been treated with antibiotic regimens that did not include clindamycin. The response rate was 36.5%, as compared to the 68% response rate of the 63 patients treated with regimens that included clindamycin. The opposite trend was noted when examining those with an increase in mass size. Forty-two patients required surgical extirpation of an abscess during the initial hospitalization because of failure to respond to antimicrobial therapy alone. Of these, 64% had been treated with regimens not containing clindamycin, as compared to the 36% that received clindamycin-containing regimens. Of the patients treated with antibiotics alone, 134 returned for follow-up 2–4 weeks after discharge. In 46.4% of the

Table 12.2
Recent Investigations of TOAs Treated with Conservative Medical Therapy

Author (reference)	No. of TOAs treated	No. with response (%)	No. with subsequent pregnancy of patients with follow-up (%)
Landers and Sweet (15)	217	175 (81)	8/58 (13.8)
Franklin et al (19)	120	110 (90)[a]	10/108 (9.3)
Ginsberg et al (20)	110	76 (69)	9/95 (9.5)
Edelman and Berger (21)	318	175 (55)	NS
Scott (75)	33	24 (73)	NS
Manara (76)	26	11 (42)	1/26 (3.8)
Hager (17)	32	5 (16)	4/8 (50)
Total	856	576 (67)	32/295 (10.8)

[a] Includes some patients treated with colpotomy drainage.

Table 12.3
Comparison of Clindamycin-containing Regimens and Nonclindamycin Regimens in the Treatment of TOAs[a]

Antibiotic regimen	No. with reduction of TOAs size at hospital discharge (%)	No. with further reduction of TOA size at 2–4 wk postdischarge (%)
Antimicrobial regimens that included clindamycin	43/63 (68.3)	43/50 (86)
Antimicrobial regimens that excluded clindamycin	38/104 (36.5)	39/84 (46.4)

[a] From Landers DV, Sweet RL: Tubo-ovarian abscess: contemporary approach to management. *Rev Infect Dis* 5(suppl):876, 1983.

patients treated with nonclindamycin regimens, the masses were decreased in size or absent, whereas 86% of clindamycin-treated patients showed a similar response (15).

This improved response with the use of clindamycin-containing regimens may be the result of some distinctive features separating clindamycin from the other treatment regimens used in the above cited studies. One of these features is its superior activity against resistant gram-negative anaerobes like *B. fragilis*.

The abscess is an unique environment. It is characterized by a low level of oxygen tension, and this low redox potential allows anaerobes to proliferate, which leads to tissue destruction and circulatory compromise, thus preventing many antibiotics from reaching the area. The combination of these forces and the poor phagocytosis by neutrophils in this environment are all important factors in the resistance of these infections to antimicrobial therapy. There are 10^7–10^9 bacteria per ml in an abscess, and thus an inoculum effect can occur in which the laboratory standard of 10^5 organisms is sensitive to an antibiotic, but the tremendous numbers of organisms in the abscess are resistant. In addition, the high levels of enzymes produced by bacteria within the abscess aid in the destruction of many antibiotics like penicillin, ampicillin, first generation cephalosporins, ticarcillin, carbenicillin, and chloramphenicol. Many anaerobic bacteria, including *B. fragilis*, are often resistant to the penicillins and many cephalosporins. Included in these are the newly recognized strains, *B. disiens* and *B. bivius*, which are especially prevalent in the female genital tract (85). The role of *B. fragilis* as an important pathogen in these infections is evident, based on recovery of this organism from abscess aspirates (15, 35), serologic studies demonstrating an antigenic response in patients with abscesses (86), and experimental work in animals showing that *B. fragilis* promotes abscess formation (87).

As research continues to reveal the characteristics of clindamycin and other antibiotics, such as cefoxitin, metronidazole, and third generation cephalosporins, which are active against these resistant gram-negative anaerobes, we have an explanation for the improved response of TOAs to some antimicrobial treatment regimens. The extracellular antimicrobial activity of clindamycin may further explain the favorable results with this agent, but, in addition, this agent may reach especially high concentrations within the abscesses as a result of active transport into the

abscess by polymorphonuclear leukocytes (88, 89). Furthermore, in an animal model, clindamycin has been shown to enter infected encapsulated subcutaneous abscesses in mice in a higher concentration (43–63% of peak serum levels) than other antimicrobial agents, including metronidazole, cefoxitin, and moxalactam (90). However, these other antimicrobials did also enter the abscesses in significant amounts. When the activity of 10 antimicrobial agents was measured in these subcutaneous abscesses by reduction in bacterial counts, it was found that the most active antimicrobials in order of decreasing activity were metronidazole, clindamycin, moxalactam, and cefoxitin (91).

The introduction of newer betalactam agents offers additional treatment options. Moxalactam is regarded as one of the most active of the third generation cephalosporins against *B. fragilis* (92). However, all of these newer betalactam agents seem considerably less active against *B. fragilis* than currently advocated drugs such as metronidazole, clindamycin, and cefoxitin (93, 94).

In light of the many factors enhancing the activity of clindamycin against the implicated organisms, especially *B. fragilis*, it may seem surprising that there remain a significant number of TOA treatment failures. This may be explained in part by the partial inactivation of clindamycin within the abscess environment (95). In addition, there has recently been an emergence of *B. fragilis* resistance to clindamycin. This is a plasmid-mediated resistance which some strains have shown to transfer. In addition, it has been suggested that there may be two different mechanisms of resistance in *Bacteroides* species (96).

An agent more recently investigated for the treatment of upper genital tract infections is metronidazole. It has excellent bactericidal activity against anaerobic bacteria and penetrates into tissue and abscesses well. In a comparative trial of metronidazole and tobramycin versus clindamycin and tobramycin in the treatment of 47 patients with a variety of pelvic infections, the two regimens were equally efficacious (97). Metronidazole in combination with an aminoglycoside, however, does not provide coverage against aerobic streptococci, *N. gonorrhoeae*, or microaerophilic streptococci as do the clindamycin-aminoglycoside combination or the single agent cefoxitin in the parenteral treatment of upper genital tract infections. There is very little data available on the treatment of TOAs with metronidazole combinations and virtually no data comparing metronidazole-containing regimens with other regimens in the treatment of TOAs. Caution in the use of metronidazole has been emphasized in situations where other antimicrobials might suffice until the questions of mutagenicity and carcinogenicity are more fully answered (98). A theoretical advantage of metronidazole over clindamycin has been suggested in animal experiments which have shown that metronidazole was more effective than clindamycin in decreasing the counts of *B. fragilis* in an experimental animal abscess model (92). In further experiments, it was shown that there was a diminishing impact of the antibiotics on the number of bacteria with progressive delays in the initiation of treatment. This effect was more pronounced with clindamycin than with metronidazole. The latter showed a sustained effect in reducing bacterial counts at all intervals tested (99).

Experience with cefoxitin, third generation cephalosporins, or extended spectrum penicillins in the management of TOAs is very limited. Comparative clinical trials with the agents shown to have in vitro and in vivo experimental advantages in the treatment of abscesses are clearly indicated.

At the present time, we consider the combination of clindamycin with an aminoglycoside to be the most effective regimen available for the treatment of TOAs, at least until future clinical trials are performed. Possibly, in the future the aminoglycoside will be replaced with a third generation cephalosporin or one of the new monobactam agents. Of the single agents, cefoxitin appears most appropriate, based on its demonstrated activity against anaerobes, including *B. fragilis*, and its ability to penetrate into abscesses.

Surgical Management of TOA

In the preantibiotic era, the treatment for pelvic infections consisted only of bed rest, fluids, and heat. The semifowler position was encouraged in hopes that purulent material would collect via gravity in the region of the cul-de-sac and would be accessible to colpotomy drainage. The first surgical drainage of a pelvic abscess was performed in the 1800s (18). This remained the only available alternative until the mid-20th century, with the advent of antibiotic preparations beginning with sulfa drugs and eventually penicillin. Surgical removal of in-

fected pelvic organs becomes a predominant mode of therapy, in spite of the addition of antibiotics to the armamentarium. In 1959, Collins and Jansen summarized the treatment of pelvic abscesses in this way:

> In the therapy of acute pelvic infections, one operates immediately in cases of ruptured abscesses or abscesses pointing into the cul de sac or in the region of Poupart's ligament. Otherwise, medical therapy is employed ... Failure to respond to these measures is a definite indication for surgery.

They went on to suggest that most pelvic abscesses eventually require surgical drainage or removal, but if possible delaying the surgery until the infection had "cooled" was preferable (100). In recent years, with the improvement in available antibiotics and the enhanced concern about infertility, an increasing number of investigators have encouraged conservative management of the unruptured TOA (15, 19, 20).

The approach we currently use in the management of suspected TOAs is outlined in the algorhythm in Figure 12.3. If a ruptured TOA is suspected, the patient is stabilized, antibiotics are begun, and immediate surgical intervention is undertaken. The only other indication for immediate surgery is when the diagnosis is in question and there is the strong possibility of a surgical emergency. Otherwise, the patient is begun on intravenous antibiotics that include an agent effective against resistant gram-negative anaerobes such as *B. fragilis* and *B. bivius*. If, despite appropriate antimicrobial therapy, the patient does not begin to demonstrate evidence of response in a reasonable amount of time (i.e., 48–72 hr), we would then proceed with surgical intervention. This does not mean complete cure, but rather evidence of response such as decreased temperature, decreased WBC, or subjective improvement in the patient's symptoms. During the initial antibiotic therapy, the clinician must be alert to the fact that the abscess may rupture and become a surgical emergency. Once the decision to operate has been made, there should be no delay. Each case must be individualized; in young, nulliparous patients an additional 24–48 hr are often allowed in hopes that they will begin to respond.

There are a number of factors that seem to be of some predictive value in determining which patients are more likely to fail antibiotic therapy alone. Ginsberg and associates noted that adnexal masses larger than 8 cm and/or bilateral

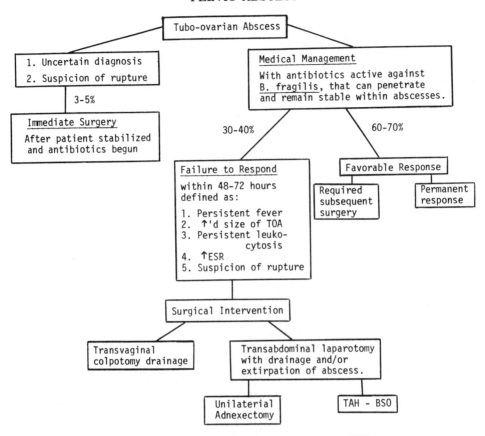

Figure 12.3. Algorhythm for management of TOAs.

adnexal involvement are predictive of failure to respond to medical therapy (20). Surprisingly, they noted that the presence of fever, the degree of leukocytosis, or the past history of PID were of no predictive value.

THE RUPTURED TOA

One of the most serious complications associated with TOAs is intraabdominal rupture, a surgical emergency for which the mortality rate is rapidly increased by unnecessary delay. In 1964, Pedowitz and Bloomfield reported on 143 cases of ruptured adnexal abscesses. Sixteen of these cases were treated prior to 1947 with a 100% mortality rate. From 1947 to 1959 127 cases were treated with a more aggressive surgical approach combined with available medical adjuvants, and the mortality was 3.1% (13). Pedowitz and Bloomfield also reported that there were 235 published cases after 1945 treated by centers using an operative approach, and in analyzing the 14 deaths that occurred, they felt that 10 cases may have been prevented from

dying. Physician delay in establishing the diagnosis was cited as the most common cause of preventable death. Collins and Jansen similarly reported an 85% mortality rate prior to 1952, but after adopting an aggressive surgical approach in addition to antibiotic therapy from 1953 to 1959, they reported 58 patients with ruptured TOAs and only 1 death. They estimated an expected recovery rate of 10–15% utilizing a medical regimen and an 85–90% recovery rate with the surgical approach (100). Subsequent investigators have continued to show improved survival with aggressive surgical management of ruptured TOAs. In 1969, Mickal and Sellmann reported a 11.1% mortality rate from 1951–1959 and 3.7% from 1959–1966 (22). Rivlin and Hunt, in 1977, reported a 7.1% mortality in 113 patients with ruptured TOAs (101). The major difference in this series was the extent of surgery performed at the time of laparotomy. In Rivlin's series, hysterectomy was performed in only 3% of the patients, with hormonal and menstrual function being retained in 73.5%. This was a surprise, considering the 70% hysterectomy rate reported by Pedowitz and Bloomfield, as well as the 80% rate in the Mickal and Sellmans series (13, 22). In addition, only 17.5% of patients in Rivlin's report required further surgery at a later date in the 1- to 5-year follow-up period. Landers Sweet recently reported four patients with ruptured TOAs that underwent unilateral adnexectomy and none required further surgery in the two to ten year follow-up, and one patient carried a subsequent intrauterine pregnancy to term (15). It appears that when aggressive surgical intervention is combined with appropriate antibiotic therapy in the treatment of ruptured unilateral TOAs, a conservative surgical approach utilizing unilateral adnexectomy and aimed at preserving hormonal and reproductive function can be safely employed.

SURGICAL APPROACH TO UNRUPTURED TOAs

No general consensus exists as to the appropriate surgical approach for the unruptured TOA. The techniques which have been used include: extraperitoneal drainage; posterior colpotomy drainage; transabdominal drainage; unilateral adnexectomy; and total abdominal hysterectomy with bilateral salpingo-oophorectomy.

Extraperitoneal drainage of TOAs has been used in the past to drain abscesses accessible to an incision just above Poupart's ligament. This procedure unfortunately requires adherence of the parietal and visceral peritoneum. We will not describe this procedure in detail, as its place in the treatment of TOAs is very limited and can probably be replaced with better results by unilateral excision.

Drainage of TOAs through a posterior colpotomy has been used for many years. This procedure is an effective mode of treatment when combined with antimicrobial therapy and restricted to patients with fluctuant abscesses in the midline which dissect the rectovaginal septum and are firmly attached to the parietal peritoneum. These requirements markedly reduce the number of TOAs that can be safely drained by this procedure. The morbidity of this procedure is significantly greater if these requirements are not met. In 1976, Rubenstein, Mishell and Ledger reported on 65 patients with pelvic abscesses that were drained by colpotomy or rectal incision. About one-third of their patients required a subsequent major operation because of residual pain or infection (102). In

1982, Rivlin and associates reported a combined series of 348 cases of colpotomy drainage, resulting in 23 cases of diffuse peritoneal sepsis (6.5%). Of these 23 cases there were six (26%) deaths (93). In 1983, Revlin reported 59 patients treated over a 20-yr span with colpotomy drainage in which there were two deaths, both related to diffuse peritonitis following septic abortion. Further surgery during the same admission was performed in 13 instances; additional surgery at a later date in 11 patients. Fourteen (58%) of these 24 repeat surgical procedures were performed as emergency operations (104). Colpotomy drainage, if appropriate, should be performed under general anesthesia, with the patient in the dorsal lithotomy position. The bladder is emptied, and an examination under anesthesia is performed to ensure that the abscess is adherent (i.e., cannot be moved out of the culdesac) and appropriate for colpotomy drainage. The vagina is then prepped with betadine and a tenaculum is used on the posterior lip of the cervix for countertraction. The vaginal mucosa is incised in a transverse manner at the junction of the posterior vaginal fornix with the cervix as recently described by Rivlin (104). The abscess cavity is entered with a kelly clamp which is then opened to enlarge the incision. Appropriate cultures are obtained, and the abscess cavity is subsequently explored, usually with the surgeon's finger to breakdown any adhesions or loculation within the abscess cavity. A mushroom catheter is inserted into the cavity for drainage. This catheter is removed 48–72 hr after drainage has stopped. Colpotomy drainage can be a useful adjuvant in the treatment of a small number of unilocular TOAs that fit the specific requirements for vaginal drainage and are resistant to treatment with antibiotics alone. There still exists some danger of diffuse peritoneal sepsis and death, but this can be minimized by carefully selecting the patients that would benefit from this form of therapy.

Vaginal colpotomy drainage is a procedure which is very rarely performed on our service. We feel it was designed for and was appropriate for use in the preantibiotic era when extraperitoneal drainage of abscesses was a paramount need. Without concurrent antibiotic therapy, a transabdominal approach to an acute abscess would most likely result in peritonitis and high mortality rates. Our lack of enthusiasm for vaginal colpotomy drainage is based on the following: (a) there is a high rate of complications and, subsequently, more definitive surgery following colpotomy drainage (102, 103, 104); (b) most TOAs do not meet the requisite requirements for the vaginal approach (i.e., midline mass which adheres to pelvic peritoneum and dissects upper one-third of rectovaginal septum; and (c) with the high incidence of unilateral abscesses being reported, it is our belief that unilateral adnexectomy with extirpation of infected tissue offers a better chance for preservation of future fertility and/or hormonal production from the contralateral adnexa.

CONSERVATIVE SURGERY VERSUS TOTAL HYSTERECTOMY WITH BILATERAL ADNEXECTOMY

There remains some controversy concerning the extent of surgery that is appropriate for the patient requiring surgical intervention in the treatment of a TOA. A number of investigators have advocated the complete removal of all reproductive organs by total abdominal hysterectomy with bilateral salpingo-oophorectomy (13, 14, 84, 100). This approach was stimulated by the report of Pedowitz and Bloomfield that in patients with only unilateral TOAs grossly, one-third had microscopic abscesses on the contralateral ovary (13). The alternative approach is a unilateral salpingo-oophorectomy for one-sided TOAs, with bilateral salpingo-oophorectomy limited to patients with bilateral disease. While it is true that complete removal of reproductive organs is most often curative, the more conservative unilateral adnexectomy offers the advantage of a hope for future fertility, maintenance of hormonal and menstrual function, and the avoidance of the physiologic and psychologic effects of hysterectomy and gonadectomy. The major question involved is whether or not these benefits outweigh the risk of requiring further surgical therapy. As antibiotic regimens continue to improve and more data accumulate on the patients treated with conservative surgery, the answer to these questions should become available.

Several investigators have reported results of conservative surgical management of patients with unilateral TOAs (13, 15, 20, 22, 25, 76, 101). These data, summarized in Table 4, indicate that approximately 17% of patients treated with unilateral adnexectomy will require additional surgery at a later date. Unfortunately, all of the data on conservative surgical treatment of TOAs is retrospective and suffers from poor long-term follow-up. Included in this group is the unique series of Rivlin and Hunt (101). They combined conservative surgery with intra- and postoperative antibiotic peritoneal lavage for the treatment of 113 patients with ruptured TOAs. They found that only four patients (3%) required hysterectomy initially. In the 83 patients treated with adnexal procedures (unilateral or bilateral) without removal of the uterus, 16 (19%) required further surgical intervention. In our recent series, 19 patients were treated with unilateral adnexectomy, and only two required subsequent surgery while three had subsequent pregnancies (15). Thus, it appears that although there is a risk that further surgery will be required, the conservative surgical approach does offer the TOA patient that fails initial antibiotic therapy another alternative to permanent sterilization and castration. Perhaps patients with unilateral TOAs that do respond to antibiotics initially but

Table 12.4
Summary of Treatment with Unilateral Adnexectomy

Study (reference)	No. treated with unilateral adnexectomy	No. requiring subsequent surgery (%)	No. with subsequent pregnancy (%)
Pedowitz and Bloomfield (13)	14	6 (43)	NS
Landers and Sweet (15)	19	2 (10.5)	3 (15.8)
Hager (17)	6	0 (0)	4 (80)[a]
Ginsberg et al (20)	5	1 (20)	NS
Mickal and Sellmann (22)	8	1 (12.5)	NS
Golde et al (35)	12	0 (0)	1 (8.3)
Manara (76)	10	0 (0)	NS
Rivlin and Hunt (101)	27	7 (26)[b]	1 (3.7)
Total	101	17 (16.8)	9/64 (14.1)

[a] Only five of the six patients treated with unilateral adnexectomy attempted to conceive.
[b] All patients had ruptured TOAs, and 10 were treated with incomplete unilateral adnexectomy.

have persistence of their mass could benefit from unilateral adnexectomy in terms of future fertility and flareups. There is likely to be a continued demand for the conservative surgical approach, especially as such techniques as in vitro fertilization and donor embryo transplantation become available. Conservative surgery, in which the uterus is left in place and any normal ovarian tissue is preserved, may be an acceptable procedure in selected cases where future fertility is desired.

Technical Aspects of TOA Surgery

Surgical extirpation of a pelvic abscess will be necessary in a significant number of patients with either ruptured abscesses or abscesses unresponsive to medical management. This type of surgery is often plagued with distorted tissue planes. The dissection may be bloody and the abscess may involve contiguous structures including bowel, bladder, and ureter.

INCISION

Considerable exposure is necessary, as these abscesses may extend laterally to involve the pelvic side wall, posteriorly to the rectum, or even superiorly toward the umbilicus. Concealed pockets of pus may also collect in the upper abdomen, which must be eliminated if present. The Pfannensteil incision would be the least appropriate incision, offering the disadvantages of limited exposure and a potential risk of subfascial infections and even necrotizing fascitis, as the fascia is separated from the underlying rectus muscle. The Mallard incision offers the advantage of greater exposure (especially to the lateral pelvic walls) and the strength of a transverse incision. A theoretic disadvantage may be that the healing edge of the cut belly muscle may serve as a further nidus for infection, although we have not found this to be a problem and have had good success with this incision. The low (subumbilical) vertical incision offers the advantages of adequate exposure as well as ease of extension if more exposure is needed, and it does not require cutting across muscle. The major disadvantage is the relative weakness of a vertical incision compared with a transverse incision, particularly in infected cases, although this may be minimized by proper surgical technique and optimal choice of suture material for closure. Of secondary concern is the lack of aesthetic appeal with the vertical incision.

PROCEDURE

Once adequate exposure is achieved and the site of the abscess is identified, the final decision can be made as to the extent of surgery that is required. Careful dissection of the distorted tissue planes is crucial in order to avoid injury to contiguous structures. The abscess and involved reproductive organs should be completely free of bowel, bladder, and ureters before adnexectomy or hysterectomy is undertaken. This may require identifying and isolating the ureters in order to avoid injury. Careful exploration of other areas of the abdomen for concealed pockets of pus is equally important. Copious irrigation with warm saline is then carried out prior to closure. Since intravenous levels of antibiotics should be maintained before, during, and after surgery, there is no advantage to irrigating with antimicrobial solutions. If hysterectomy is performed, the vaginal cuff should not be closed, but rather sutured open with a running interlocking suture around the edges of the vaginal cuff to provide hemostasis. Either a large bore Malecot drain or Jackson-Pratt drain is then placed, exiting through the vaginal cuff and connected to closed suction drainage. If the uterus is left in place and there has been rupture or leakage of the abscess, a Malecot or multiple Jackson-Pratt drain can be brought out through a posterior colpotomy incision. These drains are removed after 48–72 hr if drainage has stopped.

CLOSURE

The fascia should be closed with permanent suture, such as wire, or a synthetic nonabsorbable monofilament suture. The Smead-Jones technique is preferred for added strength when closing vertical incisions. A delayed primary closure of the skin and subcutaneous tissue is the procedure of choice. Brown and co-workers reported a significant reduction in the incidence of wound infection with use of the delayed primary closure approach. Among 146 patients at risk for wound infection in whom a delayed primary wound closure was undertaken, only 3 (2.1%) developed a wound infection. In a matched group of 146 patients undergoing immediate wound closure, 34 (23.3%) developed a wound infection (105). A pack of moist fine mesh gauze is placed in the subcutaneous tissue layers and covered with a sterile dressing for 3–4 days, at which time the incision is reinspected and, if clean, is closed with a tape or Steri-Strip closure.

Irrigation of the incision with povidone-iodine solution has been shown to be ineffective in reducing the incidence of wound infection (106, 107).

Fertility Following TOAs

The preservation of reproductive organs in the management of TOAs is in no way a guarantee of future fertility, especially in patients who may well have tubal damage from previous episodes of upper genital tract infection. Although several investigators have reported the incidence of subsequent pregnancy following TOAs, the follow-up was very limited, leaving it impossible to assess the number of patients attempting to conceive and their success rate (15, 17, 19, 20, 35, 101, 103). The pregnancy rate has been reported to range from 9.5–13.8% following conservative medical management (15, 19, 20), 3.7–16% following unilateral adnexal procedures with preoperative antibiotics (15, 20, 35), and 10–15% following antibiotics plus colpotomy drainage (101, 103). Hager recently published a series in which 50 patients treated for TOAs were evaluated (17). A total of 11 of these patients had reproductive potential following treatment, but only eight attempted to conceive. Four of the eight (50%) conceived a total of five intrauterine pregnancies. There were no ectopic pregnancies. Included in this group were five patients that underwent a unilateral salpingo-oophorectomy and attempted to conceive, of which four were successful (80%). Acknowledging that these numbers are very small, we must recognize that we may be dramatically underestimating reproductive potential following TOAs, unless we consider the number of patients attempting to conceive following conservative medical or surgical management. Furthermore, there has been very little data published on patients treated vigorously with antibiotics such as clindamycin metronidazole, cefoxitin, or moxalactam that can penetrate abscesses. More investigation is also needed to elucidate the role of unilateral adnexectomy in the enhancement of future fertility following a unilateral TOA.

Future Directions in the Management of TOAs

A relatively new technique currently being employed is the percutaneous drainage of intraabdominal abscesses guided by CT or real time ultrasound. This technique has been reported to be successful in 75–89% of abscesses (108–111). The majority of abscesses success-

fully drained by this technique have been unilocular abscesses. Mandel and associates, however, have performed percutaneous drainage on multilocular abscesses. They report success with placement of more than one drainage tube for multilocular abscesses (108).

In addition to localization and percutaneous insertion of catheters for drainage in abscess, the CT scan and ultrasound are also used to follow the response of these abscesses to the drainage technique. Repeat scans are generally performed within 48 hr after drainage to evaluate response. These catheters can also be used for irrigation of the abscess cavities, as well as injections of contrast material to assure reduction of cavity size on repeat scans. The evaluation of this technique in the treatment of TOAs in significant numbers has yet to be reported.

The role of laparoscopy in the diagnosis and management of salpingitis has revolutionized current thinking on the etiology and pathogenesis of the disease process. The laparoscope may also prove to be extremely useful in the management of TOAs. Adducci reported his experience with colpotomy drainage during laparoscopy of nine patients with PID-associated pelvic abscesses (112). All nine patients responded well to this approach. This technique offers the advantage of direct visualization of the abscess being drained, as well as confirmation of the diagnosis. Laparoscopic directed percutaneous drainage of TOAs may become a useful technique but requires additional evaluation.

SUMMARY

The incidence of tuboovarian abscesses (TOAs) is expected to increase as a result of the current epidemic of sexually transmitted diseases and their sequelae. Patients with TOAs most commonly present with lower abdominal pain and an adnexal mass(es). Fever and leukocytosis may be absent. Ultrasound, CT scans, laparoscopy, or laparotomy may be necessary to confirm the diagnosis. TOAs may be unilateral or bilateral regardless of IUD usage. The microbiology of TOAs is polymicrobial with a preponderance of anaerobic organisms.

An initial conservative antimicrobial approach to the management of the unruptured TOA is appropriate if the antimicrobial agents used can penetrate abscesses, remain active within the abscess environment, and are active against the major pathogens in TOAs, including the resistant gram-negative anaerobes such as *B. fragilis* and *Bacteroides bivius*. However, if the patient does not begin to show a response within a reasonable amount of time, i.e., 48–72 hr, surgical intervention should be undertaken. Suspicion of rupture should remain an indication for immediate surgery. Once surgery is undertaken, a conservative approach with unilateral adnexectomy for one-sided TOAs is appropriate if future fertility or hormone production is desired. The surgery may be difficult, requiring careful dissection and postoperative intraperitoneal drainage. Permanent fascial sutures and delayed primary closure can be used to decrease postoperative infectious complications.

References

1. Ledger WJ: Infections in obstetrics and gynecology: new developments in treatment. *Surg Clin North Am* 52:1447–1458, 1972.
2. Sweet RL: Management of mixed aerobic-anaerobic infections of the female genital tract. *J Antimicrob Chemother* 8(Suppl D):105–114, 1981.
3. McNamara MT, Meed PB: Diagnosis and management of the pelvic abscess. *J Reprod Med* 17:299–304, 1976.
4. Pedowitz P, Bloomfield RD: Ruptured adnexal abscess (tubo-ovarian) with generalized peritonitis. *Am J Obstet Gynecol* 88:721–729, 1964.
5. Mickal A, Sellmann AA: Management of tubo-ovarian abscess. *Clin Obstet Gynecol* 12:252–264, 1969.
6. Hevron JE, Llorens AS: Management of postoperative abscess following gynecologic surgery. *Obstet Gynecol* 47:553–556, 1976.
7. Ledger WJ, Campbell C, Taylor D, Willson JR: Adnexal abscess as a late complication of pelvic operations. *Surg Gynecol Obstet* 129:973–978, 1969.
8. Gibbs RS, Jones PM, Wilder CJ: Antibiotic therapy of endometritis following cesarean section: treatment successes and failures. *Obstet Gynecol* 52:31–37, 1978.
9. Ledger WJ, Reite AM, Headington JT: The surveillance of infection of an inpatient gynecology service. *Obstet Gynecol* 37:769, 1971.
10. Ledger WJ, Child MA: The hospital care of patients undergoing hysterectomy. An analysis of 12,026 patients from the Professional Activity Study. *Am J Obstet Gynecol* 117:423, 1973.
11. Sweet RL: Anaerobic infections of the female genital tract. *Am J Obstet Gynecol* 122:891–901, 1975.
12. Eschenbach DA: Acute pelvic inflammatory disease; etiology, risk factors and pathogenesis. *Clin Obstet Gynecol* 19:147, 1976.
13. Pedowitz P, Bloomfield RD: Ruptured adnexal abscess (tubo-ovarian) with generalized peritonitis. *Am J Obstet Gynecol* 88:721, 1964.
14. Nebel WA, Lucas WE: Management of tubo-ovarian abscess. *Obstet Gynecol* 32:381, 1968.
15. Landers DV, Sweet RL: Tubo-ovarian abscess: contemporary approach to management. *Rev Infect Dis* 5(suppl):876, 1983.
16. Burkman R, Schlesselman S, McCaffrey L,

Gupta PK, Spence M: The relationship of genital tract actinomycetes and the development of pelvic inflammatory disease. *Am J Obstet Gynecol* 143:585, 1982.
17. Hager WD: Follow-up of patients with tubo-ovarian abscess(es) in association with salpingitis. *Obstet Gynecol* 61:680, 1983.
18. Benigno BB: Medical and surgical management of the pelvic abscess. *Clin Obstet Gynecol* 24:1187, 1981.
19. Franklin EW, Hevron JE, Thompson JD: Management of the pelvic abscess. *Clin Obstet Gynecol* 16:66, 1973.
20. Ginsberg DS, Stern JL, Hamod KA, Genadry R, Spence MR: Tubo-ovarian abscess: a retrospective review. *Am J Obstet Gynecol* 138:1055, 1980.
21. Edelman DA, Berger GS: Contraceptive practice and tubo-ovarian abscess. *Am J Obstet Gynecol* 138:541, 1980.
22. Mickal A, Sellmann AH: Management of tubo-ovarian abscess. *Clin Obstet Gynecol* 12:252, 1969.
23. Clark JR, Moore-Hines S: A study of tubo-ovarian abscess at Howard University Hospital (1965 through 1975). *J Natl Med Assoc* 71:1109, 1979.
24. Vemereen J, Telinde RW: Intra-abdominal rupture of pelvic abscess. *Am J Obstet Gynecol* 68:402, 1954.
25. Filly RA: Detection of abdominal abscesses: a combined approach employing ultrasonography, computed tomography and gallium-67 scanning. *J Assoc Can Radiol* 30:202, 1979.
26. Norton L, Eule J, Burdick D: Accuracy of technique to detect intraperitoneal abscess. *Surgery* 84:370, 1978.
27. Hopkins GB, Kan M, Mende CW: Gallium-67 scintography and intraabdominal sepsis: clinical experience in 140 patients with suspected intraabdominal abscess. *West J Med* 125:425, 1976.
28. Carroll B, Silverman PM, Goodwin DA, McDougall R: Ultrasonography and Indium 111 white blood cell scanning for the detection of intraabdominal abscesses. *Radiology* 140:155, 1981.
29. Coleman RE, Black RE, Welch DM, et al: Indium-111 labeled leukocytes in the evaluation of suspected abdominal abscesses. *Am J Surg* 139:99, 1980.
30. Bicknell TA, Kohatsu S, Goodwin DA: Use of Indium-111-labeled autologous leukocytes in differentiating pancreatic abscess from pseudocyst. *Am J Surg* 142:312, 1981.
31. Taylor KJW, DeGraaft MCI, Wasson JF, Rosenfield AT, Audriole VT: Accuracy of grey-scale ultrasound diagnosis of abdominal and pelvic abscesses in 220 patients. *Lancet* 1:83, 1978.
32. Spirtos NJ, Bernstine EL, Crawford WL, Fayle J: Sonography in acute pelvic inflammatory disease. *J Reprod Med* 27:312, 1982.
33. Uhrich PC, Sanders RC: Ultrasonic characteristics of pelvic inflammatory masses. *J Clin Ultrasound* 4:199, 1976.
34. Moir C, Robins RE: Role of ultrasound, gallium scanning and computed tomography in the diagnosis of intra-abdominal abscess. *Am J Surg* 143:582, 1982.
35. Golde SH, Israel R, Ledger WJ: Unilateral tubo-ovarian abscess: a distinct entity. *Am J Obstet Gynecol* 127:807, 1977.

36. Swenson RM, Michaelson TC, Daly MJ, et al: Anaerobic bacterial infections of the female genital tract. *Obstet Gynecol* 42:538, 1973

37. Thadepalli H, Gorbach SL, Keith L: Anaerobic infections of the female genital tract: bacteriologic and therapeutic aspects. *Am J Obstet Gynecol* 117:1034, 1973.

38. Altemeier WA: The anaerobic streptococci in tubo-ovarian abscess. *Am J Obstet Gynecol* 39:1038, 1940.

39. Ledger WJ, Campbell C, Willson JR: Postoperative adnexal infections. *Obstet Gynecol* 31:83, 1968.

40. Pearson HE, Anderson GV: Genital bacteroidal abscesses in women. *Am J Obstet Gynecol* 107:1264, 1970.

41. Weinstein WM, Onderdonk AB, Bartlett JG, Gorbach SL: Experimental intra-abdominal abscess in rats: development of an experimental model. *Infect Immun* 10:1250, 1974.

42. Hammill HA, Owens WE, Ford LC, Finegold SM: A rat model of unilateral utero-tubo-ovarian abscess. *Rev Infect Dis* 6(suppl 1):96–100, 1984.

43. Bartlett JG, Louie TJ, Gorbach SL, Onderdonk AB: Therapeutic efficacy of 29 antimicrobial regimens in experimental intra-abdominal sepsis. *Rev Infect Dis* 3:535, 1981.

44. Bartlett JG: Recent developments in the management of anaerobic infections. *Rev Infect Dis* 5:235, 1981.

45. Onderdonk AB, Kasper DL, Cizneros RL, Bartlett JG: The capsular polysaccharide of *B. fragilis* as a virulence factor: comparison of the pathogenic potential of encapsulated and unencapsulated strains. *J Infect Dis* 136:82, 1977.

46. Bjornson AB, Bjornson HS: Participation of immunoglobulin and the alternative complement pathway in opsonization of *Bacteroides fragilis* and *Bacteroides thetaiotaomicorn. Rev Infect Dis* 1(2):347, 1979.

47. Kasper DL, Onderdonk AB, Cabb J, Bartlett JG: Protective efficacy of immunization with capsular antigen against experimental infection with *Bacteroides fragilis. J Infect Dis* 140:724, 1979.

48. Onderdonk AB, Markham RB, Zaleznik DF, Cizneros RL, Kasper DL: Evidence of T cell dependent immunity to *Bacteroides fragilis* in an intra-abdominal abscess model. *J Clin Invest* 69:9, 1982.

49. Zaleznik DF, Kasper DL: The role of anaerobic bacteria in abscess formation. *Annu Rev Med* 38:217, 1982.

50. Polk BF, Kasper DL, Shapiro M, Taber IB, Schoenbaum SC, Goldstein PR: Serum antibody response to *Bacteroides fragilis* in women with abscesses following hysterectomy. *Obstet Gynecol* 55:163, 1980.

51. Chow AW, Alkisian KL, Marshall JR, Guze LB: The bacteriology of acute pelvic inflammatory disease. *Am J Obstet Gynecol* 122:876, 1975.

52. Monif GRG, Welkons SI, Baer H, et al: Cul de sac isolates from patients with endometritis-salpingitis-peritonitis and gonococcal endocervicitis. *Am J Obstet Gynecol* 126:158, 1976.

53. Holmes KK, Eschenbach DA, Knapp JS: Salpingitis: overview of etiology and epidemiology. *Am J Obstet Gynecol* 138(7):893, 1980.

54. Eschenbach DA: Epidemiology and diagnosis of acute pelvic inflammatory disease. *Obstet Gynecol* 55(5-S):1425, 1980.

55. Sweet RL, Schachter J, Landers DV: Chlamydia infections in obstetrics and gynecology. *Clin Obstet Gynecol* 26(1):143, 1983.

56. Mardh P-A, Ripa KT, Svensson L, Westrom L: *Chlamydia trachomatis* in patients with acute salpingitis. *N Engl J Med* 296:1377, 1977.

57. Paavonen J, Saikku P, Vesterienen E, Aho K: *Chlamydia trachomatis* in acute salpingitis. *Br J Vener Dis* 55(3):203, 1979.

58. Treharne JD, Ripe KR, March P-A, Svensson L, Westrom L, Darougar S: Antibodies to *Chlamydia trachomatis* in acute salpingitis. *Br J Vener Dis* 55(1):26, 1979.

59. Ripa KR, Svensson L, Treharne JD, Westrom L, Mardh P-A: *Chlamydia trachomatis* infection in patients with laparoscopically verified salpingitis: results of isolation and antibody determinations. *Am J Obstet Gynecol* 138:960, 1980.

60. Paavonen J: *Chlamydia trachomatis* in acute salpingitis. *Am J Obstet Gynecol* 138:957, 1980.

61. Mardh P-A, Lind I, Svensson L, Westrom L, Moller BR: Antibodies to *Chlamydia trachomatis, Mycoplasma hominis* and *Neisseria gonorrhoeae* in sera from patients with acute salpingitis. *Br J Vener Dis* 57:125, 1981.

62. Mardh P-A, Westrom L: Tubal and cervical cultures in acute salpingitis with special reference to *Mycoplasma hominis* and T-strain mycoplasma. *Br J Vener Dis* 46:179, 1970.

63. Sweet RL, Draper DL, Schachter J, et al: Microbiology and pathogenesis of acute salpingitis as determined by laparoscopy: what is the appropriate site to sample? *Am J Obstet Gynecol* 138:985, 1980.

64. Moller BR, Freundt EA, Black FT, et al: Experimental infection of the genital tract of female grivet monkeys by *Mycoplasma hominis. Infect Immun* 20:248, 1978.

65. Thomas M, Jones M, Ray S, Andrews B: *Mycoplasma pneumoniae* in a tubo-ovarian abscess. *Lancet* 7938:774, 1975.

66. Schiffer MA, Elguezabal A, Sultana M, Allen AC: Actinomycosis infections associated with intrauterine contraceptive devices. *Obstet Gynecol* 45:67, 1975.

67. Lomax CW, Harbert GM, Thornton WN: Actinomycosis of the female genital tract. *Obstet Gynecol* 48:341, 1976.

68. Gupta PK, Erozan YS, Frost JK: Actinomyces and the IUD: an update. *Acta Cytol (Baltimore)* 22:281, 1978.

69. Schmidt WA, et al: Actinomycosis and intrauterine contraceptive devices. *Diagn Gynecol Obstet* 2:165, 1980.

70. Ward ME, Watt PJ, Robertson JN: The human fallopian tube: a laboratory model for gonococcal infection. *J Infect Dis* 129:650, 1974.

71. Carney FE, Taylor-Robinson D: Growth and effect of *Neisseria gonorrhoeae* in organ cultures. *Br J Vener Dis* 49:435, 1973.

72. Gregg CR, Melly MA, McGee ZA: Gonococcal lipopolysaccharide: a toxin for human fallopian tube mucosa. *Am J Obstet Gynecol* 138:981, 1980.

73. Hare MJ, Barnes CFJ: Fallopian tube organ culture in the investigation of bacteroides as a cause of pelvic inflammatory disease. In Phillips I,

Collier J (eds): Proceedings of the 2nd International Symposium on Metronidazole. London, The Royal Society of Medicine, 1979, pp 191–198.

74. Golditch IM, Huston JE: Serious pelvic infections associated with intrauterine contraceptive devices. *Int J Fertil* 18:156, 1973.

75. Scott WC: Pelvic abscess in association with intrauterine contraceptive devices. *Am J Obstet Gynecol* 131:149, 1978.

76. Manara LR: Management of tubo-ovarian abscess. *JADA* 81(7):476, 1981.

77. Taylor ES, McMillan JH, Green BE, Droegemueller W, Thompson HE: The intrauterine device. *Obstet Gynecol* 46:429, 1975.

78. Dawood MY, Birnbaum SJ: Unilateral tuboovarian abscess and an intrauterine contraceptive device. *Obstet Gynecol* 46:429, 1975.

79. Burnhill MS: Syndrome of progressive endometritis associated with intrauterine contraceptive devices. *Adv Planned Parent* 8:144–150, 1973.

80. Mishel DR, Bell J, Good RG, Mover DL: The intrauterine device: a bacteriological study of the endometrial cavity. *Am J Obstet Gynecol* 96:119, 1966.

81. Sparks RA, Purrier BGA, Watt PJ, Ectein M: Bacterial colonization of uterine cavity: Role of tailed intrauterine contraceptive devices. *Br Med J* 282:1189, 1981.

82. Skangalis M, Mahoney CJ, O'Leary WM: Microbial presence in the uterine cavity as affected by varieties of intrauterine contraceptive devices. *Fertil Steril* 37(2):263, 1982.

83. Saini S, Kellum JM, O'Leary MP, et al: Improved localization and survival in patients with intra abdominal abscesses. *Am J Surg* 154:136, 1983.

84. Kaplan AL, Jacobs WM, Ehresman JB: Aggressive management of pelvic abscess. *Am J Obstet Gynecol* 98:482, 1967.

85. Kirby BD, George WL, Sutter VL, Citron DM, Finegold SM: Gram negative anaerobic bacilli: their role in infection and patterns of susceptibility to antimicrobial agents. I. Little known Bacteroides species. *Rev Infect Dis* 2:914, 1980.

86. Kasper DL, Onderdonk AB, Polk BFF, Bartlett JG: Surface antigens as virulence factors in infection with *Bacteroides fragilis*. *Rev Infect Dis* 2:914, 1980.

87. Bartlett JG, Onderdonk AB, Louiee TJ, Kasper DL, Gorbach SL: A review: lessons from an animal model of intra-abdominal sepsis. *Arch Surg* 113:853, 1978.

88. Klempner MS, Styrt B: Clindamycin uptake by human neutrophils. *J Infect Dis* 144:472, 1981.

89. Prokesch RC, Hand WL: Antibiotic entry into human polymorphonuclear leukocytes. *Antimicrob Agents Chemother* 21:373, 1982.

90. Joiner KA, Lowe BR, Dzink JL, Bartlett JG: Antibiotic levels in infected and sterile subcutaneous abscesses in mice. *J Infect Dis* 143:487, 1981.

91. Joiner K, Lowe B, Dznik J, Bartlett JG: Antibiotic levels in infected and sterile subcutaneous abscesses in mice. *J Infect Dis* 143:487, 1981.

92. Bartlett JG: Recent developments in the management of anaerobic infections. *Rev Infect Dis* 5(2):235, 1983.

93. Cuchural G, Jacobus N, Gorbach SL, Tally FP, Barza M, and Gorbach SL: Penetration of clindamycin into experimental infections with *Bacteroides fragilis*. *J Antimicrob Chemother* 8:59, 1981.

94. Rolfe RD, Finegold SM: Comparative in vitro activity of new betalactam antibiotics against anaerobic bacteria. *Antimicrob Agents Chemother* 20:600, 1981.

95. Simon GL, Richmond DM, Tally FP, Barza M, Gorbach SL: Penetration of clindamycin into experimental infections with *Bacteroides fragilis*. *J Antimicrob Chemother* 8:59, 1981.

96. Guiney DG Jr, Hasegawa P, Stalker D, Davis CE: Genetic analysis of clindamycin resistance in Bacteroides species. *J Infect Dis* 147(3):551, 1983.

97. Gall SA, Kohan AP, Ayers OM: Intravenous metronidazole or clindamycin with tobramycin for therapy of pelvic infections. *Obstet Gynecol* 577:51, 1981.

98. Robbie MO, Sweet RL: Metronidazole use in obstetrics and gynecology: a review. *Am J Obstet Gynecol* 145(7):865, 1983.

99. Bartlett JG, Dezfuliun M, Joiner K: Relative efficacy and critical interval of antimicrobial agents in experimental infections involving *Bacteroides fragilis*. *Arch Surg* 118(2):181, 1983.

100. Collins CG, Jansen FW: Treatment of pelvic abscess. *Clin Obstet Gynecol* 2:512, 1959.

101. Rivlin ME, Hunt JA: Ruptured tubo-ovarian abscess: is hysterectomy necessary? *Obstet Gynecol* 50(S):518, 1977.

102. Rubenstein PR, Mishell DR, Ledger WJ: Colpotomy drainage of pelvic abscess. *Obstet Gynecol* 48(2):142, 1976.

103. Rivlin ME, Golan A, Darling MR: Diffuse peritoneal sepsis associated with colpotomy drainage of pelvic abscess. *J Reprod Med* 27(7):406, 1982.

104. Rivlin ME: Clinical outcome following vaginal drainage of pelvic abscess. *Obstet Gynecol* 61(2):169, 1983.

105. Brown SE, Allen HH, Robins RN: The use of delayed primary wound closure in preventing wound infections. *Am J Obstet Gynecol* 127(7):713, 1977.

106. Galland RB, Mosley JG, Saunders JH, Darrell JH: Prevention of wound infection in abdominal operations by preoperative antibiotics or povidone-iodine. *Lancet* 8047:1043, 1977.

107. Balle PC, Homesley HD: Ineffectiveness of povidone-iodine irrigation of abdominal incisions. *Obstet Gynecol* 55(6):744, 1980.

108. Mandel SR, Body D, Jaques PF, Mandell V, Staab EV: Drainage of hepatic, intraabdominal and mesiastinal abscesses guided by computerized axial tomography. *Am J Surg* 145:120, 1983.

109. van Sonnenberg E, Ferrucci JT, Mueller PR, et al: Percutaneous radiographically guided catheter drainage of abdominal abscesses. *JAMA* 247(2):190, 1982.

110. Gerzof SG, Robbins AH, Johnson WC, Birkett DH, Nabseth DC: Percutaneous catheter drainage of abdominal abscesses. *N Engl J Med* 305(12):653, 1981.

111. Gronvall S, Gammelgaard J, Haubek A, Holm HH: Drainage of abdominal abscesses guided by gonography. *Am J Radiol* 138:527, 1982.

112. Adducci JE: Laparoscopy in the diagnosis and treatment of pelvic inflammatory disease with abscess formation. *Int Surg* 66:359, 1981.

CHAPTER 13

Perinatal Infections

VIRUSES

Rubella

Rubella (also known as German measles) is usually a mild, viral illness with fever, postauricular or suboccipital lymphadenopathy, arthralgia, and a transient erythematous rash. It has been gratifying that since 1966 the incidence rate of reported rubella cases has fallen dramatically from 28 cases/100,000 population to approximately 1 case/100,000 in 1982 (1). Since Gregg, an Australian ophthalmologist, observed in 1941 that rubella in early pregnancy was teratogenic, this disease has been of concern to the obstetrician.

EPIDEMIOLOGY

Wild rubella virus is spread by droplets or direct contact with infected persons or articles contaminated with nasopharyngeal secretions. Although it is considered primarily a disease of childhood, in the past few years more than half the cases have occurred in patients over age 9. Only on rare occasions have serious sequelae such as central nervous system involvement of thrombocytopenia developed. By reproductive age, about 75–85% of the population has had rubella, and about half are subclinical infections. Once wild virus infection occurs (even if subclinical), immunity is life-long.

Before vaccination became available in 1969, rubella occurred at 6- to 9-yr cycles, but the last major epidemic was in 1964. The main problem is infection during the early pregnancy when primary maternal rubella may lead to involvement of the embryo or fetus. Overall, the risk of congenital rubella syndrome is generally quoted to be about 20% when primary maternal infection occurs in the first trimester of pregnancy (Table 13.1). The risk ranges from 50% in the 1st month to 10% by the 3rd month. In a recent survey, the estimate has been higher in England when there has been symptomatic maternal infection (2). Cataracts, patent ductus arteriosus, and deafness are the most common abnormalities. When these children have been followed for a few years, additional disorders such as diabetes have occurred more frequently than expected. Congenital rubella syndrome has not been eliminated from the United States, but progress is being made. In 1979, 55 cases were reported by the National Congenital Rubella Syndrome Registry. In 1980, only 14 cases were reported, and in 1981 and 1982, there were 9 cases reported each year (1).

DIAGNOSIS

The clinical diagnosis of rubella is often difficult, since it resembles a number of other exanthemas. With rubella infection, the virus can be isolated from the bloodstream and throat 7–10 days after exposure. Shedding of virus from the throat continues for about a week. The rash, which typically starts in the face, develops commonly 16–18 days after exposure.

The diagnosis of rubella should never be based solely on clinical criteria. To confirm rubella infection, a variety of antibody tests are available.

Hemagglutinating Inhibition Antibody (HI)

This IgG class antibody is most commonly used for screening. It reaches a peak within a few weeks, and after wild virus infection HI titers usually remain positive for life. From 5 to 15% of normal women with remote rubella infection have stable HI titers >1:256. A titer of >1:8 (i.e., ≥ 1:16) is conclusive evidence of immunity. Recently there has been controversy as to the interpretation of a titer equal to 1:8. In such cases, HI test should be repeated. If a titer equal to 1:8 is again reported, then this most probably indicates long lasting immunity. On the other hand, if the repeat titer shows titer rise ≥4 fold, then this is evidence of acute rubella infection. Because of variations between laboratories and day-to-day variations within one

Table 13.1
Risk of Congenital Rubella after Maternal Infection with Rash at Successive Stages of Pregnancy[a]

Gestational age (wk)	No. followed up	Overall risk (%)
<11	9	90
11–12	4	33
13–14	12	11
15–16	14	24

[a] Adapted from Miller E, Cradock-Watson JE, Pollock TM: Consequences of confirmed maternal rubella at successive stages of pregnancy. *Lancet* 2:781, 1982.

laboratory, it is essential that paired serum samples be tested on the same day, in the same laboratory.

Complement Fixation Test (CF)

Also an IgG class antibody, CF antibody appears later than HI and may be useful in some diagnostic situations, such as patients with high HI or patients first seen 1–5 weeks after exposure. It may thus be possible to demonstrate a significant rise in CF antibody when it is too late to demonstrate this change in HI antibody. The CF test has to be requested as it is not performed routinely.

Rubella Specific IgM

IgM antibodies appear early and last for only a few weeks. This test may be helpful in some diagnostic situations, but is available in few laboratories. Although a positive rubella-IgM titer is indicative of recent primary rubella infection, its absence does not necessarily exclude it, as in some patients IgM may disappear in less than 4–5 weeks.

Others

Other serologic responses are detectable by radioimmunoassay, neutralization, or enzyme-linked immunosorbent assay (ELISA). At present, these have little clinical utility. When a patient is first seen having an elevated HI titer, it is not always possible to determine whether there has been acute primary rubella infection, even though these other tests are properly used.

COUNSELING AND MANAGEMENT

In pregnant women with confirmed rubella infection, there must be proper counseling re-

garding the risks and types of congenital anomalies. At present, culturing amniotic fluid for rubella virus is not advised, as this is not able to distinguish reliably the infected fetus from the uninfected one among pregnancies at risk. Counseling should also consider the small, but known, risks of pregnancy termination to the mother.

Use of immune globulin (IG) after exposure has been recommended by some authors. However, the Advisory Committee to the Centers for Disease Control notes that IG given after exposure prevents neither infection nor viremia, although it may alter symptoms (3). Further, infants with congenital rubella have been born to women who received IG shortly after exposure. Thus, they do not recommend IG for routine use for postexposure prophylaxis. Yet, they suggest that IG might be useful in a susceptible, exposed pregnant women for whom pregnancy termination would be acceptable. In this case, IG might offer some protection against fetal infection (3).

PREVENTION

When rubella vaccine became available in 1969, the strategy in the United States was to control rubella in preschool and young school-aged children who were known reservoirs. It was believed that this approach would prevent exposure of susceptible, pregnant women to the wild virus. By 1977, however, 10–20% of women of childbearing age still were susceptible; this proportion was similar to that in the prevaccine years. Even more important, there had been a continuation of endemic congenital rubella syndrome cases at its low incidence. Accordingly, public health authorities subsequently increased efforts to vaccinate older teenagers and military recruits (1).

In January 1979, the rubella vaccine RA 27/3 replaced HPV-77 vaccine in the United States. All rubella vaccines contain live, attenuated virus. RA 27/3 is administered subcutaneously. After vaccination, approximately 95% of susceptible individuals develop HI antibodies, which provide long-term (probably life-long) protection. Among adults who did not show a positive HI titer after vaccination, nearly all show detectable antibody when a more sensitive test is used. According to the Centers for Disease Control, any detectable rubella antibody or a history of rubella vaccination is presumptive evidence of immunity.

Vaccines may shed the attenuated virus from the nasopharynx for a few weeks, but there is no evidence that the vaccine virus can be transmitted. Thus, there appears to be no risk to susceptible, pregnant women, who contact recently vaccinated children or adults.

Rubella-susceptible women who are of reproductive age should be considered candidates for immunization, but it is recommended that pregnancy be avoided for 90 days. The immediate postpartum period is often suggested as an excellent time for immunization. Vaccinated women may breast-feed without fear of adverse effect to the newborn, and Rh-negative women may receive RhD immune globulin, if indicated, as well as the rubella vaccine.

To eradicate congenital rubella syndrome, it has been suggested that efforts should be increased to ensure that patients are either immune to rubella or vaccinated as part of routine medical and gynecologic care. For reproductive age women, recommendations have included determining rubella immunity or vaccinating women in family planning clinics, during any hospitalization, at the time of premarital serology testing, or at college entry examinations.

Recent reports of rubella outbreaks in hospitals have led to the recommendation to screen for rubella immunity and vaccinate susceptible hospital employees who may have contact with pregnant women (4, 5).

It is recommended that rubella vaccine not be given to pregnant women and that pregnancy be avoided for 90 days. Nevertheless, many rubella-susceptible pregnant women have received rubella vaccine within 3 months after the time of conception. As of late 1980, 101 of these women delivered at term (3). After vaccination with HPV-77 preparation, the virus has been isolated from the products of conception in about 20% of the cases. With the RA 27/3 vaccine, cases are fewer, but this virus appears to be isolated less frequently. Even though the virus may be isolated in the products of conception, none of these 101 infants had any anomalies consistent with the congenital rubella syndrome. Although the risk of teratogenicity from the vaccine virus is uncertain, the risk is considerably less than that of the wild virus and has been estimated by the Centers for Disease Control at 0–4%. The risk estimate was derived by the binomial distribution.

Side effects of the vaccine include arthralgias, but true arthritis occurred in less than 1%. In susceptible adult women, joint symptoms are more frequent and tend to be more severe than in children, but adults have not usually had to disrupt work. Other complaints such as pain or parethesias have been rare.

Besides pregnancy, contraindications to vaccination are febrile illnesses and immunosuppression. Precautions are necessary in rare individuals with neomycin allergy.

Genital Herpes Infection in Pregnancy

Herpes simplex virus may cause infection in the adult, the newborn, or on rare occasion, the fetus. In the adult, typical lesions of genital herpes consist of vesicles or ulcers, which are small, multiple, and painful. Usually the disease is self-limited, but in a small percent of cases (4–8%) (1) of primary genital herpes, more widespread infection including viral meningitis occurs. In the newborn infant, however, systemic, frequently lethal, disease is a serious and common problem.

EPIDEMIOLOGY

In adults, the herpes virus commonly causes infection of the mouth and lips and less commonly of the genital tract and skin. In the past, herpes simplex virus, type 1, was said to be responsible for infection of the mouth and of the skin above the waist, and type 2 virus was responsible for infection of the genitalia of the skin below the waist. The majority of infections still follow the pattern, but either type may cause infection at either site. In Seattle, 10% of first episode of genital herpes infections are caused by type 1 virus (1).

Adult genital herpes may present as primary infections (first episode) or as recurrent episodes. In addition, patients with prior antibody to HSV-1 may acquire genital infection with HSV-2. Because this infection has a shorter course than occurs with a true primary HSV-2 infection, Corey has referred to this condition as a nonprimary first episode genital herpes (1). There are general distinguishing features between true primary and recurrent genital herpes infection, as shown in Table 13.2.

Although there are no complete data on the national incidence of genital herpes, there is evidence at many clinics that its incidence is rising (1). The Centers for Disease Control also estimated recently that there had been a ninefold increase in private patient visits for genital herpes in the United States between 1966 and 1979 (2).

In surveys of adult females, herpes simplex

Table 13.2
Characteristics of True Primary and Recurrent Genital Herpes Infection

Features	True primary	Recurrent
Incubation period	2–10 days	
Prodrome		1–2 days
Fever	+	
Regional lymphade-nopathy	+	
Malaise	+	
Duration of genital symptoms (mean)	Approx. 15 days	Approx. 7 days
Duration of viral shedding (mean)	Approx. 12 days	Approx. 5 days
Number of lesions	Greater	Fewer

has been isolated from the genitalia of 0.02–4%. In high risk populations, such as women attending a venereal disease clinic, the rate is reported at the higher end of the range (1). Among pregnant women, recent surveys have found positive cultures in from 0.01 to 4% of *asymptomatic* women (3–6). Of all patients with positive cultures, those without symptoms have been reported to account for between approximately one-third and two-thirds (5–10). Pregnancy probably does not lead to any increase in frequency or in severity of genital herpes infections. Serologic surveys show that 30–90% of women have antibody to HSV-2, but it may be difficult to differentiate specific serum antibodies of type 2 from type 1 as there is extensive cross-reactivity (1).

Some have reported that maternal infection has adverse effects in early pregnancy, reporting a three-fold increase in abortion. Infants with neonatal herpes infections have a high rate of prematurity (7). Both abortion and prematurity were reported to be more common with primary maternal infection than with recurrent infection. Transplacental infection of the fetus resulting in congenital infection is a rare sequel to maternal infection. Only a few documented cases have been reported.

The major perinatal problem is neonatal herpes infections. Exact estimates of its frequency are subject to error, since up to 50% of infants with culture-proved, fatal disease may *not* show typical lesions on the skin or mucous membranes. Thus, the viral infection may not be recognized. In addition, viral laboratories have not been widely available, and recent treatment recommendations have probably decreased the incidence of neonatal disease. It is estimated that neonatal herpes occurs in 1 of every 5000 to 20,000 neonates in the United States (8).

Neonatal herpes is acquired perinatally from an infected, lower maternal genital tract, most commonly during vaginal delivery. Other cases have occurred in newborns delivered by cesarean birth performed a number of hours after labor has begun or after the membranes have ruptured. If genital herpes is present at term in the mother, the risk of neonatal herpes infection among infants delivering through the vagina is approximately 40–60% (9–10). Among infected infants, the risk of death or serious sequalae is about 50%. The risk of neonatal herpes is probably greater among infants delivered of women with clinically evident lesions, but neonatal disease clearly may occur in infants born vaginally of women with recurrent or with asymptomatic infection (7). Indeed, Whitley and co-workers reported in 1980 that 70% of mothers delivering HSV-infected newborns had asymptomatic genital infection. Maternal antibodies thus do not offer complete protection to the neonate.

DIAGNOSIS

The clinical diagnosis of genital herpes is based upon typical, painful crops of vesicles and ulcers in various stages of progression. With primary infection, there is apt to be regional lymphadenopathy, fever, and other more marked constitutional symptoms. The course of primary genital herpes usually lasts 2–3 weeks. Clinically detectable recurrences occur variably, but about 50% of patients will have recurrent disease within 6 months (11). Further, likelihood of recurrence depends of serotype of HSV. Reeves and co-workers noted a recurrence risk after first episode of 14% with HSV-1, but of 60% with HSV-2 genital herpes (11). Recurrences are more mild, with fewer lesions, fewer constitutional symptoms, and a shorter course (usually 7–10 days) (Table 13.2).

One-third to two-thirds of women with genital culture positive for HSV do not have typical clinically evident lesions. For screening procedures, cytological and culture techniques have been used. While HSV infection may be suggested by rather typical changes seen in Papanicolaou smear (intranuclear inclusions and multinucleated giant cells), the sensitivity of this test is only about 50% (i.e., about 50% false-negative). Other direct staining techniques such as indirect immunoperoxidase and direct immunofluorescence have been found to be about

20% more sensitive, but still should not be used as the sole screening test for pregnant patients at term or in labor (1). Development of monoclonal antibodies may lead to rapid, more sensitive and more specific staining techniques (1). At present, the best diagnostic test to rule out the presence of herpes virus infection is the viral culture. For clinical use, it is fortunate that this virus grows rapidly, with most positive cultures identifiable at 48–72 hr. The virus is also hearty and can be transported on ice, when necessary, for up to 72 hr without difficulty (1).

Neonatal herpes infection may be limited to the skin or may have systemic involvement, either with or without cutaneous involvement. Typically, clinical disease begins at the end of the 1st week of life. Since findings depend upon the organ system involved, the presentation may include: skin lesions, cough, cyanosis, tachypnea, dyspnea, jaundice, seizures, or disseminated intravascular coagulopathy. In infants at risk for, or suspected of having neonatal herpes, the only reliable diagnostic test is the viral culture. One cannot rely upon clinical exam or cytologic changes.

A few infants have been recognized with congenital (transplacental) herpes infection. Congenital infection has been manifest by typical cutaneous lesions apparent within 24–48 hr of life as fetal infection presumably occurs within a few days of birth. In other cases, there have been less specific clinical signs (microcephaly and spasticity) with serologic evidence of intrauterine infection. Transplacental infection presumably results from maternal viremia, which occurs only with primary maternal infection.

In the individual patient, serologic techniques have no practical utility because of cross-reactivity with antibodies. For the present, clinical management should be the same whether the maternal disease is primary or recurrent.

TREATMENT

For many years, clinical trials had reported the value of various therapies such as heterocyclic dyes and 2 deoxy-D-glucose, but these suggested agents did not hold up in more extensive trials.

Acyclovir

Within the past few years, the first effective antiviral chemotherapeutic agent for genital herpes has become available. Acyclovir (Zovirax) interferes selectively with viral thymidine kinase. Acyclovir is concentrated in HSV infected cells and is converted to the active derivative, acyclovir triphosphate. Acyclovir is not concentrated in uninfected cells. The active form of the drug is a competitive inhibitor of viral DNA polymerase and is a DNA chain terminator. Thus, its mechanism of action is inhibition or viral DNA synthesis, and it has a high margin of safety in view of its selectivity for HSV-infected cells.

The optimal approach to therapy with acyclovir is being actively investigated. As of this writing, the only approved uses of acyclovir in genital herpes are as (a) a 5% *ointment* in a polyethylene glycol base for primary episodes and (b) a powder for intravenous administration for *severe* primary herpes. A double-blind, placebo-controlled trial has shown that topical acyclovir led to significant shortening of mean duration of pain (6.2 versus 8.8 days), of mean viral shedding (4.1 versus 7.0 days), and of mean time to healing (10.6 versus 12.3 days). However, in women with recurrent infection, acyclovir did not facilitate healing, and topical acyclovir had no effect in preventing recurrences (12, 16).

This topical preparation was applied every 3 hr, 6 times daily, for 7 days to external lesions. The patient should use a glove or finger cot in order to avoid spread of infection to her fingers. Also, because the polyethylene glycol base is irritating, this topical preparation should not be applied in the vagina.

Topical acyclovir does not have FDA approval for use in pregnancy. Yet, because of its specificity for viral infected cells, the likelihood of an adverse effect on the fetus seems remote.

It is possible that topical acyclovir may have some value in recurrent episodes *if* the patient initiates treatment during the prodrome (13) or if a cream base is used. However, the presently available topical preparation should not be used in recurrent infections.

Intravenous acyclovir sodium (5 mg/kg every 8 hr for 5 days) has also been evaluated in a double-blind, placebo-controlled trial of 30 patients with primary genital herpes. In patients given the IV acyclovir, there was a significant reduction in median healing time (9 versus 15 days), duration of vesicles (2.5 versus 5 days), duration of symptoms (6.3 versus 8.8 days), and duration of viral shedding (2.0 versus 8.8 days) (14). Although there has been no direct comparison of the topical versus IV preparations, some authorities advise the use of the IV for those who have primary herpes which requires hospitalization (15).

Oral use of acyclovir has attracted much attention for both treatment and prevention. The oral preparation would offer the advantage of convenience and ease of administration. In a double-blind study of 48 adults with first episode genital herpes infection, Bryson and colleagues found that oral acyclovir (200 mg, 5 times/day for 10 days) significantly reduced duration of virus shedding (in women, 4.9 versus 14.7 days), time to healing (in females, 10 versus 16.2 days), occurrence of new lesions after 48 hr (in females, 0/16 versus 8/15), and duration and severity of symptomatology. No toxicity was seen, but recurrence rates were similar (15).

Use of oral acyclovir to prevent recurrences in patients with frequent episodes (approximately 1 per month) has also been evaluated recently. In double-blind, placebo-controlled trials, recent results have shown that oral acyclovir (either 200 mg or 400 mg b.i.d.) for 3 or 4 months significantly decreases recurrences (16, 17). Douglas and colleagues noted that in a 4-month trial 65% of patients taking acyclovir b.i.d. had no recurrences compared to only 6% of patients taking placebo (p < 0.001). After enrollment, patients taking oral acyclovir had the first clinical recurrence at a mean of 120 days. For patients taking placebo, the interval was 18 days (p < 0.001) (16). After the oral acyclovir was stopped, there was no influence on subsequent rate of recurrence (16).

Vaccination

Most recurrent HSV infections are caused by reactivation of an endogenous latent virus, which probably has been dormant in neural tissue. Individuals who have recurrent HSV infections usually have circulating antibody, often in high titers. Thus, antibody by itself does not prevent recurrences, and prevention or amelioration of recurrent HSV by vaccines has not been viewed with enthusiasm (18). Live virus vaccines are often preferred because they induce better immune response. However, some investigators have also hypothesized that HSV-2 may be oncogenic, further decreasing interest in a live HSV vaccine (18). Recently, however, work at the University of Washington has led to an immunogenic vaccine, which appears safe at least in short-term follow-up (19). Studies of its clinical efficacy are awaited. The vaccine uses α-glycoprotein units of the HSV-2 for antigenic stimulation and thus avoids concern of oncogenicity of the line virus vaccines. In 23 volunteers,

22 showed cell-mediated immune response, and most had humoral response. Mild local erythema, pain, or itching occurred in less than half the patients.

Supportive Treatment

Additional measures such as frequent sitzbaths, topical anesthetics, and treatment of secondary yeast infections are also of benefit in decreasing symptomatology.

PREVENTION OF NEONATAL HERPES INFECTION

Because of the severity of neonatal herpes infection and the lack of satisfactory chemo- or immunotherapy, the only present means of preventing neonatal infection is avoiding contact between the fetus and the infected maternal lower genital tract by means of cesarean section. Accordingly, recommendations are for delivery by cesarean section when there is clinical or culture evidence of active infection at the time of labor. In the original studies of Amstey and Monif (9) and Nahmias and colleagues (10), the risk of neonatal herpes increased markedly when cesarean section was performed after the membranes had been ruptured for 4 or more hours. Accordingly, it has been a widely held position that with membrane rupture of this duration or greater, there was no advantage in preventing neonatal herpes by performing a cesarean section (20). Yet, many of the cesarean sections carried out after 4 hr of membrane rupture may have been performed after many vaginal examinations, many hours of labor, and much longer intervals of membrane rupture. Accordingly, many have recently reconsidered the value of cesarean section to prevent neonatal herpes even when the interval of membrane rupture has been over 4 hr. Grossman and colleagues performed six cesarean sections in patients with ROM for 6 to 30 hr and found no cases of neonatal herpes (22), but these cases are too few in number to determine the correct management of this difficult situation. These recommendations should be applied to women with either primary or recurrent, clinical or subclinical, infection, although the risk of neonatal disease is undoubtedly not equal in all these situations. If at all possible, cytologic evidence of herpes infection should not be used to make such important decisions. Rather, presence of infection should be determined by cultures.

Accordingly, patients with previous history of

genital herpes or with genital herpes in a given pregnancy should be screened for recurrent herpes of the genital tract at term. In general, weekly cultures should be initiated at 35 or 36 weeks. If premature delivery is anticipated, then screening should be started earlier. For patients with recurrent herpes and a lesion in late pregnancy, repeat cultures may be taken every 3–4 days to determine when the culture becomes negative. If the last two cultures taken prior to birth have been negative and if there are no new lesions, then it is safe to assume that there is no active infection in the maternal genital tract. Accordingly, the patient may be treated normally (21–24).

If cultures taken in late pregnancy are positive, then the patient should be informed to contact the physician immediately upon beginning labor or upon rupturing her membranes. When labor seems likely in a patient with active herpes at term, a planned cesarean delivery is appropriate. However, it is not necessary to perform a cesarean section in all patients with active herpes in late pregnancy, since infections of the genital tract resolve before the onset of labor. Management can be individualized by the use of repeated cultures, repeated every 3–4 days when necessary.

Previous recommendations included use of amniocentesis to exclude transplacental herpes prior to performing a cesarean section in a mother with genital herpes (2). However, most experts no longer favor this step in the management as the risk of transplacental infection is low (probably lower than the risk of amniocentesis), and the amniotic fluid tests may be problematic. Block and Goodner noted a case in which amniocentesis at 38 weeks revealed "herpetic changes" upon cytologic examination of fetal cells, but 7 days later the viral culture was negative. An electively scheduled cesarean section was performed yielding an uninfected neonate (25). At Cornell Medical Center, Zervoudakis and colleagues reported that a woman who had a history of recurrent genital herpes was delivered by cesarean section because HSV was isolated from her cervix at term. Amniotic fluid, which was collected mainly to assess fetal maturity, was also cultured for HSV and was positive. The infant was unaffected and remained healthy at 18 months follow-up. Fetal immunoglobulin levels did not suggest infection (26). Despite these problems, some authors have suggested that amniocentesis may be offered to patients with primary herpes in pregnancy (22).

USE OF FETAL SCALP ELECTRODES

A few cases have been reported in which neonatal HSV infection may have been introduced or worsened because of use of a scalp electrode (27). In most cases (4 of 6), the mothers have had subclinical infection. Yet it is difficult to evaluate the relative importance of the electrode insertion in the ultimate course and outcome. If proper screening is carried out, the physician should know whether HSV is present in the cervix at the time of delivery, and if so, vaginal delivery should be avoided.

MANAGEMENT OF THE NEWBORN AT RISK FOR HERPES

Kibrick has recently provided reasonable guidelines (28). In the nursery, infection control measures include isolation of the newborn, gown and glove precautions, and double-bagging of contaminated materials. The newborn may be brought to the mother provided she observes supervised, thorough handwashing, is not in bed, and is wearing a clean gown.

Newborns of mothers with nongenital herpes do not require any special precautions during labor and delivery. However, after the mother has contact, then the newborn is considered suspect for herpes and is handled as above.

Suspected infants should be cultured for herpes virus and observed closely by examination. Kibrick suggests that infants at risk be considered for prophylactic use of ophthalmic idoxuridine or vidarabine (28). If the parents are reliable, it is not necessary to delay the infant's discharge. Rather the parents may be informed of signs and symptoms of possible neonatal infections and contacted regularly by telephone. The alternative is to keep the infant hospitalized through the first 10–12 days of life. This approach might be preferable in selected situations, such as poor parent compliance and long distances of travel.

MANAGEMENT OF THE INFECTED MOTHER DURING HOSPITALIZATION

Whether the delivery has been by the vaginal or abdominal routes or if antepartum admission is necessary, women with active genital herpes infections should be given a private room. Gown and glove precautions and vigorous handwashing are advised for persons having contact with the patient. Bed linens, perineal pads, hospital gowns, and other possible contaminated items should be placed in double plastic bags prior to disposal. Kibrick recommends that the infected mother may handle her infant, with the precautions cited above. The baby must be brought to her; the mother should not enter the nursery.

It is not known whether breast-feeding by a woman with active genital herpes poses any clear risk to the newborn.

Since women with nongenital herpes at delivery may also infect their newborn, many of the precautions advised for control of genital herpes are recommended in this situation. Accordingly, the following measures are in order: private room, gown and glove for contacts, and the proper disposal of linen and dressings. In addition, Kibrick advises topical applications of agents such as ethyl ether, povidone-iodine (betadine), or tincture of benzoin to hasten crusting of the lesions. Then, after the lesions have become encrusted, he permits the mother to handle and feed her infant, provided the precautions used for women with genital herpes are followed. In these cases, he also requires that the lesions be covered by a dressing or face mask.

Because herpes infection may result in serious untoward effects in newborns, it is essential to educate the mother fully regarding the reasoning behind these precautions.

HOSPITAL PERSONNEL WITH HERPATIC LESIONS ON EXPOSED BODY SURFACES

Nursery and labor and delivery personnel should not be permitted to handle newborns until their lesions are gone. Topical agents, such as ether benzoin, may be applied to hasten clearing. However, Kibrick notes

If a choice must be made between inadequate nursery coverage and using knowledgeable, trained personnel with dried (crusted) lesions the latter alternative is preferable. Careful handwashing and glove changes before handling each infant should be stressed. The lesions should not be crusted, but should be covered appropriately with a face mask or dressing.

Cytomegalovirus

Cytomegalovirus (CMV), a DNA virus of the herpes virus group, causes cytomegalic inclusion disease. Characteristic large cells with prominent intranuclear inclusion bodies have been identified with this disease since the early 20th century, but the virus was not isolated until 1956. Initially, CMV was considered to be rare

because only the classic clinically severe form of the disease was appreciated. Recent studies utilizing viral cultures have identified the frequent presence of "silent" CMV in which no clinical manifestations are present. CMV is now recognized as the most common cause of intrauterine infection (1, 2). It has been estimated that there are 50,000 infants born annually in the United States with congenital infection, and 5–10% of these children will develop neurologic sequelae.

Indeed, absence of detectable infection at birth may not be innocuous. The persistent and progressive nature of these inapparent congenital infections may result in CNS pathology and neurologic sequelae, which represent the major impact of CMV infection (31).

The teratogenic potential of CMV is unsettled. Although the virus can cause a reduction in the absolute number of cells in various organs, whether this is due to a direct effect on the cells or whether it is secondary to endothelial and vascular damage is not known. Malformations such as cataracts or congenital heart lesions are seldom seen with CMV. Thus, congenital CMV bears a closer resemblance to congenital toxoplasmosis, in which defects are secondary to destruction of tissue, than to congenital rubella.

EPIDEMIOLOGY

Approximately 50% of females in the United States and Europe are susceptible to CMV by the time they reach the reproductive age group, and the highest rate of seroconversion occurs between the ages of 15 and 35 (Table 13.3).

In a recent study from Alabama, Hunter and colleagues found 30–40% of pregnant women

Table 13.3
Prevalence of Cytomegalovirus Infection

	Usual rate (%)
Asymptomatic CMV infection of the cervix in pregnancy	4
Previous infection with CMV (seropositivity)	50–60
Maternal seroconversion in pregnancy	1–2.5
Congenital infection (transplacental acquisition)	0.2–2
Perinatal infection (acquisition) from vaginal secretions, milk, etc.)	3–5 (10–13 in infants with >30 days hospitalization)

were susceptible to CMV. Primary CMV infection, as evidenced by seroconversion, occurred in 1.6% of 8,000 pregnancies (4). CMV infection is more likely in lower socioeconomic groups. Although CMV infection is widespread, it produces serious illness only in fetuses, immunodeficient individuals, and patients receiving immunosuppressive therapy. Most adult infections are subclinical, and the remainder (approximately 10%) cause a mononucleosis-like illness.

CMV has developed a remarkably successful form of parasitizing humans. It is persistently excreted and is communicable for long periods of time. In addition, it does not interrupt the line of transmission by causing the infected host to die. Infants infected congenitally excrete CMV on an average of 4 yr. Those acquiring CMV at the time of birth excrete the virus for 2 hr. Many seropositive young adults shed CMV intermittently. Recurrent excretion of CMV in asymptomatic persons may be due to several possible mechanisms. Following primary infection, a low-grade chronic infection might be established in which viral excretion periodically reaches detectable levels. Reinfection could occur in immune persons due to antigenic and genetic disparity among CMV strains. Also, like herpes simplex virus, CMV may become latent during the primary infection and in later life be reactivated by various stimuli.

Asymptomatic CMV infection and excretion is common during pregnancy. The cervix is involved in 3–18%, urinary tract in 3–9%, breast milk in up to 27%, and the pharynx in 1–2%. The incidence of CMV infection is highest in low income, young, primiparous, lower educational status, and unmarried women. Longitudinal studies have demonstrated that the average incidence of cervical excretion of CMV in pregnancy increases from 1.5% in the first trimester to 13.5% near term. These asymptomatic infections occur mainly in seropositive women whose antibody status does not change in spite of viral shedding. Pregnancy itself may either increase a woman' susceptability to CMV infection or reactivate latent infection.

In addition to those fetuses infected by vertical transmission from mother, an additional 3–5% of live-born infants acquire CMV peripartum, presumably as a result of exposure to infected cervical secretions, ingestion of infected milk, or oral to oral contact with mother. In infants with prolonged hospital study (>30 days), perinatal acquisition of CMV has been reported as 13% (4). If a maternal genital CMV infection is present at the time of birth, 30–50% of the neonates will acquire the virus.

The infections transmitted in utero are the major concern, especially as they relate to infant development. Congenital infections may occur following either primary or recurrent maternal infection. The occurrence of a demonstrably high rate (3.4–6%) of congenital infection in infants born to previously immune mothers suggests that recurrent maternal CMV is an important cause of intrauterine transmission of CMV. In fact, the birth of an infant with congenital CMV infection does not ensure that a subsequent fetus will not become infected in utero. Congenital CMV has been reported in consecutive pregnancies, up to 3 yr apart. As previously noted, primary CMV infection may occur in pregnancy. The exact means by which pregnant women acquire primary CMV is not known. CMV is a sexually transmitted disease, and pregnant women may be infected by their sexual partners. It has not been established whether transmission of CMV to the fetus in mothers with documented humoral immunity is due to reactivation of endogenous latent CMV or reinfection with an antigenically different strain.

There are multiple potential sources of perinatal infection with CMV. Transplacental vertical transmission from mother to fetus has been confirmed. In addition, in utero infection may possibly be due to ascending infection across intact membranes from an infected cervix. The frequent presence of CMV in the cervix and birth canal is an obvious source for acquired neonatal CMV infection, similar to that seen with herpes simplex virus. Although CMV has been isolated in breast milk, no correlation between breast-feeding and CMV excretion in infants has been demonstrated. Another potential source of infection is sibling contact.

It is not clear whether the long-term prognosis for the fetus is different in primary or recurrent maternal CMV infection. In general, primary maternal infection is viewed as potentially more dangerous for the fetus, but not all fetuses of mothers with primary CMV infection became infected (5, 6). Hunter reported that 46% (17 of 37) of infants born to women with primary CMV infection were infected in utero. Only 2 of these 17 (11%) congenital infections were clinically detected in the nursery (4). Despite the high prevalence of CMV infection in pregnant women (documented by cervical excretion or viruria), infection in the mother is three to four times greater than that in neonates. Of more significance is the timing of infection in gestation. Monif et al have shown that the more severely affected infants are those who acquire CMV infection in the first or second trimester of pregnancy (6). Those born after third trimester maternal infection were normal at birth, but had positive cord sera for CMV IgM antibodies, suggestive of "silent" congenital CMV infection. Stern and Tucker have shown that 50% of infants whose mothers developed a primary infection during pregnancy were excreting cirrus after delivery (5). Of the eight women who had reactivation of CMV infection during pregnancy, none of their infants were excreting virus after delivery. Thus it appears that primary CMV infection is more important than reactivation of latent infection in pregnancy, and primary infection during the first two trimesters presents a greater risk for resulting in fetal infection than infection occurring in the third trimester.

The prognosis is poor for babies with clinically apparent disease at birth. CNS and perceptual disabilities usually result in severe mental retardation. The major site for this chronic morbidity is the brain and perceptual organs, with resultant seizures, spastic diplegia, optic atrophy, blindness, and sensorineural deafness. With recent emphasis shifting from the obviously diseased infant, the major focus of interest is on the prognosis of the 90–95% of congenitally infected neonates who appear normal at birth. These children may not develop normally, as significant neurologic sequelae may become apparent with time. Long-term longitudinal follow-up studies have documented progressive sensorineural hearing loss and apparently subtle brain damage resulting in lowered IQ and school-associated behavioral problems, which develop over several years following delivery of infants with subclinical CMV (2). The prevalance of CMV infection suggests that this agent may be a leading cause of deafness, a major contributor to school-related learning disabilities, and a significant public health problem (7).

DIAGNOSIS

Clinical Manifestations

Over 90% of maternal infections with CMV, primary or recurrent, are asymptomatic. Occasionally, CMV infection presents as a heterophile-negative mononucleosis syndrome with leukocytosis, with relative and absolute lymphocytosis, abnormal liver function tests, abrupt onset of spiking temperature, and constitutional symptoms such as malaise, myalgias, and chills. The mildness of the pharyngitis, minimal lymphadenopathy, and absence of hepatosplenomegaly and jaundice help to differentiate CMV from the infectious mononucleosis syndrome.

The spectrum of disease caused by CMV in the fetus and neonate is very broad. Of the congenitally infected infants, 90–95% are completely asymptomatic at birth. Clinically apparent disease ranges from isolated organ involvement to the classic multiorgan system disease. In the severely infected neonates, the clinical features include hepatosplenomegaly, jaundice, thrombocytopenia, purpura, microcephaly, deafness, chorioretinitis, optic atrophy, and cerebral calcifications. The cerebral calcifications of CMV are characteristically periventricular in the subependymal region. A characteristic tetrad of findings has been described in the infants who have survived fulminant clinically apparent CMV infection. These are: (a) mental retardation; (b) chorioretinitis; (c) cerebral calcifications; and (d) micro- or hydrocephaly.

Laboratory

Maternal Infection. Because maternal infection is almost always asymptomatic, the diagnosis is rarely suspected or confirmed in pregnancy. Even when clinical disease occurs, it is generally mild, and CMV is usually overlooked as a diagnostic possibility.

Several antibody tests are available for CMV. The complement fixation (CF) method is no longer preferred because of considerable cross-reactivity with other herpes viruses. Indirect hemagglutination (IHA), enzyme-linked immunosorbent assay (ELISA), indirect fluorescent antibody, and neutralization tests are available for epidemiologi. studies. Since approximately 50% of adults have antibody, a single positive test does not necessarily indicate recent or current infection. Demonstration of seroconversion is the best documentation that a primary infection has occurred. If infection has occurred within the previous 60 days, IgM-specific antibody can be detected in the serum.

The best way to establish the presence of CMV infection is by isolating the virus. Virus isolation does not differentiate primary infection from recurrent. On the other hand, diagnosis of asymptomatic recurrent CMV is dependent on viral isolation from urine or cervix, because no change in antibody levels occurs in normal hosts with recurrent infection. CMV from swabs or urine may require 2–6 weeks before cytopathic effects of the virus are seen in tissue culture.

Infections in Neonates. The small percentage of clinically apparent infections in neonates is similar in presentation to other congenital infections, such as toxoplasmosis, rubella, syphilis, and herpes. The characteristic periventricular calcifications may be helpful in clinically differentiating congenital CMV infection from these other infections, but laboratory confirmation is necessary to document CMV infection. While serology can be used as an aid in diagnosis of congenital CMV infection, virus isolation is more sensitive and direct. As in adults, the newer methods have replaced the CF test.

The great majority of neonates with congenital CMV have antibody to CMV when tested with the newer methods. Approximately 80% of congenitally infected infants have IgM-specific antibody in their serum during the first few months of life. This test is rather sophisticated and available from only a few medical research laboratories.

Virus isolation is the best method available for documenting newborn CMV infection. Specimens can be taken from the urine, nasopharynx, conjunctiva, and spinal fluid.

Characteristic cytomegalic inclusions may be seen in tissues collected at autopsy or by biopsy, for example, of the kidney.

TREATMENT

There is no known treatment of CMV infection. In mothers with the infectious mononucleosis-like illness, treatment is symptomatic. No satisfactory therapy is available for the treatment of congenital CMV infection. Attempts have been made at using antiviral agents such as adenosine arabonaside (Ara-A) and cytosine arabonaside (Ara-C) for neonates with severe, clinical infection, but these drugs are quite toxic. Further, although they temporarily suppress the excretion of CMV, virus shedding resumes when the drugs are stopped. Because of their toxicity, these antiviral agents are not used in asymptomatic CMV infection.

The clinician is faced with a dilemma when dealing with maternal CMV. The overwhelming majority of maternal infections are undiagnosable, and serologic screening programs for maternal CMV infection are very limited. Thus counseling patients about CMV is practically impossible. If a primary CMV infection is documented in the first 20 weeks of pregnancy (for example, after presentation as a heterophile-negative mononucleosis syndrome), a therapeutic termination of pregnancy should be considered. Counseling a mother who has already given birth to an infected infant is even a bigger problem. In such a situation, the incidence of recurrence is unknown, and it is not clear whether subsequent congenital infections have the same prognostic significance as the initial episode.

The development of a CMV vaccine has been suggested as a means of preventing congenital CMV infection, with its associated morbidity and mortality. However, the fact that CMV persists in the host even in the presence of high levels of specific antibody and the demonstration that existing maternal antibody does not invariably protect against congenital infection suggests that such an approach is unlikely to be successful. Other methods of prevention and control will probably be required.

Because large quantities of CMV are excreted by infected neonates, it has been suggested that pregnant pediatric health care workers might be at high risk to develop CMV infection. However, Dworsky and co-workers recently reported that the annual primary CMV infection rate (as determined by seroconversion) was no more common among pediatric house staff (2.7%) and pediatric nursing staff (3.3%) than it was among young women in the community (2.5% during pregnancy and 5.5% between pregnancy) (8). The higher than expected rate of conversion between pregnancies suggested that exposure to young infants by family or other social exposure may be the most important factor in horizontal transmission. Thus these authors conclude that standard infection control measures for handling potentially contaminated material in pediatric units would seem to provide sufficient protection from CMV infection. Further, other isolation measures in infants known to have CMV infection would be "useless or even dangerous."

Hepatitis

Acute viral hepatitis is a systemic infection predominately affecting the liver. Distinct hepatotropic viral agents cause hepatitis types A, B, and non-A/non-B (termed HA, HB and NANB, respectively). Laboratory diagnosis can be made by testing immunologic responses to the viral agents of HA and HB, whereas NANB is established only be exclusion. Synonyms for hepatitis A include infectious hepatitis and short incubation hepatitis. Hepatitis B has been referred to as serum hepatitis, long incubation hepatitis, hepatitis B surface antigen (HBsAg)-positive, or Australia antigen-positive hepatitis. Other transmissible agents causing secondary hepatitis include cytomegalovirus, Epstein-Barr, varicella zoster, coxsackle B, herpes simplex, and rubella viruses. Since the major impact of hepatitis on the fetus and neonate relates to hepatitis B, the major emphasis of this discussion will be on the epidemiology, mode of transmission, and clinical aspects of hepatitis B.

Maternal infection during pregnancy with the hepatitis B virus is increasingly recognized as a threat to the fetus and/or neonate. In addition, it is apparent that clinically apparent icteric hepatitis is only a part of the disease spectrum and that "silent" infections (carrier state) may result in chronic and progressive disease in the mother and her offspring.

EPIDEMIOLOGY

The nomenclature of hepatitis antigens and antibodies is summarized in Table 13.4. Hepatitis B infection is related to the presence of three morphologically distinct viral like particles as seen by electron microscopic studies (1, 2, 3). The 42 nm HB virus (or Dane particles) is a DNA virus. A 27-nm core contains the double stranded DNA and is completely enveloped by the surface antigen (HBsAg). Excessive amounts of DNA-free HBsAg are synthesized by the liver cells of infected individuals and circulate freely in the serum as 20-nm spheres and tubules. It is now possible to isolate these various particles and produce antibodies to the antigens present. The HBsAg which is present on the tubular and spherical particles and on the surface of the Dane particle, can be measured and is specific for hepatitis B; the corresponding antibody is hepatitis B surface antibody (anti-HBs). The core of the Dane particle contains the hepatitis B core antigen (HBcAg); its specific antibody is anti-HBc.

An additional antigen antibody system, the e system has been described in HBV infection (4, 5, 6). The antigen is distinct from all known antigenic determinants of HBsAg and HBcAg but appears to be associated with the intact virus (Dane particle and high serum levels of hepatitis B viral-specific DNA-polymerase activity). The e antigen appears early in almost all patients during the acute phase of hepatitis B infection and may persist in patients in whom the infection progresses to chronic active hepatitis. Most importantly, several important prognostic and epidemiologic observations have been made with the e system. Persistent carriers of HBsAg who are e antigen-positive have a greater chance of developing chronic active hepatitis. Secondly, it has been demonstrated that HBsAg-positive blood that lacked e antigen but contained anti-e antibody did not cause posttransfusion hepatitis, whereas e antigen-positive blood carried a significant risk for development of posttransfusion hepatitis B. The third finding relates to pregnancy and vertical transmission of hepatitis

Table 13.4
Nomenclature of Hepatitis Antigens and Antibodies

Hepatitis type	Description	Antigen	Antibody	Comments
B	Dane particle; 42-nm size represents intact virus (surface and core)	1. Hepatitis B surface antigen (HBsAg)	Anti-HBs	DNA-type virus
		2. Hepatitis B core antigen (HBcAg)	Anti-HBc	
	Core of Dane particle; 27-nm size	HBcAg core antigen (HBcAg)	Anti-HBc	Contains DNA-polymerase in hepatocytes but not serum
	Spherical and filamentous forms which are 22-nm size have same antigen properties as surface of Dane particle.	HBsAg	Anti-HBs	HBsAg denotes hepatitis B infection; anti-HBs is probably protective antibody
A	Spherical virus particle; 27-nm size	Hepatitis A antigen (HAAg)	Anti-HA	RNA virus

B from mother to offspring. Mothers with e antigen-positive blood uniformly transmitted HBsAg to their children, while those with HBsAg-positive, e antigen-negative blood appeared not to transmit HBsAg to their offspring (7). Thus, it seems likely that the presence of e antigen identifies the group which is highly infectious and at greater risk of transmitting hepatitis B virus.

Recently, the properties of hepatitis A virus (HAV) have become better understood. The HA virus is a 27-nm RNA virus and may be classified as an enterovirus (8). It commonly produces acute hepatitis but is usually a mild self-limited disease without any chronic sequelae. The presence of IgM anti-HA in the serum suggests current or recent infection(9). IgG anti-HA indicates infection occurring in the past and confers immunity to hepatitis A. Mild and clinically unrecognized infections with HA virus commonly occur in childhood and account for the high incidence of IgG anti-HA in adult populations, a finding reflected in the adequate antibodies present in normal immune serum globulin (ISG).

The ability to identify the antigens and their antibody responses in both hepatitis A and B has led to the belief that all clinical cases of acute hepatitis infection are not due to these agents. As a result, the concept of non-A, non-B viral hepatitis has been developed (10, 11). Recent studies have documented that 90% of posttransfusion hepatitis is related to non-A, non-B virus. Approximately 20% of sporadic cases of acute hepatitis are due to a non-A, non-B agent. This form of hepatitis is a particular problem in dialysis and renal transplantation units. The incubation period of non-A, non-B hepatitis is similar to hepatitis B, and a 10–30% incidence of chronic hepatitis occurs following infection with this agent(s).

The comparative clinical and epidemiologic features of hepatitis A and B are shown in Table 13.5. It has become clear that distinction between hepatitis A and B cannot be made solely on epidemiologic and clinical grounds. Detection of serum HBsAg has become the important diagnostic tool in distinguishing between the two. HBsAg is present in approximately 1 per 1000 adults in the United States and Europe (12). However, it is present in 2–25% of adults in tropical areas and Southeast Asia (3).

Epidemiological studies have demonstrated an increasing incidence of hepatitis B in the general population and in hospitalized patients with acute hepatitis. Hepatitis B is often a more

Table 13.5
Clinical and Epidemiologic Features of Acute Viral Hepatitis

	Hepatitis A	Hepatitis B
Epidemiologic features:		
Onset	Acute	Acute and insidious
Age group	Children and adults	All ages
Season	Fall and winter	All year
Parenteral transmission	Rare	Common
Nonparenteral transmission	Common	Common
Incubation period	15–45 days	45–160 days
Clinical Features:		
Prodrome	Common	Common
Severity	Mild	Mild to severe
Prognosis	Benign	More severe in older age group
Chronic hepatitis	No	Occasionally
Prophylaxis with conventional gamma globulin (ISG)	Partial protection	Low rate of protection unless is recent lot with high levels of anti-HBs
Hepatitis B immune globulin (HBIG)		Probably protective
Abnormal SGOT	Transient, 1–3 weeks	Usually more prolonged, 1–8 months.
Immunity		
Previous infection	Protects	Protects

severe infection than hepatitis A. Hepatitis B virus infection is transmitted predominantly by sexual contact, parenteral exposures, and vertical transmission from mother to newborn during the birth process (13). HBsAg has been identified in urine, feces, seminal fluid, saliva, intestinal fluid, and gastric juice. Asymptomatic persistence of HBsAg, without abnormalities of liver function tests, is the commonest form of hepatitis B virus infection. Asymptomatic carriers of hepatitis B are estimated to number about 900,000 in the United States and 150 million worldwide are believed to serve as an epidemiologic reservoir for hepatitis B infection (13). During childbearing age, 70% of women in the United States are susceptible to hepatitis B. Approximately two cases of overt hepatitis and one chronic carrier of hepatitis B are encountered per 1000 pregnant women in the general United States population. This risk for infection varies greatly depending on occupation, socioeconomic status, history of drug abuse, or geographic factors.

A chronic carrier state and chronic liver disease of more than 6 months duration are recognized only for infection with hepatitis B or non-A, non-B hepatitis. Nearly 10% of acute hepatitis B patients have unresolved hepatitis, frequently persisting for years, and often progressing to a form of chronic hepatitis. A large percentage of patients with primary hepatocellular carcinoma is positive for HBsAg (14). The hepatitis B virus is suspected to be oncogenic, and recently the integration of viral DNA with cellular DNA of human hepatocellular carcinoma has been demonstrated.

Hepatitis A virus is excreted in large quantities in stool immediately prior to the onset of clinical symptoms. This accounts for the predominant spread by oral-fecal route of transmission.

Maternal-infant transmission can occur via four routes. These include: (a) transplacental; (b) intrapartum; (c) postpartum; and in breast milk or colostrum (15, 16). Recent investigations have demonstrated several important epidemiologic and clinical aspects of hepatitis B infection in the neonate (15–17). Approximately 75% of newborns of mothers with acute hepatitis B during the third trimester of pregnancy or during the first 2 months postpartum will become HBsAg-positive. Biochemical and histologic abnormalities often are present but are usually mild. Persistence of HBsAg has been associated with chronic hepatitis and cirrhosis. The mode

of transmission is considered to be oral contamination of the neonate during delivery with maternal blood and/or feces. When maternal hepatitis occurs in early pregnancy HBsAg is detected much less often in the neonate (14).

The frequency of transmission is also relatively low when the mother is an asymptomatic carrier of HBsAg. In the United States and other Western industrialized countries, hepatitis is documented in approximately 10% of neonates born to mothers who are chronic carriers of HBsAg. In areas of the world (Taiwan and Japan) where maternal asymptomatic carriers are more common, higher rates of neonatal transmission occur (17, 18).

Thus, in Asia 30–40% of chronic carriers transmit HBV to their newborn infants (19). Schweitzer and associates in the United States reported that only 1 of 21 infants born to HBsAg-positive mothers become HBsAg-positive themselves (16). Studies form Denmark (20) and Greece (21) have confirmed this low risk of transmission for Western societies. However, in Taiwan, Stevens and colleagues (17) demonstrated that 63 infants born to 158 HBsAg carrier mothers were HBsAg-positive. Okada et al provided similar high rates of transmission in their study of Japanese HBsAg carriers (18).

Several studies have documented that the crucial determinant of vertical transmission from mother to newborn is the presence of e antigen (7, 17, 22, 23). HBeAg-positive mothers have high levels of virus and are more likely to transmit it to their offspring. Lee and co-workers reported that 26 of the 37 infants (70.3%) born to HBeAg-positive mothers were HBsAg-positive by 5 months of age (23). Beasley et al noted that all the infants who were chronic HBsAg carriers were born to HBeAg-positive mothers (24). In addition, nearly all babies born to HBeAg-positive mothers became infected with HBV during the 1st year of life, and 85% became chronic HBsAg carriers.

In a well-nourished normal population, mortality from hepatitis is low and no greater in pregnant than nonpregnant individuals (12). Where malnutrition is a problem, the mortality is much higher but still is similar in pregnant and nonpregnant women. The incidence of spontaneous abortion during the first trimester in patients with acute viral hepatitis has been reported to be increased. Similarly, when viral hepatitis occurs during the third trimester there is a reported increased incidence of preterm labor (15). However, the incidence of spontaneous abortion and preterm delivery is probably no higher with hepatitis than with other febrile illnesses. Although transplacental passage of hepatitis virus has been established, teratogenic damage has never been demonstrated for hepatitis B or A (3).

CLINICAL MANIFESTATIONS

The incubation period for hepatitis A is usually 15–45 days and that of hepatitis B is 45–160 days. Fever, headache, and abdominal pain may be the initial symptoms. In several days the fever subsides, the urine becomes dark, and jaundice is present. The liver is usually enlarged and tender. As the jaundice clears, the patient feels better, and recovery rapidly occurs. However, about 10% of patients with hepatitis B develop chronic disease; 7% progress to chronic persistent hepatitis, and 3% develop chronic active hepatitis. Rare cases of acute fulminant fatal hepatitis occur; these patients usually present in hepatic coma. The combination of a rapidly shrinking liver, rapidly rising bilirubin, and prolongation of the prothrombin time with clinical signs of encephalopathy and ascites should suggest impending hepatic failure in any patient with acute hepatitis. The mortality rate is greater than 80% in fulminant hepatitis.

In the neonate the most frequent presentation of hepatitis B infection is asymptomatic chronic hepatitis with histologic evidence of unresolved hepatitis. (15). Clinical illness is relatively infrequent with congenital hepatitis infection. About 10% of newborns with asymptomatic disease become icteric at 3–4 months of age.

DIAGNOSIS

Specific diagnosis of hepatitis depends upon laboratory confirmation. A laboratory guide to the differential diagnosis of viral hepatitis is provided in Table 13.6. Hepatitis B surface antigen is the primary diagnostic tool for differentiating hepatitis A from hepatitis B. The diagnosis of acute hepatitis A relies on the use of IgM specific anti-HAV. Non-A, non-B hepatitis is diagnosed by excluding hepatitis A and hepatitis B. HBsAg is present in the blood 30–50 days after exposure and 7–21 days before the onset of jaundice. The antigen may disappear with the onset of jaundice, or it may persist for many weeks. Chronic HBsAg carriers occur in 1% of patients in the United States. The SGPT levels rise about 50 days after exposure and are increased at the time jaundice appears. The elevated SGPT levels persist for 30–60 days.

Hepatitis Be antigen appears early in the disease and persists days to weeks and, in some cases, indefinitely. When HBeAg is present the patient is likely to be infectious. When anti-HBe antibody is present, the patient is much less likely to be infectious.

Infected newborns can be diagnosed by demonstrating the presence of HBsAg in the blood. These infants have mild to moderate elevations of the serum transaminase levels. Liver biopsy of infectious children may show unresolved hepatitis.

TREATMENT

Most pregnancies complicated by acute viral hepatitis can be managed on an outpatient basis.

Table 13.6
Practical Laboratory Guide for the Differential Diagnosis of Viral Hepatitis

Clinical intepretation	IgM Anti-HA	HBsAg	HBeAg	Anti-HBe	Anti-HBc	Anti-HBs
Acute HA	+	–	–	–	–	–
Incubation period or early acute HB	–	+	+	–	–	–
Acute HB	–	+	+	–	+	–
Fulminant HB	–	+	–	–	+	+/–
Convalescence from acute HB	–	–	–	+	+	+/–
Chronic HB	–	–	–	+	+	+/–
Persistent HB carrier state	–	+	–	+	+	–
Past infection with HB virus	–	–	–	–	+	+
Infection with HB virus without detectable (excess) HBsAg	–	–	–	–	+	–
Immunization without infection	–	–	–	–	–	+
Non-A/non-B hepatitis by exclusion of markers for HA and HB	–	–	–	–	–	–

No specific treatment exists for hepatitis. Increased bedrest and a high-protein, low-fat diet is recommended (12). Indications for hospitalization in patients with viral hepatitis include severe anemia, diabetes, intractable nausea and vomiting, a prolonged prothrombin time, low serum albumin level, and a serum bilirubin greater than 15 mg/100 ml (12).

Prevention is the best management for the child. No treatment is recommended for the asymptomatic carrier neonate. In the rare symptomatic neonatal hepatitis case supportive care is all that is required.

PREVENTION

Pregnant women and children with household or other short-duration exposure to hepatitis A infection should be given immune serum globulin (ISG) in a dose of 0.02–0.05 ml/kg to modify the disease. For prolonged exposure, the dose should be 0.06–0.14 ml/kg.

The risk of acquiring hepatitis B is greatest for those exposed to hepatitis patients or blood containing HBsAg and especially HBeAg; examples included household contact, hospital exposures and inoculation with contaminated needles. Women with definite exposure to hepatitis B virus should be given hepatitis B immune globulin (HBIG). This is given in a dose of 0.05–0.07 ml/kg as soon as possible within a 7-day period after exposure, with a second, identical dose given 30 days after the first.

Children born to women who have acute hepatitis B during pregnancy or who are HBeAg-positive at term should be given HBIG the day of birth in a single dose of 0.5 ml, and this is repeated twice at 3 months and 6 months. Preliminary studies indicate that this approach may prevent the development of infection in some children. Beasely and co-workers reported that although the 3-dose regimen of HBIG only reduced the HBV infection rate from 94.3 to 75%, it decreased the chronic carrier rate in newborns to 22.5% compared to 91.4% in the placebo group (24). In an attempt to further reduce the chronic HBsAg carrier state beyond the 75% prevention obtained with HBIG, the hepatitis B vaccine has been used in clinical trials in neonates born to e antigen-positive mothers. The hepatitis B vaccine (Heptavax-B) has been demonstrated to produce an appropriate immune response in neonates as well as children and infants (25). Currently a combined approach to prophylaxis is being investigated. This approach includes HBIG at birth to provide immediate passive immunization while the newborn develops an antibody response to the hepatitis B vaccine which provides long-term protection against repeated exposure to the chronic maternal carrier of HBV.

PRECAUTIONS INTRAPARTUM AT DELIVERY, AND POSTPARTUM

Patients with acute HAV excrete the virus in their stool. Enteric precautions should be instituted, but a private room and isolation are not necessary (26). For patients who have HBsAg-positive blood, precautions should be employed (26). Dressings and linen soiled with amniotic fluid, lochia, or wound exudates must be handled as contaminated material.

During delivery of HBsAg-positive (especially HBeAg-positive) mothers, gloves should be worn and masks and glasses or goggles worn to keep infectious fluids away from the mouth, nose, and eyes. Needless to say, precautions should be taken with needles and syringes. The neonate is rarely infectious during the initial few days after delivery and does not require isolation. Oxman et al have suggested that breast-feeding may be allowed by the HBsAg-positive mother (27). However, if there are bleeding fissures around the nipple, nursing should be discontinued.

Varicella-Zoster Infection

Varicella-zoster (V-Z) virus is a member of the herpes virus group. Similar to other members of the herpes group, V-Z is a DNAa virus and exhibits viral latency (1). Initial (primary) infection with V-Z virus results in varicella (chickenpox). This common childhood disease is usually marked by typical skin lesions, which progress from macules and papules to vesicles that occur in successive crops and evolve into pustules which form crusts and scabs (2). A highly contagious disorder, it is acquired by most persons in the United States prior to reproductive age and is generally self-limited. Among adults who contract the disease, constitutional and pulmonary symptoms may be more severe. Zoster (shingles) is the result of reactivation of the latent virus. It generally occurs in the older adult population or immunocompromised patients. Characteristically zoster presents as painful vesicular lesions which occur in a pattern of distribution that follows segmental dermatomes.

This discussion will be limited to the effects of V-Z virus in pregnancy and the management and prevention of V-Z infections during the perinatal period. Two major problems exist when V-Z infection occurs in pregnancy. First, the infection itself poses a risk for significant morbidity and mortality for mother and neonate. Secondly, V-Z virus has a teratogenic effect, and infection early in pregnancy may result in congenital anomalies.

EPIDEMIOLOGY

In 1982, over 167,000 cases of chickenpox were reported in the United States (3), and this disease remains second only to gonorrhea as the most frequently reported infectious disease in the United States (3). Because of extensive underreporting, it has been estimated that 2–3 million cases of chickenpox occur annually in the United States (4, 5). However, because V-Z is endemic in the United States and extremely contagious, over 90% of the population have been infected before they reach adulthood (4). Consequently, the occurrence of chickenpox among women of childbearing age and thus in pregnancy is uncommon. In the Collaborative Perinatal Research Study prospective analysis of 30,059 pregnancies, there were 20 V-Z infections diagnosed of which 14 were confirmed; thus, at a minimum there were 5 V-Z cases/10,000 pregnancies (6). A lower attack rate of 1 case/10,000 pregnancies was noted by Siegel and Fuerst in New York City (7).

CLINICAL PRESENTATION

The incubation period of varicella ranges from 10 to 20 days but usually is 13–17 days. In children fever and rash occur simultaneously, while in adults fever and generalized malaise precede the rash by several days (8). Characteristically, the rash begins on the face and scalp and spreads to the trunk. The extremities tend to be minimally involved. Skin lesions begin as macules which progress to vesicular stage followed by pustules, crusts, and scabs). Itching is common and a prominent feature of the disease. For 2–5 days new crops of lesions occur, and the various stages (i.e., vasicles, pustules, scabs) are present simultaneously.

The most common complications of chickenpox is secondary bacterial infection of the skin lesions (2). Rarely, encephalitis, meningitis, myocarditis, glomerulonephritis, and arthritis occur. The most serious complication of chicken-

pox is varicella pneumonia. It occurs most often in adults and is associated with a significant mortality risk.

VARICELLA IN THE MOTHER

Varicella is an unusual infection among adults and probably occurs with no greater frequency among pregnant women. In the past pregnant women were believed to be at greater risk to develop severe or fatal varicella than nonpregnant adults. However, the current consensus holds that while adults are at increased risk to develop varicella pneumonia, this risk is no greater among pregnant women (4, 9, 10). Recently, Young and Gershon, in a review of the literature on varicella pneumonia in pregnancy, reported that among 77 cases of chickenpox in pregnant women, 22 (29%) developed varicella pneumonia (2). All 10 deaths occurred in the pneumonia group for a pneumonia mortality rate of 45% (overall mortality rate for varicella was 13%). Thus, it seems clear that uncomplicated chickenpox poses no severe risk to the pregnant women. While pneumonia (in the past) was associated with a significant mortality rate, pneumonia is an uncommon complication, and our current ability to manage severe respiratory distress and failure is much enhanced. In fact, over the past decade no cases of mortality with varicella during pregnancy have been reported.

The major point for the clinician is to maintain a high index of suspicion that pneumonia may complicate varicella in pregnant women. Pulmonary symptoms begin on the 2nd–6th day after appearance of the rash and usually consist of a mild nonproductive cough. If the disease is more severe, there may be additional symptoms of pleuritic chest pain, hemoptysis, dyspnea, and frank cyanosis. Physical examination reveals fever, rales, and wheezes. The chest x-ray characteristically reveals a diffuse nodular or miliary pattern, especially in the perihilar regions. In the rare event of varicella in pregnancy, the patient should be warned to contact the physician *immediately* if even mild pulmonary symptoms develop. Hospitalization with full respiratory support should then be made available.

EFFECTS OF VARICELLA IN EARLY PREGNANCY

Congenital anomalies due to varicella in early pregnancy were not recognized until LaForet and Lynch (in 1947) reported the birth of an infant, exposed to V-Z virus during the first trimester, who had limb hypoplasia, cicatrical skin lesions, atrophic digits, bilateral cortical atrophy, severe psychomotor retardation, and growth retardation (11). It is now appreciated that maternal varicella infection in the first trimester of pregnancy can produce a congenital varicella syndrome, which consists of cutaneous scars, limb hypoplasia, rudimentary digits, ocular abnormalities (optic atrophy, microopthalmia, cataracts), cerebral cortical atrophy, mental retardation, and growth retardation. Because both gestational varicella and the reported cases of varicella congenital syndrome are uncommon, the risk of a fetus developing congenital anomalies if the mother acquired chickenpox during the first trimester has not been quantitated. In general, it is believed the risk is small (1, 2, 4).

Although the risk of the congenital varicella syndrome is small, a number of authorities have recommended administration of varicella immune globulin (also called zoster immunoglobulin, ZIG) to pregnant women with a negative history of varicella as soon as possible but within 3 days of exposure, as this may protect the fetus during the viremia. Once the mother has the rash, there would be no reason to administer the ZIG, as viremia would have already occurred. ZIG is available through the American Red Cross at regional distribution centers. Recently, varicella zoster immune globulin (VZIG) has become available. VZIG is prepared from donors with high antibody titers to V-Z virus and will replace the use of ZIG.

VARICELLA IN THE NEWBORN

Acquisition of maternal antibody usually protects the fetus. However, if an infant is born after the maternal viremia but before the mother has developed an antibody response, then the fetus is at high risk for life-threatening, neonatal varicella infection. Meyers noted that infants at risk are those whose mothers contract varicella within 5 days of birth or within the first 5 days after delivery (12). Congenital varicella infection has been reported in 17% of term infants born to mothers with varicella within 4–5 days of delivery, and the case fatality was 31% (4/13). Infants born 5 or more days after maternal illness onset develop either mild varicella or no infection at all.

Both ZIG and VZIG have been shown to modify or prevent varicella in normal children, and Brunell has recommended their use in preventing severe neonatal varicella (10). Thus, infants at risk (born 1 day before or 4 days after the

onset of maternal varicella) should receive ZIG or VZIG as passive immunization. The dose is 1.25 ml.

Recently, Weibel et al reported excellent results with a live attenuated varicella vaccine (13). There was a 94% seroconversion rate, and the vaccine was 100% efficacious in preventing varicella. In the placebo-control group 39/446 childen developed varicella. Further studies are awaited, and if they confirm these findings, the vaccine given to young children could well eliminate varicella as a source of morbidity and/or mortality to pregnant women and their offspring.

EFFECT OF ZOSTER ON PREGNANCY

Herpes zoster is caused by the same virus as is varicella. It occurs very rarely in pregnancy. Because it is reactivation of latent V-Z virus and maternal antibodies are present in normal, healthy women, zoster poses no threat to the fetus or neonate.

Measles (Rubeola)

Rubeola is an acute illness which most commonly occurs in childhood. It is the most communicable of the childhood exanthems (1). Rubeola is characterized by fever, coryza, conjunctivitis, cough, and a generalized maculopapular rash that usually appears 1–2 days after the pathognomonic Koplik's spots in the oral cavity. The rubeola virus is a paramyxovirus which contains RNA as its nuclear protein.

EPIDEMIOLOGY

The virus is spread chiefly by droplets expectorated by an infected person and gains access to susceptible people via the nose, oropharynx, and conjunctival mucosa. The incubation time is between 10 and 14 days. Measles is most communicable during the prodrome and cattarrhal stages of the infection. Approximately three-fourths of exposed susceptible contacts acquire rubeola (1).

Prior to the availability of live measles vaccines, epidemics of measles occurred at intervals of 2–3 yr in the United States. The use of attenuated measles vaccine since 1963 has had a major impact on the epidemiology of this disease. In the United States there has been a decline in reported cases from 480,000 in 1962 to 22,000 in 1968. However, a cutback in the vaccination program led to a reversal of this trend, and in 1971, 75,000 cases were reported.

With reinstitution of the vaccination program in 1972 the trend turned downward again. In 1982, the incidence of measles reached an all time low with only 1,714 cases reported (0.7/ 100,000 population) (2). It appears that virtual elimination of measles in the United States is an obtainable goal in the near future.

Measles occurs less frequently during pregnancy than chickenpox or mumps. Prior to the introduction of the measles vaccine, there were 0.4–0.6 cases of measles per 10,000 pregnancies (3, 4). This figure is probably even lower since the measles vaccine was introduced.

CLINICAL MANIFESTATIONS

The prodrome of fever and malaise begins 10 to 11 days postexposure and is followed within 24 hr by coryza, sneezing, conjunctivitis, and cough. This cattarrhal phase is exacerbated over the next several days, and a marked conjunctivitis and photophobia occur. The pathognomonic Koplik's spots appear at the end of the prodrome. These are tiny, granular, slightly raised white lesions surrounded by a halo of erythema which is located on the lateral buccal mucosa. The rash appears 12–14 days after exposure. It begins on the head and neck, especially postauricular, and subsequently the maculopapular rash spread to the trunk, upper extremities, and finally the lower extremities (5).

The respiratory tract is the most frequent site for complications of measles. Otitis media and croup are frequent occurrences, but bacterial pneumonia is the complication which most frequently is associated with mortality. The most common bacterial organisms involved in rubeola pneumonia are *Streptococcus pneumoniae, Haemophilus influenzae, Staphylococcus aureus*, and *Streptococcus pyogenes* (5). Encephalitis, a less common but serious complication, is estimated to occur with a frequency of 1 per 1000 cases of measles. LaBoccetta and Tornay noted that death occurs in about 11% of encephalitis cases (6). Other complications of measles include thrombocytopenic purpura, myocarditis, and subacute sclerosing panencephalitis, which is a progressive neurologic disease associated with chronic rubeola infection of the central nervous system.

MATERNAL EFFECTS OF MEASLES

It is unclear whether pregnant women with measles are at greater risk for serious complications and death than nonpregnant adults. Several studies of large measles epidemics have reported an increased mortality among pregnant women. The deaths were usually related to pneumonia (7). More recent studies in the United States and Australia have noted that measles in pregnant women is only rarely associated with pneumonia or other complications (8).

FETAL EFFECTS OF MEASLES

Young and Gershon (5) and Sever and colleagues (8) have summarized the results of reports in the literature concerning measles in pregnancy as suggesting that there is an increased rate of prematurity in pregnancies complicated by measles, especially when the disease occurs late in gestation. However, no clear evidence exists, suggesting that maternal measles is associated with an increased risk for spontaneous abortion.

Because of the rarity of measles in pregnancy no statement can be made regarding the teratogenic potential of gestational measles for the fetus. No particular constellation of abnormalities has been found among the sporadic instances of congenital defects that have been reported in association with maternal measles (9). In general, if there is any increased risk of malformations following measles, the risk is small.

PERINATAL MEASLES

Measles which becomes clinically apparent in the first 10 days of life is considered transplacental in origin (i.e., congenital), whereas those cases occurring at 14 days or after are acquired postnatally. Postnatally acquired measles is usually associated with a mild course. Congenital measles includes cases in which the disease is present at birth or infection acquired in utero appears during the first 10 days of life. The spectrum of illness in congenital measles varies from a mild illness to rapidly fatal disease. However, the presence of maternal measles immediately prior to delivery does not involve the fetus and neonate commonly (5, 7). In reported cases of congenital measles there were 7 deaths in 22 infected newborns, a mortality rate of 32% (10–13). Approximately the same case to fatality ratio (30 : 33%) was observed whether the rash was present at birth or appeared subsequently. It appears that premature infants with congenital measles have a significantly higher increased death rate (56%) than do term infants (20%). Insufficient data are available to evaluate whether transplacentally acquired antibodies to measles virus may diminish the case to fatality ratio in congenital measles when the mother's rash occurs more than 48 hr before delivery. These reported cases of mortality due to congenital measles all occurred in the preantibiotic era. With antimicrobial therapy effective against bacterial pneumonia and modern medical support systems fatal outcomes with rubeola infection are much less likely.

DIAGNOSIS

In general, the diagnosis of measles relies on a history of recent exposure and the typical clinical presentation of the disease. However, the diagnosis is more difficult during the prodrome (when the illness is most communicable) or when illness and the exanthema are attenuated by passively acquired measles antibodies. Included in the differential are (a) drug eruptions and allergies; (b) rubella; (c) scarlet fever; (d) meningococcemia; (e) roseola; (f) Rocky Mountain spotted fever; (g) toxoplasmosis; (h) enterovirus; and (i) infectious mononucleosis.

TREATMENT AND PREVENTION

The treatment of uncomplicated measles is symptomatic. When otitis media or pneumonia develop, appropriate antibiotic therapy should be instituted on the basis of a gram stain and culture.

Passive immunization is recommended for the prevention of measles in susceptible exposed pregnant women, neonates, and their contacts in the delivery room or nursery. Immune serum globulin (ISG) in a dose of 0.25 ml/kg administered as soon as possible after exposure may prevent or at least modify the infection (14). Children born to women who have measles in the last week of pregnancy or the first week postpartum should be given ISG as soon as possible in a dose of 0.25 ml/kg (14).

Mumps

Mumps is an acute generalized infection with a predilection for the parotid and salivary glands, but also may affect the brain, pancreas, and gonads. There is no associated rash. The mumps virus is a member of the paramyxovirus family and is thus an RNA virus.

EPIDEMIOLOGY

Mumps virus is transmitted by saliva and droplet contamination. The virus has been re-covered from saliva and respiratory secretions from 7 days prior to the onset of parotitis until 9 days afterwards. The usual incubation period is 14–18 days.

Mumps is primarily a disease of childhood, and only 10% of cases occur after the age of 15. Many adults are immune as a result of clinical or subclinical infection (one-third of cases). However, mumps is much less contagious than measles or chickenpox, and even among susceptible subjects exposed to household members, the attack rate is low. Mumps occurs more frequently in pregnant women than measles or chickenpox. The incidence in prospective studies has been variously reported as ranging from 0.8–10 cases per 10,000 pregnancies (1, 2).

CLINICAL MANIFESTATIONS

The prodrome of mumps consists of fever, malaise, myalgia, and anorexia. Parotitis occurs within 24 hr and is characterized by a swollen and tender parotid gland. The orifice of Stenson's duct is usually red and swollen. In most cases parotitis is bilateral. The submaxillary glands are involved less often and almost never without parotid gland involvement. The sublingual glands are rarely affected. Mumps is generally a self-limited and complication-free disease. However, it can be a significant cause of morbidity.

Orchitis occurs in about 20% of postpubertal males and is the most common manifestation other than parotitis in this group. Oophoritis is far less common. The most common neurologic complication of mumps is aseptic meningitis. However, the course of mumps-associated aseptic meningitis is almost always benign and self-limited. In addition, mumps may cause pancreatitis, mastitis, thyroiditis, myocarditis, nephritis, or arthritis.

MATERNAL EFFECTS OF MUMPS

Mumps in pregnancy is generally benign and not more severe than in nonpregnant patients (3–5). Aseptic meningitis in pregnant patients is neither more frequent nor more severe. Mortality in association with mumps is extremely rare in both pregnant and nonpregnant women.

FETAL EFFECTS OF MUMPS

Retrospective studies have suggested that mumps during the first trimester of pregnancy is associated with a two-fold increase in the incidence of spontaneous abortion (6). No significant association between maternal mumps infection and prematurity, intrauterine growth retardation, or perinatal mortality has been demonstrated.

The role of mumps virus in congenital disease remains controversial. Despite animal studies in which mumps virus induced congenital malformations, definite evidence of a teratogenic potential for mumps virus in humans has not been presented. Siegal, in a controlled prospective study, noted that the rate of congenitally malformed neonates among women who had mumps during pregnancy (2 of 117) was essentially the same rate as in infants born to uninfected mothers (2 of 123) (7).

The predominant concern during the past 15 yr has been the postulated association between maternal mumps infection and the development of subsequent congenital cardiac abnormalities, specifically endocardial fibroelastosis (EFE). Initial studies noted that a high proportion of children diagnosed as having EFE had positive mumps skin tests, although they lacked circulating humoral antibody, and proposed an association between mumps and EFE (8–10). Moreover, St. Gene and associates reported that mumps virus produced lesions in chicken embryos similar to EFE (11). Subsequent studies have failed to verify such an association between a positive mumps skin test and EFE (12–14). Resolution of this controversy can only occur with use of carefully controlled prospective studies. However, the low incidence of mumps in pregnancy precludes such data from being obtained in the near future. Moreover, even if such an association exists, the low incidence of mumps in pregnancy would make such an occurrence very infrequent.

DIAGNOSIS

The diagnosis of mumps is usually made on clinical grounds. When there is acute, bilateral painful parotitis with a history of recent exposure the diagnosis is straightforward. It may be more difficult when disease is unilateral or confined to organs other than the parotid gland. In these cases, diagnosis depends upon virus isolation or more usually by demonstration of a rising CF, HI, or neutralizing antibody titer in paired acute and convalescent serum.

TREATMENT

The treatment of mumps is symptomatic in pregnancy as well as in the nonpregnant patients. Analgesics, bed rest, and application of cold or heat to the parotids are useful. Maternal mumps is not an indication for termination of pregnancy.

The live-attenuated mumps vaccine has been effective in preventing primary mumps. In susceptible subjects, 95% develop antibodies without clinically adverse reactions. The duration of protection afforded by immunization is not known. Immunization with the mumps live virus vaccine in pregnancy is contraindicated on the theoretical grounds that the developing fetus might be harmed. Although the risk to the fetus seems negligible, the innocuous nature of mumps in pregnancy suggests that any risk from vaccination is unwarranted.

Influenza

Influenza is an epidemic disease which has been known since antiquity. The influenza viruses are myxoviruses. Three antigenically different influenza viruses have been identified (1). Type A influenza is responsible for most epidemics and is associated with severe cases. Less frequently, type B is involved in epidemics, but tends to cause milder clinical disease. The third, type C, is the least frequent.

EPIDEMIOLOGY

Both the frequency and severity of influenza epidemics have been related to antigenic changes in the virus (1). The major antigenic changes which occur at 10- to 30-yr intervals are associated with severe infection, while the minor antigenic changes that occur annually are not.

Two major pandemics with influenza have occurred in this century. The pandemic of 1918 was responsible for 20 million deaths worldwide (2). More recently, the Asian influenza pandemic of 1957–1958 caused considerable morbidity and mortality.

CLINICAL PRESENTATION

The incubation type for influenza is 1–4 days. Influenza presents clinically with an abrupt onset of a respiratory infection associated with fever, malaise, myalgias, and headache. The severity of the diseases varies from mild to severe with pneumonia present. The major portion of the clinical disease lasts, on the average, 3 days.

Definitive diagnosis is made by virus isolation from throat washings during the acute illness or by serologic confirmation of a four-fold rise in antibody with paired acute-convalescent serum.

Either compliment fixation or hemagglutination inhibition tests may be done.

MATERNAL EFFECTS OF INFLUENZA

The major concern during pregnancy is the increased likelihood for life-threatening pneumonia as a complication of influenza among pregnant women. Reports from the epidemics of 1918, as well as from 1957, all indicate that pregnant women were disproportionately represented in individuals dying of influenza. The maternal mortality rate associated with influenza during the 1918 pandemic was approximately 30% (3, 4). Moreover, Harris reported that while the overall maternal mortality rate was 27%, in those cases complicated by pneumonia the mortality rate rose to 50% (4). Finland noted that during the 1918 pandemic the worldwide mortality rate was 10% in the general population but that in some areas the mortality rate in pregnant women was 80% (5). During the 1957 pandemic, in Minnesota 50% of all deaths from Asian influenza among women occurred during pregnancy (6). It is not clear that pregnant women are more likely to develop influenza or that they are more likely to develop influenza pneumonia. However, if influenza pneumonia develops in pregnancy, then it appears to be more severe. Deaths among pregnant women with influenza may result from secondary bacterial infection (such as with *S. aureus*, *S. pneumoniae*, or *Klebsiella* species), but also from primary influenza pneumonia without bacterial superinfection.

FETAL EFFECTS OF INFLUENZA

The effect of influenza upon rates of abortion, prematurity, and congenital anomalies is difficult to determine because the evidence is contradictory. In part, confusion may arise from variations of the virus itself from epidemic to epidemic and from lack of well-controlled studies. Studies that did not include serologic confirmation of influenza infection have noted an increased risk for developmental anomalies in pregnancies with a history of influenza. Coffey and Jessup (in Ireland) noted that women who gave birth to infants with malformations (neural tube defects primarily) were more likely to have a history of influenza during pregnancy (18.4%) than mothers delivering normal babies (3.6%) (7). In a subsequent prospective study these investigators reported that the malformation rate was more than doubled in pregnancies with

a history of influenza at the time of the 1957 Asian flu pandemic (8). Similarly, Doll et al (in Scotland) noted that congenital anomalies occurred at a higher rate among infants born to women with histories of influenza infection during pregnancy (9). Hakosalo and Saxen confirmed this association among Finnish women (10). However, studies using serologic confirmation of influenza infection were not used. Hardy and co-workers noted a 5.3% incidence of congenital anomalies among women infected during the first trimester; cardiac anomalies were the most common (11). Griffiths et al also noted an increase in anomalies, but they all occurred in pregnancies with second and third trimester infection with influenza (12). Wilson and co-workers noted no increase in anomalies associated with early pregnancy influenza infection (13). Similarly, neither the Collaborative Perinatal Research Study (14) nor the study by Brown (15) revealed any association between maternal influenza infection and congenital anomalies among offspring. In summary, the vast majority of women who have influenza in pregnancy have normal outcomes, and there seems to be little influence upon congenital anomalies, intrauterine growth, prematurity, or stillbirth.

MANAGEMENT AND PREVENTION

Management of the uncomplicated pregnant women with influenza consists of symtpomatic relief (1) with bed rest, analgesia, liberal fluid intake, and fever control with acetaminophen. The physician must be alert to the development of pneumonia. If pneumonia occurs in pregnant women with influenza, prompt hospitalization is indicated and broad spectrum antibiotic coverage for bacterial superinfection pneumonia is required.

Use of amantadine, which blocks the replication of influenza A virus, has been efficacious in nonpregnant patients—both to prevent symptoms, shorten the clinical course, and improve pulmonary function (16). However, the drug has been associated with teratogenic effects in animals and is not recommended for use in pregnancy (17).

In years of epidemics, it is generally considered advisable to vaccinate pregnant women. During the 1977 Swine flu vaccination program, however, pregnancy was not considered among the high risk conditions, such as rheumatic heart and chronic lung disease. Flu vaccines are as immunogenic in pregnant women as in other adults, and no unusual complications have been encountered in pregnant women. The vaccines are killed virus preparations and, thus, safe for use during pregnancy.

Enteroviruses

The enteroviruses consist of three major groups, the polio viruses, Coxsackie viruses, and echoviruses. These viruses are a subgroup of the picornaviruses. Enteroviruses are small viruses (18–30 nm) with an RNA core. They occur worldwide, both in sporadic and epidemic form, and cause a variety of illnesses (2–6). Congenital and neonatal infections have been associated with polio viruses, echoviruses, and Coxsackie viruses (1–8). Cherry noted that enterovirus infections of the fetus and newborn are more severe than similar infections in older age groups (2). He felt that the relatively immature neonatal immune system may be the explanation for this phenomenon.

Polio Viruses

Following the introduction of polio vaccines, poliomyelitis is an uncommon disease in Western industrialized nations. Only a brief review of the effects of polio viruses on pregnancy and the neonate is presented. Investigations in the prevaccine era clearly demonstrated that polio virus infections during pregnancy could result in spontaneous abortion, stillbirth, low birth weight infants and neonatal poliomyelitis (1, 9–11). Although it is documented that polio virus can be transmitted across the placenta to the fetus, the majority of pregnant women (nearly two-thirds) with clinically apparent poliomyelitis delivered normal, full-term babies (1). Finally, there is no evidence that polio viruses are teratogens, and no increase in congenital malformations has been noted (9–11).

Echoviruses

A total of 33 echoviruses have been identified (several of these have been reassigned to other groups of viruses). The echoviruses are responsible for a variety of illnesses in adults and children, including respiratory disease, rashes, gastroenteritis, conjunctivitis, aseptic meningitis, and pericarditis (12).

Echovirus infection in pregnancy has not been associated with spontaneous abortions, premature delivery, stillbirths, or congenital malfor-

mations (1, 2, 12–15). There have been reports of neonatally acquired infections caused by many of the echoviruses. The clinical findings associated with echovirus neonatal infection include fever with splenomegaly and lymphadenopathy, mascular rashes, diarrhea and vomiting, pneumonitis, otitis media, jaundice, coryza with cough, and septic meningitis (1, 2, 12). However, it has been demonstrated that congenital echovirus infection can produce severe disease and damage to the neonate. Echovirus 14 has been reported to be the cause of a febrile illness that developed at 3 days of life and progressed to cyanotic episodes, hypothermia, hepatomegaly, bradycardia and purpura, with resultant death at 7 days of life (15). Echovirus 19 has been reported to be the cause of hepatic necrosis and massive hemorrhage in three infants (17). No specific treatment or vaccines are available for echovirus infections.

Coxsackieviruses

The coxsackieviruses are divided into two major groups. Group A coxsackievirus contains 23 types, and group B coxsackievirus includes 6 types. Group A coxsackieviruses do not cause significant perinatal illness, except in rare cases.

Group B coxsackieviruses can cause pleurodynia, meningoencephalitis, and myocarditis. Hepatitis, the hemolytic-uremic syndrome, and pneumonia are infrequent but severe manifestations of group B coxsackievirus infection. Transplacental transmission of group B coxsackievirus has been demonstrated (18–21). However, the magnitude of the risk to the fetus has not been defined. The great majority of maternal group B coxsackievirus infection results in no demonstrable adverse effects on the fetus. No evidence exists that demonstrates a role for coxsackieviruses in spontaneous abortion (15) or preterm labor and delivery. Brown and Karunas in a study involving nearly 23,000 pregnancies reported that coxsackieviruses B-2, B-3, B-4, and A-9 had a positive correlation between maternal infection and neonatal anomalies (13). The coxsackie B-4 virus in the first trimester has been associated with urogenital malformations, such as hypospadias, epispadias, and cryptorchidism. Coxsackievirus A-9 maternal infection was associated with digestive tract anomalies, and types B-3 and B-4 were associated with cardiovascular defects. There was an association between the B1–B5 coxsackievirus group and congenital heart disease. In addition,

Brown and Karunas noted that there was no correlation between reported maternal illness and serologic evidence of infection in the offspring (13). Thus, even asymptomatic maternal coxsackievirus infection may result in fetal maldevelopment.

Congenital coxsackievirus infection within 48 hr of birth is a rare occurrence (1). Neonatal infection with coxsackievirus can be acquired from mother, nursing personnel, or infected babies in the nursery. A large number of studies have documented the variety and severity of neonatal coxsackievirus infection, especially types B1–B5. The majority have focused on myocarditis and CNS infection (1, 2). Myocarditis seems to be a particularly prominent manifestation of group B coxsackievirus infection in the neonate.

Diagnosis of coxsackievirus infection is based on virus isolation from throat or rectum and serologic evidence of increasing antibody titer during the convalescent period. Hemagglutination-inhibition (HI) or complement fixation (CF) may be performed.

Miscellaneous Viruses

WESTERN EQUINE ENCEPHALITIS

Western equine encephalitis is a member of the arbovirus group and is transmitted by mosquitoes. Most human infection is subclinical, but clinically recognized disease does occur in the Western and Southwestern United States. The disease presents as an influenza-like disease or meningoencephalitis.

Transplacental transmission of Western equine encephalitis virus has been reported (1, 2). In these cases, the mother experienced a febrile illness with headache, malaise, and lethargy 3–10 days prior to delivery, and serologic titers several weeks later were positive for Western equine encephalitis. Although at birth the children appeared well, by 5–6 days of life they had evidence of meningitis. In some instances the neonates were severely ill, but only a single case of permanent neurologic damage has been reported.

Thus, in occasional cases, Western equine encephalitis can be transmitted to the fetus when maternal infection with the agent occurs late in pregnancy. Treatment is symptomatic. No vaccine is clinically available.

VENEZUELAN EQUINE ENCEPHALITIS

The Venezuelan equine encephalitis virus is transmitted by mosquitoes, and horses and small mammals are the usual hosts. However, human cases have been reported, and they present as an influenza-like disease or with the signs of encephalitis.

Maternal infection can result in abortion or congenital malformations (1, 2). The virus primarily affects developing brain tissue. Infection during the first trimester has been associated with stillbirth, microcephaly, microopthalmia, and severe hypoplasia of the medulla. In two cases with infection at 20 weeks of gestation, the children were born without a cerebellum and almost no cortical tissue. In addition, there have been three reported cases of Venezuelan equine encephalitis infection during the 8th month of gestation. The children at birth had massive destruction of cerebral and cerebellar tissue.

Treatment for Venezuelan equine encephalitis is symptomatic. No vaccine is available.

BACTERIA

Syphilis

The epidemiology, clinical presentation, diagnosis, and treatment of syphilis is discussed in detail in Chapter 3. In this section only the perinatal consequence of syphilis will be addressed.

EPIDEMIOLOGY

As the number of reported cases of early syphilis have increased, the incidence of congenital syphilis has paralleled this rise. From a low point in 1958 of 200 cases of congenital syphilis, nearly 250 cases are now reported annually in the United States (1, 2). Traditionally, it was believed that the spirochete, *Treponema pallidum*, was incapable of crossing the placenta and infecting the fetus prior to 16–18 weeks of gestation. Langhans layer, which disappears at 16–18 weeks of pregnancy, was the supposed barrier to placental penetration (3, 4, 5). This initial impression was based upon pathologic studies which failed to identify the anatomic lesions of syphilis in fetuses less than 16–18 weeks of gestation (6). However, recent work suggests that spirochetes are capable of penetrating the placenta at any time during pregnancy, and the lack of evidence for fetal syphilitic infection prior to 16–18 weeks of gestation is a reflection of fetal immunoincompetence rather than lack of exposure (7).

In general, the major determinants of fetal infection with *T. pallidum* are the quantity of spirochetes in the maternal bloodstream and the stage of syphilis in the pregnant woman. Paley reported that with untreated syphilis of less than 2 yr duration only half of the babies were normal, while 38% had syphillis, 8.7% were stillbirth, and 4.4% died within 2 months of birth (8). With maternal syphilis of 2–5 yr duration the corresponding figures were 75, 14, 7, and 4%, respectively. If syphilis had been present for more than 5 yr, 81% were normal, 6% had syphilis, 6% were stillbirths, and 7% died during the first 3 months of life. More recently, Fiumara and co-workers noted that with untreated primary or secondary maternal syphilis, half the babies were stillborns, prematures, or neonatal deaths, and 50% had congenital syphilis (9). With early latent syphilis there were 20% premature, 16% stillbirth, 4% neonatal death, 40% congenital syphilis, and only 20% normal term infants. In cases of late syphilis, there was a 10% rate for congenital syphilis, but no increase in prematurity or perinatal mortality.

CLINICAL PRESENTATION

The clinical manifestations of syphilis in pregnant women is similar to that of nonpregnant patients and are discussed in Chapter 3. The overwhelming majority of pregnant women diagnosed to have syphilis are asymptomatic, in the latent stage, and have had syphilis for more than 1 year's duration. Congenital syphilis is divided into two stages. Early congenital disease is when clinical manifestations of syphilis appear within the first yr after birth. Late congenital syphilis refers to the occurrence of clinical findings after 2 yr of life.

In early congenital syphilis, the infant is usually asymptomatic at birth, and the only evidence of syphilis is a positive blood serology (4, 5). The early skin lesions which are similar to those seen during the secondary stage of acquired syphilis appear between 2–6 weeks following delivery (5). The skin lesions tend to be circumoral, in the anogenital area, and on the palms and soles. Typically, the rash is maculopapular or papulosquamous, but, unlike adult disease, may be vesicular or bullous. Mucosal and/or mucocutaneous lesions (i.e., condyloma latum or mucous patches) are more common than skin lesions and are darkfield exam-positive for *T. pallidum*. A mucopurulent rhinitis or snuffles is present. Fissures at the lips and anogenital area are very common and on healing produce the scars known as rhagades. By 4 months of age the pseudoparalysis of Parrot may be evident as a result of osteochondritis, osteitis, and periostitis of the long bones (5). As reported by Peterson approximately two-thirds of infants with early congenital syphilis demonstrate hepatosplenomegaly, and nearly half have symptomatic meningitis (10). Additional manifestations of early congenital syphilis include anemia, fever, lymphadenopathy, pneumonia alba, iritis, and saddle nose (5).

Late congenital syphilis includes two major groups of manifestations (11). The stigmata of syphilis refer to the clinical findings that result from the scarring of the early lesions and developmental changes caused by early syphilis. These stigmata include perforation of the nasal septum, saddle nose, bossae (overgrowth of frontal bones), Hutchinsonian teeth (tapering or notching of the permanent incisors), mulberry molars (hypoplastic cusps and poor enamel), saber shins, and rhagades (5, 12). The second group of clinical manifestations represent the product of ongoing active inflammation. Examples of this category include interstitial keratitis, neurosyphilis, neural deafness, Clutton's joints (bilateral hydrathrosis), and gummas (5, 12).

DIAGNOSIS

The diagnosis of acquired syphilis is described in Chapter 3. A diagnosis of early congenital syphilis should be suspected in any infant with unexplained hydrops fetalis, a large placenta, persistent rhinitis (snuffles), and intractable diaper rash, unexplained jaundice, and hepatosplenomegaly or anemia of undetermined cause (11). The mucocutaneous lesions and snuffles contain spirochetes, and the diagnosis can be made with a darkfield examination for *T. pallidum.*

As for late congenital syphilis, the only manifestations that are specific enough to suggest the diagnosis are the Hutchinson triad (Hutchinson's teeth, interstitial keratitis, and 8th nerve deafness), mulberry molars, and Clutton's joints.

Ingall and Musher have suggested criteria for the diagnosis of congenital syphilis (11). A definitive diagnosis relies upon darkfield or histologic confirmation of spirochetes. Presumptive diagnosis requires either: (a) rising or persistently reactive serologic tests for syphilis (VDRL or FTA-ABS); or (b) serologic test positive in presence of snuffles, condyloma latum, or bone lesions; or (c) serologic test positive in the presence of two or more of the following clinical findings (hepatosplenomegaly, lymphadenopathy, anemia, nonimmunologic hydrops fetalis, mucocutaneous manifestations, pseudoparalysis of Parrot, glomerulonephritis, or CNS involvement). A possible diagnosis for congenital syphilis exists when the VDRL or FTA-ABS are reactive with the absence of evidence for clinical disease. Because cord blood and neonatal serum may reflect the presence of maternally derived VDRL and FTA-ABS levels, if they are positive without additional signs and symptoms of syphilis either serial specimens must be obtained (rising level or persistent reactivity strongly support a diagnosis of congenital syphilis), or measurement of specific IgM against syphilis should be tested for. The presence of IgM confirms neonatal syphilis.

TREATMENT

Penicillin is the drug of choice for the treatment of syphilis in nonpregnant as well as pregnant patients. The recommended treatment schedule suggested by the Centers for Disease Control is presented in Table 13.7. Erythromycin is the drug of choice for penicillin-allergic pregnant patients with syphilis. However, this antimicrobial does not cross the placenta well, and treatment of the fetus is not guaranteed with the use of erythromycin. Thus, many pediatricians will routinely treat the newborn of a mother whose syphilis was treated with erythromicin, as if it has never been treated, with penicillin. Any infant suspected of having congenital syphilis should have a spinal tap prior to therapy. If the spinal fluid is negative, a single intramuscular injection of benzathine penicillin G (50,000 units/kg) should be given. If the spinal fluid is abnormal or a spinal tap is not performed, the infant should receive aqueous crystalline penicillin G (50,000 units/kg/day for 10 days) (13).

Group B Streptococcal Infection

The hemolytic streptococci cause a variety of infectious syndromes and are significant causes of perinatal morbidity and mortality. Lancefield in 1933 used serologic techniques to subdivide β-hemolytic streptococci into specific groups, which she named A, B, D, and E (1). In Table 13.8 the various groups of streptococci, their taxonomic designations, and hemolytic reactions on blood agar are depicted. On blood agar, a β reaction is clear or complete hemolysis around the bacterial colony, the α reaction is a greenish discoloration or partial hemolysis around the colony, and the γ reaction refers to a absence of hemolysis around the colony. Most microbiology laboratories report groups C and

Table 13.7
Centers for Disease Control Recommended Treatment of Syphilis (1982)

Early syphilis (primary, secondary, latent syphilis of 1 year's duration)
  1. Recommended regimen:
     benzathine penicillin G: 2.4 million units total, IM, at a single session
  2. Penicillin-allergic patients:
     tetracycline HCl: 500 mg, by mouth, 4 times a day for 15 days
                          or
erythromycin: 500 mg, by mouth, 4 times a day for 15 days
Syphilis of more than one year's duration
  1. Recommended regimen:
     benzathine penicillin G: 2.4 million units, IM, once a week for 3 successive weeks (total 7.2 million units)
  2. Penicillin-allergic patients:
     tetracycline HCl: 500 mg, by mouth, 4 times a day for 30 days
                          or
erythromycin: 500 mg, by mouth, 4 times a day for 30 days
Syphilis in Pregnancy
  1. Recommended regimens:
     for patients who are not allergic to penicillin, penicillin should be used in dosage schedule appropriate for the stage of syphilis as recommended for nonpregnant patients.
  2. Penicilin-allergic patients:
     If compliance and serologic follow-up can be assured, administer erythromycin in dosages appropriate for the stage of syphilis.
     If compliance and follow-up cannot be assured, consider hospitalization and penicillin desensitization.
Neurosyphilis
Aqueous crystalline penicillin G: 12–24 million units, IV, per day for 10 days, followed by benzathine penicillin G, 2.4 million units, IM, weekly for 3 dose
                          or
Aqueous procaine penicillin G: 2.4 million units, IM, daily plus probenecid 500 mg by mouth, 4 times a day, for 10 days, followed by benzathine penicillin G, 2.4 million units, IM, weekly for 3 doses
                          or
Benzathine penicillin G: 2.4 million units, IM, weekly for 3 doses.

G "as" β-hemolytic streptococci, not groups A, B, or D."

S. pyogenes (group A β-hemolytic streptococcus) has long been recognized as a major path-

Table 13.8
The Aerobic Streptococci: Taxonomic Classification and Reaction on Blood Agar[a]

Group	Common species designation	Reaction on blood agar
A	*S. pyogenes*	β, rarely α
B	*S. agalactiae*	Usually β, rarely α or γ
C	*S. equi, S. zooepidemicus, S. equisimilis, S. dysgalactiae*	Usually β, except *s. dysgalactiae* is α
D, enterococcus	*S. faecalis, S. faecium*	Usually γ, occasionally α or β
D, not enterococcus	*S. bovis, S. equinus*	Usually γ, occasionally α or β
G	*S. anginosus*	Usually β
Viridans, not group D	Many species	α or γ
	S. pneumoniae	α

[a] Adapted from Buchanan RE, Gibbon NE: *Bergey's Manual of Determinative Bacteriology*, ed 8. Baltimore, Williams & Wilkins, 1974.

ogen in perinatal sepsis. Prior to the introduction of penicillin, this organism was the major cause of puerperal sepsis and was responsible for 75% of maternal mortality due to infection.

While group B streptocci (GBS) have been recognized in veterinary medicine for many years as a cause of bovine mastitis, they were virtually ignored as human pathogens until 1964 when Eickhoff and associates noted the role of GBS in perinatal infections (2). Subsequently, an increasing number of reports in the obstetric and pediatric literature documented a growing concern with neonatal sepsis and/or meningitis due to the GBS. In fact, GBS has replaced *Escherichia coli* as the most frequent microorganism associated with bacteremia or meningitis among infants during the first 2 months of life (3). In 1977, Baker estimated that there were 12,000–15,000 newborns with GBS infection annually and that there is a 50% mortality rate among this group (4). Moreover, it has been pointed out that mortality is not the only concern in GBS neonatal involvement. Recently GBS has been identified as an important pathogen in obstetrical patients as well. This organism has been associated with urinary tract infections (5, 6), amnionitis and postpartum endometritis (7–10), intrapartum and/or postpartum bacteremia (7, 8, 11), and premature rupture of membranes (PROM), and/or preterm delivery (9, 12).

ORGANISM

The GBS (*Steptococcus agalactiae*) is a facultative gram-positive diplococcus. Colonies of GBS on sheep blood agar produce a characteristic appearance with narrow zones of β-hemolysis surrounding the colonies which are grey white in color, flat, and mucoid. Approximately 1% of GBS isolates are nonhemolytic or α-hemolytic. Thus, definitive microbiologic identification of GBS requires serologic techniques for the detection of the group B antigen. The GBS can be further subdivided into five serotypes based on antigenic structure. These are Ia, Ib, Ic, II, and III. The distribution of serotypes of GBS is similar for mother/neonate pairs. Approximately one-third of isolates are type IA, Ib or Ic, one-third are type II, and one-third type III (3).

EPIDEMIOLOGY

Asymptomatic vaginal colonization with GBS occurs in 4.6–40.6% of pregnant women (2, 4, 13–29). The reported prevalence of vaginal colonization with GBS in gravid women varies according to geographic locale, age, gravidity, duration of gestation, and the location and number of sites cultured. The carrier rates seem to be highest for women less than 20 yr old and caucasian. The highest isolation rates are reported from the introitus and lowest from the cervix. Pregnancy per se does not influence colonization rates (30). Among nonpregnant women, Baker and co-workers reported that GBS were recovered significantly more often from sexually active women, women wearing an IUD, and women 20 yr of age or younger (31). In addition, the choice of culture medium is a crucial determinant of the prevalence of GBS. The highest yield of GBS occurs when a selective medium such as Todd-Hewitt broth with sheep blood, nalidixic acid, and gentamicin are used. When selective media are not used, 50% of genital tract cultures may yield false-negative results for GBS.

Although the lower genital tract has been considered the primary site of GBS colonization (2, 13–15), recent work has suggested that the intestinal tract might be the primary reservoir for this organism and that the lower genital tract may be colonized in an ascending manner (similar to what is seen with urinary tract infection) (17, 32–35). As Baker has suggested, the wide variations in colonization rates are due not only to differences between study populations, but to a lack of standardization for culture methodology and specimen site (3). The highest colonization rates occur with use of sensitive culture methods such as selective broth, when both the lower genital tract and anorectum are cultured, and if sequential cultures are obtained throughout pregnancy.

The presence of GBS in the maternal genital tract is the major determinant of both infection in the neonate and colonization of the newborn (15, 17, 18, 22, 35–37). Vertical transmission from mother to fetus occurs either via an ascending route in utero through intact or ruptured membrane or by acquisition during passage through the birth canal intrapartum. The risk of transmission has been shown to range from 42 to 72% among neonates born to colonized mothers, while approximately only 8% of infants born to noncolonized mothers become colonized (Table 13.9). Based on these prospective studies, nearly two-thirds of infants born to colonized mothers will also be asymptomatic carriers of GBS. Thus, the prevalence for GBS colonization tends to be similar for both pregnant women and their offsprings in any given population. However, despite high prevalence rates for vertical transmission, the incidence of GBS infection during the first 7 days of life ranges from 1.3 to 3/1000 live births and after 7

days the range is 1 to 1.7/1000 live births (15, 17, 18, 30, 38, 39). It is apparent that only one symptomatic, clinical GBS infection occurs for approximately every 100 colonized infants.

In addition to maternal-infant transmission, nosocomial acquisition of GBS occurs (17, 22, 40–43). From 16 to 47% of nursery personnel are carriers of GBS and may be a source for neonatal transmission (3). Studies have demonstrated nosocomial transmission rates of GBS in neonates born to culture-negative mothers. In addition, cross-contamination may arise from maternally colonized infants via inappropriately washed hands of nursery personnel (3). Studies have demonstrated nosocomial transmission rates of GBS in neonates born to culture-negative mothers in the range of 13–43% (40–43). Whether late onset GBS infection is largely due to nosocomial acquisition of GBS is unclear. Both nonmaternal and maternal sources have been implicated (3).

Because of the discrepancy between colonization rates and actual infection rates with GBS in neonates, attempts have been made to identify those factors which predispose the neonate to clinical infection. In general it is accepted that colonization is unrelated to maternal age, race, parity, blood type, duration of labor, or mode of delivery (3).

Several investigators have correlated the risk of neonatal GBS infection with the density (i.e., quantitation) of maternal genital tract colonization with GBS. Bobitt (44), Anthony et al (19), Pass et al (18), and Ancona et al (28) demonstrated that neonates delivered through birth canals which are heavily colonized with GBS were significantly more likely to acquire GBS than those born to mothers with small quantities of the organisms in their vagina. For

Table 13.9
Vertical Transmission of Group B Streptococci from Colonized Mothers to Neonates

Study	Rate of maternal genital colonization	Percentage of colonized neonates born to colonized mothers	Percentage of colonized neonates born to noncolonized mothers
Baker and Barrett (15)	22.5	72	12.0
Ferrieri et al (21)	8.3	50	1.0
Aber et al (17)	28.7	71	27.0
Paredes et al (40)	27.7	65	ND
Pass et al (18)	19.0	47	3.0
Anthony et al (22)	28.0	63	9.0
Yow et al (23)	20.4	42	1.2
Ancona et al (28)	8.0	67	ND
Lewin and Amstey (29)	8.0	50	ND
Band et al (41)	23.2	58	ND

example, Anthony reported that mothers who were trace-positive had a 31% chance of delivering colonized infants, whereas, mothers with 1+ to 4+ growth had a 95% chance.

One of the most important risk factors which has been studied is prematurity. Controversy exists as to whether premature neonates (preterm, less than 37 weeks, or low birth weight, less than 2500 g) have an increased risk for vertical transmission from the maternal genital tract and an increased risk for colonization. Siegal et al in their control population of over 9000 infants found no difference in the colonization rate for infants more than 37 weeks (12%) versus those less than 37 weeks (11%) (45). Baker and Barrett, on the other hand, noted that term babies had a 27% rate of colonization, while preterm neonates had a rate of 18% (15). Studies by Pass et al (18), Anthony et al (20), and Ancona et al (28) also did not demonstrate a relationship between colonization rates and gestational age. On the other hand, Aber and co-workers (17) reported a higher colonization rate among premature than term neonates.

Less controversial is the association between gestational age and risk of symptomatic GBS infection, especially early onset disease. The majority of investigators have identified a significant association between preterm delivery and an increased risk for symptomatic early onset GBS infection, prolonged duration of ruptured membranes (more than 24 hr) before delivery, prolonged duration of labor, and maternal intrapartum or postpartum infection (2, 4, 13, 15, 18, 21, 35–37, 46–48).

Franciosi and co-workers demonstrated no association between preterm infants and an increased risk for GBS early onset infection; of 43 GBS-infected neonates, 28 (65%) were term and 36 (83%) had birth weights more than 2500 g (14). Bobitt (44), Baker and Barrett (15), Siegel et al (45), Lloyd et al (48), Boyer et (35–37), and Pass et al (18) have shown that there is a significant increase in the risk for GBS early onset infection in preterm infants. This risk is approximately a 10- to 15-fold increase. Bobitt found that in 11 consecutive cases of GBS sepsis, 5 were less than 2500 g (3 were 2000–2500 g, and 2 were less than 2000) and suggested that premature neonates were at increased risk for GBS sepsis (44). Siegal et al reported that 41% of GBS disease occurred in infants under 2500 g (45), and Baker and Barrett reported that 80% of infants with GBS disease were less than 2500 g. In Canada, Lloyd and co-workers in an 8 yr

study involving over 30,000 births, found low birth weight and prematurity to be risk factors in GBS septicemia (48). Pass and colleagues demonstrated that with preterm onset of labor the risk of symptomatic GBS sepsis in neonates born to colonized women was 15.2% rather than the usual 1–2% risk (18). Boyer and co-workers reported that as birth weight decreased, attack rates for GBS increased from 1.1/1000 in infants more than 2500 g to 26.2/1000 in infants less 1000 g, and the relative risk of developing GBS early onset disease for infants less than 2500 g was 7.3-fold higher than the risk for infants more than 2500 g (36).

The duration of membrane rupture prior to delivery has also been studied as a risk factor. In Bobbit's study, only 2 of 11 infants with GBS disease had membranes ruptured longer than 24 hr (44). Anthony reported that colonization rates were unrelated to duration of membrane rupture (57% of colonized mothers delivered colonized babies when membranes were ruptured less than 6 hr versus 50% of colonized mothers delivering colonized babies when membranes were ruptured greater than 12 hr) (22). Baker and Barrett, however, found that colonized mothers had a higher incidence of PROM greater than 24 hr (11 versus 5.8%) (15). Lloyd reported that neither PROM greater than 24 hr nor maternal fever or neonatal asphyxia aided in the identification of infants at risk for GBS disease (48). Taken together studies by Eickhoff et al (2), Hood et al (13), Pass et al (10), Baker and Barrett (15), Tseng and Randall (49), and Stewardson-Krieger and Gotoff (50) demonstrated that the presence of intraamniotic infection or a greater than 24-hr duration of membrane rupture is associated with an increased risk for neonatal early onset GBS infection among the offspring of colonized mothers (10.7% as compared to the usual 1–2% of neonates born to colonized mothers who develop GBS sepsis). Stewardson-Krieger and Gotoff reported that the GBS attack rate was directly proportional to the duration from ROM to delivery; with duration ≤19 hr, the attack rate was 0.7/1000 live births compared to a rate of 18.3/1000 live births, with durations >30 hr (nearly a 25-fold increased risk) (50). Recently, Boyer and colleagues noted that as the duration of membrane rupture increased, attack rates for GBS infection also did and rose from 0.8/1000 infants with ROM ≤6 hr to 10.8/1000 in those with duration >48 hr. In this study the relative risk of developing GBS early onset disease for infants with ROM >18 hr was 7.2-fold higher than that for infants with less than 18 hr duration of membrane rupture (36). However, it is important to recognize that fulminant early onset GBS sepsis does occur in the presence of intact membranes and in neonates delivered by cesarean section.

Of considerable interest has been the report by Regan and co-workers that suggested an association between GBS colonization of the cervix and the development of premature ruptured membranes (PROM) and preterm delivery (12). In a survey of 6706 patients, of which 877 (13.4%) had GBS isolation from the cervix, they noted that 15.3% of GBS-positive patients had PROM compared to 8.1% of the total population (p < 0.005), and 5.4% of GBS-positive mothers had a preterm delivery versus a 1.8% rate of preterm delivery in their total population (p < 0.005). Minkoff et al have confirmed a relationship between GBS colonization and PROM; among GBS positives the PROM rate was 50%, while it was 14.8% in the GBS-negative group (p < 0.01) (9).

Intrapartum fever (suggestive of amnionitis) is a perinatal risk factor associated with an increased risk for early onset GBS sepsis (15, 36, 51). Boyer and co-workers noted that attack rates for GBS were 5.6/1000 infants among mothers with intrapartum fever versus a 1.5/1000 infant rate for afebrile mothers (36). As noted by these authors, this relative risk of four is very likely to be an underestimation because the overwhelming majority of patients with an intrapartum fever received antimicrobial therapy during labor. Farco documented that neonates born to mothers with postpartum GBS bacteremia are also at increased risk to develop early onset GBS sepsis (7).

Additional risk factors have been suggested. Baker and Kasper proposed that the offspring of mothers who lack antibodies to group B streptococci type III have a greater risk of acquiring type-specific disease (52). Hemming and co-workers confirmed this association with very low levels of maternally acquired antibody and the development of type II and III early onset GBS disease (53). Baker and Edwards suggested two mechanisms which result in low levels of neonatal antibody to GBS (3). Either it reflects low maternal levels and lack of acquired immunity in the mother or failure for adequate concentrations of these IgG antibodies to be transplacentally transported to the fetus. The very small preterm infant (less than 30 weeks) may be significantly compromised by the second explanation because nearly two-thirds of maternally derived IgG is actively transported from mother to fetus in the last 10 weeks of pregnancy. In support of this concept is the work of Shigeoka et al who demonstrated that infants with early onset GBS sepsis who received exchange transfusion with fresh donor blood containing type III opsonins were more likely to survive than those transfused with blood from donors without type III opsonins (54). Recently Baker and colleagues noted low levels of antibody to type III capsular polysaccharide in all 32 infants with early onset, type III GBS sepsis. A significant correlation was observed between the levels in the mother and infant. Moreover, mothers with type III GBS colonization whose infants were well had antibody levels < 2 μg/ml significantly more often (73%) than those whose infants developed early onset GBS disease (17%) (55). Such data have stimulated interest in and hope for a vaccine approach to the prevention of GBS disease. Whether such an approach will work must be determined in large scale prospective clinical trials.

A possible association with the use of invasive fetal monitoring (i.e., use of fetal scalp electrode and intrauterine pressure catheter) and the development of early onset GBS has been suggested. Bobitt and Ledger noted that 95% of GBS neonatal infection occurred in the 40% of patients with invasive fetal monitoring at Los Angeles County Hospital (44). However, it is important to recognize that those monitored were a high risk population and thus may have also been at increased risk for GBS.

Despite the above controversy over risk factors for GBS disease, it seems clear that GBS infection among prematures is more serious than that occurring in term infants. Combining data from published series indicates that the greatest threat of GBS infection is indeed to the premature (Table 13.10). The risk of an infected premature baby dying was 66%, whereas the risk of death for term infants was only 17%.

The major epidemiologic question in early onset GBS infection revolves around whether most cases are acquired in utero (prepartum or intrapartum) or during delivery and the subsequent postdelivery period (36). As described above, an association between GBS maternal colonization and PROM and/or preterm delivery has been reported (9, 12). In addition to these suggestive studies, additional data have been published that strongly point to a major

Table 13.10
The Effect of Prematurity on Survival of Infants with Early Onset Group B Streptococcal Infections

| Study | No. of cases | Premature | | Term | | Total deaths |
		GBS infection	Mortality	GBS infection	Mortality	
Eickhoff et al (2)	10	4	2	6	2	4
Berggvist et al (46)	7	0	0	7	1	1
Hey et al (56)	6	3	3	3	3	6
Echeverria (57)	16	9	4	7	1	5
Horn et al (58)	6	1	1	5	2	3
Quirante et al (47)	17	17	16	0	0	16
Reid (25)	7	7	4	0	0	4
Bobitt and Ledger (44)	11	6	3	5	0	3
Hemming et al (59)	15	12	9	3	3	12
Boyer et al (36)	61	30	15	31	1	16
Stewardson-Krieger and Gottof (50)	32	21	15	11	0	15
Total	188	110	72/110	78	13/78	85
Percent		59	66	41	17	

role for ascending infection from the colonized lower genital tract in the pathogenesis of early onset GBS sepsis. Studies which documented the presence of bacteremia at birth in a large proportion of neonates with early onset GBS disease indicate that most cases of GBS early onset disease have an intrauterine pathogenesis (18, 36, 60). Pass et al noted that six (67%) of their nine infants with early onset GBS infection were ill at or within 1 hr of delivery (18). Pyati and colleagues reported that 21 (88%) of the 24 neonates with early onset GBS sepsis were bacteremic at birth (61). Most recently, Boyer and colleagues demonstrated that 41 (67%) of the 61 neonates with early onset GBS sepsis were bacteremic either at birth or within 1 hr of age (36). Thus, it appears that GBS infection is often well established before birth. This has major implications for both prevention and treatment plans as will be discussed subsequently.

The epidemiology and pathogenesis of late onset GBS infection (occurring more than 7 days after birth) is not as clear as for early onset disease (3). Serotype III strains account for the majority of late onset GBS infection. The GBS organisms responsible for late onset disease are acquired by maternal neonatal vertical transmission or from nosocomial sources. Anthony and Okada reported that approximately one-third of infants with GBS infection had the onset of their symptoms beyond 1 week of age (38). Similarly, Pass and co-workers noted that

nearly 32% of infants with GBS infection had late onset of symptoms (18). Although survival rates are much improved for late onset as compared to early onset GBS infection, a high rate of neurologic sequelae occur among survivors with meningitis, which tends to be the predominant form of late onset GBS disease.

Lastly, Several investigations have suggested that serum complement and circulating polymorphonuclear leukocytes either independently or in conjunction with serum antibodies may play a significant role in the pathogenesis of group B streptococcal infection in neonates. In vitro studies have demonstrated that components of both the classical and alternative complement pathways are necessary for efficient opsonization of GBS. Whether the immaturity of the complement system in prematures predisposes them to severe GBS infection is an unproven, but attractive hypothesis (3). Similarly, the role of leukocyte abnormalities in GBS infection requires investigation.

Interestingly, investigators in the 1960s and 1970s noted a clinical similarity between early onset GBS infection in the neonate and septic shock with endotoxin in the adult (61, 63). Recently, Schlievert et al reported that group B streptococcal cells enhanced host susceptibility (in an animal model) to lethal shock by endotoxin as much as 40,000-fold (64). They postulated that such enhancement may be the mechanism responsible for death in the neonate with early onset GBS sepsis.

CLINICAL MANIFESTATIONS

Neonatal Infection with GBS

Although Eickhoff et al described GBS sepsis as a fulminent illness in early neonatal life, it was not until the reports of Baker and Barrett (15) and Franciosi and co-workers (14) that two clinically distinct neonatal GBS infections were identified. Early onset GBS disease appears within the 1st week of life, usually within the initial 48 hr. In 60% early onset GBS sepsis presents within 24 hr of birth (30, 38), and Stewardson-Kreiger and Gotoff noted that 56% of their early onset cases were symptomatic at birth (50). Early onset GBS infection is characterized by rapid clinical deterioration and high mortality. It predominantly occurs in preterm and/or low birth weight infants born to mothers with a variety of obstetric complications associated with an increased risk for GBS neonatal infection (see discussion in Epidemiology section). These risk factors include genital tract colonization with GBS (especially heavy growth), preterm labor, prolonged duration between ruptured membranes and delivery, and presence of maternal intra- or postpartum infection.

The three major presentations in early onset GBS infection include septicemia (bacteremia and clinical signs of sepsis), pneumonia, and meningitis. Respiratory symptoms and signs such as grunting, tachypnea, apnea, and/or cyanosis are usually the earliest clinical findings (3). Hypotension occurs in 25%. Additional symptoms and signs similar to those associated with any bacterial infection are present (lethargy, poor feeding, hypothermia or fever, pallor, and jaundice). Meningitis is present in approximately 30% of early onset GBS infections (30, 38). Pneumonia is present in 40% of infants with early onset GBS infection, and almost all of these present with grunting, tachypnea, and apnea (31).

In the fulminant form, early onset GBS disease presents as septic shock accompanied by respiratory distress leading to death within several hours despite appropriate antibiotic therapy. The mortality rate in early studies ranged from 50 to 70%; Anthony and Okada reviewed nearly 300 cases of early onset GBS infection with a mortality rate of 55% (38). More recent studies suggest a lower rate (see table 13.3). The mortality rate correlates directly with birth weight, low birth weight and/or preterm neonates being at an increased risk for a fatal outcome.

Late onset GBS disease occurs more insidiously and usually occurs after the 1st week of life and up until 12 weeks of age. The majority of these infants (85%) have meningitis as the prominent clinical manifestation. The presenting symptoms in newborns with meningitis include fever (nearly 100%), irritability or lethargy (sometimes both), and poor feeding. In 20–30% of cases of meningitis antecedent upper respiratory tract symptoms were present. Although the mortality rate in late onset GBS disease is lower (15–20%), up to 50% of babies with meningitis subsequently demonstrate neurologic sequelae. Late onset disease may also result in localized infections involving middle ears, sinuses, conjunctiva, breasts, lungs, bones, joints, and skin.

Meningitis seems to be related to the serotype of GBS. More than 80% of early onset GBS infection with meningitis present are due to type III organisms. More than 90% of late onset disease (in which meningitis is usually present) are due to type III GBS. These findings are in contrast to the distribution of GBS serotypes among asymptomatic maternal carriers, where one-third have type Ia, Ib, Ic, one-third have type II, and the final one-third have type III organisms.

While early onset disease has been associated with transmission from the mother's genital tract either prior to labor or during parturition, such a route of transmission is thought to occur less frequently in late onset disease. Nosocomial transmission of GBS can occur in the nursery from colonized nursing staff or by cross-colonization from other infants.

Maternal Infection with Group B Streptococci

Although GBS have been recognized as a major cause of neonatal morbidity and mortality, they have not been considered a significant cause of puerperal infection. Several recent investigations have identified GBS as an important cause of maternal infections as well. Initially studies by Ledger et al and Baker noted that GBS isolates were recovered from 11 and 21%, respectively, of bacteremic patients on obstetric services (11, 30). More recent studies have firmly established the GBS organism as an important putative agent for postpartum endomyometritis (especially following cesarean section) and as an organism likely to be recovered in bacteremic patients (7, 8, 10) (Table 13.11). In these reports, bacteremia occurred in 31–35% (usual rate in obstetrics is 10%), 56–

Table 13.11
Group B Streptococci and Puerperal Infections

Study	No. of cases	Cases of bacteremia	Number of C-sections	Incidence of GBS puerperal infection/ 1000 deliveries
Faro (7)	40	14 (35%)	38 (95%)	1.3
Gibbs and Blanco (8)	48	48[a]	31 (68%)	NS[b]
Pass et al (10)	68	21 (32%)	38 (56%)	6.5

[a] Bacteremia was index for study.
[b] NS, not stated.

95% of the patients had been delivered by cesarean section, and the incidence of GBS puerperal sepsis ranged from 1.3 to 6.5/1000 deliveries. Characteristically, women with GBS puerperal infection develop high spiking fever within 12 hr of delivery. Other clinical features include tachycardia, chills, and tender uterine fundus and parametrium.

As described in Chapter 18, GBS also cause maternal urinary tract infection—both bacteriuria and symptomatic disease. GBS urinary tract infections will not be discussed in this section.

DIAGNOSIS OF GROUP B STREPTOCOCCAL INFECTION

Maternal asymptomatic genitourinary or gastrointestinal colonization with GBS can be diagnosed only by culture, preferably using a selective medium. The optimal media for cultivation of group B *Streptococcus* is a selective broth media, Todd-Hewitt broth, which contains gentamicin, colistin (or polymyxin B), and nalidixic acid. These antibiotics inhibit the growth of gram-negative enterobacteriaceae and other bacteria in the normal genital tract flora that could interfere with the recovery and identification of group B streptococci. Symptomatic maternal genitourinary tract infection with GBS may present with fever, chills, uterine tenderness, dysuria, urgency, and pyuria. Because none of these is specific for GBS, the diagnosis must be confirmed by isolation of the GBS. However, in certain clinical situations, empiric therapy should provide coverage against GBS because of its frequency (i.e., intraamniotic infection and early onset puerperal sepsis following a cesarean section).

The great majority of colonized neonates are asymptomatic, and diagnosis requires culture identification of GBS. In the neonate sampling should include the umbilicus, throat, external auditory canal, and rectum. The symptomatic neonatal infections are divided into early and late onset, and the clinical manifestations have

been described above. None of the clinical manifestations of neonatal disease is sufficient to diagnose GBS disease in the absence of a positive culture. In the neonate a diagnosis of GBS should be suspected when these clinical manifestations occur in association with a gram stain of amniotic fluid, gastric aspirate, or tracheal aspirate, which has a predominance of gram-positive cocci.

Despite appropriate concern over the emergence of the GBS as a significant pathogen for neonatal sepsis and meningitis and the postulated role for this organism in the etiology of PROM and preterm labor and delivery, controversy exists over the need for routine screening of all prenatal patients for GBS. In fact, the general consensus is that such a practice is not appropriate. Rather, efforts have focused on two alternate approaches. First an attempt has been made to perform selective maternal culturing for GBS. Pasnick et al noted that all their cases of early onset GBS infection occurred with a maternal history of preterm onset of labor and/or PROM. Using these two criteria they could limit their cultures to 13% of their obstetric population and thus decrease the ratio of infants at risk to infants actually infected from 100:1 to 20:1. Ideally, identification of genital tract GBS in women with PROM or preterm labor would facilitate attempts at prevention of neonatal GBS infection, early treatment of fetuses at risk for intrauterine acquisition of GBS, and alerting the pediatricians to the possibility of GBS infection. In addition, it would simplify the economic and logistic problems associated with universal routine GBS screening.

However, this selective approach is only practical if the second approach, methods of rapid diagnosis, becomes widely available. Several rapid diagnostic tests have been developed to make a presumptive diagnosis based on detection of group B or type-specific polysaccharide antigens in serum urine or spinal fluid by means of monoclonal antibodies or hyperimmune antisera (65). To date the tests shown to have clinical potential include countercurrent immunoelectrophoresis, latex particle agglutination, staphylococcal coagglutination, and enzyme immunoassay (3). In the neonate, concentrated urine is the specimen most likely to be positive. Screening of prenatal patients for genital tract colonization must await development of rapid and accurate diagnostic tests that can be performed on vaginal and/or cervical specimens.

TREATMENT AND PREVENTION OF GROUP B STREPTOCOCCAL INFECTION

Penicillin remains the drug of choice for symptomatic GBS infection in mother or neonate if the infecting organism has been identified. However, in most instances treatment must be empirically begun prior to the availability of culture results. Maternal infections such as amnionitis or postpartum endomyometritis tend to be polymicrobic in nature with aerobic and anaerobic bacteria present. Thus, treatment of these infections requires a broad spectrum approach as discussed in Chapter 9. In these instances, a broader spectrum approach for empirically treating the mother is required. Ampicillin is a frequently used and very effective agent in such situations and provides adequate treatment for GBS. The new semisynthetic penicillins (piperacillin, mezlocillin, ticarcillin) and first and second generation cephalosporins have very good in vitro activity. Erythromycin and clindamycin also provide very good coverage. However, a high degree of resistance occurs with tetracyclines. Although GBS are resistant to aminoglycosides, addition of gentamicin or tobramycin to one of the penicillins results in a synergistic action against GBS. Because ampicillin is capable of crossing meninges into the CSF, the most common pediatric recommendation for GBS neonatal infection is an ampicillin-aminoglycoside combination.

Among the multitude of new third generation cephalosporins, cefotaxime has activity against GBS comparable to penicillin G. However, moxalactam is much less active against GBS than penicillin G. Cefoperazone and ceftazidime have activity that falls in between that of cefoxtamine and moxalactam (66).

As a result of the severity of early and late onset GBS neonatal infection and the recognition that the major method of pathogenesis is vertical transmission, major efforts have been addressed to prophylactic administration of antibiotics to gravid women whose genital tracts are colonized with GBS (Table 13.12). To date studies in the literature suggest that attempts at reducing maternal carrier rates are generally unsuccessful (67–70) (Table 5). Hall and associates noted that administration of ampicillin to gravid women with cervical colonization of GBS resulted in a significant decreased colonization rate within 3 weeks of therapy, but the women treated were often recolonized by the time of parturition (67). In addition, the infants of the treated mothers were colonized at the same rate as the control infants. Gardner et al demonstrated that oral penicillin treatment of couples in the early third trimester was not an effective means of reducing maternal colonization at the time of delivery (68). They noted that at the time of delivery 67% of the treated group were colonized which did not differ significantly from the 63% incidence of persistent colonization at delivery in the untreated controls. Lewin and Amstey treated the pregnant woman and her partner in the third trimester with an injection of 1.2 million units benzathine penicillin G plus 1.2 million units procaine penicillin G (69). Although they noted a significant reduction in GBS colonization at delivery in the treated group compared to the untreated control group, 18% of the treated mothers were positive at delivery.

To circumvent the problem of a high percentage of reacquisition of GBS following attempted prophylaxis in the early third trimester, Merenstein and co-workers evaluated the efficacy of an oral penicillin regimen at 38 weeks of gestation (70). They noted a significant reduction in maternal and infant colonization with GBS in the treatment group (mothers and sexual partners treated). However, this approach misses the group at greatest risk, the preterm pregnancy where neonatal mortality with GBS infection is much greater.

The attempt at prophylaxis against GBS is hindered by several factors. Venereal transmission of GBS allows for reinfection. Secondly, it is difficult to eradicate GBS from the rectum because of the betalactamase enzymes (which inactivate pencillin and ampicillin) produced by the Enterobacteriaceae in this locale. Thirdly, the high ratio of maternal and neonatal colonization to infection requires that 100 women (plus their sexual partners) must be treated for each possible case of GBS infection. Such widespread use of penicillins and ampicillin imposes a risk for severe allergic reactions to these drugs.

Table 13.12
Effect of Antibiotic Prophylaxis in Maternal Carriers of Group B *Streptococcus*

Study	Method used for prophylaxis	Treatment group		Placebo group	
		Mother	Newborn	Mother	Newborn
Hall et al (67)	Third trimester: oral ampicillin for 7 days[a]	8/15	6/21	13/16	10/24
Gardner et al (68)	Third trimester: oral penicilin[a]	27/40		12/19	
Lewin and Amstey (69)	Third trimester: bicillin 1.2 million units plus procaine penicilin G 1.2 million units IM[a]	2/11	1/11	9/12	4/12
Merenstein et al (70)	Oral penicillin q.i.d. 38 weeks to delivery[a]	0/19	0/20	12/22	8/24
Yow et al (71)	Intrapartum IV ampicillin	34/34	0/34	24/24	14/24
Allardice et al (72)	Intrapartum IV ampicillin	28/28	3/28 0/28[b]	136/136	62/136 9/136[b]
Boyer et al (37)	Intrapartum IV ampicillin		1/43[c] 1/31[d] 7/46[e]		13/37[c] 80/327[d] 43/96[e]

[a] Partners also treated.
[b] Infection with GBS.
[c] Randomized trial.
[d] Nonrandomized, no risk factor.
[e] Nonrandomized, preterm labor, prolonged ROM, intrapartum fever.

Finally, the sporadic nature of GBS colonization of the vagina, with spontaneous clearing and recolonization in combination with failure to document eradication of the GBS from the genital tract with antibiotic prophylaxis suggests that maternal antepartum treatment is not the proper approach to prevent GBS neonatal disease.

More recently attempts to prevent vertical transmission of GBS infection have focused on the use of intrapartum antimicrobial treatment. Yow and colleagues reported that the use of intravenous ampicillin (500 mg/dose) during the intrapartum period in GBS-positive mothers prevented neonatal GBS colonization and disease (71). Although this was not a prospective, randomized, and controlled study, the authors recommended routine screening of all pregnant women at 34–36 weeks of gestation and intrapartum ampicillin for all GBS-positive parturients. Allardice and co-workers in Canada confirmed the efficacy of intrapartum ampicillin in preventing vertical transmission of GBS from colonized mothers to neonates (72). Once again such an approach fails to provide prophylaxis for neonates born at less than 34 weeks. Also it requires large numbers (10–35%) of pregnant women to receive parenteral penicillins and

thus be exposed to their potential adverse reactions. Boyer and co-workers have suggested a practical and interesting approach to the use of intrapartum ampicillin for prevention of neonatal early onset GBS sepsis (35–37). They reported that increased attack rates for GBS infection were associated with birth weights <2500 g, prolonged ROM, and intrapartum maternal fever. Forty-five (74%) of the 61 affected infants and 15 (94%) of the 16 neonates with fatal outcome had one or more of these maternal risk factors (36). In addition, these workers reported that 67% of prenatal GBS carriers retained carriage at delivery, while only 8% of women with negative prenatal cultures acquired carriage by the time of delivery (35). Finally, Boyer et al examined the effect of intrapartum ampicillin treatment on vertical transmission of GBS (37). Ampicillin virtually eliminated vertical transmission of GBS in the treatment group without perinatal risk factors and in the treatment groups with premature labor and/or prolonged ruptured membranes. GBS colonization occurred in the neonates born to women with intrapartum fever or less than 1 hr of ampicillin treatment prior to delivery. Thus, combining a single antepartum screening culture for GBS with intrapartum intravenous ampicillin treatment for mothers with suspected amnionitis, preterm labor, and/or PROM who are GBS carriers would result in a significant reduction in the vertical transmission of GBS from mother to infant.

Additional attempts to antibiotic prophylaxis have focused on the neonate itself. Steigman and co-workers reported that at Mt. Sinai Hospital not a single case of early onset GBS disease was seen in over 132,000 deliveries since 1952 (73). At Mt. Sinai a single intrasmuscular injection of 50,000 units of aqueous penicillin is routinely given at birth for the prevention of gonococcal opthalmia; they hypothesized that their lack of GBS disease was a "fringe benefit" of this policy. Such an observation was surprising in view of the report by Paredes which documented the failure of penicillin to eradicate the carrier state of GBS in neonates (74). However, Siegel's prospective study on more than 18,000 infants supports the Mt. Sinai hypothesis (45). Single IM injections of aqueous penicillin were given within 60 min of delivery to over 9,000 infants. The control group consisted of over 9,000 infants who received topical tetracycline for the prevention of gonococcal opthalmia. The incidence of GBS colonization fell from 11% to 4% in full-term infants, and from 12 to 1% in prematures. The incidence of early onset GBS disease fell from 1.29/1000 in the control group, to 0.11/1000 in the penicillin-treated group. In the initial study year there was a slight, but significant, increase in mortality from penicillin-resistant organisms in the penicillin-treated group. The later finding has not persisted in the subsequent study years. Similarly, Lloyd et al demonstrated that penicillin prophylaxis in neonates less than 2500 g reduced the colonization rate and the attack rate of GBS (48). In addition, they noted no increase in the mortality rate from other infections.

The major drawback to this approach is the recent recognition that the overwhelming majority of neonates with early onset GBS sepsis are bacteremic at birth or within 1 hr of delivery (18, 36, 60). Although a single injection of penicillin can sterilize a blood culture, it is not adequate therapy for bacteremia. Pyati et al provided excellent data suggesting that effective prophylaxis against GBS infection must be aimed at prevention of vertical transmission from mother rather than targeting the neonate at birth (60). In this study, infants were randomized to receive 50,000 units of penicillin G within 90 min of birth and every 12 hr for 72 hr or only

routine new born care. In the treatment group of 589 infants, there were 10 with GBS bacteremia, and 6 of these died. There were 14 cases of GBS bacteremia with 8 (57%) deaths among the 598 control patients. Most importantly bacteremia was present in 90% of treated and 86% of controls. Very clearly this study demonstrates that penicillin prophylaxis in the neonate is ineffective at preventing bacteremia or reducing the mortality rate.

Baker and Edwards recommended that chemoprophylaxis should be routinely considered for the nonaffected sibling of a twin with early onset GBS disease and for the pregnant woman who has delivered a previous infant with GBS disease (3).

The final approach to prevention relates to attempts at purifying the type-specific group B streptococcal antigens and then measuring maternal antibodies. In those mothers who are colonized but have a deficiency in antibody levels, vigorous antibiotic therapy would be instituted. Alternately, development of a vaccine would allow development of maternal antibodies which would be passively transferred to protect the fetus and neonate.

At the present time, we do not recommend routine screening for GBS in gravid patients. In women with PROM or preterm labor, cultures for GBS should be obtained. The colonized mother with PROM or gestation less than 37 weeks should receive intravenous ampicillin 1 g every 6 hr intrapartum. Such a regimen results in therapeutic levels in the fetus, and adequate levels can be detected in the neonate for about 8 hr following delivery; additionally, this approach has been shown to be effective at preventing vertical transmission and limits therapy to the high risk group for early onset GBS sepsis.

Listeriosis

Listeriosis is an infection caused by *Listeria monocytogenes*, a motile, microaerophilic, non-spore-forming, gram-positive bacillus. Maternal infection may lead to preterm labor and fetal infection. High perinatal morbidity and mortality rates are associated with listeriosis (1–5).

EPIDEMIOLOGY

The epidemiology of *Listeria* infections is poorly understood (1, 2, 5). Based on serologic testing, four serovars of *L. monocytogenes* have been identified. In the United States and Canada the majority of isolates are serovar IVb. Similar to group B streptococcal infection, neonatal listeriosis has been divided into two serologically and clinically distinct entities (2).

Early onset listeriosis is most commonly associated with serotypes Ia and IVb. This form is a diffuse sepsis with pulmonary, hepatic, and central nervous system involvement. The stillbirth rate and neonatal mortality rate are very high. *Listeria* of the early onset type tends to occur in low birth weight babies. Early onset disease is much more common in Europe than in the United States (2).

Late onset listeriosis manifests as meningitis and is associated with serotype IVb. The neonates are normal birth weight and usually are born to mothers with uneventful prenatal courses. Forty percent of late onset disease infants die, and hydrocephaly and/or mental retardation are not uncommon sequelae (6).

Reiss et al have described the pathogenesis of *Listeria* infection in neonates (7). They proposed that maternal infection results in placental infection which leads to fetal septicemia and multiorgan involvement in the fetus. Amniotic fluid becomes infected with *L. monocytogenes* secondary to excretion of the organism in fetal urine. Aspiration and swallowing of infected amniotic fluid results in respiratory tract involvement in the infection. Alternately, an ascending route of infection from cervical colonization with *L. monocytogenes* (even across intact membranes) has been proposed (1).

CLINICAL PRESENTATION

MATERNAL INFECTION

Unfortunately, no specific clinical manifestations exist which distinguish listeriosis from other infectious diseases that occur during pregnancy. Many pregnant women with *Listeria* remain asymptomatic. When symptomatic they present with a flu-like syndrome characterized by fever, chills, malaise, myalgias, back pain, and upper respiratory complaints. In general, maternal infection is mild and innocuous. Rarely, maternal infection is associated with diffuse sepsis.

NEONATAL INFECTION

With early onset *Listeria* infection the neonate is severely ill at or shortly after birth (1–3, 5). The infant presents with severe respiratory distress, cyanosis, and hypothermia. A papular skin rash and/or purulent conjunctivitis may occur. However, unlike GBS, neonates with early onset *Listeria* pneumonia do not have radiologic resemblance to hyaline membrane disease (3).

The late onset form of *Listeria* usually affects healthy, term infants. These infants develop meningitis between 1 to 6 weeks after delivery. Clinically, *Listeria* meningitis presents a picture similar to that seen with any bacterial meningitis of the newborn.

DIAGNOSIS

Because neonatal *Listeria* infection (both early and late onset) is associated with a high mortality rate, clinicians must maintain a high index of suspicion that any febrile illness in pregnancy may well be listeriosis. In such instances, cervical and blood cultures should be promptly obtained for *L. monocytogenes*. It is critical to communicate with the microbiologist that *Listeria* is a concern; colonies of *L. monocytogenes* can be easily mistaken for diptheroids and ignored. A gram stain revealing gram-positive pleomorphic rods with rounded ends is very suggestive of *L. monocytogenes*.

Serologic testing is available for the diagnosis of *Listeria*. These include agglutination reactions, complement fixation (CF), fluorescent antibody test (FA), indirect hemagglutination test, and ELISA (5).

MANAGEMENT

Although penicillin G and ampicillin are usually effective in vivo, current opinion holds that optimum therapy against *L. monocytogenes* is a combination regimen of ampicillin plus an aminoglycoside (8). Maternal treatment consists of ampicillin (1–2 g IV, every 4–6 hr) and gentamicin (2 mg/kg IV every 8 hr). For the newborn, the ampicillin dosage is 200–300 mg/kg/day administered in 4–6 divided doses. Treatment is given for 3 weeks.

PROTOZOA

Toxoplasmosis

Toxoplasmosis is a widely distributed illness, caused by *Toxoplasma gondii*, an intracellular parasite. Knowledge of the disease's natural history, diagnosis, treatment, and prevention are necessary for the obstetrician because of the impact of this disease on the fetus.

EPIDEMIOLOGY

Although *T. gondii* is found in many mammalian species, the cat is the only definitive host. This parasite may exist in three forms (trophozoite, cyst, or oocyst). Trophozoites are the invasive forms, and the cysts are the latent forms. The oocysts are found only in cats. Human infection may be acquired by consuming raw or undercooked meat of infected animals (especially mutton and lamb) or by contact with oocysts from the feces of an infected cat. The oocysts may be spread to humans or to food by hand or by insects. Cats acquire toxoplasmosis by eating infected mice or other animals. Oocysts in cat feces do not become infective for 4–5 days. Once infected by oocysts from cat feces or by cysts from infected meat, persons may experience a parasitemia during which fetal involvement may occur. Later, *T. gondii* cysts appear in tissues, especially striated muscle and brain, where they persist indefinitely.

Among pregnant women, serologic evidence of past infection with *T. gondii* is present commonly. In New York and Alabama, the prevalence of *Toxoplasma* antibodies was 20–40% (1), while in Paris the prevalence was 84% (2).

Seroconversion during pregnancy was noted in approximately 2/1000 pregnant women in New York in the early 1970s (1). In Alabama in the 1980s, maternal toxoplasmosis was noted in only 0.06%, a marked decrease from the 0.6% rate noted in the same area a decade earlier. In Oslo, Norway, the rate of seroconversion is 2/1000 pregnancies (3), while in Paris the rate of seroconversion among young married women was higher (10/1000 per year). Note that the rates in Paris are expressed as cases per year not per pregnant women.

Earlier data had indicated that when primary toxoplasmosis was acquired during pregnancy, there was approximately a one-third chance of fetal infection. Of those fetuses infected, one-third again had clinically detectable illness, and two-thirds had subclinical disease (4, 5). However, a reanalysis of expanded data by Desmonts and Couvreur has revealed a change in distribution. Of 145 women with acquired toxoplasmosis in pregnancy (without spiramycin treatment), 85 (59%) gave birth to congenitally infected infants. Of these 85 infants, 64 (75%) had subclinical infection (5). The rate of fetal infection is higher when maternal infection occurs in the third trimester than when it occurs in the second or first trimester (59% versus 29% versus 19%), but the *severity* of fetal infection is greater when maternal infection occurs in the first trimester (6). Among 126 women with first trimester toxoplasmosis, 8 had children with clinical disease (7 severe, 1 mild); and there were 6 perinatal deaths (total clinical disease of 11%). Among 128 women with third trimester toxoplasmosis, 8 had children with clinical disease (all mild), and there were no perinatal deaths (total clinical disease of 4.5%) (6). In Alabama, the incidence of congenital toxoplasmosis decreased in the last decade from 1/1000 to 1/8500 less births. Congenital infection does not affect more than one infant in a particular mother (6). The role of toxoplasmosis in chronic abortion remains unresolved after 20 yr of study.

DIAGNOSIS

Subclinical disease is the rule with toxoplasmosis. When it is apparent clinically in a normal host, the most common manifestation is lymphadenopathy (most commonly cervical). Fever, fatigue, sore throat, maculopapular rash, and occasionally hepatosplenomegaly may also be noted. Examination of the peripheral blood shows lymphocytosis or an occasional atypical lymphocyte. According, this disease is often thought to be "flu" or infectious mononucleosis. An occasional adult may have mainly ocular symptoms including haziness of vision, pain, and photophobia. In these cases, opthalmologic examination shows clusters of yellow-white patches in the optic fundus, representative of a focal necrotizing retinochoroiditis. In healthy adults, clinical toxoplasmosis is mild and self-limited; only in immunosuppressed individuals does it lead to serious pulmonary or central nervous system involvement.

As noted, most infants with congenital toxoplasmosis have only serologic abnormalities. Of those with clinical disease, few have the commonly suggested triad of intracerebral calcifications, chorioretinitis, and hydrocephaly in the past. Rather, common findings in symptomatic infants were chorioretinitis (80%), abnormal spinal fluid (69%), anemia (64%), splenomegaly (56%), jaundice (54%), fever (51%), lymphadenopathy (43%), convulsions (34%), and vomiting (32%). Thus, there is wide spectrum of disease. Acute, primary toxoplasmosis in pregnancy has also been associated with abortion, prematurity, and growth retardation.

Serologic techniques are used mainly to confirm toxoplasmosis. IgG antibodies are detected by the indirect fluorescent-antibody test, Sabin-Feldman dye test, indirect hemagglutination inhibition test, and complement fixation test (7). Acute infection is diagnosed by a serial two-tube (i.e., four-fold) rise in titer of any of these tests, but as with rubella the specimens should be tested in parallel. Titers resulting from recent infection nearly always rise to >1:512 or 1:1000 with the indirect fluorescent-antibody and the dye tests. These antibodies peak within 1–2 months of the onset of infection, and low titers persist for years.

IgM antibodies may be detected by an indirect fluorescent-antibody technique. They appear within a week and usually last for a few months.

For pregnant patients with possible exposure, Krick and Remington advise use of IgM indirect fluorescent-antibody test when the IgG test (conventional indirect fluorescent-antibody or dye test) is positive at any titer (7). The combination of a negative IgM with an IgG test of >1:1000 suggests remote infection. Conventional (IgG) and IgM indirect fluorescent-antibody tests are available at the Centers for Disease Control through state laboratories.

Histologic techniques for diagnosis may be used in some circumstances (e.g., lymph node biopsy), but in general these are too cumbersome for widespread detection.

PREVENTION

To prevent toxoplasmosis in pregnancy, most authorites advise: (a) avoiding undercooked meat; (b) handwashing after handling a cat, especially before eating; (c) having someone else change the litterbox daily; (d) not permitting indoor cats to go outside, where they may attack an infected mouse; (e) not allowing stray cats in the house; and (f) not feeding raw meat to cats. Based on their data in Alabama, Hunter and colleagues did not favor routine serologic screening programs in view of the expense of screening large numbers of women who are susceptible and the low attack rate. Alternatively, patient education is recommended by Frenkel (8). Wilson and Remington, however, note that regional programs are needed in the United States to provide data pertinent in this country (9).

TREATMENT

For women with confirmed first trimester toxoplasmosis, the physician should offer counseling regarding the risk of serious congenital infection and regarding pregnancy termination.

In the United States, the only effective medical therapy is a combination of sulfadiazine (or triple sulfonamide) with pyrimethamine. Because of marrow toxicity of this regimen, folinic acid or baking yeast should be given as well. Spiramycin has been used extensively in Europe but is not available in the United States. Based on studies in France, treatment of primary toxoplasmosis in pregnancy with spiramycin decreases, but does not eliminate, the risk of congenital infection in the fetus. In a study of 542 women with acquired toxoplasmosis in pregnancy, 77% of those treated versus 39% of those without treatment gave birth to uninfected infants. Further, clinically infected infants accounted for 5% of those born to women with treatment and for 14% of those born to women without treatment (6). However, in the United States, there has been no agreement on treatment in pregnancy to control fetal infection. Those who emphasize the lack of efficacy studies and the teratogenicity of pyrimethamine have concluded that pregnant women should not be treated except in the rare instance of serious maternal disease. Others would avoid pyrimethamine, but use sulfadiazine in women with first trimester toxoplasmosis if the mother does not choose abortion.

All authorities agree that symptomatic infants with congenital toxoplasmosis should be treated with sulfadiazine, pyrimethamine, and folinic acid supplementation. Details of the treatment regimens are available (6). In the infant with asymptomatic toxoplasmosis at birth, late central nervous sequelae are possible. Thus, some treat all newborns with toxoplasmosis, and others suggest treatment of newborns with proved toxoplasmosis of abnormal cerebrospinal fluid examination.

References

Rubella

1. Centers for Disease Control: Rubella and congenital rubella—United States, 1980–1983. *MMWR* 32:505, 1983.
2. Miller E, Cradock-Watson JE, Pollock TM: Consequences of confirmed maternal rubella at successive stages of pregnancy. *Lancet* 2:781–1982.
3. Centers for Disease Control: Rubella prevention. *MMWR* 30:37, 1981.
4. Polk BF, White JA, DeGirolomi PC, et al: An outbreak of rubella among hospital personnel. *N Engl J Med* 703:541, 1980.
5. Centers for Disease Control: Rubella in hospitals—California. *MMWR* 32:37, 1983.

Genital Herpes Infection in Pregnancy

1. Corey L: The diagnosis and treatment of genital herpes *JAMA* 248:1041, 1982.

2. Genital herpes infection—United States, 1966–1979. *MWR* 31:137, 1982.
3. Bolognese RJ, Cosen SL, Fuccillo DA, et al: Herpes virus hominis type II infections in asymptomatic pregnant women. *Obstet Gynecol* 48:507, 1976.
4. Tejani N, Klein SW, Kaplan M: Subclinical herpes simplex genitalis infections in the perinatal period. *Am J Obstet Gynecol* 135:547, 1979.
5. Scher J, Bottone E, Desmond, E, Simons, W: The incidence and outcome of asymptomatic herpes simplex genitalis in an obstetric population. *Am J Obstet Gynecol* 144:906, 1982.
6. Nahmias AJ, Roczman, B: Infection with herpes simplex virus I and II. *N Engl J Med* 289:781, 1973.
7. Whitley RJ, Nahmias AJ, Visintine AM, et al: The natural history of herpes simplex virus infection of mother and newborn. *Pediatrics* 66:489, 1980.
8. Sever JL, Larsen JW, Grossman JH: *Handbook of Perinatal Infections.* Boston. Little Brown, 1979.
9. Amstey MS, Monif GR: Genital herpes virus infection in pregnancy. *Obstet Gynecol* 44:394, 1974.
10. Nahmias AJ, Josey WE, Naib ZM, et al: Perinatal risk associated with maternal genital herpes simplex virus infection. *Am J Obstet Gynecol* 110:825, 1971.
11. Adam E, Kaufman RH, Mirkovic RR, et al: Persistence of virus shedding in asymptomatic women after recovery from herpes genitalis. *Obstet Gynecol* 54:171, 1979.
12. Reeves WC, Corey L, Adams H, et al: Risk of recurrence after first episodes of genital herpes. *N Engl J Med* 305:315, 1981.
13. Corey L, Nahmias AJ, Guinan ME, et al: A trial of topical acyclovir in genital herpes simplex virus infections. *N Engl J Med* 306:1313, 1982.
14. Hirsch MS, Schooley RT: Treatment of herpes virus infections. *N Engl J Med* 309:1034, 1983.
15. Mindel A, Adler MW, et al: Intravenous acyclovir treatment for primary genital herpes. *Lancet* 1982:697.
16. Bryso YJ, Dillon M, Lovett M, et al: Treatment of first episodes of genital herpes simplex virus infection with oral acyclovir. *N Engl J Med* 308:916, 1983.
17. Douglas J, Critchlow D, Benedetti J, et al: Trial of prophylactic oral acyclovir for frequent recurrences of genital herpes. Efficacy and long-term followup. 23rd Interscience Conference on Antimicrobial Agents and Chemotherapy, October, 1983, Las Vegas, abstracts no. 561.
18. Larsen T, Dillon M, Goldman L, et al: Double-blind, placebo-controlled study of acyclovir prophylaxis in frequently recurrent genital herpes simplex virus infection. 23rd Interscience Conference on Antimicrobial Agents and Chemotherapy, October 1983, Las Vegas, abstract no. 562.
19. Wise TG, Pavan PR, evans FA: Herpes simplex virus vaccines. *J Infect Dis* 136:706, 1977.
20. Mertz GJ: Western Society for Clinical Investigation. Medical World News. March 14, 1983. Carmel, CA, 1983.
21. Amstey MS: Management of pregnancy complicated by genital herpes virus infection. *Obstet Gynecol* 37:515, 1971.
22. Grossman JH, Wallen WC, Sever JL: Management of genital herpes simplex virus infection during pregnancy. *Obstet Gynecol* 58:1, 1981.
23. Boehm FH, Estes W, Wright PF, Growdon JF: Management of genital herpes simplex virus infection occurring during pregnancy. *Am J Obstet Gynecol* 141:735, 181.
24. Harger JH, Pazin GJ, Armstrong JA, Breinig MC, et al: Characteristics and management of pregnancy in women with genital herpes simplex virus infection. *Am J Obstet Gynecol* 145:784, 1983.
25. Block BSB, Goodner DM: False-positive amniotic fluid cytology in a parturient with active genital herpes infection at term. *Obstet Gynecol* 54:658, 1979.
26. Zervoudakis IA, Silverman F, Senterfit LB, et al: Herpes simplex in the amniotic fluid of an unaffected fetus. *Obstet Gynecol* 55:16S, 1980.
27. Goldkrand JW: Intrapartum inoculation of herpes simplex virus by fetal scalp electrode. *Obstet Gynecol* 59:263, 1982.
28. Kibrick S: Herpes simplex infection at term. What to do with mother, newborn, and nursery personnel. *JAMA* 253:157, 1980.

Cytomegalovirus

1. Hanshaw JB: Congenital cytomegalovirus infection: a 15 year prospective study. *J Infect Dis* 123:555–561, 1971.
2. Hanshaw JB: Cytomegalovirus. In Remington JS, Klein JO (eds): *Infectious Diseases of the Fetus and Newborn Infant.* Philadelphia, WB Saunders, 1983, pp 104–142.
3. Hanshaw JB, Scheiner AP, Moxley AW, et al: School failure and deafness after "silent" congenital cytomegalovirus. *N Engl J Med* 295:468–470, 1976.
4. Hunter K, Stagno S, Capps E, Smith RJ: Prenatal screening of pregnant women for infections caused by cytomegalovirus, Epstein-Barr virus, herpesvirus, rubella and *Toxoplasma gondii.* *Am J Obstet Gynecol* 145:269, 1983.
5. Stern J, Tucker SM: Prospective study of cytomegalovirus infection in pregnancy. *Br Med J* 2:268, 1973.
6. Monif GRG, Egan EA, Held B, et al: The correlation of maternal cytomegalovirus infection during varying stages in gestation and neonatal involvement. *J Pediatr* 80:17, 1972.
7. Reynolds DW, Stagno S, Stubbs KG, et al: Inapparent congenital cytomegalovirus infection with elevated cord IgM levels: causal relation with auditory and mental deficiency. *N Engl J Med* 290:291, 1974.
8. Dworsky ME, Welch K, Cassady G, Stagno S: Occupational risk for primary cytomegalovirus infection among pediatric health care workers. *N Engl J Med* 309:950, 1983.

Hepatitis

1. Bayer ME, Blumberg BS, Werner B: Particles associated with Australia antigen in the sera of patients with leukemia, Down's syndrome, and hepatitis. *Nature* 218:1057–1059, 1968.
2. Dane DS, Cameron CH, Briggs M: Virus-like particles in serum of patients with Australia antigen-

associated hepatitis. *Lancet* 1:695–698, 1970.
3. Crumpacker CS: Hepatitis. In Remington JS, Klein JO (eds): *Infectious Diseases of the Fetus and Newborn*. Philadelphia, WB Saunders, 1983, pp 591–618.
4. Nielsen JO, Dietrichson O, Juhl E: Incidence and meaning of the "e" determinant among hepatitis B antigen positive patients with acute and chronic liver disease. *Lancet* 2:913–915, 1974.
5. Fay O, Tanno H, Roncoroni M, et al: Prognostic implications of the "e" antigen of hepatitis B virus. *JAMA* 238:2501–2503, 1977.
6. Alter HJ, Seeff LB, Kaplen PM, et al: Type B hepatitis: the infectivity of blood positive for "e" antigen and DNA polymerase after accidental needle stick exposure. *N Engl J Med* 295:909–913, 1976.
7. Okada K, Kamiyama, I, Inomata M, et al: "e" antigen and anti-e in the serum of asymptomatic carrier mothers as indicators of positive and negative transmission of hepatitis B virus to their infants. *N Engl J Med* 294:746–749, 1976.
8. Provost PJ, Wolanski BS, Miller WJ: Physical, chemical and morphologic dimensions of human hepatitis A virus. *Proc Soc Exp Biol Med* 148:532–536, 1975.
9. Denhardt F: Predictive value of markers of hepatitis virus infection. *J Infect Dis* 141:299–305, 1980.
10. Tabor E, Geraty RJ, Dickes JA, et al: Transmission of non-A, non-B hepatitis from man to chimpanzee. *Lancet* 1:463–466, 1978.
11. Kabin M, TAbor E, Gerety RJ: Antigen-antibody system associated with non-A, non-B hepatitis detected by indirect immunofluorescence. *Lancet* 2:221–224, 1979.
12. Sever JL, Larsen JW Jr, Grossman JH III: *Handbook of Perinatal Infections*. Boston, Little, Brown, 1979, p 37–43.
13. Centers for Disease Control: Inactivated hepatitis B virus vaccine. Recommendations of the Immunization Practices Advisory Committee. *Ann Intern Med* 97:379–383, 1982.
14. Szmuness W: Hepatocellular carcinoma and the hepatitis B virus: evidence for a causal association. *Prog Med Virol* 24:40, 1978.
15. Schweitzer IL, Dunn AEG, Peters RL, Spears RL: Viral hepatitis B in neonates and infants. *Am J Med* 55:762–771, 1973.
16. Schweitzer IL, Mosley JW, Aschcavai M, et al: Factors influencing neonatal infection by hepatitis B virus. *Gastroenterology* 65:277–283, 1973.
17. Stevens CE, Beasley RP, Tsui J, Lee WC: Vertical transmission of hepatitis B antigen in Taiwan. *N Engl J Med* 292:771–774, 1975.
18. Okada K, Yamada T, Miyakawa, Mayumi M: Hepatitis B surface antigen in the serum of infants after delivery from asymptomatic carrier mothers. *J Pediatr* 87:360–363, 1975.
19. Derso A, Boxall EH, Tarlow MJ, Flewett TH: Transmission of HBsAg from mother to infant in four ethnic groups. *Br Med J* 1:949, 1978.
20. Skinhoj P, Sardemann H, Cohen J: Hepatitis associated antigen (HAA) in pregnant women and their newborn infants. *Am J Dis Child* 123:380–381, 1972.
21. Papaevangelou GJ: Hepatitis B in infants. *N Engl J Med* 288:972–975, 1973.
22. Stevens CE, Neurath RA, Beasley RP, Szmuness W: HBeAg and anti-HBe detection by radioimmunoassay: correlation with vertical transmission of hepatitis B virus in Taiwan. *J Med Virol* 3:237, 1979.
23. Lee AKY, Ip HMH, Wong VCW: Mechanisms of maternal-fetal transmission of Hepatitis B virus. *J Infect D* 138:668–671, 1978.
24. Beasley P, Trapco C, Stevens CE, Szmuness W: The "e" antigen and vertical transmission of hepatitis B surface antigen. *Am J Epidemiol* 105:94–98, 1977.
25. Barin F, Goudeau A, Denis F, et al: Immune response in neonates to hepatitis B vaccine. *Lancet* 1:251–253, 1982.
26. Favero MS: Guidelines for the care of patients hospitalized with viral hepatitis. *Ann Intern Med* 91:872–, 1979.
27. Oxman MN, Richman DD, Spector SA: Management at delivery of mother and infant when herpes simplex, varicella-zoster, hepatitis, or tuberculosis have occurred during pregnancy. In Remington JS, Swartz MN (eds): *Current Clinical Topics in Infectious Diseases*. New York, McGraw Hill, 1983, pp 224–280.

Varicella-Zoster Virus

1. Charles D: Infections. In: *Infections in Obstetrics and Gynecology*. Philadelphia, WB Saunders, 1980, pp 162–166.
2. Young NA, Gershon AA: Chicken pox, measles, and mumps. In Remington JS, Klein JO (eds): *Infectious Diseases of the Fetus and Newborn*. Philadelphia, WB Saunders, 1983, pp 375–402.
3. Centers for Disease Control: Annual summary 1982. Reported morbidity and mortality in the United States. *MMWR* 31:21–22, 1983.
4. Hermmann KL: Congenital and perinatal varicella. *Clin Obstet Gynecol* 25:605–609, 1982.
5. Preblud SR, D'Angelo LJ: Chickenpox in the United States 1972–1977. *J Infect Dis* 140:257–, 1979.
6. Sever J, White LR: Intrauterine viral infections. *Annu Rev Med* 19:471, 1968.
7. Siegel M, Fuerst HT: Low birth weight and maternal virus disease. A prospective study of rubella, measles, mumps, chickenpox, and hepatitis. *JAMA* 197:88–1966.
8. Christie AB: Chickenpox. In Christie AB (ed): *Infectious Diseases. Epidemiology and Clinical Practice*. London, E and S Livingston, 1969, pp 238–255.
9. Pearson HE: Parturition varicella-zoster. *Obstet Gynecol* 32:21–27, 1964.
10. Brunell PA: Varicella-zoster infections in pregnancy. *JAMA* 199:315, 1967.
11. LaForet E, Lynch CL: Multiple congenital defects following maternal varicella. *N Engl J Med* 236:534–537, 1947.
12. Meyers JD: Congenital varicella in term infants: risk considered. *J Infect Dis* 129:215–217, 1974.
13. Weibel RE, Neff BJ, Kuter BJ, et al: Live attenuated varicella virus vaccine. Efficacy trial in healthy children. *N Engl J Med* 310:1409–1415, 1984.

Rubeola (Measles)

1. Hope-Simpson RE: Infectiousness of communicable diseases in the household (measles, mumps, and chicken pox). *Lancet* 2:549, 1952.
2. Centers for Disease Control: Annual Summary 1982: Reported morbidity and mortality in the United States. *MWR* 31:48–51, 1983.
3. Sever J, White LR: Intrauterine viral infection. *Annu Rev Med* 19:471–486, 1968.
4. Siegal M, Fuerst HT: Low birth weight and maternal virus diseases. A prospective study of rubella, measles, mumps, chicken pox, and hepatitis. *JAMA* 197:88, 1966.
5. Young NA, Gershon AA: Chicken pox, measles and mumps. In Remington JS, Klein JO (eds): *Infectious Diseases of the Fetus and Newborn Infant.* Philadelphia, WB Saunders, 1983, pp 375–427.
6. LaBoccetta AC, Tornay AS: Measles encephalitis. Report of 61 cases. *Am J Dis Child* 107:247, 1964.
7. Christensen PE, Schmidt H, Ban HO, et al: An epidemic of measles in Southern Greenland, 1951. Measles in virgin soil. II. The epidemic proper. *Acta Med Scand* 144:431–440, 1953.
8. Sever JL, Larsen JW Jr, Grossman JH III: *Handbook of Perinatal Infections.* Boston, Little, Brown, 1979, pp 63–64.
9. Siegel M: Congenital malformations following chicken pox, measles, mumps, and hepatitis. Results of a cohort study. *JAMA* 226:1521–1524, 1973.
10. Nouvat JR: Rougeole et grossesse. Thesis 113, Bourdeaux, 1904 (as described in Young NA, Gershan AA: Chicken pox, measles and mumps. In Remington JS, Klein JO (eds): *Infectious Diseases of the Fetus and Newborn Infants.* Philadelphia, WB Saunders, 1983, pp 375–427.
11. Dyer I: Measles complicating pregnancy. Report of 24 cases with 3 instances of congenital measles. *South Med J* 33:601, 1940.
12. Kohn JL: Measles in newborn infants (maternal infection). *J Pediatr* 3:176, 1933.
13. Richardson DL: Measles contracted in utero. *RI Med* 3:13, 1920.
14. American Academy of Pediatrics: Report of the Committee on Infectious Diseases, ed 17. Evanston, 1974, pp 74–82.

Mumps

1. Sever J, White LR: Intrauterine viral infections. *Annu Rev Med* 19:471–486, 1968.
2. Siegel M, Fuerst HT: Low birth weight and maternal virus diseases. A prospective study of rubella, measles, mumps, chicken pox, and hepatitis. *JAMA* 197:88, 1966.
3. Bowers D: Mumps during pregnancy. *West J Surg Obstet Gynecol* 61:72, 1953.
4. Schwartz HA: Mumps in pregnancy. *Am J Obstet Gynecol* 60:875, 1950.
5. Hardy JB: Viral infection in pregnancy. A review. *Am J Obstet Gynecol* 93:1052, 1965.
6. Siegal M, Fuerst HT, Peress NS: Comparative fetal mortality in maternal virus disease. A prospective study on rubella, measles, mumps, chicken pox, and hepatitis. *N Engl J Med* 274:768, 1966.

7. Siegal M: Congenital malformations following chicken pox, measles, mumps, and hepatitis. Results of a cohort study. *JAMA* 226:1521, 1973.
8. Noren GR, Adams P Jr, Anderson RC: Positive skin reactivity to mumps virus antigen in endocardial fibroelastosis. *J Pediatr* 62:604, 1963.
9. St. Gene JW, Jr, Noren GR, Adams P: Proposed embryopathic relation between mumps virus and primary endocardial fibroelactosis. *N Engl J Med* 275:339, 1966.
10. Vosburgh JB, Diehl AM, Liu C, et al: Relationship of mumps to endocardial fibroelastosis. *Am J Dis Child* 109:60, 1965.
11. St. Geme JW Jr, Peralta H, Farias E, et al: Experimental gestational mumps virus infection and anocardial fibroelastosis. *Pediatrics* 48:82, 1971.
12. Gersony WM, Katz SL, Nadas AS: Endocardial fibroelastosis and the mumps virus. *Pediatrics* 37:340, 1966.
13. Guneroth WG: Endocardial fibroelastosis and mumps. *Pediatrics* 38:309, 1966.
14. Nahmias AJ, Armstrong G: Mumps virus and endocardial fibroelastosis. *N Engl J Med* 275:1449, 1966.

Influenza

1. Sever JL, Larsen JW Jr, Grossman JH III: *Handbook of Perinatal Infections.* Boston, Little, Brown, 1980, pp 45–50.
2. Weinstein L: Influenza—1918: a revisit? *N Engl J Med* 294:1058–1060, 1976.
3. Bland PB: Influenza in relation to pregnancy and labor. *Am J Obstet Dis Woman* 79:184–197, 1919.
4. Harris JW: Influenza occurring in pregnant women. A statistical study of thirteen hundred and fifty cases. *JAMA* 72:978–980, 1919.
5. Finland M: Influenza complicating pregnancy. In Charles D, Finland M (eds): *Obstetrics and Perinatal Infections.* Philadelphia, Lea & Febiger, 1973, pp 355–398.
6. Freeman DW, Barno A: Deaths from Asian influenza associated with pregnancy. *Am J Obstet Gynecol* 78:1172–1175, 1959.
7. Coffey VP, Jessup WJE: Congenital abnormalities. *Ir J Med Sci* 349:30, 1955.
8. Coffey VP, Jessup WJE: Maternal influenza and congenital deformities: a prospective study. *Lancet* 2:935–938, 1959.
9. Doll RA, Hill AB, Sakula J: Asian influenza in pregnancy and congenital defects. *Br J Prev Soc Med* 14:167–172, 1960.
10. Hakosalo J, Saxen L: Influenza epidemic and congenital defects. *Lancet* 2:1346–1347, 1971.
11. Hardy JMB, Ararowicz EN, Mannini A, et al: The effect of Asian influenza on the outcome of pregnancy, Baltimore, 1957–58. *Am J Public Health* 51:1182–1188, 1961.
12. Griffiths PD, Ronalds CJ, Heath RB: A prospective study of influenza infections during pregnancy. *J Epidemiol Commun Health* 34:1224, 1980.
13. Wilsohn MG, Heins HL, Imagawa DT, et al: Teratogenic effects of Asian influenza. *JAMA* 171:638–641, 1959.
14. Elizan TS, Ajero-Froehlich L, Labiyi A, Ley A, Sever JL: Viral infection in pregnancy and congenital CNS malformations in man. *Arch Neurol* 20:115, 1969.

15. Brown GC: Maternal virus infection and congenital anomalies. A prospective study. *Arch Environ Health* 21:362, 1970.
16. Amantadine for high risk influenza. *Med Lett Drugs Ther* 20:25, 1978.
17. Larsen JW Jr: Influenza and pregnancy. *Clin Obstet Gynecol* 25:599–603, 1982.

Enteroviruses

1. Hanshaw JB, Dudgeon JA: *Viral Diseases of the Fetus and Newborn*. Philadelphia, WB Saunders, 1978, pp 182–191.
2. Cherry JD: Enteroviruses. In Remington JS, Klein JO (eds): *Infectious Diseases of the Fetus and Newborn Infant*. Philadelphia, WB Saunders, 1983, pp 290–334.
3. Cherry JD, Nelson DB: Enterovirus infections: their epidemiology and pathogenesis. *Clin Pediatr* 5:659, 1966.
4. Kibrick S: Current status of Coxsackie and ECHO viruses in human disease. *Prog Med Virol* 6:27, 1964.
5. Grist NR, Bell EJ, Assad F: Enteroviruses in human diseases. *Progr Med Virol* 24:114, 1978.
6. Cherry JD: Nonpolio enteroviruses: coxsackie viruses, echoviruses and enteroviruses. In Feign RD, Cherry JD (eds): *The Textbook of Pediatric Infectious Diseases*. Philadelphia, WB Saunders, 1981.
7. Hardy JB: Viral infections in pregnancy. A review. *Am J Obstet Gynecol* 93:1052, 1965.
8. Horstmann DM: Viral infections in pregnancy. *Yale J Biol Med* 42:99, 1969.
9. Horn P: Poliomyelitis in pregnancy. A twenty year report from Los Angeles County, California. *Obstet Gynecol* 6;121, 1955.
10. Bates T: Poliomyelitis in pregnancy, fetus and newborn. *Am J Dis Child* 90:189, 1955.
11. Siegel M, Greenberg M: Poliomyelitis in pregnancy: effect on fetus and newborn infant. *J Pediatr* 49:280, 1956.
12. Sever JL, Larsen JW Jr, Grossman JH III: Handbook of Perinatal Infections. Boston, Little, Brown, 1979, pp 64–66.
13. Brown GC, Karunas RS: Relationship of congenital anomalies and maternal infection with selected enteroviruses. *Am J Epidemiol* 95:207–217, 1972.
14. Kleinman H, Prince JT, Mathey WE, et al: ECHO 9 virus infection and congenital abnormalities: a negative report. *Pediatrics* 29:261–269, 1962.
15. Landsman JB, Grist NR, Ross CAC: ECHO 9 virus infection and congenital malformations. *Br J Prev Soc Med* 18:152–156, 1964.
16. Hughes J, Wilfert CM, Moore M, et al: ECHO virus 14 infection associated with fatal neonatal hepatic necrosis. *Am J Dis Child* 123:61–67, 1972.
17. Philip AGS, Larsen EJ: Overwhelming neonatal infection with ECHO 19 virus. *J Pediatr* 82:391–397, 1973.
18. Kibrick S, Benirschke K: Acute septic myocarditis and meningoencephalitis in the newborn child infected with Coxsackie virus group B, type 3. *N Engl J Med* 255:883–884, 1956.
19. Brightman VJ, Scott TFM, Westphal M, Boggs TR: An outbreak of Coxsackie B-5 virus infection in the newborn nursery. *J Pediatr* 69:179–192, 1966.

20. Benirschke K, Pendleton ME: Coxsackie virus infection. An important complication of pregnancy. *Obstet Gynecol* 12:305–309, 1958.
21. McLean DM, Donohue WL, Snelling CE, Wyllie JC: Coxsackie B-5 virus as a cause of neonatal encephalitis and myocarditis. *Can Med Assoc J* 85:1046, 1961.

Other Viruses

Western Equine Encephalitis

1. Cops SC, Giddings LE: Transplacental transmission of western equine encephalitis. Report of a case. *Pediatrics* 24:31–33, 1959.
2. Shinefield HR, Townsend TE: Transplacental transmission of western equine encephalomyelitis. *J Pediatr* 43:21–25, 1953.

Venezuelan Equine Encephalitis

1. Spertzel RO, Crabbs CL, Vaughn RE: Transplacental transmission of Venezuelan equine encephalomyelitis virus in mice. *Infect Immun* 6:339–343, 1972.
2. Wenger F: Venezuelan equine encephalitis. *Teratology* 16:369, 1977.

Bacteria

Syphilis

1. Centers for Disease Control: Annual summary 1982: Reported morbidity and mortality in the United States. *MWR* 31:77–82, 1983.
2. Centers for Disease Control: Syphilis trends in the United States. *MWR* 31:441–444, 1981.
3. Dippel AL: The relationship of congenital syphilis to abortion and miscarriage, and the mechanism of intrauterine protection. *Am J Obstet Gynecol* 47:369, 1944.
4. Fiumara NJ: Veneral disease. In Charles D, Finland M (eds): *Obstetric and Perinatal Infections*. Philadelphia, Lea & Febiger, 1973.
5. Kampmeier RH: Late and congenital syphilis. *Dermatol Clin* 1:23–42, 1983.
6. Benirschke K: Syphilis—the placenta and the fetus. *Am J Dis Child* 128:142, 1974.
7. Harter CA, Benirschke K: Fetal syphilis in the first trimester. *Am J Obstet Gynecol* 124:705–711, 1976.
8. Paley PS: Syphilis in pregnancy. *NY State J Med* 37:585, 1937.
9. Fiumara NJ, Fleming WL, Downing JG, Good FL: The incidence of prenatal syphilis at the Boston City Hospital. *N Engl J Med* 247:48, 1952.
10. Peterson JC: In Kumpmeier RH (ed): *Essentials of Syphiology*. Philadelphia, JB Lippincott, 1943.
11. Ingall D, Musher D: Syphilis. In Remington JS, Klein JO (eds): *Infectious Diseases of the Fetus and the Newborn*. Philadelphia, WB Saunders, 1983.
12. Fiumara NJ, Lessel S: Manifestations of late congenital syphilis: an analysis of 172 patients. *Arch Dermatol* 102:78, 1970.
13. Sexually Transmitted Diseases Treatment Guidelines 1982. *MWR* 31:(S), 1982.

Group B *Streptococcus*

1. Lancefield RC: A serological differentiation of human and other groups of hemolytic streptococci. *J Exp Med* 57:571–595, 1933.

2. Eickhoff TC, Klein JO, Daly AL, et al. Neonatal sepsis and other infections due to group B beta-hemolytic streptococci. *N Engl J Med* 271:1221–1228, 1964.

3. Baker CJ, Edwards MS: Group B streptococcal infections. In Remington JS, Klein JO (eds): *Infectious Diseases of the Fetus and Newborn Infant.* Philadelphia, WB Saunders, 1983, p 820.

4. Baker CJ: Summary of the workshop on perinatal infections due to group B streptococcus. *J Infect Dis* 136:137, 1977.

5. Wood EG, Dillon HC Jr: A prospective study of group B streptococcal bacteriuria in pregnancy. *Am J Obstet Gynecol* 140:515, 1981.

6. Mead PJ, Harris RE: The incidence of group B beta hemolytic streptococcus in antepartum urinary tract infections. *Obstet Gynecol* 51:412, 1978.

7. Faro S: Group B beta hemolytic streptococci and puerperal infections. *Am J Obstet Gynecol* 139:686–689, 1981.

8. Gibbs RS, Blanco JD: Streptococcal infections in pregnancy. A study of 48 bacteremias. *Am J Obstet Gynecol* 140:405–411, 1981.

9. Minkoff HL, Sierra MF, Pringle GF, Schwarz RH: Vaginal colonization with group B beta hemolytic streptococcus as a risk factor for post-cesarean section febrile morbidity. *Am J Obstet Gynecol* 142:992–995, 1982.

10. Pass MA, Gray BM, Dillon HC Jr: Puerperal and perinatal infections with group B streptococci. *Am J Obstet Gynecol* 143:147–152, 1982.

11. Ledger WJ, Norman M, Gee C, Lewis W: Bacteremia on an obstetric-gynecologic service. *Am J Obstet Gynecol* 121:205–212, 1975.

12. Regan JA, Chao S, James LS: Premature rupture of membranes, preterm delivery, and group B streptococcal colonization of mothers. *Am J Obstet Gynecol* 141:184–186, 1981.

13. Hood M, Janney A, Dameron G: Beta-hemolytic streptococcus group B associated with problems of perinatal period. *Am J Obstet Gynecol* 82:809–818, 1961.

14. Franciosi RA, Knostman JD, Zimmerman RA: Group B streptococcal neonatal and infant infections. *J Pediatr* 82:707–718, 1973.

15. Baker CJ, Barrett FF: Transmission of group B streptococci among parturient women and their neonates. *J Pediatr* 83:919–925, 1973.

16. Schauf V, Hlaing V: Group B streptococcal colonization in pregnancy. *Obstet Gynecol* 47:719, 1976.

17. Aber RC, Allen N, Howell JT, et al: Nosocomial transmission of group B strep. *Pediatrics* 58:346–353, 1976.

18. Pass MA, Gray BM, Khare S, Dillon HC Jr: Prospective studies of group G streptococcal infections in infants. *J Pediatr* 95:437–443, 1979.

19. Anthony BF, Okada DM, Hobel CJ: Epidemiology of group B streptococcus: longitudinal observations during pregnancy. *J Infect Dis* 137:524, 1978.

20. Anthony BF, Eisenstadt R, Carter J, et al: Genital and intestinal carriage of group B streptococci during pregnancy. *J Infect Dis* 143:761–766, 1981.

21. Ferrieri P, Cleary PP, Seeds AE: Epidemiology of group B streptococcal carriage in pregnant women and newborn infants. *J Med Microbiol* 10:103–114, 1977.

22. Anthony BF, Okada DM, Hobel CJ: Epidemiology of the group B streptococcus: maternal and nosocomial sources for infant acquisitions. *J Pediatr* 95:431–436, 1979.

23. Yow MD, Leeds LJ, Thompson PK, et al: the natural history of group B streptococcal colonization in the pregnant woman and her offspring. I. Colonization studies. *Am J Obstet Gynecol* 137:34–38, 1980.

24. Sokol RJ, Walker RS: B-hemolytic streptococcus in a population of antepartum patients. *Obstet Gynecol* 42:227–232, 1973.

25. Reid TMS: Emergence of group B streptococci in obstetric and perinatal infection. *Br Med J* 2:533–535, 1975.

26. MacDonal NE, MacKenzie AMR: Maternal and neonatal colonization with group B streptococci in Ottawa. *Can Med Assoc J* 120:1100–1111, 1979.

27. Beachler CW, Baker CJ, Kasper DL, et al: Group B streptococcal colonization and antibody status in lower socioeconomic parturient women. *Am J Obstet Gynecol* 133:171–173, 1979.

28. Ancona RJ, Ferrieri P, Willimas PP: Maternal factors that enhance the acquisition of group B streptococci by newborn infants. *J Med Microbiol* 13:273–280, 1980.

29. Lewin EB, Amstey MS: Natural history of group B streptococcus colonization and its therapy during pregnancy. *Am J Obstet Gynecol* 139:512–515, 1981.

30. Baker CJ: Group B streptococcal infections. *Adv Intern Med* 25:475–501, 1980.

31. Baker CJ, Goroff DK, Alpert S, et al: Vaginal colonization with group B streptococcus: a study in college women. *J Infect Dis* 135:392–397, 1977.

32. Badri MS, Zawaneh S, Cruz AC, et al: Rectal colonization with group B streptococcus: relation to vaginal colonization of pregnant women. *J Infect Dis* 135:308–312, 1977.

33. Dillon HC Jr, Gray E, Pass MA, Gray BM: Anorectal and vaginal carriage of group B streptococci during pregnancy. *J Infect Dis* 145:794–799, 1982.

34. Hoogkamp-Korstanje JAA, Gerrards LJ, Cats BP: Maternal carriage and neonatal acquisition of group B streptococci. *J Infect Dis* 145:800–803, 1982.

35. Boyer KM, Gadzala CA, Kelly PD, et al: Selective intrapartum chemoprophylaxis of neonatal group B streptococcal early onset disease. II. Predictive value of prenatal cultures. *J Infect Dis* 148:802–809, 1983.

36. Boyer KM, Gadzala CA, Burd LI, et al: Selective intrapartum chemoprophylaxis of neonatal group B streptococcal early onset disease. I. Epidemiologic rationale. *J Infect Dis* 148:795–801, 1983.

37. Boyer KM, Gadzala CA, Kelly PD: Selective intrapartum chemoprophylaxis of neonatal group B streptococcal early onset disease. III. Interruption of mother-to infant transmission. *J Infect Dis* 148:810–816, 1983.

38. Anthony BF, Okada DM: The emergency of group B streptococci in infections of the newborn infant. *Annu Rev Med* 28:355–369, 1977.

39. Wilkinson HW: Group B streptococcal infection

in humans. *Annu Rev Microbiol* 32:41–57, 1978.

40. Paredes A, et al: Nosocomial transmission of group B streptococci in a newborn nursery. *Pediatrics* 59:670, 1977.

41. Band JD, Clegg HW, Hayes PS, et al: Transmission of group B streptococci. *Am J Dis Child* 135:355–358, 1981.

42. Steere AC, Aber RC, Warford LR, et al: Possible nosocomial transmissino of group B streptococci in a newborn nursery. *J Pediatr* 87:784–787, 1975.

43. Easmon CSF, Hasting MJG, Clare AJ, et al: Nosocomial transmission of group B streptococci. *Br Med J* 283:459–461, 1981.

44. Bobitt JR, Ledger WJ: Obstetric observations in eleven cases of neonatal sepsis due to the group B hemolytic streptococcus. *Obstet Gynecol* 47:439, 1975.

45. Siegal JD, McCracken GH, Threlkeld N, et al: Single-dose penicillin prophylaxis against neonatal group B streptococcal infections. *N Engl J Med* 45:685, 1978.

46. Berggvist G, Hurvell B, Thal E, Valcavincova V: Neonatal infections caused by group B streptococci: relationship between the occurrence in the vaginal flora of term pregnant women and infection in the newborn infant. *Scand J Infect Dis* 3:209–212, 1971.

47. Quirante J, Ceballos R, Cassady G: Group B B-hemolytic streptococcal infections in the newborn. *Am J Dis Child* 128:659–665, 1973.

48. Lloyd DJ, Scott KE, Aterman K, et al: Prevention of group B beta hemolytic streptococcal septicemia in low birth weight neonates by penicillin administered within two hours of birth. *Lancet* 1:713, 1979.

49. Tseng PI, Randall SR: Group B streptococcal disease in neonates and infants. *NY State J Med* 74:2169–2173, 1974.

50. Stewardson-Krieger PB, Gotoff SP: Risk factors in early onset neonatal group B streptococcal infections. *Infection* 6:50–53, 1978.

51. Franciosi RA: Infants at risk for early onset group B streptococcal infection. *Minn Med* 62:801–804, 1979.

52. Baker CJ, Kasper DL: Correlation of maternal antibody efficiency with susceptibility to neonatal group B streptococcal infection. *N Engl J Med* 294:753–756, 1976.

53. Hemming VG, Hall RT, Rhodes PG, et al: Assessment of group B streptococcal opsonins in human and ribbit serum by neutrophil chemiluminescence. *J Clin Invest* 58:1379–1387, 1976.

54. Shigeoka AO, Hall HT, Hill HR: Blood transfusion in group B streptococcal sepsis. *Lancet* 1:636–638, 1978.

55. Baker CJ, Edwards MS, Kasper DL: Role of antibody to native type III polysaccharide of group B streptococcus in infant infection. *Pediatrics* 68:544–549, 1981.

56. Hey DJ, Hall RT, Burry VT, et al: Neonatal infections caused by group B streptococci. *Am J Obstet Gynecol* 116:43, 1973.

57. Echeverria P: Observations concerning infection with B-hemolytic streptococci, not group A or D, in neonates. *J Pediatr* 83:499, 1974.

58. Horn KA, Meyer WT, Wyrick BC, et al: Group B streptococcal neonatal infection. *JAMA* 230:1165, 1974.

59. Hemming VG, McCloskey DW, Hill HR, et al: Pneumonia in the neonate associated with group B streptococcal septicemia. *Am J Dis Child* 130:1231, 1976.

60. Pyati SP, Pildes RS, Jacobs NM, et al: Penicillin in infants weighing two kilograms or less with early onset group B streptococcal disease. *N Engl J Med* 308:1383–1389, 1983.

61. Fenton LJ, Strunck RC: Compliment activation and group B streptococcal infection in the neonate: similarities to endotoxin shock. *Pediatrics* 60:901, 1977.

62. Jeffrey H, Michison R, Wigglesworth JS, et al: Early neonatal bacteremia. Comparison of group B streptococci, other gram positive and gram negative infection. *Arch Dis Child* 52:683, 1977.

63. Maher E, Irwin RC: Group B streptococcal infection in infancy: a case report and review. *Pediatrics* 38:659, 1966.

64. Schlievert PM, Varner MW, Galask RP: Endotoxin enhancement as a possible etiology of early onset group B beta hemolytic streptococcal sepsis in the newborn. *Obstet Gynecol* 61:588–592, 1983.

65. Polin RS, Kennet R: Use of monoclonal antibodies in an enzyme immunoassay for rapid identification of group B streptococcus types II and III. *J Clin Microbiol* 11:332–336, 1980.

66. Jacobs MR, Kelly F, Speck WT: Susceptibility of group B streptococcus to 16 B-lactan antibiotics, including new penicillin and cephalosporin derivatives. *Antimicrob Agents Chemother* 22:897–900, 1982.

67. Hall RT, Barnes W, Krishman L, et al: Antibiotic treatment of parturient women colonized with group B streptococci. *Am J Obstet Gynecol* 124:630, 1976.

68. Gardner SW, Yow MD, Leeds LJ, Thompson PK, Mason EO, Clark DJ: Failure of penicillin to eradicate group B streptococcal colonization in the pregnant woman. *Am J Obstet Gynecol* 135:1062–1065, 1979.

69. Lewin EB, Amstey MS: Natural history of group B streptococcus colonization and its therapy during pregnancy. *Am J Obstet Gynecol* 139:512–515, 1981.

70. Merenstein GB, Todd WA, Brown G, et al: Group B beta hemolytic streptococcus: randomized controlled treatment at term. *Obstet Gynecol* 55:315–318, 1980.

71. Yow MD, Mason EO, Leeds LJ, et al: Ampicillin prevents intrapartum transmission of group B streptococcus. *JAMA* 241:1245–1247, 1979.

72. Allardice JG, Baskett TF, Seshia MMK, et al: Perinatal group B streptococcal colonization and infection. *Am J Obstet Gynecol* 142:617–620, 1982.

73. Steigman AJ, Bottone EJ, Hanna BA: Control of perinatal group B streptococcal sepsis: efficacy of single injection of aqueous penicillin at birth. *Mt Sinai J Med NY* 45:685–693, 1978.

74. Paredes A, et al: Failure of penicillin to eradicate the carrier state of group B streptococcus in infants. *J Pediatr* 89:191, 1976.

Listeriosis

1. Charles D: *Infections in Obstetrics and Gynecology.* Philadelphia, WB Saunders, 1980, pp 192–197.

2. Sever JC, Larsen JW Jr, Grossman JH III: Lis-

teriosis. In *Handbook of Perinatal Infections*. Boston, Little Brown, 1980, pp 141–144.

3. Ahlfors C, Goetzman BW, Halsted CC, et al: Neonatal listeriosis. *Am J Dis Child* 131:405–408, 1977.

4. Anderson G: *Listeria monocytogenes* septicemia in pregnancy. *Obstet Gynecol* 46:102–104, 1975.

5. Seeliger HPR, Finger H: Listeriosis. In Remington JS, Klein JO (eds): *Infectious Diseases of the Fetus and Newborn Infant*. Philadelphia, WB Saunders, 1983, pp 264–289.

6. Kalis P, LeFrock JL, Smith W, et al: Listeriosis. *Am J Med Sci* 271:159–169, 1976.

7. Reiss HJ, Potal J, Krebs A: Granulomatosis infanti septica. Eine durch Einen sepzifischen erreger hervorgerufene fetale sepsis. *Klin Wochenschr* 29:29–32, 1951.

8. Moellering RC, Medoff G, Leech I, et al: Antibiotic synergism against *Listeria monocytogenes*. *Antimicrob Agents Chemother* 1:30–34, 1972.

Protozoa

Toxoplasmosis

1. Fuchs F, Kimball AC, Kean BH: The management of toxoplasmosis in pregnancy. *Clin Perinatol* 1:407, 1974.

2. Desmonts G, Couveur J: Toxoplasmosis in pregnancy and its transmission to the fetus. *Bull NY Acad Med* 50:146–159, 1974.

3. Stray-Pedersen B: A prospective study of acquired toxoplasmosis among 8,043 pregnant women in the Oslo area. *Am J Obstet Gynecol* 136:399, 1980.

4. Beverely JKA: Toxoplasmosis. *Br Med J* 2:475, 1973.

5. Desmonts G, Couvreur J: Congenital toxoplasmosis. A prospective study of 378 pregnancies. *N Engl J Med* 290:1110, 1974.

6. Remington JS, Desmonts G: Toxoplasmosis. In Remington JS, Klein JO (eds): *Infectious Diseases of the Fetus and Newborn Infants*. Philadelphia, WB Saunders, 1983, pp 143–263.

7. Krick JA, Remington JS: Current concepts in parasitology. Toxoplasmosis in the adult—an overview. *N Engl J Med* 298:550, 1978.

8. Frenkel JK: Congenital toxoplasmosis: prevention or palliation? *Am J Obstet Gynecol* 141:359, 1981.

9. Wilson CB, Remington JS: What can be done to prevent congenital toxoplasmosis? *Am J Obstet Gynecol* 138:357, 1980.

10. Beverely JKA: Toxoplasmosis. *Br Med J* 2:475, 1973.

11. Desmonts G, Couvreur J: Congenital toxoplasmosis. A prospective study of 378 pregnancies. *N Engl J Med* 290:1110, 1974.

12. Remington JS, Desmonts G: Toxoplasmosis. In Remington JS, Klein JO (eds): *Infectious Diseases of the Fetus and Newborn Infants*. Philadelphia, WB Saunders, 1983, pp 143–263.

13. Krick JA, Remington JS: Current concepts in parasitology. Toxoplasmosis in the adult—an overview. *N Engl J Med* 298:550, 1978.

14. Frenkel JK: Congenital toxoplasmosis: prevention or palliation? *Am J Obstet Gynecol* 141:359, 1981.

15. Wilson CB, Remington JS: What can be done to prevent congenital toxoplasmosis? *Am J Obstet Gynecol* 138:357, 1980.

CHAPTER 14

Parasitic Diseases in Pregnancy

Significant parasitic infestations occur during pregnancy with a worldwide distribution (1). Such agents are generally more common in tropical and underdeveloped areas of the world. The range of protozoans and helminths that infest humans is vast. Table 14.1 lists those infestations which are either common or have a potentially adverse effect on pregnancy outcome. While the prevalence of parasitic diseases during pregnancy is much lower in the United States and other Western industrialized nations, the wide accessibility to rapid foreign travel has resulted in a rather large "at risk" pool of tourists (2) exposed to a multitude of protozoan and helminth infections during their travels. Ironically, the response to parasitic infection by nonresident visitors to endemic areas may be more severe than that of the local inhabitants who have acquired immunity to these agents (1). Additionally, the recent influx of immigrants into the United States from South and Central America and Southeast Asia has led to the presence of a population with a very high prevalence of parasitic infestation. Finally, there are areas in the United States where the environmental, economic, and sanitary conditions are appropriate for the maintenance of endemic parasites (2). Epidemics of giardiasis and amebiasis have occurred in the United States, schistosomiasis is endemic in Puerto Rico, and hookworm is endemic in the Southeastern United States.

Lee (2) has suggested that parasitic infestation may adversely affect fertility and/or reproductive capacity in three ways (see Table 14.2). First, the infecting organism can result in sufficient debilitation and/or anatomic damage to the genital tract so that either conception is impossible or normal implantation does not occur. Secondly, parasitic infestations may be severe enough to adversely affect the mother's health to the point where medical intervention to terminate the pregnancy is required. Thirdly, protozoan parasites may infect placenta and cross the placenta to produce adverse fetal af-

fects such as abortion, fetal infection, stillbirth, intrauterine growth retardation, and congenital infection. Additional mechanisms for producing adverse effects upon pregnancy outcome have been proposed (3). The nutritional status of pregnant women in the tropics and underdeveloped areas is borderline. Parasitic disease may significantly interfere with the nutrition of these women and may result in a worsening of the already critical nutritional status with resultant impaired fetal growth. Another factor leading to poor outcome may be that malnutrition is associated with immunodeficiency, and thus the susceptibility of pregnant women to bacterial and viral infections and their recognized consequences for the fetus and newborn is increased.

PROTOZOAN INFECTIONS

Amebiasis

Amebiasis is an ulcerative and inflammatory disease of the colon caused by the protozoan *Entamoeba histolytica*. In addition, the organism may occur in extraintestinal sites, most commonly, the liver. *E. histolytica* occurs throughout the world, with its prevalence being highest in tropical areas and countries with low levels of sanitation and personal hygiene (4). Over 40% of the population are infected in many tropical countries, while in the United States the prevalence rate is 3–4%. However, as noted in Chapter 3, among the male homosexual population in the United States, prevalence rates of 40% have been reported (5).

Infection is acquired by ingestion of the cyst form of *E. histolytica*. The cysts, which contain eight trophozoites, rupture in the small bowel to release the trophozoites. The trophozoites migrate to the colon, with binary fission occurring every 8 hr. If environmental conditions are not appropriate for continued multiplication, encystment occurs, and the life cycle is complete (6). However, the trophozoite, under the influence of poorly understood environmental fac-

Table 14.1
Parasitic Infestations Which May Occur in Pregnant Women

Protozoan agents	
Entamoeba histolytica	*Leishmania donovani*
Giardia lamblia	*Leishmania tropica*
Plasmodium falciparum	*Leishmania braziliensis*
Plasmodium vivax	*Leishmania mexicana*
Plasmodium malariae	*Trypanosoma cruzi*
Plasmodium ovale	*Trypanosoma brucei*
Trichimonas vaginalis	*Toxoplasma gondii*
Pneumocystis carinii	*Babesia* species

Helminths	
Intestinal nematodes	Trematodes (flukes)
(roundworms)	*Schistosoma mansoni*
Ascaris lumbricoides	*Schistosomiasis japonicum*
Trichuris trichuria	*Schistosomiasis haematobium*
Enterobius vermicularis	Cestodes (tapeworms)
Ancyclostoma duodenale	*Taenia saginata*
Necator americanus	*Taenia solium*
Strongyloides stercoralis	*Diphyllobothrium latum*
Tissue nematodes	*Hymenolepis nana*
Trichinella spiralis	*Echinococcus granulosis*
Wuchereria bancrofti	
Brugia malayi	

Table 14.2
Adverse Effect of Parasitic Diseases on Fertility and Pregnancy Outcome

	Impaired fertility secondary to maternal debilitation	Impaired fertility secondary to direct damage to reproductive organs	Adversely affect maternal health during pregnancy	Affect fetus and neonate
Protozoan infection				
Amebiasis	+	+	+	+[a]
Giardiasis	+		±	
Leishmaniasis	+		+	?
Malaria	+		+	+[b]
Trypanosomiasis	+		+	+[a, b]
P. carinii				
infection				+[a, b]
Toxoplasmosis				+[b]
Trichimoniasis				+[a]
Helminthic Infection				
Intestinal nematodes				
Ascaris	+	+		
Trichuriasis	+		+	
Enterobiasis		+		+[a]
Hookworm			+	
Tissue-invading nematodes				
Filariasis		+		
Trichinosis			+	
Trematodes				
Schistosomiasis		+		
Cestodes				
Diphyllobothriasis			+	
Echinococcosis		+	+	

[a] Infection acquired postdelivery from mother.
[b] Congenital infection.

tors, may invade the mucosal wall of the colon (7). The trophozoites are facultative anaerobes, and once they gain access to submucosal areas they are capable of maintaining an ideal environment for their survival by producing tissue anoxia, necrosis, and a low pH. It is this large area of necrosis in the submucosa that produces the characteristic flask-shaped ulcer of amebiasis.

CLINICAL PRESENTATION

Clinical findings associated with *E. histolytica* infestation range from the asymptomatic carrier state to fulminant dysentery. The asymptomatic carrier state is the most common manifestation of this infection. It has been estimated that clinical disease may occur in 10–50% of asymptomatic carriers (2). Immunosuppression, malnutrition, steroid therapy, and pregnancy have been noted to result in the development of clinical disease in the asymptomatic carrier (2, 3).

The clinical disease of amebiasis may be mild and characterized by colonic irritation with colicky lower abdominal pain and altered bowel habits; stool may be loose with mucus and/or blood present. With more extensive colonic disease the patient presents with bloody frequent diarrheal stools, abdominal pain and tenderness, right upper quadrant pain and tenderness, and hepatomegaly. In the extreme an acute abdomen can be present secondary to bowel perforation and acute amebic peritonitis. This serious complication occurs in 3–4% of patients with severe amebic dysentery and is associated with a high mortality rate (8). Following an acute episode of amebiasis, a chronic irritative bowel syndrome may be present for several months.

In addition to peritonitis secondary to bowel perforation, extraintestinal amebiasis may also occur by metastasis of trophozoites via the portal vein system of lymphatics, usually to the liver initially. As noted by Adams and McLeod, the majority of patients with amebic liver abscesses have no history of antecedent of current bowel disease (9). Patients with amebic liver abscess present with right upper quadrant pain, fever, tender hepatomegaly, rapid weight loss, and pallor. Amebic liver abscesses may extend into adjacent organs, most commonly the pleural cavity, but ruptures into the pericardium or peritoneum may occur (9).

DIAGNOSIS

The diagnosis of intestinal amebiasis is made by demonstrating *E. histolytica* in stool. Either the presence of trophozoites or cysts confirms the diagnosis. Stool specimens are best examined fresh. Sigmoidoscopy is an excellent approach for making the diagnosis. Amebic colitis appears as punctate hemorrhagic areas or small ulcers with exudative centers and hyperemic borders. Aspiration of these lesions provides a reliable specimen for identification of motile, erythrocyte-containing *E. histolytica*.

Patients with amebic liver abscess often do not have concurrent intestinal involvement, and thus stool specimens are negative for *E. histolytica*. These patients have leukocytosis, elevated alkaline phosphatase levels, radioisotopic scanning or computerized tomography demonstration of a solitary (usually) defect in the right lobe of the liver, and a positive serologic test for amebiasis. In general, aspiration of the cyst is not necessary to make the diagnosis.

EFFECTS OF AMEBIASIS ON PREGNANCY

Several reports have suggested that amebiasis during pregnancy may be more severe and may be associated with a higher mortality rate than occurs in nonpregnant women (2, 10, 11). Abioye noted that 68% of fatal cases of amebiasis in females occurred in association with pregnancy (11). On the other hand, only 17.1% of fatal typhoid cases and 12.5% of other fatal enterocolitis cases among females occurred during pregnancy. Reinhardt described several factors that may account for this increased susceptibility during pregnancy (3). These included: (a) increased levels of free plasma cortisol during pregnancy; (b) increased levels of serum cholesterol in early pregnancy; and (c) malnutrition and anemia which are commonly present in pregnant women living in areas endemic for amebiasis. It has also been suggested that amebiasis during pregnancy may result in an adverse effect upon the fetus (12). Czeizel et al noted that women with spontaneous abortions had a significantly higher incidence of positive stool cultures for *E. histolytica*, as compared to women having term births (12). In addition, these workers demonstrated an increased incidence of amebiasis in women with stillbirths, preterm deliveries, and infants having congenital anomalies than in those with normal term deliveries (12). It is important to recognize that asymptomatic or mild amebiasis may develop into severe amebic dysentery during pregnancy and the puerperium. Thus, consideration must be given to treatment of these milder forms of amebiasis in pregnant women.

There is no evidence that *E. histolytica* is associated with intrauterine fetal infection. However, the newborn may acquire the disease secondary to person-to-person transmission, usually from its mother. Neonates with amebiasis present with sudden onset and are seriously ill with bloody diarrhea, hepatic abscess, gangrene of the colon, and colon perforation with peritonitis (13).

TREATMENT

Because the cyst stage of *E. histolytica* is resistant to physical and chemical agents, antimicrobial therapy is directed against the trophozoite stage. A variety of drugs is available, and the treatment regimen should be based on both the location (intestinal and/or visceral) and severity of amebiasis (2). In addition, it is very important that pregnant women with amebiasis be treated during pregnancy because of the reported increased incidence of severe disease in pregnancy (10, 11).

In the asymptomatic patient or in those with mild intestinal amebiasis, the agent of choice is diiodohydroxyquin or diloxanide furoate (available through the Centers for Disease Control only). However, during pregnancy these drugs should not be employed because their effects upon pregnancy are unclear. In pregnant women paromomycin (Humatin) is the drug of choice for asymptomatic or mild intestinal disease. This agent is an aminoglycoside antimicrobial which is poorly absorbed and is active against lumenal *E. histolytica*. Treatment consists of paromomycin (25–35 mg/kg/day in 3 daily doses for 5–10 days).

Patients with symptoms of colitis and passage of mucus and blood should be treated with two agents, one effective against intralumenal trophozoites and a second which is active against trophozoites invading the colon wall and/or involving extraintestinal sites. The luminal agent can be diiodohydroxyquin, diloxanide, or paromomycin, which is the preferred agent during pregnancy. Metronidazole is the recommended extralumenal agent and is given in a dose of 750 mg three times/day for 5 days. The concern over potential teratogenic effects with metronidazole use is discussed in detail in Chapter 19, but it has been widely used in pregnancy without ill effect.

Extraintestinal amebiasis such as amebic abscess is treated with metronidazole in a dose of 750 mg three times/day for 10 days. Chloroquine is an alternative choice in a dosage of 500 mg/day for 2–3 weeks. Emetine is an additional agent for extralumenal disease, but its cardiac toxicity limits its use to situations associated with critically ill patients with complications such as peritonitis or ruptured amebic abscess.

Giardiasis

Giardia lamblia is a protozoan parasite that has a trophozoite and cystic stage and inhabits the duodenum. Giardiasis is a ubiquitous disease with worldwide distribution. Areas of increased risk include Southeast and South Asia, West and Central Africa, South America, Mexico, Korea, and the Soviet Union. In addition, large scale epidemics of giardiasis have occurred in the United States, and the disease is prevalent among male homosexuals (1, 2). *G. lamblia* is the most commonly identified pathogenic intestinal parasite in the United States, occurring in 3–9% of stool specimens (3).

It is the resistant cyst stage which is transmitted by the fecal-oral route. In the duodenum the cysts rupture to release trophozoites, which firmly attach via their suckling disc to the intestinal epithelium. The cysts develop as liquid feces is dehydrated as it transits the colon.

CLINICAL PRESENTATION

Giardiasis may range from an asymptomatic carrier state to severe diarrhea with malabsorption. Characteristically, giardiasis presents with sudden onset of explosive, watery, foul-smelling, bulky diarrhea. Anorexia, nausea, vomiting, belching of sulfuric material, abdominal cramps, low grade fever, chills, and malaise also occur. There is an absence of blood or mucus in the stool.

DIAGNOSIS

In the early acute stage giardiasis can be diagnosed by immediate examination of a stool wet smear which demonstrates trophozoites. Alternately, stool can be preserved in formalin or polyvinyl alcohol for later examination. Later in the disease process, the stool is more formed and contains the cyst form. Concentration techniques are usually necessary to demonstrate the cysts. Duodenal aspirates will contain trophozoites. No serologic test is available for the diagnosis of giardiasis.

EFFECT ON PREGNANCY

In general, giardiasis has minimal adverse effects upon pregnancy outcome (2). However, significant malabsorption may impair fertility and adversely affect pregnancy. Kreutner et al recently described three cases of severe giardiasis in pregnant women and suggested that the disease is more severe in pregnancy with significant weight loss and debility (3).

TREATMENT

The treatment of choice in giardiasis is quinacrine hydrochloride (Atabrine) in a dosage of 100 mg three times/day for 7 days. Alternate agents include metronidazole in a dose of 250 mg three times/day for 7 days or furazolidone (Furoxone) 100 mg four times/day for 7 days. Because all three of these drugs may adversely affect the fetus, the recommended treatment of symptomatic giardiasis in pregnancy is paromomycin (Humatin) (25–30 mg/kg/day in divided doses three times daily for 5–10 days) (3).

Leishmaniasis

Leishmaniasis is a group of clinical diseases produced by protozoan organisms of the genus *Leishmania*. The four species which are human pathogens include: *Leishmania donovani; Leishmania tropica; Leishmania braziliensis*; and *Leishmania mexicana*. There are three distinct clinical forms of leishmaniasis (3). Kala-azar (visceral or systemic leishmaniasis) is caused by *L. donovani*. Cutaneous leishmaniasis is produced by *L. tropica*. American leishmaniasis (mucocutaneous disease) is due to *L. braziliensis* and *L. mexicana*. These various species of *Leishmania* are transmitted by the bite of sandflies (*Phlebotomus*).

Kala-azar is widely distributed throughout the world, with its greatest prevalence in India and China (2). Cutaneous leishmaniasis (Oriental sores) occurs in tropical and subtropical areas of the Eastern and Western hemispheres, especially China, Asia Minor, Africa, and Central and South America. The mucocutaneous form of the disease is seen in Central and South America.

CLINICAL PRESENTATION

Kala-azar has a slow insidious onset following an incubation period of up to 18 months (2). It characteristically presents as prolonged fever, progressive weight loss, weakness, hepatosplenomegaly, anemia, leukopenia, hypoalbuminemia, and hyperglobulinemia (2). Cutaneous leishmaniasis initially appears as a pruritic red papule that occurs at the site of inoculation. This lesion slowly progresses to a shallow ulcer with seropurulent discharge. Tender regional lymphadenopathy is present. The ulcer generally heals spontaneously over several months.

While the mucocutaneous form of leishmaniasis begins similarly as a small papule which progresses to an ulcerative stage, this disease is progressive in nature, with development of new ulcerations involving the mucocutaneous borders of the nose and mouth (2). Extensive tissue destruction and scarring occur as these lesions slowly heal over several years.

DIAGNOSIS

The diagnosis of kala-azar is suggested by the characteristic clinical presentation occurring in an endemic area and is confirmed by demonstrating leishmania bodies within cells of the reticuloendothelial system, usually by marrow aspiration. Culture can be performed on this specimen. Similarly, cutaneous leishmaniasis is suspected when the typical ulcer appears in an endemic area. The diagnosis is confirmed by demonstrating the organism in smears obtained from the borders of the lesion. The Montenegro skin test is positive in this form of leishmaniasis.

EFFECT ON PREGNANCY

Kala-azar, caused by *L. donovani*, is the only form of leishmaniasis in which a parasitemia occurs (1). Consequently, it is the only leishmaniasis that has been reported to cause intrauterine fetal infection (3). If kala-azar is acquired during pregnancy, Lee has suggested that it is associated with increased fetal loss (1).

TREATMENT

The treatment of all three forms of leishmaniasis relies on the use of either pentavalent organic antimonials (Pentostan, Neostibosan, or Glucantime) or aromatic diamidines such as pentamidine isethionate. The latter group are the most effective drugs against leishmaniasis but are associated with frequent side effects and are thus reserved for resistant cases (2).

The use of these drugs in pregnancy is limited, and their effects are not clear. They should be used with caution, and only treatment of kala-azar seems appropriate during pregnancy.

Trypanosomiasis

There are two forms of human trypanosomiasis. Chagas's disease is caused by *Trypanosoma cruzi* and African sleeping sickness by *Trypanosoma brucei gambiense* and *Trypanosoma bru-*

cei rhodesiense. These two diseases differ in their geographic distribution, mode of transmission, pathogenesis, and clinical course (1).

CHAGAS'S DISEASE (AMERICAN TRYPANOSOMIASIS)

Chagas's disease is caused by *T. cruzi* and occurs in Central and South America where Reinhardt has estimated that 7 million people are infected with this protozoan parasite (2). *T. cruzi* is transmitted by triatomid bugs which live in the cracks and holes of the primitive dwellings in urban shanty towns (1–3).

The triatomid bug feeds by sucking blood. Its bites occur around the mouth and nose, and metacyclic forms of *T. cruzi* are deposited as the triatomid feeds. The trypanosomes penetrate through the bite wound or mucous membranes (2). *T. cruzi* is capable of penetrating into mammalian cells, where it develops into an amastigote (*Leishmania*) form. Here the organism multiplies and forms a pseudocyst which ruptures with release of protozoan organisms which enter the blood stream or invade adjacent cells (1).

Acute Chagas's disease generally occurs in children. Only 1% of inhabitants of endemic areas who become infected develop clinically apparent acute disease. The most common site for the bite is the face. Urticaria often develops at the bite site, followed by an inflammatory nodule, the chagoma (3). The bite is often associated with Romana's sign, which is unilateral nonpurulent edema of the palpebral folds and an ipsilateral regional lymphadenopathy (1, 3). After 2 or 3 weeks, parasitemia occurs with widespread dissemination, fever, lymphadenopathy, malaise, and peripheral edema (3, 4). *T. cruzi* invades cells, resulting in the typical involvement of the heart, liver, gastrointestinal tract, and central nervous system. The cardiac disease is characterized by tachycardia, arrhythmia, hypotensions, cardiomegaly, and congestive heart failure (3). The mortality rate in the acute phase of Chagas' disease is 10–20% with most deaths secondary to cardiac disease or encephalitis.

Chronic Chagas's disease, which occurs generally in patients with no history of acute disease, has a slow and insidious onset (1). Cardiac involvement occurs in 20–40% of patients with chronic disease and presents as progressive cardiac enlargement in association with electrocardiographic abnormalities. Involvement of chronic gastrointestinal disease is characterized by progressive development of megaesophagus or megacolon. Mortality rates of nearly 20% have been reported in association with chronic Chagas's disease, approximately half the deaths being due to congestive heart failure (3).

Diagnosis in the acute stage of Chagas's disease can be made by demonstrating the protozoan *T. cruzi* on thin or thick smears of the blood or buffy coat. Xenodiagnosis, which is performed by allowing laboratory-bred triatomids to feed on the patient and examining the fecal contents of the bugs for trypanosomes in 30–60 days, is available in endemic areas. Serologic tests, indirect-hemagglutination or complement-fixation, are available. Chronic Chagas's disease is suggested by the characteristic clinical picture and confirmed by serologic tests and/or by biopsy demonstration of *T. cruzi* in tissue.

In South America 1–10% of spontaneous abortions are attributed to Chagas's disease (5). Infection of the placenta usually can be demonstrated in these cases (3). Congenital infection with Chagas's disease is well documented and is reported to occur in 1–4% of deliveries in women with serologic evidence of Chagas's disease (5, 6). The congenitally infected neonates tend to be preterm and/or small for gestational age. Bettencourt noted that approximately 36% of congenitally infected infants died prior to 4 months of life. In addition, *T. cruzi* may be found in breast milk (4). Edgcomb and Johnson reported that the cardiac involvement associated with acute Chagas's is often more severe in pregnant and puerperal women than in nonpregnant women (5).

Acute Chagas's disease may be treated with Nifurtimox (Lampit) in a daily dose of 8–10 mg/kg given in three doses for 90 days. This drug is available from the Centers for Disease Control. In pregnant women with evidence of cardiac or CNS disease, treatment should be started promptly. No effective treatment is available for chronic Chagas's disease.

AFRICAN SLEEPING SICKNESS (AFRICAN TRYPANOSOMIASIS)

African trypanosomiasis is caused by *Trypanosoma gambiense* (West African disease) and *Trypanosoma rhodesiense* (East African disease). Infection is transmitted to humans by the bite of the tsetse fly (7). These trypanosomes remain extracellular and accumulate in connective tissue (8).

West African trypanosomiasis initially presents as a local lesion, the trypanoma, at the bite site which ulcerates and spontaneously resolves over several weeks (1). Characteristically, lymphadenopathy occurs in the initial hematolymphatic stage which lasts 6 months to 5 years and progresses insidiously to the later meningoencephalitic stage. In this stage the patient develops increasing indifference and somnolence. The disease is usually fatal.

East African trypanosomiasis is a much more acute disease and is associated with more severe symptoms. The disease usually begins within a few days of the bite and presents with high fever, malaise, and headache. No lymphadenopathy occurs. Central nervous system involvement occurs early and is associated with rapid clinical deterioration (1). The disease is rapidly progressive, with death occurring in weeks to months.

The diagnosis of African trypanosomiasis should be suspected in patients with unexplained febrile illnesses occurring among inhabitants of or visitors to endemic areas for the causative agents. West African trypanosomiasis is characterized by Winterbottom's sign, which is lymph gland enlargement (usually posterior cervical) that is not tender and has the consistency of ripe plums. The optimum diagnostic test is lymph gland puncture to provide a wet smear for detection of trypanosomes (1). East African trypanosomiasis should be suspected in patients recently returned from or residing in Central Africa who develop fever, headache, and weight loss. Diagnosis is confirmed by demonstrating trypanosomes on a wet or stained thick smear of blood or after concentration procedures (1). Serologic tests are available, and high levels of serum IgM are considered pathognomonic while the presence of IgM in the CSF is diagnostic (9).

As noted by Lee (4), African trypanosomiasis usually produces such severe and progressive disease that pregnancy does not occur. However, if the disease is acquired during pregnancy, abortion, preterm labor and delivery, and/or stillbirth may occur (10). East African trypanosomiasis has such a fulminant course that is usually kills the infected patient before gestation can be completed.

Treatment of African trypanosomiasis is provided with suramin, pentamidines, and arsenicals. However, suramin and pentamidine do not penetrate the central nervous system well, and the arsenicals should be included in the treatment of disease with nervous system involvement. Suramin is given intravenously, starting with 100 or 200 mg, followed within a few days by weekly injections of 1 g. Pentamidine is given by daily injections of 3 mg/kg for a total of 10 injections. Melarsoprol is the arsenical most commonly employed as a daily dose of 3.6 mg/kg in three or four injections IM or SC. The usually fatal outcome of African trypanosomiasis supports the need for aggressive therapy with potentially toxic agents even in pregnant women (4).

Malaria

Malaria remains a major health problem in many areas of the world and has a significant impact on maternal, fetal, and neonatal health (1–4). The overwhelming majority of human malaria is caused by four species of the obligate intracellular protozoan parasite *Plasmodium*. These are: *Plasmodium falciparum*; *Plasmodium vivax*; *Plasmodium malariae*; and *Plasmodium ovale*. Each of these species has its own morphologic characteristics and life cycle.

Malaria is transmitted by the bite of infected female anopheline mosquitoes. While asexual reproduction occurs in humans, sexual reproduction occurs in the mosquito. Following sexual reproduction sporozoites, which are the infective form of *Plasmodium* species, are stored in the salivary glands of the mosquito. After the sporozoites are inoculated by the mosquito bite into subcutaneous capillaries, they migrate to the liver, where they invade hepatic cells (Fig. 14.1). In the liver, parasites exist as exoerythrocytic forms and multiply to form hepatic schizonts. Mature schizonts contain 7500–40,000 merozoites, depending upon the type of *Plasmodium* species. Following rupture of the schizonts (after 1–2 weeks) the merozoites enter the bloodstream and invade erythrocytes. This invasion of the red blood cells (RBC) initiates the cycle of growth and multiplication known as schizogony and ultimately leads to destruction of the parasitized RBC (2, 5).

With *P. falciparum* and *P. malariae*, all of the exoerythrocytic schizonts rupture at about the same time, and thus none persist in a latent form in the liver. For *P. vivax* and *P. ovale* there are both primary exoerythrocytic forms which rupture to cause the initial episode of parasitemia and latent exoerythrocytic forms that remain in the liver for long periods of time prior to rupturing. Rupture of the latent hepatic schizonts is responsible for recurrent parasitemia and erythrocytic infection. Once *Plasmodium*

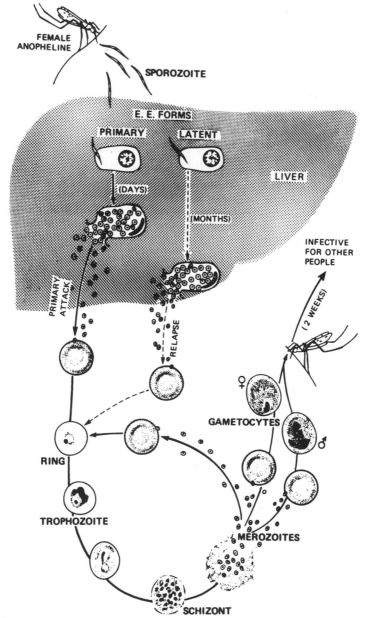

Figure 14.1.   Life cycle of plasmodia in man. (From Wyler DJ, Miller LH: Plasmodium species. In Mandell GL, Douglas RG, Bennett JE (eds): *Principles and Practice of Infectious Disease.* New York, John Wiley & Sons, 1979.)

organisms enter the erythrocytic stage they never reinvade the liver.

After entering the RBC, merozoites acquire a signet ring appearance, thus becoming ring forms. With an increase in cytoplasm as development of the asexual organism occurs, the parasites are called trophozoites. Nuclear division then occurs, producing the schizont. Upon completion of asexual reproduction 6–24 individual merozoites (depending upon the species) are

present in each schizont. Rupture of the schizont releases the merozoites into the bloodstream, where they rapidly attach to and invade new RBCs. This complete process requires 72 hr for *P. malariae* and 48 hr for *P. falciparum, P. vivax,* and *P. ovale.* Male and female gametocytes develop from a subpopulation of merozoites and are then ingested by female anopheline mosquitos during feeding (5). Sexual reproduction occurs in the mosquito gut and the fertilized zygotes invade the gut wall, where they develop into oocysts which contain thousands of sporozoites and migrate to the salivary glands.

In addition to human-to-human transmission via a mosquito vector, malaria may be transmitted by transfusion of blood products and shared syringes and needles among drug abusers.

P. falciparum infection is the most serious and life-threatening form of malaria. This organism parasitizes RBC of any age and reaches very high concentrations in the bloodstream. As noted by Lee (5) the large numbers of parasitized RBC with altered rheologic and immunologic properties associated with *P. falciparum* infection are responsible for the development of the life-threatening complications such as black water fever, pulmonary edema, and cerebral malaria that occur almost exclusively with *P. falciparum* infection. Recently, infection with *P. falciparum* has been complicated by the emergence of strains resistant not only to chloroquine but also to sulfonamides and pyrimethamine (6). Resistance to chloroquine is found among *P. falciparum* strains occurring in Southeast Asia, Africa, South America, and the Pacific Islands.

CLINICAL PRESENTATION

The classic finding of acute malarial infection is the malaria paroxysm which is characterized by high fever, chills, and rigors (2). Initially patients present in the "cold period" with cold pale skin, cyanotic lips and nail beds, and "goose bumps." Within a few minutes to 2 hr the "hot phase" commences, with high temperatures and warm dry skin. In addition, tachycardia, tachypnea, headache, backache, abdominal pain, nausea, vomiting, and delirium are present. The marked peripheral vasodilatation produces a decrease in intravascular volume and results in orthostatic hypotension. Although there is often a regular recurrence pattern to these malarial paroxysms, they may occur at irregular levels.

Patients often have hepatosplenomegaly. In *P. vivax* infection the spleen is prone to rupture, and care must be taken during examination of the patient. In addition jaundice, petechiae, retinal vasospasm and hemorrhage, and chest rales are present. With *P. falciparum* infection, neurologic abnormalities may occur. Malarial patients also demonstrate a normochromic normocytic hemolytic anemia, leukopenia, monocytosis, and thrombocytopenia.

In endemic areas initial malaria infection occurs during childhood. Repeated clinical infections tend to be reduced in severity as a result of acquired cellular and humoral immunity (5). Nonimmune visitors to malaria endemic areas will have more severe clinical disease than the immune local residents. Similarly, in pregnancy, the immune woman acquiring malarial infection suffers less severe infection than the nonimmune woman.

DIAGNOSIS

The diagnosis of malaria is made by demonstrating the *Plasmodium* parasites in stained peripheral blood smears obtained from patients with the characteristic malaria paroxysm. The thick smear is useful to detect the presence of parasites, and then a thin smear may be utilized to make a species diagnosis. Quantitation of parasitemia is utilized for evaluation of response to therapy.

EFFECT ON PREGNANCY

Bruce-Chwatt (7) and Gilles et al (8) have demonstrated that malaria is more frequent during pregnancy than in nonpregnant patients. In addition, Bruce-Chwatt (7) and Reinhardt (9) have suggested that there is an increased susceptibility to malaria during the first pregnancy. Several clinical investigations have documented that malarial attacks, especially with *P. falciparum* during pregnancy, are likely to be more severe than in nonpregnant women (7, 9–11).

As noted by Lee (5) a gradient of clinical illness with malaria in pregnancy exists. Those pregnant women not immune to drug-resistant *P. falciparum* develop the most severe illness. Moderately severe malaria with fever and anemia occurs in nonimmune women with species of *Plasmodium* susceptible to chloroquine. These patients are also at risk for congenital malaria and intrauterine growth retardation. Reactivated latent disease occurring in an immune pregnant woman is associated with mild illness and placental infection but not fetal infection. The other extreme—acquisition of malaria in the nonimmune mother—can result in life-threatening disease and a high risk for fetal loss.

Reinhardt demonstrated that mothers with low birth weight infants (<2500 g), preterm deliveries (<37 weeks), and small-for-gestational age infants had significantly higher antibody titers against *Plasmodium* than did control patients (5). This association between maternal malaria and low birth weight offspring has been confirmed by several reports (7, 12–16). Low birth-weight occurs more frequently in pregnancies in which the placenta has been infected with the parasites (5, 12, 16). Cannon (16) postulated that placental infestation with parasites and the associated infiltration of lymphocytes and macrophages interfere with placental circulation and result in diminished transplacental transport of oxygen and nutrients to the fetus.

Fetal mortality rates (predominantly spontaneous first trimester abortions) have ranged from 14–60% (17, 18). In addition malarial infection during pregnancy increases the risk for stillbirth, prematurity, and neonatal mortality (5, 15, 19). Reinhardt has suggested several mechanisms by which congenital malaria occurs (1). These include: (a) transplacenta passage of parasites; (b) inoculation of parasites from maternal into fetal blood via skin abrasions at time of delivery; and (c) passage of parasites into amniotic fluid. In the neonate, congenital malaria presents within 48–72 hr after delivery with fever, hepatosplenomegaly, jaundice, and anemia. Finally, malaria may interfere with immune defense mechanisms and subject mother and fetus to an increased risk of bacterial or viral infection (1).

TREATMENT

Oral chloroquine phosphate is the drug of choice for all malarial infections not due to chloroquine resistant. *P. falciparum.* The dosage is 1 g orally, followed by 500 mg in 6 hr and then 500 mg/day for 2 days. Chloroquine alone treats only the erythrocytic stage of malaria. Thus patients with mosquito transmitted *P. vivax* and *P. ovale* require additional treatment for the latent exoerythrocytic hepatic schizonts. These forms are eradicated by primaquine phosphate (26.3 mg by mouth each day for 14 days). Patients receiving primaquine should first be screened for G-6-PD deficiency.

Mild to moderate malaria due to chloroquine-resistant *P. falciparum* is treated with a combination of quinine sulfate (650 mg t.i.d. by mouth for 10 days, pyrimethamine 25 mg b.i.d. by mouth for 3 days, and sulfadiazine or sulfisoxazole 500 mg q.i.d. by mouth for 5 days. Severe infection with *P. falciparum* should be treated with quinine dihydrochloride given as a slow intravenous drip over 60 min.

In nonimmune pregnant women, clinical episodes of malaria should be treated promptly. This is true even though all the antimalarial agents have potentially adverse effects upon the fetus (5). Chloroquine may produce retinal and cochleovestibular damage; quinine is ototoxic; primaquine may cause hemolysis in glucose-6-phosphate dehydrogenase (G-6-PD)-deficient patients, as well as methemoglobinemia, and pyrimethamine may be teratogenic. Essentially, the treatment regimens for malaria are similar for pregnant women to those for nonpregnant patients. Malaria with *P. falciparum* should be viewed as a medical emergency in pregnancy, and patients from Southeast Asia and South America should be treated with multiple drug regimens including quinine and pyrimethamine, sulfonamides, or dapsone.

Chemoprophylaxis should be provided for travelers to endemic malarial areas. The usual prophylactic regimen is chloroquine phosphate (500 mg by mouth once per week, beginning 1 week prior to departure and continuing for 8 weeks after leaving the endemic area). The use of mosquito netting and insect repellant is also crucial to prevention programs. Pyrimethamine is required for prophylaxis against *P. falciparum* strains resistant to chloroquine. Concomitant use of folinic acid should be considered. However, the ideal prophylaxis for pregnant women is not to travel to endemic malarial areas.

Toxoplasmosis

Toxoplasmosis is the infection caused by the protozoan parasite *Toxoplasma gondii.* This disease is discussed in Chapter 13.

Trichomoniasis

Trichomoniasis is a vaginal infection caused by the anaerobic protozoan parasite *Trichomonas vaginalis.* This entity is discussed in Chapter 3.

HELMINTHS

Helminths, or worms capable of parasitizing humans, are ubiquitous organisms occurring with a wide geographic distribution (especially prevalent in tropical regions) and are unique organisms among the infectious agents (1, 2). *Ascaris* and *Enterobius* account for 1 billion infections each, *Trichuris* and hookworms 500 million each, and schistosomes and filariae 250 million each (1). Warren estimated that over 50 million helminth infections are present in the United States (3).

There are several unique characteristics of the helminths as infectious agents (1, 2). They are large enough to be seen by the naked eye, and their reproduction requires completion of the life cycle outside the human host. Thus, with but rare exception, helminths do not multiply in the human host, and the infestation size is determined by the number of worms initially acquired. There is a strong association between helminthic infestation and the eosinophil.

As noted by Lee (2), complex mechanisms of disease production in the human exist for helminthic infection; they may be caused by the adult worm or its ova or larvae. Schistosomes produce disease secondary to inflammation produced by eggs or cercaria. Filariae obstruct lymphatic channels, and other helminths produce disease during migration of the adult worms or larvae. The intestinal helminths may produce disease by competing with the host for nutrition or by causing anemia secondary to blood loss.

Two major groups of parasitic helminths infect man: (a) Nematoda (roundworms) and (b) Platyhelminthes (flatworms). The flatworms include the trematodes (flukes) and cestodes (tapeworms).

Nematoda (Roundworms)

ASCARIASIS

Ascariasis is the most common helminthic infection of man, with an estimated 1 billion cases. *Ascaris lumbricoides* is the causative agent. This organism is most abundant in tropical areas, especially in areas with contamination of the soil by human feces. However, Warren estimates that nearly 4 million cases exist in the United States particularly in the Southeast (3). Transmission of ascaris is usually hand-to-mouth. Ascaris is asymptomatic in the overwhelming majority of cases but may produce serious disease on occasion.

Adult forms of *A. lumbricoides* inhabit the lumen of the small intestine. Female worms lay 200,000 ova daily which pass with feces. Following passage, fully developed infective embryos are formed within the eggs in 5–10 days (4). Following ingestion of infective embryonated eggs, the eggs hatch in the small intestine, where the larvae penetrate through the mucosal lining to enter the portal vein system or intestinal lymphatics (3, 4). They then migrate via the venous system to the lungs, where the larvae penetrate into the alveolus and migrate up the bronchi and trachea and are swallowed. Maturation into the adult worm occurs in the small intestine with a life span of 10–24 months.

Only a few worms are present in the vast majority of *Ascaris* infections, and in these instances infection is not clinically apparent (5). On occasion a single worm may produce clinical disease by migrating to an important anatomic location such as the biliary duct or appendix. When heavy infestation is present, the chance for adult worms to migrate is greater, and thus the risk for clinically apparent disease is increased (2). Intestinal obstruction is a rare serious complication caused by a bolus of worms. If many eggs are ingested, larval migration produces symptomatic pulmonary disease with nocturnal cough and eosinophilia. Fever, rales, persistent cough, and transient radiographic infiltrates may be present as well. Adult *Ascaris* has been reported to invade the female genital tract to cause tuboovarian abscess (6). Similarly, Sterling and Guay reported invasion of the female genital tract by *A. lumbricoides* (7). Congenital *Ascaris* infection is rare, although Chu and coworkers described an infant who delivered in association with 12 adult *Acaris* worms (8).

The diagnosis of ascariasis is made by demonstrating *Ascaris* eggs in the stool, by recovery of an adult worm, or by seeing larvae on sputum or gastric aspirates (2).

In nonpregnant patients with ascaris, mebendazole (Vermox) is the treatment of choice in a dosage of 100 mg b.i.d. for 3 days (Table 14.3). This drug is poorly absorbed from the gastrointestinal tract and thus is free of toxicity. However, it is teratogenic in animals and should not be used in pregnancy (9). When intestinal or biliary obstruction is present, piperazine (Antepar) should also be administered (150 mg/kg initially, followed by six doses of 65 mg/kg at 12-h intervals).

During pregnancy pyrantel pamoate (Antiminth) (75 mg/kg/day for 2 days) is the recommended therapy. Treatment in early pregnancy should be given to mothers with heavy worm infestation. The lightly infected mother should be treated immediately before or after delivery because of the risk of neonatal infection (2).

ENTEROBIASIS

Enterobius vermicularis, the pinworm, is a highly prevalent worm widely distributed throughout the world. It has a simple life cycle in which ingested infective eggs hatch into larvae in the doudenum and mature into adults within the gut lumen (2). The fertilized female pinworm contains over 10,000 eggs and at night-

Table 14.3
Recommended Therapy for Common Helminth Infections

Parasite	Infective stage	Mode of transmission	Drug of choice nonpregnant patient	Treatment indications in pregnancy	Drug of choice in pregnancy
Nematodes (roundworms)					
Ascaris lumbricoides	Mature egg	Ingestion	Mebendazole, 100 mg, orally, single dose	Obstruction secondary to worms; risk neonatal infection	Pyrantel pamoate, 75 mg/kg/day for 2 days (maximum dose 3.5 g)
Enterobius vermicularis	Egg	Ingestion	Mebendazole, 100 mg, orally, single dose	None	Pyrantel pamoate, 11 mg/kg as single dose
Hookworm					
Necator americanus Ancylostoma duodenale	Larvae	Skin penetration	Mebendazole, 100 mg, orally, bid × 3	Heavy infestation with anemia or malnutrition not responding to iron and rest	
Strongyloides stercoralis	Larvae	Skin penetration or colon penetration	Thiabendazole 25 mg/kg, bid × 2 days	Presence of infection (even asymptomatic)	Thiabendazole, 25 mg/kg, bid × 2 days
Trichuris trichiuria	Egg	Ingestion	Mebendazole, 100 mg, orally, bid × 3 days	Blood loss or rectal prolapse	Mebendazole, 100 mg, orally, bid (delay until after delivery if possible)
Filariasis					
Wuchereria bancrofti Brugia malayi	Microfilaria	Mosquito bite	Diethylcarbamazine, 3 mg/kg tid × 3 weeks, surgery for obstructive elephantiasis	Severe disease, otherwise do not treat until after delivery	Diethylcarbamazine, 3 mg/kg tid × 3 weeks, surgery for obstructive elephantiasis of birth canal
Trichinella spiralis	Larval cysts	Ingestion of uncooked infected meat	Thiabendazole 25 mg/kg, bid × 5 days if begun within 24 hr of ingesting contaminated meat; steroids to suppress inflammation	Ingestion of contaminated meat Severe illness (myositis, myocarditis)	Thiabendazole, 25 mg/kg, bid × 5 days within 24 hr of ingesting contaminated meat. Steroids

Parasite	Infective form	Mode of transmission	Treatment	Treatment	Contraindication
Trematodes (flatworms) Schistosomiasis *Schistosoma mansoni Schistosoma japonicum Schistotoma haematobium*	Cercarieae	Skin penetration	Niridazole, 25 mg/kg, evenly divided over 7 days	Niridazole, 25 mg/kg, evenly divided over 7 days	Severe disease
Cestodes (tapeworms) *Taenia saginata*	Larvae	Ingestion of raw or undercooked meat containing larvae	Niclosamide 2 g as a single dose	Niclosamide 2 g as a single dose	Best to withhold treatment until after delivery unless severe disease
Taenia solium Diphyllobothrium latum Hymenolepis nana	Egg	Ingestion	Nicosamide 2 g/day × 5 days	Niclosamide 2 g/day × 5 days	Treatment delayed until postdelivery unless severe disease
Echinococcus granulosus	Egg	Ingestion	Surgical excision	Surgical excision of hydatid cyst	Presence of hydatid cyst

time migrates to the perianal area, where the eggs are deposited. The eggs are infective within a few hours, and thus autoinoculation may occur. In addition, eggs remain viable and infective for 7–10 days and are widely disseminated in the local environment. Thus pinworm infestation occurs in multiple family members.

The vast majority of pinworm infections are asymptomatic (2, 4). Clinical findings are generally limited to perianal and perineal pruritis. Frequently, the itching occurs at nighttime. Migrant pinworms have been noted to ascend the vagina, producing vaginitis (6) and on occasion pelvic inflammatory disease (10). Lee (2) suggested that pregnancy may exacerbate symptoms of vaginitis and/or pruritis vulvae. No congenital infection has been described.

Diagnosis depends upon demonstrating the presence of pinworms on adhesive cellophane tape applied to the perianal region first thing in the morning. Mebendazole (Vermox) is the drug of choice in nonpregnant patients but should not be used during pregnancy. Pyrantel pamoate (Antiminth), in a dosage of 11 mg/kg up to 1 g as a single dose, is the preferred drug during pregnancy. The treatment is repeated after a 2-week interval (9).

HOOKWORM

Hookworm infection has a widespread geographic distribution in tropical and subtropical regions of the world (2, 4). Hookworm is caused by infection of the small intestine by *Ancyclostoma duodenale* (Old World hookworm) or *Necator americanus* (New World hookworm), which is fairly prevalent in the Southeastern United States (3).

Human infection occurs when hookworm larvae penetrate through the skin (2). At least 5–10 min of contact with contaminated soil is required for such penetration to take place. The larvae enter the bloodstream and are then carried to the lungs. Here they emerge into alveoli, ascend up the bronchi and trachea, and then are swallowed. Larvae mature into adult worms in the small intestine, and the adult forms live attached to the mucosa of the small intestine. The female worm produces 6000–20,000 eggs/day which are passed in the feces. Under suitable soil conditions the eggs hatch into larvae which molt to become infective for humans.

The clinical presentation in hookworm infection depends upon the stage of infection and the number of invading worms (2). In the initial stage a pruritic vesiculopapular rash may be associated with skin invasion by infective larvae. Migration of larvae via the lung may result in cough, wheezing, fever, and eosinophilia. The major chronic manifestations of hookworm disease are related to the number of parasites present and include iron deficiency anemia and hypoalbuminemia due to blood loss caused by the hookworms. Each adult worm can extract 0.03–0.26 ml of blood per day; in a light infection with 50–100 worms a 30-ml blood loss per day occurs, and with a heavy infection of 300 worms, blood loss of 80 ml/day occur (2). Langer and Hung (11) noted that previously asymptomatic hookworm infection may become clinically manifest in situations associated with increased iron needs, such as pregnancy and lactation. The diagnosis of hookworm disease depends upon demonstration of eggs in direct fecal smears.

Hookworm infection in pregnancy without anemia or malnutrition does not require treatment. Replacement of iron, vitamins, and protein often suffices. However, if this nutritional support is not adequate, specific hookworm treatment is necessary. Mebendazole is the drug of choice in nonpregnant patients in a dose of 100 mg b.i.d. for 3 days. However, it is teratogenic in animals and is best not used in pregnancy (2). Pyrantel pamoate is the recommended antihookworm drug for pregnant patients in a dose of 11 mg/kg up to 1 g in a single dose.

STRONGYLOIDIASIS

Strongyloides stercoralis is capable of producing severe, potentially fatal infection because of its ability to cause overwhelming autoinfection, especially with alterations in the host immune system (2, 4). Pregnancy is an example of such an occurrence. *Strongyloides* is widely distributed in the tropics but has been estimated to exist in up to 4% of people in the Southern United States (3, 4).

S. stercoralis survives and reproduces in man or in suitable soil (4). It is the only common nematode parasite which can complete its life cycle in the human host (2). The parasites are acquired from infected soil, where the filariform larvae penetrate the skin. They then enter the bloodstream and migrate the lungs. The larvae break into alveoli, ascend the trachea, and are swallowed. The adult form resides in the duodenum and upper jejunum, where the females deposit ova as they burrow into the intestinal

mucosa. The eggs may mature into infective filariaform larvae in the intestine and then penetrate the mucosa to restart the life cycle via autoinfection. This repetitive autoinfection and migration results in large numbers of adult worms inhabiting the small bowel.

Approximately one-third of humans with *S. stercoralis* infestation are symptomatic (4). Skin invasion produces a pruritic papular erythematous rash. Migration of larvae through the lungs is associated with a Loeffler-like syndrome of chest symptoms, diffuse opacities on x-ray, and eosinophilia in sputum and blood (2, 4). Most commonly seen are the signs and symptoms associated with the intestinal phase of *Strongyloides* infection. Diarrhea, abdominal pain, and eosinophilia are characteristic findings. In addition the large numbers of intestinal worms may produce malabsorption, protein-losing enteropathy, and iron deficiency anemia (2).

Diagnosis depends upon demonstrating *S. stercoralis* larvae in feces or in aspirated duodenal fluid. The only effective drug is thiabendazole (Mintezol) and is given in a dose of 25 mg/kg twice per day for 2 days. Because of the risk for hyperinfection associated with immunosuppression, even asymptomatic pregnant patients with *Strongyloides* infection should be treated. The mortality rate is very high in cases of overwhelming autoinfection, and prompt diagnosis and treatment may be life-saving (2, 4).

TRICHURIASIS

Trichuris trichuria, the whipworm, is one of the most prevalent helminth infestations (1, 2, 4). In the United States approximately 2 million people are infected with *Trichuris* (3). This parasite resides in the cecum and ascending colon. Man is the principal host, and infection is acquired by ingesting embryonated eggs (2). No extraintestinal migration of larvae occur in the life cycle of *T. trichuria*.

The majority of infected persons have low numbers of *Trichuris* and are asymptomatic (2, 4). However, heavy infestation can occur (especially in children) and is associated with anemia, bloody diarrhea, abdominal pain, and malaise. Severe infection with dysentery and tenesmus may result in rectal prolapse (12). Other than iron deficiency anemia or malnutrition in association with heavy infestations of whipworms, *Trichuris* is not a significant threat to pregnant women or their fetuses.

Diagnosis is made by demonstrating the characteristic lemon-shaped ova on a smear of fecal material. The treatment of choice is mebendazole (Vermox) (100 mg twice per day for 3 days). However, unless severe infection with significant anemia, malnutrition, and/or rectal prolapse is present, treatment of pregnant women should be delayed until after delivery (2).

Tissue Nematodes

FILARIASIS

The two major groups of filarial infection are bancroftian filariasis caused by *Wuchereria bancrofti* and malayan filariasis caused by *Brugia malayi*. These are similar clinical infections which are transmitted to man by mosquitoes (4). *W. bancrofti* is widely distributed throughout tropical and subtropical areas, while *B. malayi* is found only in South and Southeast Asia (4). It is estimated that worldwide, 250 million people are infected with these two parasitic helminths.

Following the bite of an infected mosquito, infective larvae pass into the lymphatics and lymph nodes, where they mature into adult worms. Fertilized female filarias discharge microfilariae into the bloodstream. With the exception of *W. bancrofti* in patients from the South Pacific, a surge of microfilariae into the blood stream occurs at nighttime. Microfilariae can invade the placenta and fetus (13, 14), especially in deliveries occurring during nighttime (13). Carayon et al have reported the presence of chronic bancroftian filariasis in the Fallopian tubes or ovaries, with resultant infertility (15).

The clinical findings in filariasis are due to either acute inflammation or to chronic lymphatic obstruction. Lymphadenopathy may be the only manifestation of the infection, or edema and ultimately elephantiasis may occur (2, 4). If lymphatics rupture into body cavities, the patient may present with chyluria, chylothorax, or chylous ascites. If elephantiasis involves the breast, it may interfere with lactation, and if the vulva is involved, labor may be obstructed (2).

Diagnosis depends on demonstration of the parasite in either blood or tissue. Blood samples should be obtained at nighttime for smear to identify the microfilariae. Adult worms can be demonstrated at times in lymph node biopsy specimens. Serologic tests are available for use but if the parasite is not seen, diagnosis relies on clinical findings and the presence of eosinophilia (2, 4).

No completely satisfactory treatment for filariasis exists. Diethylcarbamazine (Heterazan), in a dosage of 3 mg/kg three times daily for 3 weeks, reduces the number of microfilariae in the blood and may kill the adult worms (2, 4). The treatment may precipitate an acute inflammatory response around the dead worms. Anti-inflammatory drugs may be used to treat this reaction. Treatment during pregnancy is best withheld until after delivery.

TRICHINOSIS

T. spiralis, the parasite that causes trichinosis, is widespread throughout temperate areas of the world, especially where pork is a major component of the diet. Trichnosis occurs when inadequately cooked meat contaminated with infective larvae of *T. spiralis* is eaten (2, 4). The larvae are ingested in an encystic form in muscle and are freed from the cyst by acid-pepsin digestion in the stomach. Once the larvae reach the duodenum and jejunum, they attach to the mucosa and mature into adult worms. The adult forms of *Trichinella* penetrate the intestinal mucosa to begin discharging larvae (2, 4). The newborn larvae enter the bloodstream from where they invade striated muscles. After burrowing into the muscle the larvae encyst and become infective. Over the next several months the cyst calcifies.

The major reservoir for *T. spiralis* is the pig. Restrictions on methods of feeding used by commercial hog feeders has significantly decreased this source, and recent epidemics of trichinosis in the United States have been traced to meat obtained from game animals such as bears (2).

The most common type of trichinosis infection is asymptomatic infestation. With larval invasion of the intestinal wall, nausea, vomiting, diarrhea, and abdominal pain occur. During the period of larval migration, fever and eosinophilia develop. With larval invasion of muscle patients present with fever, myalgia, periorbital edema, splinter hemorrhages, and rash.

Diagnosis of trichinosis should be suspected in patients presenting with periorbital edema, myositis, and elevated creatine phosphokinase (CPK) and lactic dehydrogenase levels present secondary to muscle involvement (4). Serologic tests are available (bentonite flocculation) but are not positive during the early stages of disease (2, 4). Demonstration of encysted larvae in a muscle biopsy is diagnostic (2).

There is no completely effective therapy for

trichinosis. Thiabendazole (25 mg/kg twice per day for 5 days) is effective against ingested larvae, and if given within 24 hr of ingestion of meat contaminated with *T. spiralis* may prevent trichinosis or reduce its clinical severity (2). For later stages, supportive care with rest and salicylates is recommended. In severe disease, corticosteroids may be used to depress the inflammatory response.

Trematodes (Flatworms or Flukes)

SCHISTOSOMIASIS

There are three human blood flukes—*Schistosoma mansoni*, *Schistosoma japonicum*, and *Schistosoma haematobium*—which cause schistosomiasis. They have complex life cycles which involve aquatic snails as intermediate hosts. The schistosomes differ from other trematodes in that they exist as separate sexes and infect man by free-living cercariae (2).

The geographic distribution of the schistosomes is determined by the snail host. *S. mansoni* occurs in Africa, Middle East, northern South America, and Puerto Rico. *S. haematobium* is limited to Africa and the Middle East. *S. japonicum* occurs in the Far East. Man is the principal definitive host for these parasites (16). Following mating of adult worms, eggs are passed outside via host excreta. The eggs hatch in fresh water, where they release ciliated motile miracidia that penetrate into the body of their intermediate host—the snail. For each species and geographic strain there is a specific snail host. These miracidia multiply asexually inside the snail and emerge as motile cercariae which are the infective form. The cercariae penetrate human skin when they come into contact with it. Subsequently, they change into schistosomula and migrate to the lungs and liver. They then mature into adult schistosomes and descend via the venous system to their final habitat (16). *S. mansoni* localizes in the mesenteric and hemorrhoidal veins, *S. japonicum* in the mesenteric and portal veins, and *S. haematobium* in the hemorrhoidal, pelvic, and bladder venous plexuses. In these locations adult worms produce eggs that migrate to the bladder or intestinal tract lumen.

Acute schistosomiasis first presents as a dermatitis within 24 hr of skin penetration by the cercariae. It is a pruritic papular skin rash commonly called "swimmer's itch" (16). With commencement of ova production, schistosomiasis is manifested by urticaria, fever, and malaise. *S.*

mansoni and *S. japonicum* produce diarrhea with blood and mucos, weight loss, abdominal pain, and hepatosplenomegaly. The chronic disease is characterized by Banti's syndrome or polyposis of the colon. The end stage of hepatic schistosomiasis presents with jaundice, ascites, and liver failure. Infection with *S. haematobium* is characterized by hematuria during the acute phase, and the chronic stage is associated with polyposis and malignant changes in the bladder (2, 16).

The female genital tract can be infected with eggs of *S. mansoni* and *S. haematobium* (17–19). Rosen and Kim have noted that acute and chronic schistosomiasis inflammation of the Fallopian tube can result in ectopic pregnancies and infertility (20). Inflammation of the cervix, vagina and vulva may also occur and interfere with coitus, fertility or ability to deliver vaginally (16, 21). The frequency of placental infection is high in endemic areas, but the infestations are light and are associated with little inflammatory reaction (22, 23). There is no evidence that placental schistosomiasis is associated with intrauterine growth retardation or preterm delivery (22).

Diagnosis of schistosomiasis should be suspected in patients with the characteristic clinical findings and a history of travel to an endemic area. A definitive diagnosis requires demonstration of schistome eggs in feces or urine or in tissue obtained by biopsy of the rectum, bladder, or liver.

The majority of schistosomiasis cases are infected with few worms and have minimal or asymptomatic disease. Niridazole is effective against *S. mansoni* and *S. haematobium* and reduces the egg counts in *S. japonicum* infection (16). It is dosed in evenly divided doses of 25 mg/kg for 7 days. Alternative therapy includes antimony compounds which are associated with significant cardiac and renal toxicity. If possible, these drugs should not be given during pregnancy.

Cestodes (Tapeworms)

Tapeworms are capable of producing human disease in either stage of their life cycle (24). The adult stage produces signs and symptoms related to the gastrointestinal tract, where the adult worm lives. The larval stage produces signs and symptoms secondary to enlarging larval cysts in various tissues.

Humans are the definitive hosts for the tapeworms causing gastrointestinal symptoms. There are four of these worms: *Taenia saginata* (beef tapeworm), *Taenia solium* (pork tapeworm), *Diphyllobothrium latum* (fish tapeworm), and *Hymenolepis nana*. The only larval stage man supports, among the cestodes, is *Echinococcus granulosus*. Human infection occurs when raw or undercooked meat containing the larvae of the tapeworms is ingested.

Taenia saginata (BEEF TAPEWORM)

Man is the only definitive host of *T. saginata*. Following ingestion, the larva is released, develops into an adult worm, and attaches to the intestinal wall. This tapeworm can grow to over 30 feet in length. Symptoms due to *T. saginata* are limited and involve abdominal cramps and hunger (24). The diagnosis is made by examining the stool for proglottids. Treatment is available with niclosamide (Yomesan) in a dose of 2 g. Alternate drugs include paromomycin (Humetin) (1 g every 4 hr for four doses) or Quinacrine hydrochloride (1 g, single dose). During pregnancy, treatment may be withheld until after delivery.

Taenia solium (PORK TAPEWORM)

Man is the only definitive host for this parasite which is acquired by ingesting inadequately cooked infected pork. *T. solium* reaches a length of 10–20 feet. Clinical manifestations of intestinal pork tapeworm infection are mild or nonexistent (24). The treatment of choice is niclosamide (Yomesan) as a single 2-g dose. In pregnant women, treatment can be delayed until after delivery.

Diphyllobothrium latum (FISH TAPEWORM)

The adult fish tapeworm reaches lengths of 40–50 feet. *D. latum* has the greatest chance to adversely affect pregnancy (2). It competes with its human host for folic acid and vitamin B_{12}; in pregnancy this may result in megaloblastic anemia. Diagnosis is made by demonstrating proglottids or eggs in feces. Pregnant women with anemia due to *D. latum* should receive vitamin B_{12} and folic acid. Niclosamide (Yomesan) as a 2-g single dose is the treatment of choice. Paromomycin or quinacrine are alternatives. In pregnancy, treatment can be delayed until after delivery.

Hymenolepis nana (DWARF TAPEWORM)

Man acts as both the definitive and intermediate host for *H. nana*. The adult worm is 1–2 inches in length, thus the name of dwarf tapeworm. The clinical symptomatology manifests as abdominal cramps and diarrhea. Diagnosis is confirmed by demonstrating the eggs of *H. nana* in stool. Treatment of *H. nana* is with niclosamide (Yomesan) (2 g/day for 5 days). The 5-day course is necessary because recently encysted larvae may release eggs for up to 4 days. During pregnancy, treatment may be delayed until after delivery.

Echinococcus granulosis (HYDATID DISEASE)

Humans are accidental intermediate hosts of. *E. granulosus*, the carnivore tapeworm. Following ingestion of eggs, larvae penetrate into the mesenteric vessels and are carried to multiple organs. The liver and lungs are the most common sites for the development of large hydatid cyst(s). Diagnosis is suggested by the presence of a cystic mass and eosinophilia in a patient from an endemic area (2). The Casoni skin test and serologic tests are useful. Treatment of the hydatid cyst is surgical.

References

Amebiasis

1. Trussell RR, Beeley L: Infestations. *Clin Obstet Gynecol* 8:333–340, 1981.
2. Lee RV: Parasitic infestations. In Burrow GN, Ferris TF (eds): *Medical Complications during Pregnancy.* Philadelphia, WB Saunders, 1982, pp 386–404.
3. Reinhardt MC: Effects of parasitic infections in pregnant women. In *Perinatal Infections.* Ciba Foundation Symposium 77. Amsterdam, Excerpta Medica, 1980, pp 149–170.
4. Elsdon-Drew R: The epidemiology of amoebiasis. *Adv Parasitol* 1:62, 1968.
5. Schmerin MJ, Gelston A, Jones TA: Amebiasis: an increasing problem among homosexuals in New York City. *JAMA* 238:1386, 1977.
6. Jones TC: Entamoeba histolytica (amebiasis). In Mandell GL, Douglas RG, Bennett JE (eds): *Principles and Practice of Infectious Disease.* New York, John Wiley & Sons, 1979, pp 2087–2094.
7. Perez-Tamayo R, Brandt H: Amebiasis. In Marcial-Rojas RA (ed): *Pathology of Protozoal and Helminthic Diseases.* Baltimore, Williams & Wilkins, 1971, p 145.
8. Adams EB, MacLeod N: Invasive amebiasis. I. Amebic dysentery and its complications. *Medicine* 56:315–324, 1977.
9. Adams EB, MacLeod N: Invasive amebiasis. II. Amebic liver abscess and its complications. *Medicine* 56:325, 1977.
10. Armon PJ: Amoebiasis in pregnancy and the puer-

perium. *Br J Obstet Gynecol* 85:264, 1978.
11. Abioye AA: Fatal amoebic colitis in pregnancy and the puerperium: a new clinico-pathological entity. *J Trop Med Hyg* 76:97–100, 1973
12. Czeizel E, Hancsok M, Palkowich I, et al: Possible relation between fetal death and *E. histolytica* infection of the mother. *Am J Obstet Gynecol* 96:264, 1966.
13. Yeager AS: Protozoan and helminth infections. In Remington JD, Klein JO (eds): *Infectious Diseases of the Fetus and Neonate.* Philadelphia, WB Saunders, 1983.

Giardiasis

1. Wolfe MS: Current concepts: Giardiasis. *N Engl J Med* 298:319, 1978.
2. Lee RV: Parasitic infestations. In Burrow GN, Ferris TF (eds): *Medical Complications during Pregnancy.* Philadelphia, WB Saunders, 1982, pp 386–404.
3. Kreutner AK, Del Bene VE, Amstey MS: Giardiasis in pregnancy. *Am J Obstet Gynecol* 140:895–899, 1981.

Leishmaniasis

1. Lee RV: Parasitic infestations. In Burrow GN, Ferris TF (eds): *Medical Complications during Pregnancy.* Philadelphia, WB Saunders, 1982, pp 386–404.
2. Rocha H: Leishmania species (kala-azar). In Mandel GL, Douglas RG, Bennett JE (eds): *Principles and Practice of Infectious Diseases.* New York, John Wiley & Sons, 1979, p 2110.
3. Low GC, Cook WE: A congenital case of kala-azar. *Lancet* 211:1209, 1926.

Trypanosomiasis

1. Eyckmans LUC: Trypanosoma species (sleeping sickness and Chagas' disease). In Mandel GL, Douglas RG, Bennett JE (eds): *Principles and Practice of Infectious Diseases.* New York, John Wiley & Sons, 1979, p 2118.
2. Reinhardt MC: Effects of parasitic infection in pregnant women. In *Perinatal Infections.* Ciba Foundation Symposium 77. Amsterdam, Excerpta Medica, 1980, p 149.
3. Yaeger AS: Protozoan and helminth infections. In Remington JD, Klein JO (eds): *Infectious Diseases of the Fetus and Neonate.* Philadelphia, WB Saunders, 1983.
4. Lee RV: Parasitic infestations. In Burrow GN, Ferris TF (eds): *Medical Complications during Pregnancy.* Philadelphia, WB Saunders, 1982, pp 386–404.
5. Edgcomb JH, Johnson CM: American trypanosomiasis (Chagas' disease). In Binford CH, Connor OH (eds): *Pathology of Tropical and Extraordinary Disease,* vol 1. Washington, DC, Armed Forces Institute of Pathology, 1976, pp 244–251.
6. Bittencourt AL: Congenital Chagas' disease. *Am J Dis Child* 130:97–103, 1976.
7. Mahmoud AAF, Warren KS: Algorithms in the diagnosis and management of exotic disease. XI. African trypanosomiasis. *J Infect Dis* 133:487, 1976.
8. Goodwin LG: The pathology of African trypanosomiasis. *Trans Soc Trop Med Hyg* 64:797, 1970.

9. Weitz BGF: Infection and resistance. In Mulligan HW (ed): *The African Trypanosomiases.* London, Allen & Union, 1970, p 97.
10. Apted FIC: In Mulligan HW (ed): *The African Trypanosomiases.* London, Allen & Union, 1970, p 661.

Malaria

1. Reinhart MC: Effects of parasitic infection in pregnant women. In *Perinatal Infections.* Ciba Foundation Symposium 77. Amsterdam, Excerpta Medica, 1980, p 149.
2. Wyler DJ, Miller LH: Plasmodium species (malaria). In Mandel GL, Douglas RG, Bennett JE (eds): *Principles and Practice of Infectious Diseases.* New York, John Wiley & Sons, 1979, p 2097.
3. Yaeger AS: Protozoan and helminth infectious. In Remington JD, Klein JO (eds): *Infectious Diseases of the Fetus and Neonte.* Phildelphia, WB Saunders, 1983.
4. Young MD: Malaria. In Hunter GW III, Swartzwelder JC, Clyde DF (eds): *Tropical Medicine.* Philadelphia, WB Saunders, 1976, pp 353–396.
5. Lee RV: Parasitic infestations. In Burrow GN, Ferris TF (eds): *Medical Complications during Pregnancy.* Philadeliphia, WB Saunders, 1982, pp 386–404.
6. Bascom S, Hanson K, Thompson W, et al: *Plasmodium falciparum* malaria contracted in Thailand resistant to chloroquine and sulfonamide-pyrimethamine. *MMWR* 29:493, 1980.
7. Bruce-Chwatt LJ: Malaria in African infants and children in Southern Nigeria. *Ann Trop Med Parasitol* 19:173–200, 1957.
8. Gilles HM, Lawson JB, Sibelas M, et al: Malaria, anemia and pregnancy. *Ann Trop Med Parasitol* 63:245–263, 1969.
9. Reinhardt MC: A survey of mothers and their newborns in Abidjan (Ivory Coast). *Helv Paediatr Acta* 41(suppl):1–132, 1978.
10. Smith AM: Malaria in pregnancy. *Br Med J* 4:793, 1972.
11. Taufa T: Malaria and pregnancy. *Papua New Guinea Med J* 21:197, 1978.
12. Jelliffe EFP: Low birth-weight and malarial infection of the placenta. *Bull WHO* 38:69, 1968.
13. Archibald HM: The influence of malarian infection of the placenta on the incidence of prematurity. *Bull WHO* 15:842, 1956.
14. MacGregor JD, Avery JG: Malaria transmission and fetal growth. *Br Med J* 3:433, 1974.
15. Menon R: Pregnancy and malaria. *Med J Malaysia* 27:115, 1972.
16. Cannon DSH: Malaria and prematurity in the western region of Nigeria. *Br Med J* 2:877, 1958.
17. Torpin R: Malaria complicating pregnancy with a report of 27 cases. *Am J Obstet Gynecol* 41:882, 1941.
18. Hung LV: Paludisive at grossesse a Saigon. *Rev Palud Med Trop* 83:75, 1951 as reported in Yaeger AS: Protozoan and helminth infections. In Remington JD, Klein JO (eds): *Infectious Diseases of the Fetus and Neonate.* Philadelphia, WB Saunders, 1983.
19. Jelliffee EFP: Placental malaria and foetal growth. In *Nutrition and Infection.* Ciba Foundation Study Group no. 31. J&A Churchill, 1967, pp 18–40.

Helminthic Infections

1. Warren KS: Diseases due to helminths: Introduction. In Mandel GL, Douglas RG, Bennett JE (eds): *Principles and Practice of Infectious Diseases.* New York, John Wiley & Sons, 1979, pp 2155–2157.
2. Lee RV: Parasitic infestations. In Burrow GN, Ferris TF (eds): *Medical Complications during Pregnancy.* Philadelphia, WB Saunders, 1982, pp 386–404.
3. Warren KS: Helminthic diseases endemic in the United States. *Am J Trop Med Hyg* 23:723, 1974.
4. Mahmoud AEF: Intestinal nematodes (roundworms). In Mandel GL, Douglas RG, Bennett JE (eds): *Principles and Practice of Infectious Diseases.* New York, John Wiley & Sons, 1979, pp 2157–2173.
5. Piggott J, Hansbarger EA, Neafie RC: Human ascariasis. *Am J Clin Pathol* 52:223, 1970.
6. Garud MA, Saraiya U, Paraskar M, Khohhawalla J: Vaginal parisitosis. *Acta Cytol* 24:34, 1980.
7. Sterling R, Guay AJL: Invasion of the female generative tract by *Ascaris lumbricoides. JAMA* 107:2046–2047, 1936.
8. Chu W, Chen P, Huang C, Hsu C: Neonatal ascaris. *J Pediatr* 81:783–785, 1972.
9. Keusch GT: Antihelmithic therapy: the worm has turned. *Drug Ther* 1982, pp 55–64.
10. Brooks TJ, Goetz CC, Plauche WC: Pelvic granuloma due to *Enterobius vermicularis. JAMA* 179:492, 1962.
11. Langer A, Hung CT: Hookworm disease in pregnancy with severe anemia. *Obstet Gynecol* 42:564–567, 1973.
12. Lynch DM, Green EA, McFadzen JA, et al: *Trichuris trichuria* infestations in the United Kingdom and treatment with difetarsone. *Br Med J* 4:73, 1972.
13. Neves HA, Scaff LM: Comprovacao da microfilaremia congenita de *Wuchereria bancrofti. Rev Bras Malariol Doencas Trop* 6:283–284, 1954.
14. Bloomfield RD, Suarez JR, Malangit AC: Transplancental transfer of Bancroftian filariasis. *J Natl Med Assoc* 70:597–598, 1978.
15. Carayon A, Brenot G, Camain R: Vingt lesions tubo-ovariennes de la bilharziose et de la filariose de Bancroft. *Bull Soc Med Afr Noire Lang Fr* 12:464–473, 1967.
16. Mahmoud AAF: Trematodes (schistosomiasis, flukes). In Mandel GL, Douglas RG, Bennett JE (eds): *Principles and Practice of Infectious Diseases.* New York, John Wiley & Sons, 1979, pp 2173–2183.
17. Arean VM: Manson's schistosomiasis of the female genital tract. *Am J Obstet Gynecol* 72:1038, 1956.
18. Cowper SG: A synopsis of African Bilharziasis. London, HK Lewis, 1971.
19. Gelfand M, Ross MD, Blair DM, Weber MC: Distribution and extent of schistosomiasis in female pelvic organs with special reference to the genital tract, as determined by autopsy. *Am J Trop Med Hyg* 20:846, 1971.
20. Rosen Y, Kim B: Tubal gestation associated with *Schistosoma mansoni* salpingitis. *Obstet Gynecol* 43:413, 1974.
21. Bullough CHW: Infertility and bilharziasis of the female genital tract. *Br J Obstet Gynecol* 83:819, 1976.
22. Renaud R, Brettes P, Castanier C, Loubiere R: Placental bilharziasis. *Int J Gynecol Obstet* 10:25, 1972.
23. Bittencourt AL, deAlmeida MAC, Iunes MAF, daMotta LDC: Placental involvement in *Schistosomiasis mansoni. Am J Trop Med Hyg* 29:571, 1980.
24. Jones TC: Cestodes (tapeworms). In Mandel GL, Douglas RG, Bennett JE (eds): *Principles and Practice of Infectious Diseases.* New York, John Wiley & Sons, New York, 1979, pp 2183–2191.

CHAPTER 15

Premature Rupture of the Membranes

Although premature rupture of the membranes (PROM) is a common problem, at present there is little understanding of its basic pathophysiology and no agreement of the most favorable management. Indeed, the problem is intricate; major variables influencing the outcome of a study are gestational age, date of the study, and population features. New variables added within the last 10 yr include use of corticosteroids, tocolytics, and more potent antibiotics. Of major importance is the marked improvement in survival of low birth weight infants. In this chapter, we will provide a summary of the topic, with emphasis on works published since 1970. The literature of the former period was extensively reviewed by Gunn et al (1).

DEFINITIONS

An obstacle to an understanding of PROM is the lack of a standard and specific terminology. Nearly all recent publications are in agreement by defining PROM as rupture *at any time before the onset of contractions*. In this chapter, we shall use this definition. In early reports, some authors use rupture for intervals of up to 12 hr before diagnosing PROM. Unfortunately, "premature" also carries the connotation of preterm pregnancy. To avoid confusion, we shall use the word "preterm" to refer to gestational age of less than 37 weeks. Terminology is still further confused because others have used the expression "prolonged rupture of the membranes" and have used the same abbreviation, PROM (2, 3).

The *latent period* is defined as the time from membrane rupture to onset of contractions. It is to be distinguished from a similar term, "latent phase," designating the early phase of labor before the active phase.

Respiratory distress syndrome (RDS) requires careful definition. Commonly used criteria include early onset after birth; tachypnea, expiratory grunting, and retractions; cyanosis and hypoxia; and a chest radiograph showing a reticulogranular pattern with air bronchograms. Most studies use these criteria, but some do not define RDS. In one other, RDS is interpreted as "any breathing difficulty," and "hyaline membrane disease" is reserved for the more specific findings, noted immediately above (4).

Various terms have been used recently to describe presumed *maternal or perinatal infections* related to PROM. During labor, designations have included: "fever in labor," "intrapartum fever," "chorioamnionitis," "amnionitis," and "intrauterine infection." Whereas the first two terms are objective, they are also nonspecific, and the degree of temperature used to define "fever" is selected arbitrarily. The latter three terms are usually presumptive, based upon combinations of maternal fever, uterine irritability or tenderness, leukocytosis, or purulent cervical discharge. After delivery, maternal infection is referred to as "endometritis" or "postpartum infection." These diagnoses are usually based upon fever, uterine tenderness, and exclusion of other sources of fever. In few recent studies, though, were presumed maternal infections confirmed by reports of blood or genital tract cultures.

In neonates, the most common term used to report infection was *neonatal sepsis*, but this may mean strictly a positive blood culture or simply clinical signs or symptoms of sepsis. Neonatal meningitis and pneumonia were also noted in a few studies. Administration of antibiotics prophylactically to the mother, as in many reports, would be likely to influence detection of bacteremia in the newborn.

INCIDENCE

The incidence of PROM ranges from 4.5 to 7.6% of total deliveries in several recent reports (5–7). PROM in preterm patients occurred in approximately 1% of all pregnancies (8–10), but many authors do not provide overall incidence. Gunn and colleagues noted the incidence in earlier reports ranged from 2.7 to 17%, with an average of about 10% (1). In view of the wide range in older studies, the absence of incidence data from many recent studies, and the differences in populations studied, it would be inappropriate to conclude that there has been any decrease in the incidence of PROM. Approximately 70% of cases of PROM occur in pregnancies at term (5, 7), but, in referral centers, more than 50% of cases may occur in preterm pregnancies (11).

ETIOLOGY
Clinical Variables

In the vast majority of instances, the etiology is not understood. Evaldson and colleagues found associations between a number of clinical variables, including previous genital operations, cervical operations and lacerations, and heavy smoking (9), and Eggers and co-workers reported that a number of their cases occurred in women with cervical incompetence, multiple pregnancies, polyhydramnios, and antepartum hemorrhage (12). Naeye and Peters found no association between the frequency of PROM and parity, maternal weight, or type of work (13). Earlier studies had reported no relationship of PROM to maternal age, parity, fetal weight, and position or trauma (1). A novel observation was that PROM occurred more commonly when the barometric pressure was lower (14).

Physical Properties of the Membranes

In the last decade, there has been continued interest in the physical properties of membranes which rupture prematurely. In 1981, Skinner and colleagues reported that the collagen content of amnion normally decreases in late pregnancy, even in patients without PROM, but that these changes occur earlier in gestation in patients with PROM (15). However, Al Zaid and co-workers found no significant difference in the collagen content of fetal membranes among patient groups with term spontaneous ROM, with term artificial ROM, and with preterm PROM (16). Yet, there were important differences in methods. The former investigators measured collagen content in micrometers per milligram dry weight of amnion, whereas the latter workers measured it a micrometer per square centimeter of "fetal membranes."

Other recent reports have shown that membranes from cases with PROM are thinner (17, 18). Using in vitro techniques to measure rupturing pressure, three groups of investigators have found that the membranes from patients with PROM require either the same or higher pressure than do membranes from those without PROM (16, 17, 19). Such observations have suggested that there might be a local defect at the site of rupture, rather than a diffuse weakening, in membranes which rupture before labor. Yet, these studies of physical properties should be interpreted cautiously because of differences in measuring techniques, possible deterioration of membrane preparations, and need for proper controls.

Infection

There is substantial evidence that subclinical infection may be a cause of PROM, not merely its result. In their continuing analysis of data from the Collaborative Perinatal Project (1959–1966), Naeye and Peters point out that acute inflammation of the placental membranes is twice as common when membranes rupture within 4 hr before labor than when they rupture after the onset of labor. They suggest that this "infection" may be the cause of PROM (13). In an additional analysis of the data, Naeye (20) recently considered two successive singleton pregnancies in each of 5230 women (10,460 pregnancies). Successive pregnancies were selected in order to "minimize the influences of heredity and other undefined factors." Data on placental examination, coitus since the last clinic visit, and cervical surgery or instrumentation were available in 56%, 61%, and 76% of the cases, respectively. Naeye found that preterm PROM occurred in only 2% of 773 pregnancies when recent coitus and histologic chorioamnionitis were absent, but in 23% of 96 pregnancies when both of these features were present. Although this study shows an impressive increase in preterm PROM associated with these two features, a causal role cannot be established because there may be other factors which were not considered. Evaluation of successive pregnancies would not necessarily eliminate these additional factors.

Naeye and Ross (21) have provided also an interesting prospective study of coitus, histologic chorioamnionitis, and adverse pregnancy outcome in South African blacks. They found that histologic chorioamnionitis and PROM were increased when coitus had occurred within the last 7 days, after which no effect of coitus was noted. Use of a condom during coitus resulted in less placental inflammation. In addition, PROM was more frequent (p < 0.01) when there had been orgasm during coitus and with histologic chorioamnionitis than when these factors were absent.

Cederqvist and colleagues investigated cord blood immunoglobulins and noted two patterns of onset of infection after PROM (22). In one, there was clinical and immunologic evidence of infection within 12 hr of PROM. This observation suggests that infection occurred before rupture and may have been the cause.

Further evidence is provided by recent bacteriologic studies. Creatsas and colleagues found that patients with PROM prior to term were more likely to have anaerobes in endocervical cultures than were women without PROM at term (23). This observation may be interpreted to show that subclinical anaerobic "infection" leads to PROM. It has been demonstrated that subclinical bacterial amnionitis may develop with intact membranes (24, 25). However, the increased likelihood of anaerobes in cervical cultures may reflect hormonal or other influences at different stages of gestation or perhaps an inhibitory effect of leaking amniotic fluid on aerobes at term (26). This latter possibility is interesting in light of the observation of Del-Bene and colleagues that anaerobes were found more commonly in the cervices of women with ROM greater than 12 hr (27). In an uncontrolled study, Christensen and co-workers found potentially pathogenic bacteria in the lower genital tract of 19 of 20 women with PROM before term. The most common isolates were *Ureaplasma urealyticum, Escherichia coli*, and groups D and B streptococci (8).

In view of the implications of these studies linking subclinical infection, coitus, and adverse pregnancy outcome, a well-designed clinical, microbiologic, and histologic study to determine whether such relationships exist in current populations in the United States is needed.

DIAGNOSIS

In the majority of instances, PROM is readily diagnosed by history, physical findings, and simple laboratory tests. These diagnostic tests have been summarized recently (28, 29). Standard tests are based upon determination of pH (nitrazene test) or detection of a "ferning" pattern or of fetal cells. Although these tests are accurate in approximately 99% of cases, they each have well-known false-positive and false-negative results, especially in cases with small amounts of amniotic fluid in vagina. Newer approaches to diagnosing PROM in such equivocal cases include biochemical and histochemical tests and intraamniotic injection of various dyes.

In studies utilizing the former techniques, investigators have reported good results with activity of diamine oxidase (30, 31), detection of glucose and fructose (32), fluorescence induced by 3:4-benzylpyrene (33), rapid strip tests for pH and protein (34), and α-fetoprotein (35).

In 1970, Atlay reported a technique to diagnose PROM by injecting Evans blue dye intraamniotically and then observe the dye egress through the cervix (36). He felt that this technique correctly diagnosed the membrane status in seven equivocal cases of PROM prior to term. The authors acknowledged that the infants might be stained if delivered within 48 hr, but felt that the dye could be readily washed off. However, Morrison and Wiseman noted, in two neonates, intense bluestaining which gradually faded over 6 weeks (37). Evans blue dye itself is innocuous and is used to determine blood volume in newborns. When methylene blue dye has been injected intraamniotically, neonatal hemolysis and marked hyperbilirubinemia have been noted (38, 39). Since the effect may be dose-related, Plunkett suggested use of a dose of only 1.6 mg of dye (39). Smith has recently reported intraamniotic injection of sodium fluorescein for detection of PROM (29).

In cases where the diagnosis of PROM is uncertain, one may question use of various dye injection, since this technique carries a small risk of trauma and infection from the amniocentesis and possible risk from some of the dyes themselves. Second, there may be false-positives because of extraovular leakage of dye. Third, amniocentesis may occasionally result in rupture of previously intact membranes. Fourth, in equivocal cases, the accuracy of such tests is unknown, as there is no definitive test against which they may be compared. Fifth, patients with small or transient leaks of fluid may not be at the same risk for complications as patients with frank PROM. Finally, once the diagnosis appears established by these invasive techniques, the results may not make any major difference in management.

Ultrasound examination has also been mentioned as a diagnostic technique, since a finding of oligohydramnios might suggest PROM (40), but oligohydramnios is hardly specific and perhaps not sensitive for this diagnosis.

LABOR

Onset

At term, the onset of labor occurs within 24 hr after membrane rupture in 80–90% of patients (1). In one recent study, Kappy and co-workers found in patients at term that the latent period exceeded 24 hr in 19%. In another study, they noted that the latent period exceeded 48 hr in 12.5% (11, 41). Only 3.6% of patients did not go into labor within 7 days (41). Among patients with PROM prior to term, latent periods are longer. Again confirming older studies, more recent investigations have shown latent periods greater than 24 hr in 57–83% (11, 42), greater than 72 hr in 15–26% (6, 43, 44), and greater than or equal to 7 days in 19–41% (8, 11, 12) (Fig. 15.1). Johnson showed an inverse relationship between gestational age and the proportion of patients with latent periods greater than 3 days (43). For pregnancies between 25 and 32 weeks, 33% had latent periods greater than 3 days, whereas for pregnancies 33–34 and 35–36 weeks, the corresponding values were 16% and 4.5%, respectively.

Tocolysis

In a few studies, investigators have given tocolytic agents, either with or without steroids, to patients with PROM before term (12, 42, 45–50). In some, tocolytics were used to delay delivery for approximately 48 hr after steroid administration, while in others no limit was placed on duration of tocolytic therapy. Christensen reported that ritodrine was able to delay delivery significantly for up to, but not beyond, 24 hr (46).

Nochimson noted a greater percentage of patients delivering after 24 hr when he used magnesium sulfate, but this was not a well-controlled observation (42). Eggers was able to delay delivery for at least 6 days in 38.5% of 13 patients (12). Recently, Stubblefield and Heyl reported that they delayed delivery for 3 days in 52.6% of 19 patients, but for 7 days in only 10.5% (48).

Cesarean Delivery

In recent reports, the percentage of patients delivered by cesarean birth ranges from 7 to 44% (Tables 15.1 and 15.2) and is markedly higher than the range of 1–7% reported before 1970 (1). This increase is important as cesarean birth is both the major risk factor for puerperal infection and a risk factor for RDS. Kappy and co-workers recently reported a significantly higher rate of cesarean delivery when induction was attempted (39%) compared to when an expectant policy was followed (12%) among patients at term with PROM and an unfavorable cervix (41). However, this was not a randomized study, and the criteria for cesarean delivery in the latent phase of labor were not clear.

In a prospective, randomized study, Duff and colleagues also found a lower rate of cesarean delivery among term patients with PROM and unfavorable cervices when an expectant policy was followed (12/59 (20%) in the induction group versus 6/75 (8%) in the expectant group, p <0.05) (51). In patients managed by induction, 58% of cesarean sections were the result of failed induction, defined in this study as no cervical change after 8 hr of regular uterine activity or after a total of 12 hr of oxytocin administration. Management schemes which urge induction in either term or preterm pregnancies with unfavorable cervices are likely to have higher cesarean delivery rates.

COMPLICATIONS

The risks of PROM have generally been viewed as those of infection versus those of prematurity. Analysis of data published since 1970 is difficult because of the complexity of these studies and differences in study design. Tables 15.1 and 15.2 and Figure 15.2 summarize the results of recent works. Direct comparisons of data from one study to another require ex-

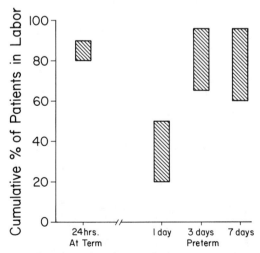

Figure 15.1. Onset of labor after premature rupture of membranes in seven studies since 1970. Column on *left* shows data for patients at term. The three columns on the *right* show data for all preterm pregnancies.

Table 15.1.
Outcome in Studies of Premature Rupture of Membranes Published in 1980–1983

Author, yr, location	Gestational age or birth weight	No. of patients	Cesarean delivery	PNM[a]	Complications RDS[b]	Infection(%)[c]
Schutte et al, 1983 (52) Amsterdam, Netherlands	16 weeks to term	321 mothers 334 infants	NR[d]	10% for 28–38 weeks; 2.6% for ≥37 weeks	NR	Neonates: Preterm 16, Term 3; Maternal: ("fever on day of delivery") 15
Brame and MacKenna, 1983 (53) North Carolina	26–35 weeks	214	7%	7%	23%	Maternal 3, Neonatal 4
Wilson et al, 1982 (54) Virginia	<37 weeks	143 mothers 145 infants	22%	15%	85% (used ventilator therapy)	Maternal 10, Neonatal 7
Kuhn et al, 1982 (49) Melbourne, Australia	25–33 weeks	216	NR	NR for group with PROM	"Severe" 18.6%	Maternal 18, Neonatal 20
Barrett and Boehm, 1982 (50) Tennessee	26–34 weeks	89 mothers 93 infants	NR	11%	23%	Amn 32, Neonatal 2
Graham, 1982 (10) Texas	<34 weeks	109	NR	21–41%	41–76%	NNS 15–28 (includes clinical diagnosis)
Kappy, 1982 (41) Massachusetts	>36 weeks	150	12–100%	0		Overall, "febrile morbidity" 13, NNS 0
Perkins, 1982 (4) New Mexico	<2001 g	133 infants 125 mothers	29%	10%	20%	"Fever" 23, NNS 0
Garite et al, 1981 (55) California	28–34 weeks	160 mothers	25–35%	2–6%	17–21%	Amn 14, Endo 14–29, NNS 0.5
Stedman et al, 1981 (45) Arizona	28–36 weeks	55	16%	7%	9%	Amn 14, NNS 2
Varner and Galask, 1981 (65) Iowa	28–36 weeks	127 infants 116 mothers	7%	3%	25%	Amn 9, Endo 7, NNS 7

Study	Gestational age	No.	PNM[a]	RDS[b]	Infection	Infection[c]	
Daikoku, 1981 (5) Maryland	≥37 weeks	454	Approx 8%	0.2%	NR	Maternal: "Fever" NNS	2.0 0.5
	<37 weeks	203	Approx 13%	32 weeks 33%; 33–36 weeks 4%	NR	Maternal: "Fever" NNS	6.9% 0.5%
Johnson et al, 1981 (43) Maryland	25–36 weeks	447	NR	25–28 weeks 43.5%; 29–32 weeks 11.3%	NR	NR	
Collaborative Group, 1981 (78)	26–37 weeks	288	NR	NR	10–12%	NR	14–15
Young et al, 1981 (58)	27–33 weeks	73	NR	NR	45–71%	NNS	4.1
Miller et al 1980 (44) North Carolina	26–34 weeks	95	24%	15%	NR	Amn Endo NNS	4.1 4.1 10.1
Christensen et al, 1980 (46) Sweden	29–35 weeks	30	10%	3.0%	10%	Amn Endo NNS	7 7 0
Evaldson et al, 1980 (9) Sweden	29–35 weeks	30	17%	18%	9%	Amn Endo NNS	20 7 12
Nochimson et al, 1980 (42) Connecticut, New York	27–34 weeks	42 (1977–1979) 61 (1974–1977)	17% 10%	5% 10%	12% 31%	Maternal: "Fever" Maternal: "Fever"	7
Schreiber and Benedetti 1980 (66) California	<2500 g	90	24%	13%	24%	Amn Endo NNS	25 27 10 18 (includes clinical diagnosis

[a] PNM, perinatal mortality.
[b] RDS, respiratory distress syndrome (see text).
[c] Infection: NNS, neonatal sepsis (positive blood culture unless otherwise noted); Amn, amnionitis; Endo, endometritis.
[d] NR, Not reported.

Table 15.2.
Outcome in Studies of Premature Rupture of Membranes Published in 1976–1979[a]

Author, yr, location	Gestational age or birth weight	No. of patients	Cesarean delivery	PNM	Complications RDS	Complications Infection (%)	Infection (%)
Kappy et al, 1979 (11) Massachusetts	24–40	78 (≥37 weeks)	36%	1%		Maternal infect. at delivery:	23
		110 (<37 weeks)	31%	10%	10%	NNS	0.5
Garite et al, 1979 (56) California	28–35 weeks	30	NR	0% (Mature group)	17%	Amn Endo (after vaginal delivery)	23 13
Eggers et al, 1979 (12) Australia	20–34 weeks	93	NR	24%	58% (25–34 weeks)	Maternal Fetal	19 17
Miller et al, 1978 (67) North Carolina	1000–2500 g	151	7%	1000–1500 g (29%) 1501–2500 g (2%)	1000–1500 g (42)% 1500–2500 g (7%)	Amn Endo NNS	8 7 2
Fayez et al, 1978 (6) Missouri	>34 weeks	59 (observed) 53 (induced)	0 6%	0 0	0 0	Amn NNS Amn	12 4 4
Berkowitz et al, 1977 (80) Connecticut	<36 weeks	340	NR	21%	41%	NN deaths related to sepsis	1.7
Bada et al, 1977 (7) Kentucky	All	963 total 270 <38 weeks	NR	Term, 0.1% Preterm, 13%	Preterm, 13%	Amn NNS (clinical diagnosis)	11 5
Mead and Clapp, 1977 (47) Vermont	27–32 weeks	43	38–48%	15–50%	22–81%	Endo Neonatal infection	15–19 26–50
Worthington et al, 1977 (85) Ontario	30–36 weeks	65	8%	8%	14%	NR	

	Gestational age	No.					
Thibeault and Emmanouilides, 1977 (2) California	25–34 weeks	153	19–34%	29%	ROM <24 hr (60%) ROM >72 hr (0%)	Amn NNS	4–33 / 3
Christensen et al, 1976 (8) Sweden	<36 weeks	24	NR	12%	30%	Endo NNS (clinical diagnosis)	12 / 8

a Abbreviations are the same as in Table 15.1.

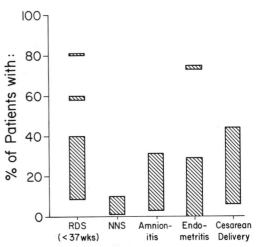

Figure 15.2. Ranges of complications in pregnancies with premature rupture of membranes in 22 studies since 1970. *RDS*, respiratory distress syndrome in pregnancies 37 weeks. *NNS*, neonatal sepsis.

treme caution. These wide ranging differences may be attributed to major differences from study to study in populations at risk, gestational age, definitions employed, and management used.

The most common complication among pregnancies with PROM before 37 weeks is RDS, which in general is found in from 10 to 40% of neonates. A small number of studies reported RDS in 60%–80% of newborns. Bona fide neonatal sepsis was documented in less than 10%, and amnionitis based always on clinical criteria occurred in from approximately 3–31%. Endometritis developed in from 0 to 29% in most groups, but it is not clear whether patients with amnionitis may also have been included in the endometritis category. In selected groups such as patients with cesarean section after PROM, endometritis has been reported in up to 70% of cases.

Causes of perinatal death may be determined by analysis of large series. four studies published since 1970 included more than 20 deaths (Table 15.3). Two of these studies were performed from the obstetrical viewpoint and included all women admitted with PROM (included those delivering stillbirths). The other two were performed from the neonatologist's viewpoint and excluded stillbirths. RDS, was, in general, the leading cause of death, especially among liveborn infants. Deaths were usually attributed to anoxia when there was an ante- or intrapartum

Table 15.3.
Effect of Corticosteroid Administration upon Respiratory Distress Syndrome and upon Infection in Patients with Premature Rupture of the Membranes

Author, yr	Design of study; agent	Gestational age range	Number of patients with PROM		Effect of steroids on:	
			With steroids	Without steroids	Respiratory distress syndrome	Infection
Studies of PROM						
Barrett and Boehm, 1982 (50)	Prospective; betamethasone use if L/S immature and gram stains of AF negative	26–34 weeks	36	53	No significant decrease, (14% steroid vs 29% no steroid group)	No increase
Kuhn et al, 1982 (49)	Prospective; partially randomized use of betamethasone	25–33 weeks	72	145	Significant decrease (p < 0.2)	Increase in fetuses, when cervical suture in place (p = 0.06)
Garite et al, 1981 (55)	Prospective; randomized use of betamethasone	28–36 weeks	80	80	None	Increased endometritis, mainly after vaginal delivery (p < 0.05)
Stedman et al, 1981 (45)	Prospective; betamethasone use not randomized	28–36 weeks	12	18	None	Not stated
Miller et al, 1980 (44)	Retrospective; -betamethasone use not randomized	26–34 -weeks	52	43	Not stated.	None
Nochimson et al, 1980 (42)	Retrospective; betamethasone use not randomized; historical controls	27–34 weeks	42	61	Apparent decrease	Apparent increase in fever *without* steroids
Kappy et al, 1979 (11)	Betamethasone use not randomized	24–37 weeks	44	45	None	None
Eggers et al, 1979 (12)	Bethamethasone use not randomized	25–34 weeks	38	55	None	Possible increase in cases with incompetent cervix (p = 0.06)
Mead and Clapp, 1977 (47)	Retrospective; betamethasone use not randomized	27–32 weeks	27	16	Marked decrease	None
Studies of Steroid Efficacy						
Caspi et al, 1981 (57)	Dexamethasone use not randomized	<34 weeks	73[a]	27[a]	Decreased (p = 0.08)	No comment

Study	Steroid protocol	Gestational age/weight			RDS outcome	Infection comment
Young et al, 1981 (58)	Dexamethasone use	27–33 weeks	38	35	Decreased (p < 0.05)	No increase in neonatal infections. No comment about maternal subgroup with PROM. Overall, maternal infection increased but "not related to steroid therapy."
Collaborative Study, 1981 (78)	Double-blind administration of dexamethasone or placebo	26–37 weeks	153	135	No significant decrease	Not reported for subgroup with PROM, but no increase overall.
Papageorgiou et al, 1979 (59)	Double-blind administration of betamethasone or placebo	25–34 weeks	17[a]	19[a]	Decreased (p < 0.039)	No increase
Ballard et al, 1979 (60)	Retrospective: betamethasone use not randomized	750–1750 g	37	43	Decreased (p = 0.005)	No comment
Taeusch et al, 1979 (61)	Double-blind administration of dexamethasone or placebo	<33 weeks	17[a]	24[a]	Not significantly decreased	Increase in maternal infection when ROM >48 hr (p < 0.008)
Morrison et al, 1978 (62)	Double-blind administration of hydrocortisone or placebo	<34 weeks	24	23	No comment about subgroup with PROM.	No increase
Block et al, 1977 (63)	Double-blind administration of betamethasone, methylprednisolone, or placebo	32–37 weeks	43	26	No significant difference	None apparent
Liggins, 1976 (64)	Double-blind administration of betamethasone or cortisone acetate ("relatively inactive" steroid)	<37 weeks	118[a]	94[a]	Decreased (p = 0.07)	No increase in "deaths with pneumonia"

[a] In these reports, the number of patients with PROM is not published. Numbers listed are patients with rupture of membranes >24 hr; these patients probably all had PROM.

death of a very small infant. Congenital anomalies and infection were each responsible for a distinct minority of deaths. Thus, in terms of both frequency and severity, RDS was a greater threat than infection to the preterm fetus.

Interaction of Treatment and Outcome

INFECTION

As noted in Figure 15.2, there are wide ranges in maternal and fetal infection. The effect of different management plans on infections is discussed below.

Effect of Steroids on Infection

A number of workers have used steroids in at least some patients with PROM. A summary of the effects in 18 studies is provided in Table 15.3. Three groups found evidence for an increased likelihood of infection after administration of steroids. In the work of Garite et al, there was a significant increase in maternal postpartum infection, mainly after vaginal delivery (55), but these infections were mild. Taeusch and colleagues also found a significant increase in maternal infection when ROM was more than 48 hr. In nonrandomized studies, the results are variable (61). In patients with PROM and a cervical suture, Kuhn and colleagues noted a higher fetal infection when steroids were used (6/11 (55%) with steroids versus 8/30 (25%) without steroids, p = 0.06) (49).

Effect of Latent Period upon Incidence of Amnionitis

In a number of earlier studies, the incidence of amnionitis rose, with increasing length of the latent period (1). Some recent reports have found a similar relationship (2, 6, 7), but other investigators have found no increase in the incidence of amnionitis among preterm pregnancies with increasing latent periods (65, 66). Still others found a variable effect depending upon weight groups (67). In Amsterdam, Schutte and colleagues found an increase in infection when vaginal examination was performed more than 24 hr before delivery in patients with PROM (52).

Effect of Prophylactic Antibiotics

Many recent studies have employed prophylactic antibiotics for either mothers or newborns, but few did so in a standardized fashion. Two recent studies evaluated prophylaxis among infants born after membranes had been ruptured for 24 hr or more. In a study of 100 infants, Habel and colleagues concluded that prophylactic antibiotics were unnecessary because infections were few, and that they were potentially hazardous because fungal infections and colonization were increased (68). Conversely, Wolf and Olinsky found neonatal infection in 17.6% and sepsis in 10% (3). They recommended use of prophylaxis until blood culture results were available.

Interest in prophylaxis among mothers with PROM has been more limited than in the past and usually reserved for patients undergoing cesarean delivery or receiving steroids. In the latter setting, Miller and colleagues found, in a retrospective study, a decrease (from 18% to 0%) in maternal infection when prophylactic ampicillin was used (44).

Because of the great variation in risk of infection, attention has been directed at determining the infection risk of a given individual. Garite and Freeman found that observing bacteria on a smear of amniotic fluid (obtained by amniocentesis) was 78% specific and 81% sensitive for prediction of infection (56). However, amniotic fluid was available in only half the patients, and amniocentesis may be accompanied by trauma, bleeding, initiation of labor, or introduction of infection. Similar results were noted recently by Cotton and Strassner (69). Accordingly, others have looked for predictors of infection maternal serum. Using an extremely broad definition for "infectious morbidity," Evans and co-workers reported that elevated serum C-reactive protein (more than or equaling 2 mg/dl) was an excellent predictor of morbidity in 36 patients with PROM before 36 weeks gestation (70). They also noted that maternal leukocytosis was significantly associated with infectious morbidity, but, because of the wide variation, this latter measure would seem to be of little value clinically. With a small number of patients, Kochenour and colleagues also found that elevated C-reactive protein levels predicted development of amnionitis (71). Later, Hawrylyshyn and colleagues reported on the predictive value of elevated CRP (more than 1.25 mg/dl) in 52 patients with PROM before 34 weeks (72). In these patients, steroids were administered routinely. Compared to WBC count ESR, the elevated CRP was the best predictor of histologic chorioamnionitis. In the 24 patients with elevated CRPs, histologic chorioamnionitis developed in

23, but clinical chorioamnionitis developed in only 7. Farb and colleagues studied patients with PROM between 20 and 36 weeks (31), with premature labor (41), and with a variety of other pregnancy conditions and found elevated CRP (more than 1.8 mg/dl) not predictive of clinical amnionitis, histologic chorioamnionitis, or neonatal sepsis (73).

Course of Amnionitis

Two recent retrospective reviews have shown that there has been an improving perinatal outcome in the face of clinically diagnosed amnionitis (74, 75). In contrast to earlier studies which had reported perinatal mortality rates as high as 32–50% in cases of amnionitis (1), these recent studies showed PNM of 2.8–14.1%, with few deaths being attributable to infection per se. Rather, the deaths were more commonly due to problems accompanying prematurity. Maternal outcome was excellent in both recent studies, although they noted an approximately threefold increase in cesarean delivery rates. In these two recent studies the vast majority of cases occurred in term pregnancies (74, 75).

Yoder and colleagues reported a prospective, case-control study of the outcome of 67 cases of microbiologically confirmed cases of intraamniotic infection (IAI) at term. Intrapartum bacteremia was found in 12% of mothers with IAI; neonatal bacteremia was documented in 8% of their infants. Cesarean delivery was indicated in 36%. Compared to controls, mothers with IAI had longer mean postpartum hospitalizations and higher fever indexes. Although neonates of mothers with IAI had significantly longer hospitalizations than control infants, the former did not have lower Apgar scores. Among the 134 infants, there was only one death, a known stillbirth in a patient who developed clinical IAI 3 days later (76).

In a recent prospective, controlled study, Garite and Freeman reported the outcome of 47 preterm neonates (28–34 weeks) born of pregnancies complicated by chorioamnionitis (77). The perinatal death rate was 13%, significantly increased ($p < 0.05$) compared with the rate of 3% in 204 preterm infants born after PROM, but without chorioamnionitis. Infants in the amnionitis group had higher rates for total infections (17%) than did infants without amnionitis (7%; $p < .05$). The former group also had a higher rate of RDS (34% versus 16%; $p < 0.01$). Noting the clinical and radiologic similarities

between RDS and group B streptococcal pneumonia, the authors hypothesized that they may have misdiagnosed some cases of pneumonia as RDS. RDS and neonatal death were significantly more common ($p < 0.05$) when chorioamnionitis developed before the onset of labor than when it developed during labor. Specific causes of death were not identified. Thus, in preterm infants, chorioamnionitis adversely affects neonatal outcome, but for the vast majority of infants the outcome is good.

RESPIRATORY DISTRESS SYNDROME

Effect of Steroids on RDS among Patients with PROM

A summary is provided in Table 15.3. Including both randomized and nonrandomized studies, a number of studies reported significant (or nearly significant) decreases in RDS, but others found no significant decrease when steroids were used in patients with PROM. Of special note, data from the large, blinded, collaborative study on antenatal dexamethasone administration showed no significant effect of steroids in reducing RDS among patients with PROM (78). However, there are major difficulties in interpreting these studies. In some of the more rigorously designed studies of steroid use, the numbers of patients with PROM is small. Thus, real differences may have been missed (a β error). Indeed, in most studies, there are at least small decreases in RDS in the steroid group. For example, in Block's paper (63), there was no significant difference in RDS in the group treated with betamethasone compared with the group given saline (3/25 (12.0%) versus 5/26 (19.2%)). With a difference of 7% between the groups, one would need approximately 200 patients in each group to achieve $p < 0.05$ (this assumes a standard β error of 0.2). There was also a relatively wide range of gestational ages studies. The minimum number of weeks for entry into a study varied from 25 to 32, and the maximum varied from 32 to 37. Since it is unlikely that an effect of steroids on RDS will be seen at all gestational age intervals, real differences may have been missed in some gestational age intervals because of combining them with infants of other gestational ages. Finally, from experiments of the surfactant-inducing potency of steroids in rats, there may be differences in the efficacy of various steroid preparations and differences from dose to dose (79).

Effect of Latent Period on RDS

Many studies have addressed this question with conflicting results. Some studies noted that prolonged ROM decreased the incidence of RDS (2, 65, 80–84). Others noted no significant effect (7, 8, 12, 61, 64, 66, 85–88), and two noted a variable effect depending upon weight groups (4, 67). These contradictory results may be explained by differences in experimental design (such as grouping of varying gestational ages and using varying sample sizes) or differences in definitions of clinical complications

Determination of Fetal Lung Maturity

Because RDS is the single greatest threat to the infants with PROM, some investigators have determined the status of fetal pulmonary maturity and proceeded with delivery when there was lung maturity. Garite et al (56) and Cotton and Strassner (69) used amniocentesis and obtained fluid in about half of the cases. In the other half, there was no suitable site for amniocentesis, or the attempt was unsuccessful. Others have attempted to collect amniotic fluid from the vagina and have had success rates of 80 to 94% (45, 89, 90). Presence of either phosphotidyl glycerol or an L/S more than 2 in amniotic fluid collected vaginally has been reported to be a good predictor of pulmonary maturity (45, 90). However, in some of these studies (89, 90), there were few amniotic fluids from patients in the critical interval between 28 and 34 weeks. In a larger series of patients with PROM before 36 weeks, Brame and McKenna determined whether phosphotidyl glycerol (PG) was present in the vaginal pool and delivered patients when there was presence of PG, spontaneous labor, or evidence of sepsis (53). Of 214 patients, 47 had PG present initially and were delivered. Of the remaining 167, 36 (21%) developed PG and were induced or delivered by cesarean section. Evidence of maternal infection developed in 8 (5%), and spontaneous labor developed in 123 (74%) of the 167 patients. PG in amniotic fluid from the vaginal reliably predicted fetal lung maturity. However, absence of PG did not necessarily mean that RDS would develop. Of the 131 patients who did not show PG in the vaginal pool in any sample, 82 (62%) were delivered of infants who had no RDS. Then, even with PROM, delivery of a premature infant simply because its lungs showed biochemical maturity may be questioned in view of other potential hazards of prematurity and the difficulty of the induction.

OTHER COMPLICATIONS

Asphyxia, defined as an Apgar score of less than 7 at 5 min of life, was noted in from 15 to 64% of live-born infants (4, 6, 9, 66). This complication was most common among the very low birth weight infants. Other complications of PROM, especially in the preterm pregnancy, are malpresentation, cord prolapse, and congenital anomalies. In view of the long list of potential hazards, it is not surprising that surviving premature infants after PROM still are subject to prolonged hospitalization.

PERINATAL MORTALITY

In the past decade, perinatal mortality (PNM) rates have decreased considerably among low birth weight infants, both with and without PROM. Factors affecting the reported PNM in the studies are: exclusion or inclusion of stillbirths, range of gestational ages studied, size of the study, and the span of years studied as well as calendar years in which the study was performed. Thus, it is not surprising to find PNM (expressed as % of all births) ranging from 2.5 to 50%. Most series have few perinatal deaths, and others do not specify the primary causes of death (see Table 15.4 for causes of death in four large series).

MATERNAL MORTALITY

Among recent studies, there was mention of only one death among over 3,000 women with PROM. This patient died of chorioamnionitis, severe toxemia, and cardiorespiratory arrest 29 weeks' gestation. Rupture of the membranes and signs of chorioamnionitis were not recognized (91). From the same institution, there are reports from the early 1950s of four other maternal deaths from long-standing infection (43). Other citations of maternal death from sepsis complicating PROM appear sporadically (92).

MANAGEMENT OPTIONS

As shown in Table 15.5, there are numerous proposals for management. However, no single plan has gathered widespread support. Aside from some studies on use of steroids, there has been few prospective, randomized, comparative studies of management of preterm PROM. Because of major differences in populations, studies are largely noncomparable and nonconvincing.

In general, physicians following a policy of

Table 15.4
Primary Causes of Death Among Infants Born with Premature Rupture of the Membranes Before Term[a]

Author[b]	Gestational age	Perinatal deaths	Causes						
			Perinatal mortality (%)	RDS (%)	Infection (%)	Congenital anomalies (%)	Asphyxia[c] anoxia (%)	Necrotizing enterocolitis (%)	Other (%)[d]
Daikoku et al (5)[b]	20–36 weeks	28	13.8	29	14	11	46		
Eggers et al (12)[b]	20–34 weeks	22	24	36	18	27	18		
Berkowitz et al (80)[c]	21–26 weeks	21	21	43	19	9.5	4.8	9.5	14
Bada et al (7)[d]	28–37 weeks	33	12.8	70	3				27

[a] Data are from studies with more than 20 perinatal deaths and with causes of death indicated.
[b] Studies of Daikoku and Eggers include stillbirths, while the other two studies included only neonatal deaths.
[c] Includes stillbirths with birth weight between 500 and 1000 g.
[d] Includes 5 deaths from "atelectasis", 2 from erythroblastosis fetalis, and 2 from intracranial hemorrhage.

Table 15.5
Management Options Proposed by Recent Authors for Patients with PROM

Term pregnancy
  Induction if spontaneous labor does not ensue within approximately 12 hr.
  Expectant management for a woman with an uncomplicated pregnancy and a cervix unfavorable for induction

Preterm pregnancy
  Expectant management. Delivery if labor or signs of infection ensue.
  Determine fetal pulmonary status by amniocentesis or from vaginal pool. Delivery if mature.
  Determine risk of infection by amniotic fluid stains or by C-reactive protein. Delivery if evidence of infection develops.
  Administer corticosteroids, with or without delivery in 24–48 hr. Tocolytics as needed.
  Delivery after an arbitrary latent period, ex, 16–72 hr.
  Combinations of the above.

intervention (such as for fetal pulmonary maturity) must consider the risks of diagnostic procedures (e.g., amniocentesis), of difficult inductions, and of hazards of prematurity other than RDS. Those following a policy of expectancy must acknowledge that in the vast majority of cases labor or infection will ensue within 3–7 days.

CONCLUSION

Recent studies have not provided a clear understanding of the pathophysiology of PROM or a sound basis for its management. Conclusions about management of PROM must be regarded as tentative, at least in part, but a number of shifts have become evident in the last decade.

First, maternal death is extremely rare, regardless of what course of action is followed. However, there has been a marked rise in cesarean delivery rate in cases with PROM and a likely associated increase in postpartum infection.

Second, the major cause of neonatal morbidity and mortality in cases of PROM before term is RDS. Both in frequency and severity, RDS is a greater threat than is neonatal sepsis.

Third, use of tocolytics in cases of PROM does appear to delay delivery, but for a limited time only (less than 3 to 7 days).

Fourth, examination of amniotic fluid appears to allow prediction of pulmonary maturity and infection. Yet, with amniocentesis, fluid is available in only half the cases, and amniocentesis may itself be attended by hazards. Reliable information regarding fetal pulmonary status may often be obtained from amniotic fluid collected in the vagina, but gram staining or culturing of this specimen is likely to be heavily contaminated with lower genital tract bacteria. Further, it is unresolved whether evidence of pulmonary maturity warrants delivery in view of other hazards of prematurity and of difficult inductions. It is also unresolved whether there is any real advantage to delivery before infection is clinically evident (i.e., when there is only a positive gram stain of the amniotic fluid).

Fifth, despite numerous investigations, there is still no agreement regarding the effect of prolonged latent periods on the incidence of RDS.

Sixth, the value of corticosteroids in decreasing RDS in preterm infants born after PROM is uncertain. Two recent well designed studies reported no signifcant effect (55, 78), but there is also evidence suggesting some value.

To resolve these problems among preterm pregnancies from PROM, there is need for comprehensive study in various populations. In clinical practice, caution should be exercised to avoid inopportune intervention with therapeutic modalities, and complete perinatal care should be provided in tertiary centers.

References

1. Gunn GC, Mishell DR, Morton DG: Premature rupture of the fetal membranes: a review. *Am J Obstet Gynecol* 106:469, 1970.
2. Thibeault DW, Emmanouilides GC: Prolonged rupture of fetal membranes and decreased frequency of respiratory distress syndrome and patent ductus arteriosus in preterm infants. *Am J Obstet Gynecol* 12:43, 1977.
3. Wolf RL, Olinsky A: Prolonged rupture of fetal membranes and neonatal infections. *S Srf Med J* 50:574, 1976.
4. Perkins RP: The neonatal significance of selected perinatal events among infants of low birth weight. II. The influence of ruptured membranes. *Am J Obstet Gynecol* 142:7, 1982.
5. Daikoku NH, Kaltreider F, Johnson TRB, et al: Premature rupture of membranes and preterm labor: neonatal infection and perinatal mortality risks. *Obstet Gynecol* 58:417, 1981.
6. Fayez JA, Hasan AA, Jonas HS, et al: Management of premature rupture of the membranes. *Obstet Gynecol* 52:17, 1981.
7. Bada HS, Alojipan LC, Andrews BF: Premature rupture of membranes and its effect on the newborn. *Pediatr Clin North Am* 24:491, 1977.
8. Christensen KK, Christensen P, Ingemarsson I, et al: A study of complications in preterm deliveries after prolonged premature rupture of the membranes. *Obstet Gynecol* 48:670, 1976.
9. Evaldson G, Lagrelius A, Winiarski J: Premature rupture of the membranes. *Acta Obstet Gynecol Scand* 59:385, 1980.
10. Graham RL, Gilstrap LC, Haulth JC, et al: Conservative management of patients with premature rupture of fetal membranes. *Obstet Gynecol* 59:607, 1982.
11. Kappy KA, Cetrulo CL, Knuppel RA, et al: Premature rupture of the membranes: a conservative approach. *Am J Obstet Gynecol* 134:655, 1979.
12. Eggers TR, Doyle LW, Pepperell RJ: Premature rupture of the membranes. *Med J Aust* 1:209, 1979.
13. Naeye RL, Peters EC: Causes and consequences of premature rupture of fetal membranes. *Lancet* 1:192, 1980.
14. Milingos S, Messinis I, Diakonmanolis D, et al: Influence of meterological factors in premature rupture of fetal membranes. *Lancet* 2:435, 1978.
15. Skinner SJM, Campos GS, Liggins GC: Collagen content of human amniotic membranes: effect of gestation length and premature rupture. *Obstet Gynecol* 57:487, 1981.
16. Al-Zaid NS, Bou-Resli MN, Goldspink G: Bursting pressure and collagen content of fetal membranes and their relation to premature rupture of the membranes. *Br J Obstet Gynaecol* 87:227, 1980.
17. Artal R, Sokol RJ, Neuman M, et al: The mechanical properties of prematurely and non-prematurely ruptured membranes, methods and preliminary results. *Am J Obstet Gynecol* 125:655, 1976.
18. Parry-Jones E, Pruja S: A study of the elasticity and tension of fetal membranes and of the relation of the area of the gestational sac to the area of the uterine cavity. *Br J Obstet Gynaecol* 83:205, 1976.
19. Lavery JP, Miller CE: Deformation and creep in the human chorioamniotic sac. *Am J Obstet Gynecol* 134:366, 1979.
20. Naeye RL: Factors that predispose to premature rupture of the fetal membranes. *Obstet Gynecol* 60:93, 1982.
21. Naeye RL, Ross S: Coitus and chorioamnionitis: a prospective study. *Early Hum Dev* 6:91, 1982.
22. Cederqvist LL, Zervoudakis IA, Ewool LC, et al: The relationship between prematurely ruptured membranes and fetal immunoglobulin production. *Am J Obstet Gynecol* 134:784, 1979.
23. Creatsas G, Pavlatos M, Lolis D, et al: Bacterial contamination of the cervix and premature rupture of the membranes. *Am J Obstet Gynecol* 139:522, 1981.
24. Bobbit JR, Ledger WJ: Unrecognized amnionitis and prematurity: a preliminary report. *J Reprod Med* 19:8, 1977.
25. Miller JM, Pupkin MJ, Hill GB: Bacterial colonization of amniotic fluid from intact fetal membranes. *Am J Obstet Gynecol* 136:796, 1980.
26. Larsen B, Snyder IS, Galask RP: Bacterial growth inhibition by amniotic fluid. I. In vitro evidence for bacterial growth-inhibiting activity. *Am J Obstet Gynecol* 119:492, 1974.
27. DelBene VE, Moore E, Rogers M, et al: Bacterial flora of patients with prematurely ruptured membranes. *South Med J* 70:948, 1977.
28. Friedman ML, McElin TW: Diagnosis of ruptured fetal membranes. Clinical study and review of the literature. *Am J Obstet Gynecol* 104:544, 1969.
29. Smith RP: A technic for the detection of rupture

of the membranes, a review and preliminary report. *Obstet Gynecol* 48:172, 1976.

30. Elmfors B, Tryding N, Tufvesson G: The diagnosis of ruptured fetal membranes by measurement of diamine oxidase (DAO) activity in vaginal fluid. *J Obstet Gynaecol Br Commonw* 81:361, 1974.

31. Wishart MM, Jenkins DT, Knott ML: Measurement of diamine oxidase activity in vaginal fluid—an aid to diagnosis of ruptured fetal membranes. *Aust NZ J Obstet Gynaecol* 19:23, 1979.

32. Gorodeski IG, Mordekhai P, Insler V, et al: Diagnosis of rupture of the fetal membranes by glucose and fructose measurements. *Obstet Gynecol* 53:611, 1979.

33. Montanari GD, Girsmondi GL, Zonoio L: 3:4 benzpyrene-induced *in vitro* fluorescence of fetal lipids in the diagnosis of ruptured membranes. *J Obstet Gynecol Br Commonw* 77:148, 1970.

34. Steinman G, Kleiner GJ, Greston WM: Spontaneous rupture of membranes, rapid strip tests for detection. *NY State J Med* 79:1849, 1979.

35. Rochelsen BL, Richardson DA, Macri JN: Rapid assay—possible application in the diagnosis of premature rupture of the membranes. *Obstet Gynecol* 62:414, 1983.

36. Atlay RD, Sutherst JR: Premature rupture of the fetal membranes confirmed by intra-amniotic injection of dye (Evans blue T-1824). *Am J Obstet Gynecol* 108:993, 1970.

37. Morrison L, Wiseman HJ: Intra-amniotic injection of Evans blue dye (letter). *Am J Obstet Gynecol* 113:1147, 1972.

38. Cowett RM, Hakason DO, Kocon RW, et al: Untoward neonatal effect of intraamnionitic administration of methylene blue. *Obstet Gynecol* 48:74S, 1976.

39. Plunkett GD: Neonatal complications (letter). *Obstet Gynecol* 41:476, 1973.

40. Larsen JW: Premature amniorrhexis. *Obstet Gynecol Annu* 8:203, 1979.

41. Kappy KA, Cetrulo CL, Knuppel RA, et al: Premature rupture of the membranes at term. A comparison of induced and spontaneous labors. *J Reprod Med* 27:29, 1982.

42. Nochimson DJ, Petrie RH, Shah BL, et al: Comparison of conservative and dynamic management of premature rupture of membranes/premature labor syndrome. *Clin Perinatol* 7:17, 1980.

43. Johnson JWC, Daikoku NH, Niebyl JR, et al: Premature rupture of the membranes and prolonged latency. *Obstet Gynecol* 57:547, 1981.

44. Miller JM, Brazy JE, Gall SA, et al: Premature rupture of the membranes: maternal and neonatal infectious morbidity related to betamethasone and antibiotic therapy. *J Reprod Med* 25:173, 1980.

45. Stedman CM, Crawford S, Staten E, et al: Management of preterm premature rupture of membranes: assessing amniotic fluid in the vagina for phosphatidylglycerol. *Am J Obstet Gynecol* 140:34, 2982.

46. Christensen KK, Ingermarsson I, Leideman T, et al: Effect of ritodrine on labor after premature rupture of the membranes. *Obstet Gynecol* 55:187, 1980.

47. Mead PB, Clapp JF: The use of betamethasone and timed delivery in management of premature rupture of the membranes in preterm pregnancy. *J Reprod Med* 19:3, 1977.

48. Stubblefield PG, Heyl PS: Treatment of premature labor with subcutaneous terbutaline. *Obstet Gynecol* 59:457, 1982.

49. Kuhn RJP, Speiers AL, Pepperell RJ, Eggers TR, et al: Betamethasone, albuterol and threatened premature delivery: Benefits and risks. *Obstet Gynecol* 60:403, 1982.

50. Barrett JM, Boehm FH: Comparison of aggressive and conservative management of premature rupture of fetal membranes. *Am J Obstet Gynecol* 144:12, 1982.

51. Duff WP, Huff RW, Gibbs RS: Management of the term patient who has premature rupture of the membranes and a cervix unfavorable for induction. *Obstet Gynecol* 63:697, 1984.

52. Schutte MF, Treffess PE, Kloostrerman GJ, et al: Management of premature rupture of membranes: the risk of vaginal examination to the infant. *Am J Obstet Gynecol* 146:395, 1983.

53. Brame RG, MacKenna J: Vaginal pool phospholipids in management of premature rupture of membranes. *Am J Obstet Gynecol* 145:992, 1983.

54. Wilson JC, Levy DL, Wilds PL: Premature rupture of membranes prior to term consequences of nonintervention. *Obstet Gynecol* 60:601, 1982.

55. Garite TJ, Freeman RK, Linzey EM, et al: Prospective randomized study of corticosteroids in the management of premature rupture of the membranes and the premature gestation. *Am J Obstet Gynecol* 141:508, 1981.

56. Garite TJ, Freeman RK, Linzey EM, et al: The use of amniocentesis in patients with premature rupture of membranes. *Obstet Gynecol* 54:226, 1979.

57. Caspi E, Schreyer P, Weinraub Z, et al: Dexamethasone for prevention of respiratory distress syndrome: multiple perinatal factors. *Obstet Gynecol* 57:41, 1981.

58. Young BK, Klein SA, Katz M, et al: Intravenous dexamethasone for prevention of neonatal respiratory disease: a prospective controlled study. *Am J Obstet Gynecol* 138:203, 1980.

59. Papageorgiou AN, Desgranges MF, Masson M, et al: The antenatal use of betamethasone in the prevention of respiratory disease syndrome: a controlled double-blind study. *Pediatrics* 63:73, 1979.

60. Ballard RA, Ballard PL, Granbert JP, et al: Prenatal administration of betamethasone for prevention of respiratory distress syndrome. *J Pediatr* 94:97, 1979.

61. Taeusch HW, Frigoletto F, Kitzmiller J, et al: Risk of respiratory distress syndrome after prenatal dexamethasone treatment. *Pediatrics* 63:64, 1979.

62. Morrison JC, Whybrew WD, Bucovaz ET, et al: Injection of corticosteroids into mother to prevent neonatal respiratory distress syndrome. *Am J Obstet Gynecol* 131:358, 1978.

63. Block MF, Kling OR, Crosby WM: Antenatal glucocorticoid therapy for the prevention of respiratory distress syndrome in the premature infant. *Obstet Gynecol* 50:186, 1977.

64. Liggins GC: Prenatal glucocorticoid treatment: prevention of respiratory distress syndrome. Lung Maturation and the Prevention of Hyaline Membrane Disease. Report of the 70th Ross Conference on Pediatric Research, Columbus, OH, 1976,

pp 97–105.

65. Varner MW, Galask RP: Conservative management of premature rupture of the membranes. *Am J Obstet Gynecol* 140:39, 1981.

66. Schreiber J, Benedetti T: Conservative management of preterm premature rupture of the fetal membranes in a low socioeconomic population. *Am J Obstet Gynecol* 136:92, 1980.

67. Miller JM, Pupkin MJ, Crenshaw C: Premature labor and premature rupture of the membranes. *Am J Obstet Gynecol* 132:1, 1978.

68. Habel AH, Sandor GS, Conn NK, et al: Premature rupture of membranes and effects of prophylactic antibiotics. *Arch Dis Child* 47:401, 1972.

69. Cotton DB, Strassner HT: Use of amniocentesis in the preterm gestation with ruptured membranes (abstr). Society of Perinatal Obstetricians, San Antonio, TX, February, 1982.

70. Evans MI, Hajj SN, Devoe LD, et al: C-reactive protein as a predictor of infectious morbidity with premature rupture of membranes. *Am J Obstet Gynecol* 138:648, 1980.

71. Kochenour NK, Rote NS, Thurneau GR: Nephlometric measurement of maternal serum C-reactive protein (CRP) as an indication of amnionitis associated with premature rupture of membranes (PROM) (abstract no. 204). Society of Gynecologic Investigation, Dallas, March, 1982.

72. Hawrylyshyn P, Bernstein P, Milligan JE, et al: Premature rupture of membranes: the role of C-reactive protein in prediction of chorioamnionitis. *Am J Obstet Gynecol* 147:240, 1983.

73. Farb HF, Arnesen M, Geistler P, et al: C-reactive protein with premature rupture of membranes and premature labor. *Obstet Gynecol* 62:49, 1983.

74. Gibbs RS, Castillo MS, Rodgers PJ: Management of acute chorioamnionitis. *Am J Obstet Gynecol* 136:709, 1980.

75. Koh KS, Chan FH, Manfared AH, et al: The changing perinatal and maternal outcome in chorioamnionitis. *Obstet Gynecol* 53:730, 1979.

76. Yoder PR, Gibbs RS, Blanco JD, et al: A prospective controlled study of maternal and perinatal outcome after intra-amniotic infection at term. *Am J Obstet Gynecol* 145:695, 1983.

77. Garite TJ, Freeman RK: Chorioamnionitis in the preterm gestation. *Obstet Gynecol* 54:539, 1982.

78. Collaborative group on antenatal steroid therapy: Effect of antenatal dexamethasone administration on the prevention of respiratory distress syndrome. *Am J Obstet Gynecol* 141:276, 1981.

79. Anderson GC, Lamden MP, Cidlowski JA, et al: Comparative pulmonary surfactant-inducing effect of three corticosteroids in the near-term rat.

Am J Obstet Gynecol 139:562, 1981.

80. Berkowitz RL, Kantor RD, Beck GJ, et al: The relationship between premature rupture of the membranes and the respiratory distress syndrome. An update and plan of management. *Am J Obstet Gynecol* 131:503, 1978.

81. Richardson CJ, Pomerance JJ, Cunningham MD, et al: Acceleration of fetal lung maturation following prolonged rupture of the membranes. *Am J Obstet Gynecol* 118:1115, 1974.

82. Bauer CR, Stern L, Colle E: Prolonged rupture of membranes associated with a decreased incidence of respiratory distress syndrome. *Pediatrics* 53:7, 1974.

83. Yoon JJ, Harper RG: Observations on the relationship between duration of rupture of the membranes and the development of idiopathic respiratory distress syndrome. *Pediatrics* 52:161, 1973.

84. Sell EJ, Harris TR: Association of premature rupture of membranes with idiopathic respiratory distress syndrome. *Obstet Gynecol* 49:167, 1977.

85. Worthington D, Maloney AHA, Smith BT: Fetal lung maturity. I. Mode of onset of premature labor. *Obstet Gynecol* 49:275, 1977.

86. Jones MD, Burd LI, Bowes WA, et al: Failure of association of premature rupture of membranes with respiratory distress syndrome. *N Engl J Med* 292:1253, 1975.

87. Dluholucky S, Babic J, Taufer I: Reduction of incidence and mortality of respiratory distress syndrome by administration of hydrocortisone to mother. *Arch Dis Child* 51:420, 1976.

88. Quirk JG, Raker RK, Petrie RH, et al: The role of glucocorticoids, unstressful labor, and atraumatic delivery in the prevention of respiratory distress syndrome. *Am J Obstet Gynecol* 134:768, 1979.

89. Isherwood DM, McMurray JA, Campbell C, et al: Case report. Prediction of fetal pulmonary maturity from amniotic fluid obtained from the vagina after premature rupture of the membranes. *Acta Obstet Gynecol Scand* 60:83, 1981.

90. Goldstein AS, Mangurten HH, Libretti JV, et al: Lecithin/sphingomyelin ratio in amniotic fluid obtained vaginally. *Am J Obstet Gynecol* 138:232, 1980.

91. Daikoku NH, Kaltreider F, Khouzami VA, et al: Premature rupture of membranes and spontaneous preterm labor: maternal endometritis risks. *Obstet Gynecol* 59:13, 1982.

92. Jewett JF: Committee on maternal welfare. Prolonged rupture of the membranes. *N Engl J Med* 292:752, 1975.

CHAPTER 16

Intraamniotic Infections (Intrauterine Infection in Late Pregnancy)

Clinically evident intrauterine infection occurs in approximately 1% of pregnancies and leads to increased maternal morbidity and perinatal mortality and morbidity. Clinicians have applied a number of terms to this entity, including chorioamnionitis, amnionitis, intrapartum infection, amniotic fluid infection, and intraamniotic infection. We have decided to use the last designation to distinguish this clinical syndrome from bacterial colonization of amniotic fluid and from histologic inflammation of the cord or placenta.

It is possible that subclinical infection of the uterine cavity and amniotic fluid may also be important, as it may lead to substantial adverse pregnancy effects such as premature labor and premature rupture of the membranes. These latter relationships will be discussed at the end of the chapter.

PATHOGENESIS

Prior to labor and rupture of the membranes (ROM), the amniotic cavity is nearly always sterile. The physical and chemical barriers formed by the intact placental membranes and cervical mucus are usually effective in preventing the entry of bacteria. With the onset of labor or with ROM, bacteria from the lower genital tract commonly ascend into the amniotic cavity. In some patients, the numbers of bacteria increase with the interval after ROM. This ascending route is the most common pathway for development of intraamniotic infection (IAI) (1). However, the precise relationship between time-related factors (labor and ROM), bacterial kinds and numbers, and development of clinical symptoms is not at all clear.

Occasional instances of documented IAI without ROM or labor support a presumed hematogenous or transplacental route of infection in

some cases. Reports of fulminant IAI with intact membranes often note *Listeria monocytogenes* as the offending organism (2, 3). Amniotic infection with this aerobic gram-positive rod often follows a maternal flu-like illness and may result in fetal demise. Other virulent organisms, such as Group A streptococci, may lead to a similar infection (4).

Certain special situations may also predispose to IAI. In a report by Charles and Edwards, 11 of 115 (9.6%) patients developed chorioamnionitis within 4 weeks of placing a cervical cerclage, and another 17 (14.8%) developed infection 4 weeks or longer after this surgical procedure (5). Infections after cerclage may develop because of the "foreign body" (the cerclage suture), instrumentation at the time of surgery, ROM during or after the procedure, or exposure of the membranes to the vaginal flora in patients with significant cervical dilatation. Kuhn and Pepperell (6) have reported infection as a complication in 18.6% of 242 pregnancies in which a cerclage had been performed. "Intrauterine infection" was diagnosed in 8% of 52 cases with cerclage in a report from the Netherlands (7), whereas Harger noted acute chorioamnionitis in 1.2% of 251 cerclages (8).

IAI may occur as a complication of diagnostic amniocentesis or intrauterine transfusion. With diagnostic amniocentesis, amnionitis has been reported from 0 to 1% of cases in a number of reports (9). In a total of 8000 procedures, only 3 cases were noted. Because of greater manipulation with intrauterine transfusion, it is not surprising that infection has been reported more commonly. Queenan noted infection as complication in approximately 10% (58) of 584 procedures (10). Of these, 3 cases developed gas gangrene, and 14 developed sepsis.

Naeye has reported an association between

recent coitus and development of histologic chorioamnionitis (11), but this work has been criticized because it did not acknowledge decreasing coital frequency in late gestation (12). Development of histologic chorioamnionitis (regardless of its etiology and significance) appears to occur more commonly in placentas of prematurely delivered women. Rather than coitus being the cause of the inflammation, it may simply be more common at earlier gestational ages. Still other studies have been unable to demonstrate any relationship between coitus and premature ROM, premature birth, or perinatal death (13).

Microbiology

Recent studies have described more completely the microorganisms which cause IAI. As with other pelvic infections, IAI is also polymicrobial, involving both aerobic and anaerobic bacteria. In a controlled study, Gibbs and colleagues collected amniotic fluid (AF) via an intrauterine pressure catheter from patients with fever and clinical IAI (14). To minimize contamination, they discarded the first 7 ml and performed quantitative cultures within approximately 1 h of specimen collection. To interpret this study further, they also reported cultures from other patients in labor, matched for gestational age, interval from ROM to specimen collection, and interval from ROM to delivery. Cultures from 52 pairs of patients were reported. In the AF of patients with IAI, the following high virulence organisms were found: *Bacteroides* species, 25%; group B streptococci, 12%; other aerobic streptococci, 13%; *Escherichia coli*, 10%; other aerobic gram negative rods, 10%; *Clostridium sp.*, 9%; *Peptococcus sp.*, 7%; and *Fusobacterium sp.*, 6%. The mean number of isolates recovered from the AF of these patients was 2.2. Of the 52 patients with clinical IAI, 48% had aerobes and anaerobes isolated; 38%

had aerobes only; 8% had anaerobes alone; and 6% had no aerobic or anaerobic bacteria in the AF. The rate of isolation of these high-virulence isolates from AF was lower in 52 matched, uninfected patients. Twenty-three percent of the control patients had high-virulence isolates, but only 7.7% had these isolates at a concentration $>10^2$ colony-forming units/milliliter (cfu/ml). In comparison, 69% of the patients with IAI had $>10^2$ cfu of a high virulence organism per milliliter of AF. Table 16.1 shows the number of patients in each group with high- and low-virulence bacteria as well as quantitation of the isolates. The study concludes that the AF cultures from patients with IAI were more likely to have $>10^2$ cfu of any isolate per milliliter, any number of high-virulence isolates, and $>10^2$ of a high-virulence isolate per milliliter. The isolation of low-virulence organisms such as lactobacilli, diphtheroids, and *Staphylococcus epidermidis* was similar in both the IAI and control group. Miller and colleagues also found an association between isolating bacteria in concentrations $>10^2$ cfu/ml of AF and "clinical chorioamnionitis" (15).

In Seattle, Gravett and co-workers performed aerobic and anaerobic cultures on AF on 16 patients with "amniotic fluid infection" (16). The most common isolates were anaerobic cocci, 4; group B streptococci, 3; *Escherichia coli* 2; and *Bacteroides bivius*, 2. In 13 of these 16 AFs, bacteria were isolated in 2+ to 4+ growth. In comparison, AF was also cultured from 22 asymptomatic patients. Here, only 11 had bacterial growth, and in 9 of 11 growth was 1+ only.

Edwards and Charles reported a smaller series of nine patients with chorioamnionitis and intact membranes after cervical cerclage (5). In this series, amniotic fluid was collected by amniocentesis, thus avoiding the problem of contamination incurred in the transcervical collection technique. The isolates were: *E. coli*, 5; other

Table 16.1
Characteristics of Amniotic Fluid from Patients with Intraamniotic Infection and from Controls (14)

Patient characteristics	Intraamniotic infection ($N = 52$)	p	Matched controls ($N = 52$)
Mean no. of isolates	2.2		1.2
No. of anaerobes	29		13
No. with $>10^2$ cfu/ml	42	<0.001	16
No. with $>10^5$ cfu/ml	23	<0.001	2
No. with no bacterial growth	3	<0.01	13
No. with high virulence isolates	42	<0.001	12
No. with low virulence isolates	7		27

aerobic gram-negative rods, 4; *S. epidermidis*, 2; *Peptostreptococcus sp.*, 3; group D streptococci, 1; *S. faecalis*, 1; *B. bivius*, 1; *Bacteroides sp.*, 1; and *E. lentum*, 1.

In none of these studies was *Neisseria gonorrhoeae* isolated. Yet, Hansfield isolated this organism in the orogastric aspirate of 14 neonates in Seattle over a 4-year period (17). When these infants were compared to 153 infants whose orogastric aspirate contained no pathogenic bacteria, the former were found to have maternal peripartum fever and histologic chorioamnionitis more frequently. On rare occasion, *N. gonorrhoeae* may cause amnionitis (18).

The isolation of genital mycoplasmas from the AF of infected patients has been described in individual case reports, but the cultures were obtained after the initiation of antibiotic therapy, thus possibly altering the flora (19). Other investigators reported an association between the isolation of *Mycoplasma hominis* and/or *Ureaplasma urealyticum* and placental inflammation (20). Unfortunately, these studies did not correlate isolation of these genital mycoplasmas with clinical infection in the mother or neonate. In a recent controlled study of IAI, Blanco and co-workers reported that 35% of 52 AFs from patients with IAI yielded *M. hominis*, whereas only 8% of the 52 matched control fluids had *M. hominis* (p < 0.001) (21). Specimens were collected via a transcervical catheter. Of the 18 AFs positive for *M. hominis*, 15 also contained >10^2 cfu of a high-virulence bacterial isolate per milliliter. *U. urealyticum* was isolated in AF from 50% of the infected and uninfected patients. Thus, *M. hominis* is present more commonly in the AF of infected patients but usually in association with other bacteria of known virulence. Furthermore, the patients with IAI and *M. hominis* in the AF responded to antibiotic therapy not specific for this organism, and in the control patients, *M. hominis* was isolated from AF on occasion without apparent sequelae. Therefore, the pathogenic potential of *M. hominis* is still unclear. Serologic and blood culturing studies may reveal its role more clearly.

At present, the role of *Chlamydia trachomatis* in amniotic fluid infections is unknown. Although *C. trachomatis* is known to grow in untreated amniotic cell monolayers (22), the clinical significance of this data is unclear, and only recently have investigators investigated the role of *C. trachomatis* in clinically evident infection. Martin and co-workers prospectively studied perinatal mortality in pregnancies complicated by maternal chlamydial infections (23). Two of the six fetal deaths in the chlamydia-positive group were associated with chorioamnionitis, compared to 1 of 8 in the control group. Wager et al showed that the rate of intrapartum fever was higher in patients with antepartum *C. trachomatis* infection (9%) than in patients without *C. trachomatis* isolated from the cervix (1%) (24). The data are interesting but must be interpreted cautiously because of the limited numbers and because the control group may not have been similar.

Host Defense Mechanisms

Although in most pregnant patients bacteria gain access to the amniotic cavity after ROM, few patients develop IAI. Therefore, some host defense mechanism must prevent or retard infection in the amniotic cavity. Possible defense mechanisms described are: polymorphonuclear leukocytes, lysozyme, β-lysine, transferrin, immunoglobulins, and inhibitory factors.

Polymorphonuclear leukocytes commonly appear in the amniotic fluid (AF) of laboring women following ROM. Although their presence is associated with fever in labor, many women without symptoms have white cells in the AF, and fulminant amnionitis such as that caused by group B streptococci may not lead to leukocytes in the AF.

Since 1968, a group of investigators at the University of Iowa have shown that AF contains an active bacterial inhibitor (25–30). In AF, they isolated a low molecular weight (approx 600 daltons) peptide-zinc complex which inhibited bacterial replication. The inhibitory activity of AF was eliminated by increasing the "phosphate" concentration and returned by adding zinc. Initial reports showed that the "phosphate":zinc ratio in the AF was a predictor of the in vitro inhibitory activity of AF (28). In a subsequent study of patients in labor, Gibbs and colleagues found that this ratio was not found to be a predictor of either clinical infection or inhibition (31). When compared to controls, patients with IAI had elevated "inorganic phosphorus" levels in the AF, but there was no correlation between the ratio of phosphorous to zinc and amniotic fluid bacterial inhibitory activity or clinical infection.

The exact mechanism of bacterial inhibition by AF is unclear; however, electron microscopy showed that microorganisms exposed to AF continue to grow and elongate but are unable to divide. This results in the formation of aberrant forms. The effect is similar for various types of bacteria (32, 33).

While the bacterial inhibitory activity of AF is an interesting in vitro system, further investigation was needed to elucidate what role this inhibitory activity might play. In a recent study of 50 patients with IAI and 50 matched controls, Blanco and colleagues found that only 30% of the AFs from patients with IAI inhibited the growth of *E. coli* as compared to 68% of the control fluids ($p < 0.001$) (34). Subsequently, these authors found that AF inhibited group B streptococci less commonly than *E. coli*, but still AF from asymptomatic patients was significantly more inhibitory than was AF from matched controls (36% versus 18%, $p < 0.02$) (35). It is unknown as to whether the inhibitory activity of AF prevents infection or whether the numbers, virulence, or other properties of bacteria alter the inhibitory activity of AF. It is possible that in some patients, the AF has inhibitory activity initially, but as bacteria invade the amniotic cavity, they may inactivate the inhibitor. In other patients, inhibitory activity may be absent from the amniotic fluid. These patients would then be susceptible to IAI if bacteria invade the amniotic fluid. With either mechanism, the types and quantities of bacteria may play a role. In other laboratories, the inhibitory activity of AF has varied with the bacteria species analyzed. (36, 37).

The variability in the inhibitory activity of AF may be due to differences in the inhibitory system, in the assay technique, or the presence of other factors preventing bacterial growth. Furthermore, the inhibitory activity of AF does not totally explain the pathogenesis of AF infection, and other complex factors must be involved.

Immunoglobulins (IgGs) are found in low but measurable levels in AF. IgGs represent an important host-defense mechanism in many sites, but little is known of their role in AF. The mean level of IgG in the AF from patients' IAI is significantly higher than the mean level in control patients (38), but these levels are still well below levels found in normal sera. Furthermore, the higher mean IgG level in the IAI fluids may be a result of nonspecific exudation of serum proteins, including IgG, into AF. Accordingly, these IgGs may not be specific for the infecting organism and may have no role in the infection. Also, the time course of infection in most patients with IAI may be too short to mount an effective immune response. However, long before the clinical symptoms appear, patients with IAI may have subclinical infection and commencement of an immune response.

Once IAI develops, the fetus may swallow and aspirate the infected fluid and is prone to develop pneumonia, enteritis, meningitis, and sepsis, as the fetal immunologic system may not be fully developed. In the mother, endomyometritis, peritonitis, and sepsis may develop as the infection spreads outward from the amniotic cavity.

DIAGNOSIS

The diagnosis of intraamniotic infection requires a high index of suspicion because the clinical criteria are neither specific nor sensitive (39). Moreover, usual laboratory indicators of infection, such as positive stains for organisms or leukocytes and positive cultures, are found much more frequently than is clinically evident infection diagnosed.

Clinical Criteria in the Mother and Fetus

The clinical diagnosis is usually based upon a fever, maternal or fetal tachycardia, uterine tenderness, foul ordor of the amniotic fluid, and leukocytosis. Other causes of fever in the parturient include concurrent infection of the urinary tract or of other organ systems and perhaps dehydration. The differential diagnosis of fetal tachycardia consists of prematurity, medications, arrhythmia, and perhaps hypoxia, whereas for maternal tachycardia other possible causes are drugs, hypotension, dehydration, and anxiety.

In Table 16.2 are listed the diagnostic criteria for acute intraamniotic infection ("chorioamnionitis") in three recent studies (1, 40, 41). In general, the most common clinical criteria are fever, leukocytosis, and ruptured membranes; fetal and maternal tachycardia are noted in variable percentages of cases. Foul amniotic fluid and uterine tenderness, although more specific signs, occur in a minority of cases. It should be noted that in all 67 cases reported by Yoder and co-workers, the clinical diagnosis was confirmed microbiologically (41).

Laboratory Criteria in Mother

Because of the lack of specific signs, the clinician commonly turns to laboratory tests for assistance. A urine specimen should be obtained for analysis . A high specific gravity may suggest dehydration, and in a properly collected specimen, bacteriuria and pyuria would suggest urinary tract infection. A portion of the urine specimen should be sent for culture and sensitivity.

Table 16.2
Clinical Criteria Used in Diagnosis for Acute Chorioamnionitis (Intraamniotic Infection) in Three Recent Studies

Type of study	University of Texas San Antonio (1): ($N =$ 171): retrospective	University of Southern California Los Angeles (40) ($N =$ 140): retrospective	University of Texas San Antonio (41) ($N =$ 67): prospective
Feature			
Ruptured membranes	98.2%	100%	100%
Peripheral leukocytosis	86.1[a]	2.9[b]	67[c]
Maternal fever	85.3	95.7	100
Fetal tachycardia	36.8	70	58
Maternal tachycardia	32.9	70	84
Foul amniotic fluid	21.6	18.6	7
Uterine tenderness	12.9		25

[a] Leukocyte count, >10,000/ml^3.
[b] Only leukocytosis, >20,000/ml^3.
[c] Leukocyte count, >15,000/ml^3.

In patients with fever, two sets of blood cultures should be drawn, but bacteremia occurs in only about 10%. Because peripheral blood leukocytosis occurs commonly in normal labor, we must not rely solely upon this result to suggest infection.

Direct examination of the amniotic fluid may provide important diagnostic information. We have found that samples can be collected by aspiration of an intrauterine pressure catheter in more than 50% of cases with fever in labor. Alternative routes include needle aspiration of the forewaters or amniocentesis. When the specimen is collected by either aspiration of a catheter or of the forewaters, contamination is possible. Thus when aspirating a catheter, discard the first 5 to 7 ml of fluid. With any technique, it is helpful to plate the specimen promptly and quantitatively, to help distinguish mere contaminants from bacteria causing infection.

In recent studies of *selected* patients at risk for infection, investigators have found a significant association between observing bacteria in a stain of uncentrifuged amniotic fluid, on the one hand, and colony counts greater than 10^2 or 10^3/ml and clinical infection on the other hand (14, 15). However, in specimens from *unselected* patients who are in labor with ruptured membranes, bacteria may be seen very commonly. Yet, few of these patients developed clinical infection (42). Accordingly, in patients with suspected intraamniotic infection, observing bacteria on a smear of uncentrifuged fluid supports the diagnosis, but there may be either false-positive or false-negative results.

In *unselected* patients in labor with ruptured membranes, some authors have found that leukocytes observed on smear correlate with infection while others do not. Among *selected* high-risk patients, again there is a correlation between presence of leukocytes in a smear and clinical infection, but there is a wide range of counts in amniotic fluid of both infected and uninfected patients.

Although 24–72 h are required before culture reports are available, samples may be of value in confirming infection or in aiding antibiotic selection. Prior to labor and ROM, amniotic fluid is generally sterile. During labor, but prior to membrane rupture, it has been shown that bacteria may commonly be found in the amniotic fluid. After the membranes have ruptured, amniotic fluid cultures are commonly positive. Samples have been obtained for culture by either amniocentesis or aspiration of a pressure catheter. Thus, in interpreting amniotic fluid cultures, one must consider technique of collection and quantitative reports.

Clinical Criteria in the Neonate (43, 44)

Most cases of early onset neonatal sepsis originate in utero. Prolonged ROM and prematurity are high-risk factors for neonatal sepsis. Immediately after delivery, though, the diagnosis of septicemia is difficult. The neonate's response to infection is impaired, and his reaction is often nonspecific.

The earliest signs are the most subtle and include changes in color, tone, activity, and feeding, poor temperature control, or simply a feeling that the newborn is "not doing well." Other early signs may be abdominal distention, apnea, and jaundice, but they may not appear until late stages, or they may even be seen in healthy prematures. Late signs may include grunting, dyspnea, cyanosis, arrhythmias, hepatosplenomegaly, petechiae, seizures, bulging fontanelles, and irritability. In addition, focal signs of meningitis or pneumonia may develop.

Since septicemia can present with such a multiplicity of findings, the differential diagnosis is extensive. When sepsis is suspected, repeated careful examination is advised, and the noenate should have a thorough laboratory evaluation.

Laboratory Criteria in the Neonate and Placenta

Examination of gastric aspirate and external ear fluid for polymorphonuclear leukocytes has been widely used, but these tests are utilized mainly to identify infants at high risk for early sepsis. Most authorities do not make a presumptive diagnosis of sepsis solely on the basis of positive fluids.

A positive blood culture is the basis of the diagnosis of septicemia. Because it is usually not practical to obtain multiple cultures spaced over wide intervals, two sets are recommended. Even this criterion has its shortcomings, since not infrequently there is contamination in the blood culture, and occasionally there is asymptomatic bacteremia. Although cord blood cultures have also been advocated by some, others have found these too misleading (39).

Cerebrospinal fluid examination is important in infants with sepsis, as one-third also develop meningeal involvement. There is a wide range of normal values in neonatal CSF, but more than 10 total cells/ml may be considered consistent with infection. In infants born of mothers with amnionitis, positive CSF cultures have been noted infrequently, especially when antibiotics are administered to the mother before delivery (1, 40, 41).

Either leukopenia ($<4000/ml^3$) or leukocyto­sis ($>25,000/mm^3$) suggests infection in the neonate, but septicemia may certainly occur with intermediate counts. The ominous findings in septicemia in the CBC are extreme leftward shift, $>50\%$ nonsegmented granulocytes, toxic granulocytes, and $< 80,000$ thrombocytes/mm^3. Finally, peripheral smear inspection may give clues to the presence of disseminated intravascular coagulopathy.

Examination of a frozen section of the cord, placenta, or membranes for a leukocytic infiltrate has been suggested as another technique to identify infants at risk for infection (39). However, placental inflammation and/or funisitis are found far in excess of proven cases of sepsis. In addition, leukocytic infiltrates have been attributed to other causes, such as hypoxia (39). Thus, because of its lack of specificity and its relative complexity, few centers employ this means of detection.

Finally, in a stillborn who has succumbed to IAI, a heart blood sample should be obtained to attempt to isolate the infecting organism. This technique should also be employed in the evaluation of the stillbirth having no apparent cause.

MANAGEMENT

In the absence of comparative studies, suggested therapy of chorioamnionitis had been arbitrary and conflicting. In broad principle, there is agreement among authors that there is a need for delivery and for antibiotics, but specific points of management are unresolved. With regard to timing of delivery, authors have suggested that it take place from 1–12 hr after chorioamnionitis (45–47) has been diagnosed, but these suggestions have not been correlated with either maternal or neonatal outcome. The preferred route of delivery is also unclear. While abdominal delivery is often recommended in order to achieve delivery within a specific time interval, there had been few data on maternal complications of cesarean section performed during frank infection. The extraperitoneal approach avoids contamination of the abdominal cavity, but is more difficult and time-consuming than the transperitoneal approach. Inadvertent entry into the peritoneum or bladder may also occur, and the teaching of this technique has declined to the extent that many practitioners have little familiarity with it. Indeed, Yonekura and colleagues recently compared 26 extraperitoneal (Norton technique) sections to 65 transperitoneal, low-cervical cesarean sections in patients with clinical amnionitis (51). All patients received combination antibiotics. In the 26 patients with extraperitoneal section, there were 2 accidental peritoneal entries, 1 inadvertent bladder entry, and 1 case of overflow urinary incontinence. There were no significant differences in wound infections (11.5% in extra- versus 14% in transperitoneal sections), postpartum hospital stay (5.31 ± 1.35 days versus 4.81 ± 1.95 days, respectively), or Apgar scores (11% less than 7 at 5 min in both groups). There were no cases of septic pelvic thrombophlebitis or pelvic abscess. The authors concluded that there was no advantage of extraperitoneal section compared to transperitoneal section when broad spectrum antibiotics were used in patients with amnionitis. Furthermore, despite recent interest, there has been no convincing demonstration of the relative merits of routine uses of extraperitoneal cesarean section or cesarean hysterectomy, as compared to those of transperitoneal section (48–50).

There are also fundamental questions regarding antibiotic administration. Many authors give them immediately to limit maternal sepsis and to initiate therapy to the fetus while others defer their use until after delivery to obtain more interpretable cultures of the newborn infant. Comparative studies of the effectiveness of various antibiotic therapies for IAI do not exist, and a variety of regimens are used on an empirical basis. At the University of Texas at San Antonio, we prefer a combination of intravenous penicillin G (5 million units every 6 hr) and intravenous gentamicin (1.5 mg/kg every 8 hr) as soon as the diagnosis is made and cultures are obtained. If vaginal delivery is anticipated within an hour or so, antibiotic therapy is often deferred until after delivery (1). When a cesarean section is necessary, we add clindamycin to the above antibiotics because of the importance of resistant *Bacteroides* in postcesarean section infection and the high (20%) failure rate of penicillin-gentamicin after cesarean section for IAI. Chloramphenicol, which also has excellent activity against *B. fragilis*, should not be used intrapartum, as it may cause "gray baby" syndrome in the neonate. Other initial regimens, such as clindamycin plus gentamicin or ampicillin and gentamicin, may be equally effective. In the future, trials with the third generation cephalosporins, perhaps with penicillin G (to provide optimal coverage of group B streptococci), may be worthwhile, since these newer agents may enter the fetal-neonatal central nervous system better than gentamicin.

Pharmacokinetic studies in late pregnancy show that clindamycin achieves peak concentrations in maternal blood within minutes after injection and in fetal blood shortly thereafter (52). Peak clindamycin concentrations were approximately one-half of maternal peaks, but the former were still within therapeutic ranges. In early pregnancy, ampicillin concentrations in maternal and fetal sera are comparable 120 min after administration, but benzylpenicillin (penicillin G) levels in fetal sera are one-third of the maternal levels 120 min after administration

(53). For this reason, some prefer ampicillin to penicillin G in treating IAI, but transport of penicillin G in late pregnancy may be improved, and outcome after using penicillin G plus gentamicin for IAI at term has led to good results (1). In late pregnancy, gentamicin also crosses the placenta rapidly, but peak fetal levels may be low, especially if maternal levels are subtherapeutic (52). Accordingly, an initial gentamicin dose of at least 1.5 mg/kg is indicated. For the antibiotics noted above, levels in AF are usually below fetal serum levels, and peak AF concentrations may be attained only after 2–6 hr (52–53).

OUTCOME

Older studies had noted poor perinatal outcome when chorioamnionitis complicated pregnancy (54). Since 1979, reports have provided systematically collected data on the outcome of mothers and neonates in pregnancies complicated by intraamniotic infection. These results have generally shown a vastly improved perinatal outcome. Because these studies are quite different in design (retrospective versus prospective, term versus preterm versus mixed, and microbiologically confirmed versus simply clinical diagnosis), these reports will be summarized individually.

In 1980, Gibbs and colleagues reported a retrospective study of management and outcome among 171 patients with uniform treatment (1). Cultures were obtained from the newborn infant but not uniformly from the amniotic fluid. Antibiotic therapy to the mother was begun with aqueous penicillin G (20–30 million units/day) and kanamycin (1000 mg/day). In the few patients not in labor at the time of the diagnosis, induction was usually undertaken. Cesarean section was generally performed only when there were additional obstetric indications. Antibiotics were not used uniformly in the neonate. The mean gestational age was 36.7 weeks.

Maternal outcome depended mainly on route of delivery, but there were no maternal deaths. Overall, bacteremia was found in 2.3% of mothers. Among women with intraamniotic infection, the rate of cesarean delivery was increased approximately three-fold to 35%, mainly because of dystocia. Cesarean delivery was carried out by a transperitoneal, low cervical transverse technique in 57 cases and by cesarean hysterectomy in the remaining 2 (both elderly multiparas). Compared to patients delivered vaginally, those delivered abdominally had generally more complicated hospitalizations despite similar durations of ROM. Yet, in all mothers, outcome was good. One episode of septic shock was seen in a patient who had been delivered vaginally, but there was a prompt response to medical therapy. No pelvic abscesses were encountered. Septic pelvic thrombophlebitis was diagnosed clinically in 3.4% of patients having cesarean delivery and in none of patients delivering vaginally. All patients delivering vaginally responded to penicillin-kanamycin whereas 20% of patients having abdominal delivery required the addition of clindamycin or chloramphenicol for cure. Abdominal wound infection was diagnosed in only 3.4% of patients having cesarean delivery, even though the incision was closed primarily.

In a similar retrospective study, Koh and colleagues managed 140 patients in fairly similar fashion at Los Angeles Hospital (40). Specifically, antibiotic therapy was usually started intrapartum (68% of cases) and continued postpartum. The regimen was usually ampicillin, and an aminoglycoside was often added after delivery. (No dosages are provided.) Cesarean section was performed in 43% of deliveries, with the major indication being "failure to progress." The mean gestational age was 39.3 weeks.

Maternal outcome was also excellent in this study. Maternal bacteremia was reported in 6.4% of patients (9/140). There were no maternal deaths and no cases of septic shock. Cesarean section was performed by the transcervical approach. There were no cesarean hysterectomies, and only one patient had a puerperal hysterectomy because of postpartum hemorrhage. Maternal outcome was also more complicated in the women delivered by cesarean section. In the group of 79 women delivered vaginally, 11% had "infectious morbidity," as compared to 48% of 61 delivered by cesarean section. In the cesarean delivery group, the wound infection rate was 4.9%.

Regarding perinatal outcome, Gibbs and colleagues found that the perinatal mortality rate (140/1000 births) was approximately seven times the overall perinatal mortality rate for infants >499 g (i.e., 18.2/1000 births (1)). For infants >1000 g, the perinatal mortality rate in the study group (i.e., 65/1000 births) is four times that of the general population (14.6/1000 births). Yet, of the 24 perinatal deaths, none was clearly attributable to infection; among live births of infants >1000 g, none died from infection. Nine infants had perinatal infections. Five

had neonatal sepsis, and three others had a radiologic and clinical diagnosis of congenital pneumonia. One other had meningitis, which was nosocomial rather than a congenital infection. Only one of these infants weighing greater than 1000 g died, the cause of death being hyaline membrane disease (1). In the study of Koh and co-workers, the perinatal mortality was lower (28.2/1000), but the mean gestational age was greater (39.3 weeks) (40). There were no intrapartum deaths, and only four neonatal deaths. Again, none was due to infection.

Gibbs and co-workers were unable to demonstrate any critical diagnosis-to-delivery interval (1). Specifically, neither perinatal nor maternal complications correlated with more prolonged intervals. Since patients with cesarean section had more complicated courses, it was concluded that cesarean section should be reserved for patients with obstetric indications in addition to chorioamnionitis. With this plan, over 90% of deliveries were achieved within 12 hr after diagnosis of chorioamnionitis.

In 1983, Yoder and colleagues provided a prospective, case-control study of 67 patients with microbiologically confirmed intraamniotic infection at term (41). Only one perinatal death was reported. The intrauterine fetal demise was evident when the mother was admitted in early labor, but she did not develop signs of IAI until 12 hr after admission. Autopsy revealed no evidence of intrauterine fetal infection, but there was placental inflammation. In 49 neonates born of mothers with IAI, cerebrospinal fluid cultures were negative, and there was no clinical evidence of meningitis or enterocolitis. Although 20% had chest radiographs interpreted as "possible" pneumonia, only 4% had unequivocal radiologic evidence of pneumonia. Neonatal bacteremia was documented in 8%. There was no significant difference in the frequency of low Apgar scores between the IAI and control groups. This study is summarized in Tables 16.3 and 16.4.

Prior to term pregnancy, neonates have a higher frequency of complications if they are delivered of mothers with IAI. Garite and Freeman noted that the perinatal death rate was significantly higher in 47 preterm neonates with IAI (13%) than in 204 neonates with similar birth weights (3%) (55). The group with IAI also had a significantly higher number with respiratory distress syndrome (RDS) and any diagnosis of infection. The results of this study are summarized in Table 16.5.

Table 16.3
Maternal Outcome in a Prospective, Case-Control Study of Intraamniotic Infection at Term[a]

Measures of maternal morbidity	Patient group		
	Intraamniotic infection (N = 67)	p_1[b]	Control (N = 67)
Intrapartum bacteremia	6/50 (12%)		NC[c]
Postpartum hospital stay (days), mean ± SD			
Abdominal delivery (N = 24)	7.1 ± 1.7	<0.005	5.5 ± 1.9
Vaginal delivery (N = 43)	4.0 ± 1.0	<0.001	2.9 ± 1.2
p_2[d]	<0.001		<0.001
Treatment with antibiotics, No. (%)			
Abdominal delivery (N = 24)	24/24 (100)	<0.001	9/24 (37.5)
Vaginal delivery (N = 43)	43/43 (100)	<0.001	1/43 (2.3)
p_2[d]			<0.001

[a] Adapted from Yoder PR, Gibbs RS, Blanco JC, Castaneda YS, St Clair PJ: A prospective, controlled study of maternal and perinatal outcome after intra-amniotic infection at term. *Am J Obstet Gynecol* 145:695, 1983.
[b] P_1, value for comparison of intraamniotic infection and control groups.
[c] Intrapartum blood cultures were not collected.
[d] P_2, value for comparison of subgroups with abdominal or vaginal delivery.

Table 16.4
Perinatal Outcome in a Prospective Case-Control Study of Intraamniotic Infection at Term[a]

Measures of perinatal morbidity[b]	Patient group				
	Intraamniotic infection (N = 67)		p	Control (N = 67)	
	No.	%		No.	%
Meconium-stained amniotic fluid	33	49	<0.01	18	27
Apgar score					
<4 at 1 min	4	6	NS	1	2
<7 at 5 min	2	3	NS	1	2
Documented bacteremia	5/59	8		0/2	
Hospital stay (days)	6.2 ± 2.5		<0.001	3.8 ± 2.1	
Perinatal deaths	1			0	

[a] Adapted from Yoder PR, Gibbs RS, Blanco JC, Castaneda YS, St Clair PJ: A prospective, controlled study of maternal and perinatal outcome after intra-amniotic infection at term. *Am J Obstet Gynecol* 145:695, 1983.

Table 16.5
Perinatal Outcome with "Amnionitis" in Preterm Gestation (28–34 weeks) (55)

	Amnionitis (N = 47)	No amnionitis (N = 204)	p
Perinatal deaths	6 (13%)	7 (3%)	<0.05
Respiratory distress syndrome	16 (34%)	33 (16%)	<0.01
Total infections	8 (17%)	13 (7%)	<0.05

It is commonly noted that patients with amnionitis have a greater likelihood of abdominal delivery, generally from 30 to 43% in recent studies (1, 40, 41). The cause of this increase may result from some effect of the infection upon uterine function, or it may result from arbitrary decisions of concerned physicians. Duff and colleagues recently reviewed the labor records and internal fetal monitoring tracings of 65 term patients who entered labor spontaneously and then developed clinical chorioamnionitis (56). In 82% of these patients, there was a positive amniotic fluid culture with high virulence organisms. Overall, chorioamnionitis developed more commonly in patients with complicated labor. For example, decreased uterine contractility and oxytocin administration were noted in 75%, and cesarean delivery was performed in 34%. Mean interval from diagnosis of chorioamnionitis to delivery was approximately 4 hr. In the group requiring cesarean delivery, uterine activity in the 3 hr prior to delivery was 146 Montevideo units. In the group delivering vaginally, mean activity was 167 Montevideo units in this interval. Mean maximum oxytocin dose was approximately 6.5 mU for the entire group. The most common fetal heart rate abnormalities were diminished variability (77%) and tachycardia (67%). Only one infant had a 5-min Apgar score <7. The authors concluded that cesarean setions were not due simply to physician's anxiety, but that chorioamnionitis has an inhibitory effect on labor.

Intraamniotic infection has a significant adverse effect upon the mother and neonate, but vigorous antibiotic therapy and reasonably prompt delivery result in an excellent prognosis, especially for the mother and the term neonate. When the combination of prematurity and amnionitis occur, then serious sequelae are more likely for the neonate.

SUBCLINICAL GENITAL INFECTION AS A CAUSE OF ADVERSE PREGNANCY OUTCOME

Preterm birth, with its subsequent morbidity and mortality, is the leading perinatal problem in the United States. Infants born before the 37th week of gestation account for approximately 80% of all perinatal deaths. In most cases, the underlying cause of premature labor is not evident, and attempts may be made to arrest premature uterine contractions. However, this symptomatic treatment (tocolysis) is not indicated in many patients because of serious maternal disease. In others, tocolytic agents are only partially effective, especially when labor is advanced or the membranes are ruptured. It is likely that therapy directed at preventing or treating underlying causes would be more successful.

Evidence from many sources links preterm birth with symptomatic or asymptomatic genitourinary tract infections. It is well known that untreated bacteriuria in pregnancy results in acute pyelonephritis in 20–40% of such cases and that pyelonephritis has a serious increased risk of fetal morbidity and mortality. It is still unclear, however, as to whether asymptomatic bacteriuria per se results in adverse effects in pregnancy (57, 58). Others have reported a similar association with bacteriuria (59), but there are still other series (in general, smaller ones) which did not find a significant effect of either asymptomatic bacteriuria or antimicrobial treatment on birth weight (60, 61). These divergent conclusions may be explained by disparate procedures and methods, such as inadequate control for other pregnancy complications (hypertension, for example), inadequate assessment of compliance to treatment, and failure to distinguish small-for-gestational age term infants from premature infants.

In addition to urinary tract infection, infection of the genital tract—either clinically evident or subclinical—has also been implicated as a cause of premature birth or low birth weight infants. In 1966, Hawkinson and Schulman studied 574 pregnant women with cervicitis and 543 control patients (62). One hundred nine (19.0%) of the women with cervicitis delivered neonates weighing less than 2500 g, as compared to 59 (10.9%) of the control women (p < 0.01). In a placebo-controlled study, treatment with a disinfectant vaginal cream (Trib, Roche Laboratories) did not alter perinatal outcome, but the authors did not state whether the therapy eradicated the cervicitis or whether cervicitis was present at the time of delivery. Also, the disinfectant cream might not have eradicated many of the microorganisms present in the genital tract.

More recent studies have shown a relationship between isolation of mycoplasmas from the genital tract and adverse pregnancy outcome. Braun and colleagues showed that women with genital mycoplasmas in the cervix and/or urine delivered neonates with a mean birth weight 202 g less than that of neonates of women without genital mycoplasmas (63). This difference in birth weights was statistically significant, but there was not a significant difference in gestational age between the two groups. From the same group, associations were also reported between (a) neonatal colonization with genital mycoplasmas and low birth weight (64) and (b) significant rises in titer to *U. urealyticum* in pregnancy and low birth weight (p < 0.02) (65). In 1983, Quinn and colleagues reported antibiotic treatment of 62 couples with histories of pregnancy wastage and with positive genital or urinary cultures for genital mycoplasmas (66). Doxycycline treatment before conception reduced the pregnancy loss rate to 48% as compared to a loss rate of 96% in the "no treatment" group. Erythromycin (250 mg q.i.d. from the 2nd or 3rd month until the end of pregnancy) further reduced the pregnancy loss rate to 16%. However, the trial was small and poorly controlled.

Lower genital infection with *C. trachomatis* has also been implicated in adverse pregnancy outcome. In a longitudinal study, Martin and colleagues found *C. trachomatis* endocervical infection in 18 (6.7%) of 268 women at 19 weeks or less of pregnancy (23). Pregnant women with endocervical *C. trachomatis* infection were significantly more likely to deliver stillborns or infants succumbing to neonatal deaths (6 of 18, 33%) than were women not infected in early pregnancy (8 of 23, 34%). In a matched cohort analysis of this data, the authors reported a perinatal mortality risk ratio for pregnancies with versus pregnancies without antepartum chlamydial infection of 10.18 (p = 0.004, one-tail test). There was also a difference in duration of gestation between *Chlamydia*-positive women and the 238 uninfected women as determined by analysis of covariance (p < 0.001). However, these findings must be viewed cautiously because of (1) the small number of patients studied, (2) incomplete data on other genitourinary pathogens, and (3) incomplete pathological studies (23). From the same institution, it has been noted that women with antepartum *C. trachomatis* infection (at 32–36 weeks of gestation) also had a significantly higher likelihood of having intrapartum fever (clinically attributed to amnionitis) (9% of 32 *C. trachomatis* positive women versus 1% of 359 negative women, p < 0.025) (24).

The association of other microorganisms and adverse pregnancy outcome has not been well established. Maternal gonococcal infection may lead to ophthalmia neonatorum and to an occasional case of gonococcal chorioamnionitis (18). Furthermore, Handsfield et al found an association between positive cultures of the neonate's orogastric aspirate for *N. gonorrhoeae* (presumably from a maternal genital tract source) and prematurity, prolonged rupture of fetal membranes, and histologic chorioamnionitis (17). However, more complete understanding of the

effect of maternal gonorrhoea in pregnancy can only be derived from prospective studies, which would not be ethical in view of the obligation to treat all patients with this infection.

Maternal genital tract colonization with group B streptococci (GBS) leads to neonatal sepsis, especially when birth occurs prematurely or when the membranes have been ruptured for prolonged intervals. However, an association between maternal GBS colonization and premature birth has been found only in the report by Regan and co-workers (67). These investigators noted delivery at <32 weeks in 1.8% of the total population but in 5.4% of women colonized with GBS (p < 0.005). PROM was also significantly more common in the colonized group (15.3% versus 8.1%, p < 0.005).

For other genital tract microorganisms, especially enterics and anaerobes, associations with premature birth have not been carefully studied, yet these organisms are commonly involved in puerperal infections.

In view of these data, older studies of antibiotic treatment in pregnancy are especially interesting. Elder and colleagues studied perinatal outcome in women with or without bacteriuria and treated with tetracycline or a placebo (58). Rather unexpectedly, perinatal outcome was improved even in the nonbacteriuric group treated with tetracycline, as compared to the nonbacteriuric group treated with placebo. The group treated with tetracycline had a significantly longer gestation (39.1 versus 38.1 weeks), higher mean birth weight (3277 g versus 3141 g), and a lower rate of preterm live births (5.4% versus 15.2%) than did the untreated group. In view of the spectrum of activity of tetracycline, including many aerobes and anaerobes, genital mycoplasmas, and *C. trachomatis*, it is possible that these observed differences may be explained by eradication of asymptomatic genital infections.

In other treatment studies, a reduction in the percent of low birth weight deliveries was seen among women who were treated with erythromycin for 6 weeks in the third trimester, as compared to that of those given a placebo (65). The decrease was from 12% (10 of 84) in the placebo group to 3% (2 of 64) in the erythromycin group (p = 0.063). The infants in the placebo group weighed significantly less (3187 g versus 3331 g, p = 0.041). Because of a low isolation rate for *C. trachomatis* (4–6%) in the population, the authors concluded that it was unlikely that the erythromycin effect was primarily explained by an antichlamydial effect. It was interesting, however, that repeated vaginal cultures, taken during and after treatment, showed "only a slight reduction in the carriage of mycoplasmas as a consequence of treatment."

Furthermore, numerous studies in the past 20 yr have noted that placental membranes of preterm pregnancies were significantly more likely to show histologic inflammation than were membranes from term placentas (68). While it has not been established that this inflammation is specific for infection, the association is a sound one and supports the link between infection and prematurity.

Within the past 5 yr, several small studies of amniotic fluid bacteriology have given further support to this hypothesis. In three studies, amniocentesis was performed in patients in premature labor. Bobitt and colleagues found subclinical infections in 6 (24%) of 25 patients and noted that perinatal morbidity was greater among infants when the AF culture was positive (69). Gravett and colleagues recently reported the isolation of microorganisms in 10 (26%) of 39 patients. Patients with such cultures were less responsive to tocolytic agents (70). On the other hand, Wallace and colleagues found that only 1 of 30 amniotic fluid cultures was consistent with regards to infection (71). In this case, infection was already evident by clinical measures.

To complement these clinical observations, Bejar and co-workers noted that a number of common genital tract bacteria elaborate phospholipase A_2, an enzyme leading to the synthesis of prostaglandins (72). These authors postulate that premature labor may be initiated by high phospholipase A_2 activity from these bacteria involved in endocervical or intrauterine contamination or infection.

Accordingly, current indirect evidence suggests that women with certain suspect microorganisms may have higher rates of prematurity or other adverse perinatal outcomes than those women without such organisms. However, these relationships need to be clarified.

References

1. Gibbs RS, Castillo MS, Rodgers PJ: Management of acute chorioamnionitis. *Am J Obstet Gynecol* 136:709, 1980.
2. Halliday HL, Hirata T: Perinatal listeriosis: a review of twelve patients. *Am J Obstet Gynecol* 133:405, 1979.
3. Shackleford PG: Listeria revisited. *Am J Dis Child* 131:391, 1977.
4. Monif GRG: Antenatal group A streptococcal infection. *Am J Obstet Gynecol* 123:213, 1975.
5. Charles D, Edwards WR: Infectious complications of cervical cerclage. *Am J Obstet Gynecol* 141:1065, 1981.
6. Kuhn RJP, Pepperell RJ: Cervical ligation: a review of 242 pregnancies. *Aust NZ J Obstet Gynaecol* 17:79, 1977.
7. Aarnoudse JG, Huisjes HJ: Complications of cerclage. *Acta Obstet Gynecol Scand* 58:255, 1979.
8. Harger JH: Comparison of success and morbidity in cervical cerclage procedures. *Obstet Gynecol* 56:543, 1980.
9. Burnett RG, Anderson WR: The hazards of amniocentesis. *J Iowa Med Soc* 58:133, 1968.
10. Queenan JT: Modern Management of the Rh Problem, ed 2. Hagerstown, MD, Harper & Row, 1977, p 180.
11. Naeye RL: Coitus and associated amniotic-fluid infections. *N Engl J Med* 301:1198, 1979.
12. Steege JF, Jelovsek FR: Sexual behavior during pregnancy. *Obstet Gynecol* 60:163, 1982.
13. Mills JL, Harlap S, Harley EE: Should coitus late in pregnancy be discouraged? *Lancet* 2:136, 1981.
14. Gibbs RS, Blanco JD, St Clair PJ, Castaneda YS: Quantitative bacteriology of amniotic fluid from patients with clinical intra-amniotic infection at term. *J Infect Dis* 145:1, 1982.
15. Miller JM, Pupkin MJ, Hill GB: Bacterial colonization of amniotic fluid from intact fetal membranes. *Am J Obstet Gynecol* 136:796, 1980.
16. Gravett MG, Eschenbach DA, Speigel-Brown CA, Holmes KK: Rapid diagnosis of amniotic fluid infection by gas-liquid chromatography. *N Engl J Med* 306:725, 1982.
17. Handsfield HH, Hodson WA, Holmes KK: Neonatal gonococcal infection. I. Orogastric contamination with *Neisseria gonorrhoeae. JAMA* 225:697, 1973.
18. Nickerson CW: Gonorrhea amnionitis. *Obstet Gynecol* 42:815, 1973.
19. Brunnel PA, Dische RM, Walker MB: Mycoplasma, amnionitis, and respiratory distress syndrome. *JAMA* 207:2097, 1969.
20. Shurin PA, Alpert S, Rosner B, Driscoll SG, Lee, Y, McCormack WM, Santamarina BAG, Kass EH: Chorioamnionitis and colonization of the newborn infant with genital mycoplasmas. *N Engl J Med* 293:5, 1975.
21. Blanco JD, Gibbs RS, Malherbe H, Strickland-Cholmley M, St Clair PJ, Castaneda YS: A controlled study of genital mycoplasmas in amniotic fluid from patients with intra-amniotic infection. *J Infect Dis* 147:650, 1983.
22. Harrison HR, Riggin RT: Infection of untreated primary human amnion monolayers with *Chlamydia trachomatis. J Infect Dis* 140:968, 1979.
23. Martin DH, Koustsky L, Eschenbach DA, Daling JR, Alexander ER, Benedetti JK, Holmes KK: Prematurity and perinatal mortality in pregnancies complicated by maternal *Chlamydia trachomatis* infections. *JAMA* 247:1585, 1982.
24. Wager GP, Martin DH, Koustsky L, Eschenbach DA, Daling JR, Chiang WT, Alexander ER, Holmes KK: Puerperal infectious morbidity: relationship to route of delivery and to antepartum *Chlamydia trachomatis* infection. *Am J Obstet Gynecol* 138:1028, 1980.
25. Larsen B, Snyder IS, Galask RP: Bacterial growth inhibition by amniotic fluid. I. *In vitro* evidence

for bacterial growth inhibiting activity. *Am J Obstet Gynecol* 119:492, 1974.

26. Larsen B, Snyder IS, Galask RP: Bacterial growth inhibition by amniotic fluid. II. Reversal of amniotic fluid bacterial growth inhibition by addition of a chemically defined medium. *Am J Obstet Gynecol* 119:497, 1974.

27. Schlievert P, Larsen B, Johnson W, Galask RP: Bacterial growth inhibition by amniotic fluid. IV. Studies on the nature of bacterial inhibition with the uswe of place-count determinations. *Am J Obstet Gynecol* 122:814, 1975.

28. Schlievert P, Johnson W, Galask RP: Bacterial growth inhibition by amniotic fluid. V. Phosphate-to-zinc ratio as a predictor of bacterial growth inhibitory activity. *Am J Obstet Gynecol* 125:899, 1976.

29. Schlievert P, Johnson W, Galask RP: Bacterial growth inhibition by amniotic fluid. VI. Evidence for a zinc-peptide antibacterial system. *Am J Obstet Gynecol* 125:906, 1976.

30. Schlievert P, Johnson W, Galask RP: Isolation of a low molecular weight antibacterial system from human amniotic fluid. *Infect Immun* 14:1156, 1976.

31. Gibbs RS, Blanco JD, Hnilica VS: Inorganic phosphorus and zinc concentrations in amniotic fluid: correlation with intra-amniotic infection and bacterial inhibitory activity. *Am J Obstet Gynecol* 143:163, 1982.

32. Galask RP, Larsen B, Snyder IS: Amniotic fluid-induced surface ultramicrocytopathology of *escherichia coli. Am J Obstet Gynecol* 118:921, 1974.

33. Larsen B, Schlievert P, Galask RP: The spectrum of antibacterial activity of human amniotic fluid determined by scanning electron microscopy. *Am J Obstet Gynecol* 119:895, 1974.

34. Blanco JD, Gibbs RS, Krebs LF, Castaneda YS: The association between the absence of amniotic fluid bacterial inhibitory activity and intra-amniotic infection. *Am J Obstet Gynecol* 143:749, 1982.

35. Blanco JD, Gibbs RS, Krebs LF: Inhibition of group B streptococci by amniotic fluid from patients with intra-amniotic infection and from control subjects. *Am J Obstet Gynecol* 147:247, 1983.

36. Miller J, Michel J, Bercovici B, Argaman M, Sacks T: Studies on the antimicrobial activity of amniotic fluid. *Am J Obstet Gynecol* 125:212, 1976.

37. Applebaum PC, Holloway Y, Ross SM, Dhupelia I: The effect of amniotic fluid on bacterial growth in three population groups. *Am J Obstet Gynecol* 128:868, 1977.

38. Blanco JD, Gibbs RS, Krebs LF: A controlled study of amniotic fluid immunoglobulin levels in intra-amniotic infection. *Obstet Gynecol* 61:450, 1983.

39. Gibbs RS: Diagnosis of intra-amniotic infection. *Sem Perinatol* 1:71, 1977.

40. Koh KS, Chan FH, Monfared AH, Ledger WJ, Paul R: The changing perinatal and maternal outcome in chorioamnionitis. *Obstet Gynecol* 53:730, 1979.

41. Yoder PR, Gibbs RS, Blanco JD, Castaneda YS, St Clair PJ: A prospective, controlled study of maternal and perinatal outcome after intra-amniotic infection at term. *Am J Obstet Gynecol* 145:695, 1983.

42. Listwa HM, Dobek AS, Carpenter J, et al: The predictability of intrauterine infection by analysis of amniotic fluid. *Obstet Gynecol* 48:31, 1976.

43. Gotoff SP, Behrman RE: Neonatal septicemia. *J Pediatr* 76:142, 1970.

44. Siegel JD, McCracken GH: Sepsis neonatorum. *N Engl J Med* 304:642, 1981.

45. Schwarz R, Fruiterman JP: Life threatening infection in pregnancy. *Clin Obstet Gynecol* 19:561, 1976.

46. MacVicar J: Chorioamnionitis. In Charles D, Finland M (eds): *Obstetric and Perinatal Infection.* Philadelphia, Lea & Febiger, 1973, pp 491–495.

47. Friedman EH: Obstetric infection in labor. In Charles D, Finland M (eds): *Obstetric and Perinatal Infection.* Philadelphia, Lea & Febiger, 1973, pp 512–516.

48. Perkins RP: The merits of extraperitoneal cesarean section: a continuing experience. *J Reprod Med* 19:154, 1977.

49. Hanson H: Revival of the extraperitoneal cesarean section. *Am J Obstet Gynecol* 130:102, 1978.

50. Imig JR, Perkins RP: Extraperitoneal cesarean section: a new need for old skills. A preliminary report. *Am J Obstet Gynecol* 125:51, 1976.

51. Yonekura ML, Wallace R, Eglinton G: Amnionitis—optimal operative management: extraperitoneal cesarean section *vs* low cervical transperitoneal cesarean section. Third Annual Meeting, Society of Perinatal Obstetricians, Abstract 24A, San Antonio, Jan 1983.

52. Weinstein AJ, Gibbs RS, Gallagher M: Placental transfer of clindamycin and gentamicin. *Am J Obstet Gynecol* 124:688, 1976.

53. Charles D: Dynamics of antibiotic transfer from mother to fetus. *Semin Perinatol* 1:89, 1977.

54. Clark DM, Anderson GV: Perinatal mortality and amnionitis in a general hospital population. *Obstet Gynecol* 31:714, 1968.

55. Garite TJ, Freeman RK: Chorioamnionitis in the preterm gestation. *Obstet Gynecol* 59:539, 1982.

56. Duff P, Sanders R, Gibbs RS: The course of labor in term patients with chorioamnionitis. *Am J Obstet Gynecol*, in press, 1985.

57. Kass EH: The role of asymptomatic bacteriuria in the pathogenesis of pyelonephritis. In Quinn EL, EH Kass (eds): *Biology of Pyelonephritis.* Boston, Little, Brown, 1960, pp 339.

58. Elder HA, Santamarina BAG, Smith S, et al: The natural history of asymptomatic bacteriuria during pregnancy: the effect of tetracycline on the clinical course and the outcome of pregnancy. *Am J Obstet Gynecol* 111:441, 1971.

59. Williams JD, Reeves DS, Condie AP, et al: Significance of bacteriuria in pregnancy. In EH Kass, W Brumfitt (eds): *Infections of the Urinary Tract.* Chicago, University of Chicago Press, 1978. p 8.

60. Whalley PJ, Cunningham FG: Short term versus continuous antimicrobial therapy of asymptomatic bacteriuria in pregnancy. *Obstet Gynecol* 49:262, 1977.

61. Gilstrap LC, Leveno KJ, Cunningham FG: Renal infection and pregnancy outcome. *Am J Obstet Gynecol* 141:709, 1981.

62. Hawkinson JA, Schulman H: Prematurity associated with cervictis and vaginitis during pregnancy. *Am J Obstet Gynecol* 94:898, 1966.

63. Braun P, Lee Y, Klein JO, et al: Birth weight and

genital mycoplasmas in pregnancy. *N Engl J Med* 284:167, 1971.

64. Lee Y, McCormack WM, Marcy SM, et al: The genital mycoplasmas: their role in disorders of reproduction and in pediatric infections. *Pediatr Clin North Am* 21:457, 1974.

65. Kass EH, McCormack WM, Lin JS, et al: Genital mycoplasmas as a cause of excess premature delivery. *Trans Assoc Am Phys* 94:261, 1981.

66. Quinn PA, Shewchuk AB, Shuber J, et al: Efficacy of antibiotic therapy in preventing spontaneous pregnancy loss among couples with genital mycoplasmas. *Am J Obstet Gynecol* 145:239, 1983.

67. Regan JA, Chao S, James SL: Premature rupture of membranes, preterm delivery, and group B streptococcal colonization of mother. *Am J Obstet Gynecol* 141:184, 1981.

68. Driscoll SG: The placenta and membranes. In Charles D, Finaldn M (eds): *Obstetrical and Perinatal Infections* Philadelphia, Lea & Febiger, 1973, p 532.

69. Bobitt JR, Hayslip CC, Damato JD: Amniotic fluid infection as determined by transabdominal amniocentesis in patients with intact membranes. *Am J Obstet Gynecol* 140:947, 1981.

70. Gravett MG, Hummel D, Eschenbach DA, et al: Abnormal vaginal and amniotic fluid flora among women in premature labor. The Third Annual Meeting of the Society of Perinatal Obstetricians, San Antonio, January, 1983.

71. Wallace RL, Herrick N: Amniocentesis in the evaluation of premature labor. *Obstet Gynecol* 57:483, 1981.

72. Bejar R, Curbelo V, Dvis C, et al: Premature labor. II. Bacterial sources of phospholipase. *Obstet Gynecol* 57:479, 1981.

CHAPTER 17

Postpartum Infections

Four decades into the antibiotic era, puerperal infections continue to pose a common and occasionally severe threat to women after childbirth. Especially in view of the recent rise in cesarean section rates and the greater risk of infection after cesarean section, we cannot expect this problem to abate.

EPIDEMIOLOGY

Firm estimates of the incidence of postpartum infection are not readily available. Many studies have reported the incidence of "standard puerperal morbidity," which was defined by the U.S. Joint Committee on Maternal Welfare as "a temperature of 100.4°F (38.0°C), the temperature to occur in any two of the first 10 days postpartum, exclusive of the first 24 hours, and to be taken by mouth by a standard technique at least four times daily." Yet, the full criteria of the original definition can no longer be applied because of early patient discharge practices. In addition, many infected patients respond to antibiotics so quickly that they do not meet the temperature criteria for standard morbidity.

Low-grade fever ($\geq$100.4°F) or isolated higher temperature elevations occur commonly in the puerperium and often resolve spontaneously, especially after vaginal delivery (1). In a study of 1000 consecutive gravidas, Filker and Monif noted that 6.5% (65) developed a temperature greater than 38°C (100.4°F) within the first 24 hours. Half of these patients (33) delivered vaginally and accounted for 3.8% of all vaginal deliveries. Eighty percent (26) of these 33 patients resolved the fever spontaneously. The other 32 patients were delivered by cesarean section and accounted for 22.5% of all abdominal deliveries. In this group, only 30% (9) resolved the fever spontaneously. The etiology of such fevers is unclear, but they may result from dehydration or reaction to an infusion of fetal proteins. Recent data from our laboratory suggest that these transient fevers are often due to transient bacterial infection in the uterus, as detected by positive amniotic fluid cultures (2). Sources of infection in the puerperal period are genital tract infection (endometritis), urinary tract infection, mastitis, breast abscess, and complications of anesthesia.

At present, the overall rate of postpartum infection may be estimated to be from 1–8%. Although the absolute risk of death from infection is small among postpartum women, sepsis remains the second most common cause of maternal death in the United States. In 1973, there were 98 deaths from sepsis (3.1/100,000 live births), second only to toxemia (3.5/100,000) (3).

A few retrospective reports have focused on cases of maternal death from infection. In two reports from Michigan, it was concluded that the deaths were preventable in over two-thirds of the cases, with both patient and medical personnel sharing responsibility equally. Patient responsibility consisted primarily of delay in seeking medical care (for example, after prolonged rupture of the membranes); physician and hospital responsibility consisted of inadequate evaluation of symptoms, incorrect diagnosis, failure to hospitalize earlier, and inadequate institution of antibiotic therapy (4, 5). Overall, in Michigan, infection was the cause of 23% of maternal deaths from 1950–1971 (6).

Epidemic infections occur infrequently on maternity services. Lethal outbreaks of β-hemolytic streptococcal infection occurred as late as 1927 and a number of nonlethal epidemics of streptococcal infection have been reported since 1965. These were all caused by group A streptococci (usually one type) and involved from two to 20 mothers, none to 11 newborn infants, and many of the hospital staff. Although there were no maternal or neonatal deaths, a number of the patients were severely ill (7). There have been no reported epidemics of puerperal infection due to organisms other than group A streptococci.

GENITAL TRACT INFECTION

The most common cause of puerperal fever is genital tract infection, usually of the uterus; the infection is called endometritis, endomyometritis, endoparametritis, or simply metritis, depending on the extent of the disease. Criteria for endomyometritis vary, but several investigators have utilized fever, uterine tenderness and purulent or foul lochia, peripheral leukocytosis, and exclusion of another infected site. Nonspecific signs and symptoms such as malaise, abdominal pain, chills, and tachycardia may also be present. However, most patients do not have this complete clinical picture. Indeed, many febrile patients with group A or B streptococcal bacteremia have no localizing signs (8). In the vast majority of cases of uterine infection, presenting signs and symptoms develop within the first 5 days after delivery.

Although genital tract cultures are of value in patients with endometritis, obtaining a satisfactory specimen without contamination from the lower genital tract is a problem. Swabbing of the vagina and endocervix is likely to produce culture results not identical to those in the endometrial cavity. Alternative techniques with a double lumen catheter may obtain a less contaminated sample of the microbiologic flora of the endometrium (9, 10). Recently, Duff and colleagues compared four endometrial culturing techniques in 18 asymptomatic women undergoing puerperal tubal ligation (11). These techniques were a transfundal aspirate, a brush biopsy through a double lumen catheter, a lavage through a double lumen catheter, and a lower segment aspirate. There were significantly fewer isolates in the transfundal culture (0.67 ± 0.98) than in the lower segment aspirate (3.2 ± 1.7) ($p < 0.05$). In both double lumen techniques, there was an intermediate number of isolates (2.2 ± 1.8 for the brush biopsy and 2.3 ± 1.7 for the lavage). Although these results were not from symptomatic patients, it would appear that even these double lumen techniques introduce bacteria into endometrial cultures.

In the absence of a simple, contamination-free technique, we suggest that an aerobic cervical culture be performed in most clinical situations. Even though broad spectrum therapy is used, this culture may identify pathogens that require specific therapy. For example, identification of group A streptococcus should lead to isolation of the patient and should be reported to physicians in the nursery. Isolation of group B streptococci or *Neisseria gonorrhoeae* should be reported to physicians in the nursery. In addition, there may be isolates which will help direct subsequent antibiotic therapy in case of initial antibiotic failure. Examples would include enterococci in initial therapy with a cephalosporin or clindamycin plus gentamicin and *Klebsiella* sp or *Staphylococcus aureus* in initial treatment with ampicillin or carbenicillin. Then, from a surveillance viewpoint, it is necessary to determine whether kinds of organisms or their antimicrobial susceptibilities are shifting.

About 10–20% of patients may have bacteremia, and two sets of blood cultures should be obtained. Isolation of an organism from the blood does not imply that this organism is, by itself, responsible for the infection; therefore, antibiotic therapy directed solely against the isolate thus identified might be inadequate treatment.

Pathophysiology—Risk Factors (Table 17.1)

METHOD OF DELIVERY

Cesarean section is the major predisposing clinical factor for pelvic infection (12). After abdominal delivery, the frequency and severity of infection are greater than when following a vaginal delivery. In the same population, Gibbs and colleagues report the incidence of endometritis after cesarean section as 38.5%, whereas it was 1.2% after vaginal delivery (12–14). However, the former figure was from a prospective study and the latter, from a retrospective study. Although this might lead to underreporting in the vaginal delivery group, other investigators have reported similar data with the risk of endometritis being 5–10 times greater after abdominal delivery (12). Endometritis rates rarely exceed 3% after a vaginal delivery, while the rates after cesarean section have been 12–95%.

Disease severity is also increased in abdominal delivery. Antibiotic failure rates and complication rates are higher for the cesarean section group (13, 14). Serious complications such as abscess or presumed septic pelvic thrombophlebitis have been reported in 2–4% of patients with endometritis after cesarean section (13). With broader antibiotic therapy, aimed at the anaerobes, however, these complications appear to be less common (15).

Death from sepsis is undeniably increased after cesarean section (12). Recent accounts from the State of Rhode Island and from Los Angeles County Hospital found the risk of lethal, maternal sepsis to be 81 times greater after

Table 17.1
Tabulation of Risk Factors for Postpartum Infection in Recent Studies

Suggestive factor	Supporting references
Operative and obstetrical factors	
Labor	Gibbs et al (14), D'Angelo and Sokol (20), Rehu and Nilsson (24), Nielsen and Hokegard (25), Hawrylyshyn et al (26)
Rupture of membranes	Gibbs et al (14), Rehu and Nilsson (24), Nielsen and Hokegard (25), Hawrylyshyn et al (26), Ott (27)
Failure to progress in labor	Hagglund et al (28)
No. of vaginal examinations	Rehu and Nilsson (24), Hawrylyshyn et al (26)
No. of rectal examinations	Rehu and Nilsson (24)
Internal fetal monitoring	Hager (29)
Low parity	Rehu and Nilsson (24)
Anesthesia	Anstey et al (31)
Skill of operator	Rehu and Nilsson (24)
Duration of operation >60 min	Haggland et al (28)
Estimated blood loss >800 ml	Haggland et al (28)
Postoperative anemia	Ott (27), Nielsen and Hokegard (25), Hawrylyshyn et al (26)
Obesity	Nielsen and Hokegard (25)
Laboratory factors	
Positive amniotic fluid culture	Gilstrap and Cunningham (17), Blanco et al (18)
Vaginal colonization group B streptococci	Minkoff et al (33)
Low phosphate/zinc ratio in amniotic fluid	Minkoff et al (34)
S. aureus in patients	Haggland et al (28)

cesarean birth than after vaginal birth. In absolute terms, the death rate from sepsis was 1 per 1600 cesarean sections. In other institutions, though, sepsis may be less of a threat as one series of 10,000 consecutive cesarean sections has been reported at a level III hospital without a single maternal death from any cause (16).

The cause of the increased incidence of infection in cesarean section has not been systematically studied, but it is reasonable to implicate increased intrauterine manipulation, foreign body (suture) reactions, tissue necrosis at the suture line, hematoma-seroma formation, and wound infections. Several studies have recently noted that women who develop postpartum endometritis commonly have positive cultures of the amniotic fluid at the time of section (17, 18).

Older studies describe a still greater increase in maternal morbidity and mortality with upper segment incisions as compared to lower segment cesarean sections. A recent retrospective case-control study of 89 patient pairs showed no higher incidence of infectious morbidity in patients having a classical cesarean section than in those having low cervical transverse cesareans, but nearly all classical sections were performed either electively or after short periods of labor and rupture of membranes (ROM) (19). Nevertheless, we emphasize that classical cesarean section should be limited to standard indications such as dense bladder scarring from previous cesarean deliveries, back down transverse lie (and inability to convert the fetus), and an anterior placenta previa.

Clearly, not all patients undergoing cesarean section are at equal risk. Those patients with electively scheduled operations (with no labor and no ROM) have lower infection rates than those with emergency or nonelective procedures (with labor, ROM, or both). This observation has been made nearly universally in a large number of studies (Tables 17.1 and 17.2).

LABOR

Labor as well as rupture of the membranes, number of vaginal examinations, and use of internal fetal monitoring have been widely discussed as possible risk factors for puerperal infection. Table 17.1 summarizes recent studies. After eliminating confounding variables with a discriminant analysis technique, D'Angelo and

Table 17.2
Effect of Duration of Rupture of Membranes Upon Pelvic Infection Following Cesarean Section [a, b]

Duration of ROM (hr)	Rate of pelvic infection (%)			
	University Texas San Antonio (23)	University Texas Dallas (17)	Walter Reed Army Medical Center (21)	Boston Lying In (29)
18.0	35 [c]		75	58
12.0–17.9	56	85	49	45
6.0–11.9	48		31	44
0.1–5.9	41	67	28	41
0	30	29	11	27

[a] Adapted from Gibbs RS: Clinical risk factors for puerperal infection. *Obstet Gynecol* 55(S):178, 1980.
[b] In San Antonio, Dallas, and Washington, DC, infection was measured as endometritis, endomyometritis, or metritis. In Boston, infection was measured as standard morbidity.
[c] Only 16 patients in this group.

Sokol reported that the most significant event related to postpartum morbidity after cesarean section was the duration of labor (20). Other studies utilizing similar statistical techniques have confirmed this result (12). In a military population, intrauterine infection increased by 9% in patients with labor and intact membranes as compared to infection in patients with no labor and no ROM (21)

RUPTURE OF MEMBRANES AND AMNIOTIC FLUID COLONIZATION

Some reports note an association between the duration of ROM and the incidence of intrauterine infection (12). The study by D'Angelo and Sokol did not find this relationship when the duration of labor was factored out, but few patients in their study had prolonged membrane rupture (20).

With the passage of time after ROM, bacterial contamination of the amniotic cavity occurs; therefore, it is logical to expect that ROM may play a role in postpartum infection. Amniotic fluid analysis by Bobitt and Ledger showed that no amniotic fluid (AF) specimen was sterile after 12 hr of ROM, and many had colony counts exceeding 10^3 cfu(colony-forming units)/ml (22). Subsequently, Gilstrap and Cunningham showed that, at the time of cesarean section, all the AF specimens in 56 women with ROM > 6 hr contained some microorganisms, and 95% of these women developed myometritis (17). Quantitation of bacteria and categorizing them into high and low virulence types improves the predictive capacity of AF sampling at cesarean sec-

tion. In a recent study of 24 women undergoing cesarean section without labor or ROM, Blanco and co-workers found that none of the patients had $>10^2$ cfu of a high virulence organism per ml of AF specimens (a "positive" culture) (18). Twenty-five percent of these patients with ROM or labor or both had "positive" cultures. Ninety-two percent of the "positive" group developed endometritis as compared to 39% of the group without a "positive" culture. This difference was highly significant. Thus, quantitation and evaluation of bacterial virulence identified a group at 92% risk for infection, as compared to a 39% risk. Interestingly, the pathogenesis of infection for each of the two groups is probably different, as evidenced by a significantly shorter time interval from surgery to diagnosis of endometritis in the patients with a "positive" culture (18.1 versus 45.0 hr, respectively). The patients with a "positive" culture at cesarean section already appear to have subclinical infection and soon after delivery show signs and symptoms. In the group without "positive" cultures at abdominal delivery, the uterine infection appears to develop after delivery.

Although quantitative cultures of AF specimens are helpful in understanding the pathogenesis of uterine infection after cesarean section, they are not, at present, practical for predicting infection because clinical infection is usually evident before culture results become available. A rapid technique, such as gas-liquid chromatography, might be helpful, not only in predicting infection, but also in identifying the organisms, enabling selection of the appropriate antibiotic therapy.

NUMBER OF VAGINAL EXAMS

Vaginal exams carry no greater infection risk than do rectal exams in labor. In two recent studies, the number of vaginal exams correlated with risk of infection (24, 26), but in many other studies, this clinical variable was not identified as a risk factor.

INTERNAL FETAL MONITORING

Since the internal fetal monitor (IFM) is a foreign body, concern exists that its use may incease intrauterine infection. Unfortunately, it is difficult to separate the effect of IFMs alone because they are often used in patients with abnormal labor, prolonged ROM, and cesarean delivery and thus already at increased risk for infection. Although some studies have implicated internal monitoring as a risk factor (29, 30), most studies show no direct increase in infection with IFM (23, 24, 26, 27, 31, 32).

SOCIOECONOMIC STATUS

Regardless of race, indigent patients have higher puerperal infection rates than do middle-class patients. The cause is unclear, but differences in flora, hygiene, nutrition, and amniotic fluid bacterial inhibitor actively have all been postulated as reasons.

OTHER FACTORS

Anemia has been associated with postpartum infection in several studies. Rather than being a cause of infection, anemia may simply represent a marker for poor nutrition or lower socioeconomic class. Obesity has not been a consistent risk factor for genital infection, but it has been a risk factor for wound infection in general surgery. Minkoff and colleagues have also found that maternal colonization with group B streptococcus and higher phosphate-zinc ratios correlated with puerperal infection (33, 34).

Microbiology

As noted earlier, endometrial cultures free of lower genital tract contaminants are not readily available. Nevertheless, endometritis most often seems to be a mixed infection with aerobic and anaerobic bacteria from the genital tract. On the average, two to three microorganisms can be recovered from the endometrial cavity, but six to seven may be isolated in some patients. In a recent study of 198 patients with endometritis after cesarean section, 53.5% of the endometrial isolates were aerobes, while 46.5% were anaerobes (35).

Aerobic organisms are found in approximately 70% of genital cultures. The gram-negative bacilli represent the largest number of aerobic isolates. Within this group, *Escherichia coli* is the most common (found in up to 30% of patients). Gram-positive aerobes are recovered less commonly; among these and the streptococci are the most frequent gram-positive isolates. Group B streptococci are isolated in 15% or so of genital isolates from patients with endometritis. *N. gonorrhoeae* may be found rarely, usually as part of a mixed infection.

Special management is required for certain aerobic microorganisms. Identification of the group B streptococcus is important, since the neonate may be colonized and at risk for fulminant sepsis. The nursery should be notified whenever group B streptococcus is isolated in a mother. Likewise, group A streptococcal infections must be regarded with special concern, as an epidemic may develop from a point source. The patient with a group A streptococcal infection should be isolated to avoid spread. *S. aureus* is another important offender because of its resistance to penicillin and its propensity for metastatic infection; however, this organism occurs in approximately 5% of genital infections.

Anaerobic organisms clearly have major roles in postpartum infection and are found in 80% of properly collected and handled cultures. The most common isolate is often a member of the *Bacteroides* species. These gram-negative bacilli are important because of their role in intraperitoneal abscess formation and their pattern of resistance to antibiotics. Although much attention has been directed at *Bacteroides fragilis* in the last decade, a number of hospitals throughout the United States report *Bacteroides bivius* as the predominant anaerobic isolate from the genital tract. Both of these microorganisms are resistant to many antibiotics, such as penicillin. Clindamycin, chloramphenicol, metronidazole, and some of the newer penicillins and cephalosporins have good activity against these species. Other common anaerobic isolates are the anaerobic streptococci (*Peptococcus* species and *Peptostreptococcus* species), *Fusobacterium* species, and *Clostridium* species. These organisms are usually sensitive to many commonly used antibiotics, including penicillin and clindamycin.

Most patients with *Clostridium perfringens* infection (even bacteremia) do well with antibiotic therapy alone. Thus, isolation of *C. perfringens*, even from the bloodstream, should not, by itself, prompt surgical intervention. Hysterectomy should be reserved for cases with evidence of myonecrosis.

Genital mycoplasmas (*Mycoplasma hominis* and *Ureaplasma urealyticum*) have been associated with postpartum infection. McCormack and colleagues and Wallace and co-workers recovered *M. hominis* from the bloodstream of 10 postpartum women (36, 37). In a larger series, Lamey and associates isolated mycoplasmas in 12.8% (16/125) blood cultures from febrile puerperal women, and from none of 60 afebrile postpartum patients (38). Finally, Platt and co-workers reported an association between a fourfold rise in mycoplasmacidal antibody titer and fever after vaginal delivery (39). However, many patients with puerperal infection respond to antibiotics not active against the genital mycoplasmas. (Please see Chapter 7.)

Chlamydia trachomatis may also be involved in postpartum infection. Wager and colleagues found an association between positive antepartum cervical cultures for *C. trachomatis* and a late-onset, mild endometritis after vaginal delivery (40). Due to the small numbers, these findings are limited. No role has been demonstrated for *C. trachomatis* infection after cesarean section.

Diagnosis

The diagosis of endomyometritis is usually based upon symptoms of fever, malaise, abdominal pain, and purulent or foul lochia. As noted, though, not all patients have the complete picture. Appropriate specimens include a complete blood count, two sets of venous blood cultures, and a uterine culture. Gram stain of the genital culture may be helpful when hemolytic streptococci, clostridial, or other anaerobes are suspected.

Treatment

With genital supportive therapy and appropriate antibiotics, the vast majority of patients improve within a few days. Well controlled treatment studies are few and mainly are restricted to some of the newer, broader spectrum agents.

Among patients with endomyometritis after vaginal delivery, responses to antibiotic therapy with penicillin plus an aminoglycoside has been close to 95% (13). In patients with poor responses, addition of appropriate antibiotics then resulted in an overall culture rate of 98%. Examples of appropriate additional antibiotics would include clindamycin, chloramphenicol, or metronidazole for a presumed anaerobic infection. In the remaining patients, causes of persistent fever included abscesses and septic pelvic thrombophlebitis. Other potential sources of fever in these patients would conclude infection of another site or a noninfectious cause of fever, such as drug fever or collagen disease. Many trials of newer antibiotics have included some patients with endometritis after vaginal delivery, but cure rates in these subgroups cannot be ascertained. One would anticipate cure rates with clindamycin plus an aminoglycoside in excess of 95% initially and a similar high rate with newer penicillins and cephalosporins.

Among patients with endomyometritis after cesarean section, response to antibiotics is poorer. Recent prospective studies have found the cure rate to be 65–78% in response to therapy with penicillin plus aminoglycoside and penicillin plus tetracycline (14, 15, 41). In about half of the failures, the cause can be identified and includes a resistant organism (often *B. fragilis* when penicillin plus aminoglycoside is used), wound infection, pelvic hematoma or abscess, and presumed septic pelvic thrombophlebitis. As with infection after vaginal delivery, the cause of apparent failure may be infection of another site or a noninfectious source.

When initial therapy consists of clindamycin plus gentamicin, the response rate of endomyometritis after cesarean section is higher (generally 90–95%), and major infectious complications may be reduced (15, 35). Experimental work in laboratory animals provides insight regarding the improved response rate with clindamycin plus an aminoglycoside.

In 1974, Weinstein and colleagues developed a rat model to study intraabdominal infection (42). They found that placing a capsule containing bowel flora in the peritoneum resulted in two stages of infection. In the first stage, 100% of the animals developed peritonitis, and 37–43% died (probably from sepsis). This initial stage lasted 4–5 days. In the second stage, the peritonitis resolved; no deaths occurred, but 100% of the survivors developed intraperitoneal abscesses. Further studies revealed that the peritonitis stage resulted from infection with gram-negative aerobic bacilli, such as *E. coli* or *Kleb-*

siella pneumoniae, while the abscess stage was mediated by anaerobes, such as the *Bacteroides* species. Treatment with gentamicin, an antibiotic specific for gram-negative bacilli, reduced the mortality rate to 4%, but 98% of the survivors still developed abscesses. Conversely, treatment with clindamycin, which is highly active against anaerobes, did not decrease the mortality rate (35%), but only 5% of the survivors developed abscesses. Administration of both clindamycin and gentamicin resulted in a 9% mortality rate and a 6% rate of abscess formation (43).

While the *B. fragilis* group is usually resistant to penicillin and many other antibiotics, they are susceptible to clindamycin. Clindamycin has activity against the gram-positive aerobes as well; therefore, the combination of clindamycin-gentamicin has a broad spectrum of activity. From the genital flora, the enterococcus appears as the only common isolate that is resistant to this combination.

Recent clinical experience shows consistently excellent results with clindamycin-gentamicin for pelvic infection after cesarean section. In 200 patients with endometritis after cesarean section, diZerega and colleagues treated half with penicillin-gentamicin and the other half with clindamycin-gentamicin (15). The rate of clinical cures was significantly higher in the clindamycin-gentamicin group (96%) than in the penicillin-gentamicin group (64%) (p < 0.001). More importantly, no serious complications occurred in the clindamycin group, while in the penicillin group, one patient developed an abscess, two required heparin for presumed septic pelvic thrombophlebitis, and one had a wound evisceration. Other measures of morbidity, such as length of hospital stay and fever index, were significantly better in the clindamycin group. Gibbs and co-workers have also found excellent cure rates for this combination (35, 44).

The improved outcome with clindamycin-gentamicin probably results from the susceptibility of *B. fragilis*, *B. bivius*, and other anaerobes to clindamycin, whereas these organisms are usually resistant to penicillin. Therefore, initial therapy for endometritis after cesarean section should consist of broad spectrum antibiotics with activity against all the *Bacteroides* species as well as gram-positive and gram-negative aerobes. Ampicillin, penicillin-gentamicin, ampicillin-gentamicin, and cephalothin-gentamicin do not provide this spectrum. At present, the combination of clindamycin and aminoglycoside may be considered the standard for comparison for treatment in genital tract infection after cesarean section.

This combination, however, is not without problems. Both drugs have serious side effects. Clindamycin therapy may lead to diarrhea in 2–6% of patients and rarely to pseudomembranous colitis. Aminoglycoside therapy may lead to nephro- or ototoxicity, and recent studies reveal that "therapeutic" aminoglycoside levels may be difficult to achieve in obstetric patients with standard dosing regimens (45–47). Furthermore, the administation of two drugs is more time-consuming and expensive than a single agent. These concerns have led to trials of broad spectrum single agents in obstetric infections.

In recent years, the pharmaceutical industry has developed a large number of new penicillins and cephalosporins, with a broader spectrum of activity. While no single agent provides activity against the entire bacterial spectrum, most have sufficient aerobic and anaerobic activity to merit use in obstetric infections. However, clinical trials with these antibiotics have been with small numbers of patients. Serious complications (abscess, septic pelvic thrombophlebitis) occur rarely, and the limited scope of the trials prevents any conclusions about the prevention of serious complications by these single agents. Also, their effectiveness in more serious infections (septic shock) is unclear since few studies include severely ill patients. For obstetric infections, the newer penicillins and cephalosporins may have a role in mild to moderate infection. Those with high cure rates in the treatment of endometritis after cesarean section are cefotaxime, moxalactam, piperacillin, and mezlocillin. (Please see Chapter 19 for a more complete discussion.) Others exist that may yield equivalent results, and many others are being developed at this time. While some of these agents have a broader spectrum of coverage than others, the clinical significance of small differences in minimal inhibitory concentrations is not always clear. Larger trials and greater clinical experience with these agents may show one to be superior to the others, but the data, at present, are insufficient to make any conclusion.

The new penicillins and cephalosporins are usually very well tolerated and have few side effects. Also, therapeutic serum levels can be achieved easily without much concern with dosing. Administration of a single agent demands less time and equipment, but the higher cost of most newer agents must be considered also.

While these new agents have been introduced into the market, other older agents are appearing with different therapeutic indications. Metronidazole, long used for trichomoniasis, has excellent anaerobic activity and is now available in parenteral form. Since it has little activity against aerobes, its use as a single agent therapy is generally unwise. Its use in combination with gentamicin still leaves the gram-positive aerobes (notably group G streptococci) uncovered. In obstetric infections, the role of metronidazole may be to replace clindamycin, not as initial therapy, but in those patients who develop significant diarrhea. The need for aerobic coverage would depend on endometrial culture results.

New antibiotics are being formulated that may replace gentamicin as initial therapy. Some new cephalosporin derivatives, the monobactams, have exquisite gram-negative activity, but they have little activity in the rest of the bacterial spectrum. These agents have the same spectrum as the aminoglycosides and should have fewer side effects. Clinical trials of these monobactams have recently begun.

MASTITIS

No definite data are available regarding incidence, but mastitis appears infrequently after delivery. Both *epidemic* and *endemic* forms of puerperal mastitis may occur. *Epidemic* puerperal mastitis has occurred among hospitalized women in conjunction with staphylococcal nursery epidemics. This form of the disease has been described mainly as a mammary adenitis, involving mainly the lactiferous glands and ducts. *Endemic* puerperal mastitis occurs sporadically among nonhospitalized, nursing women. This type often presents as a lobular, V-shaped cellulitis of the periglandular connective tissue. Often there may be a fissure, crack, or irritation on the nipple. In recent reports, endemic mastitis has been the main form encountered.

In epidemic mastitis, *S. aureus* has been the main culprit. For endemic mastitis, *S. aureus* again is a common pathogen, in either pure or mixed culture, but other common organisms include group A or group B streptococci. *Haemophilus influenzae* and *Haemophilus parainfluenzae* have been reported as well, but in up to 50% of cases only normal skin flora are cultured from breast milk (48, 49). Further insight into the relationship of breast symptoms, milk leukocytes, and quantitative breast milk cultures has been provided by the recent work of Thomsen and colleagues (50). In 491 samples from nursing women, they noted that in women without breast symptoms leukocytic counts were less than 10^6/ml of milk, and milk was sterile or contained less than 10^3 bacterial/ml. When bacteria were present in milk from asymptomatic women, the organisms were similar to those normally present on the skin, and most milk specimens revealed mixed cultures. Samples from women with breast symptoms were divided into three groups. In one group (N = 85), leukocyte counts were less than 10^6/ml of milk, and milk cultures were similar to those from women without symptoms. Breast symptoms in this group were brief (average, 2.1 days) and resolved spontaneously. This group was said to have milk stasis.

In the remaining two groups, breast milk showed greater than 10^6 leukocytes/ml. In one of these groups (N = 22), the milk cultures were sterile or revealed less than 10^3 bacteria/ml. The average duration of symptoms was 5.3 days. This group was said to have noninfectious inflammation of the breast. In the third group (N = 39), milk cultures showed both $>10^6$ leukocytes and $>10^3$ bacteria/ml. Without therapy, approximately half the patients in this group showed complete recovery after an average of 5.9 days, but symptoms of sepsis and breast abscess developed in 22 and 11% of cases, respectively. In the 39 samples of milk in this group of women, organisms identified were *S. aureus*, 18; coagulase-negative staphylococci, 10; *Streptococcus faecalis*, 2; group A streptococci, *E. coli*, 3; *K. pneumoniae*, 2; and *B. fragilis*, 3.

Sporadic mastitis most often begins from the second or third week to a number of months after delivery. Fever commonly greater than 102°F, malaise, and localized breast signs are the usual presenting problems. In untreated patients, breast abscess develops commonly. Stasis of milk from weaning is often suggested as the precipitating event for mastitis, but, in fact, only a minority of women (perhaps 20%) with mastitis have recently stopped nursing. Culture of expressed breast milk is appropriate, although it is only in a few cases that the report will alter management.

Recent authors have noted that with early antibiotic treatment endemic mastitis resolves within 24–48 hr and that abscess is unusual. In one series of 71 cases, abscess developed in only eight (11.5%); and in six of these, treatment was not instituted for more than 24 hr (48). Based upon the organisms involved and the well-known resistance of even community-acquired staphylococci to penicillin, the choice of initial antibiotic therapy would seem to be a penicillinase-resistant penicillin (such as dicloxacillin) or a cephalosporin. However, empiric therapy with penicillin V, erythromycin, or sulfonamides has resulted in prompt responses, even when there has been in vitro resistance (49). In view of the work of Thomsen and co-workers (50), it is likely that many such cases would have resolved, even without antibiotic therapy. In most cases of mastitis, antibiotics should be given orally as there is no need for hospitalization.

In addition to antibiotic therapy, adjunctive measures such as ice packs, breast support, and analgesics have been suggested. In most cases, the mother may continue to nurse from both breasts. If the infected side is too sore, she may pump this breast gently. Regular drainage of the infected breast may be important in preventing abscess. Infants do not seem to suffer any adverse effects from suckling an infected breast, except if an abscess has developed. In the unusual case when an abscess develops, prompt incision and drainage should be instituted.

URINARY TRACT INFECTION

Urinary tract infection is a common cause of postpartum fever, as the parturient is predisposed to infection by the physiologic hydroureter of pregnancy, catheterization in labor, and antecedent, asymptomatic bacteriuria. A presumptive diagnosis of urinary infection may be based on traditional signs and symptoms (frequency, dysuria, back pain, fever, and costovertebral angle tenderness). Urinalysis and urine cultures are helpful in the diagosis. Because urine specimens from puerperal women often contain contamination from the lochia, supervision at collection is important. Pyuria is still a common indicator of urinary tract infection but may develop without infection because of bladder inflammation from trauma at labor and delivery. Traditionally, specimens had to contain more than 10^5 cfu/ml of a single organism to be considered significant; however, recent evidence in nonpregnant patients suggests that $>10^2$ cfu/ml was a more specific and sensitive diagnostic criteria of infection than $>10^5$ cfu/ml in *symptomatic* patients (51). In the majority of cases, *E. coli* is isolated, although other gramnegative aerobic bacilli, enterococci, and occasionally group B streptococci may cause urinary tract infection. Since bacteremia is possible in pyelonephritis, the initial antibiotic in febrile patients should be one able to achieve high blood and urinary levels. Parenterally administered ampicillin or a cephalosporin may be used initially with an aminoglycoside added if septic shock develops or when a resistant isolate is suspected.

ANESTHESIA COMPLICATIONS

Infections resulting from spinal or epidural anesthesia are extremely rare. In a series of 10,000 spinal and 32,000 epidural anesthesias, there were no infections due to the anesthetics (52), but there has been a report of a spontaneous puerperal epidural abscess (53). With general anesthesia, atelectasis and pulmonary infections may occur and present as a puerperal fever.

On rare occasions, infections beneath the gluteus or behind the psoas muscle develop in postpartum women (54, 55). These severe infections are characterized by persistent, spiking temperature elevations and hip pain or poorly localized pelvic pain. In the reported cases, these severe infections had one common feature—the use of paracervical or transvaginal pudendal blocks. The needle penetration may be the source of contamination. In half the cases, a radiograph documented gas in the soft tissues. These patients had extensive hospitalization, and deaths have been reported. In addition to vigorous antibiotic therapy, drainage is required for treatment.

SEPTIC PELVIC THROMBOPHLEBITIS

Pelvic vein thrombophlebitis may occur in association with pelvic surgery, operative site infection following surgery, and pelvic inflammatory disease. Although it is more likely to occur following obstetric procedures, the overall incidence of the disorder, even in this clinical setting, is low. Brown and Munsick described 10 cases of pelvic vein thrombophlebitis in 5693 deliveries, an incidence of 0.18% (56). Derrick and associates found only one case of pelvic vein thrombosis in 2372 patients followed prospectively throughout pregnancy and the puerperium (57). This figure is consistent with Josey and Staggers' reported incidence of 1 in 2000 deliveries (58).

Among patients with operative site infections, the incidence of pelvic vein thrombophlebitis is higher. In an evaluation of 160 patients with established postcesarean endometritis, Gibbs and co-workers noted a 2% incidence of pelvic vein thrombophlebitis (14). Similarly, diZerega et al noted a 1% incidence of the disorder in their series of 200 patients with operative site infections following cesarean section (15%).

Pathogenesis

In 1856, Virchow established that three principal factors predisposed to venous thrombosis: changes in circulating coagulation factors, alterations in the vein wall, and stasis of blood flow. Pregnancy and obstetric surgery represent the complete fulfillment of the conditions of Virchow's disease triad (59).

A hypercoagulable state exists during pregnancy and for at least 6 weeks postpartum. Levels of clotting factors I, II, VII, IX, and X are increased throughout gestation and the early puerperium. Platelet count and platelet adhesiveness also are increased in pregnancy. In addition, the placenta and amniotic fluid are rich sources of tissue thromboplastin (factor III), and this material may be released into the systemic circulation coincident with placental separation at delivery, thereby initiating the external coagulation pathway. Further alterations in the wall of the pelvic veins during pregnancy predispose to thrombophlebitis.

Then, vascular endothelium may be injured as a direct result of surgical trauma, and surgery may result in direct inoculation of bacteria into the pelvic vessels. Endothelial injury then may occur as a result of the inflammatory reaction to the bacteria, stimulating further platelet aggregation and clot formation.

Many microorganisms have been implicated in the pathogenesis of pelvic vein thrombophlebitis including anaerobic streptococci, *Proteus* species, aerobic streptococci, staphylococci, yeast, and *Bacteroides* species (60–62). The isolation of these microorganisms from resected venous specimens suggests that bacterial injury to the endothelium of the vein is an important step in initiation of the thrombotic process.

During pregnancy, major hemodynamic changes occur within the venous system of the pelvis that predispose to stasis of blood flow. At term, the diameter of the ovarian vein is approximately 3 times its normal diameter in the nonpregnant state, and the capacity of the vein is increased 60 times (63).

Both ovarian veins are long and unbranched. Both may have multiple valves, especially the right ovarian vein. Valve leaflets are major sites for venous pooling and thus serve as a nidus for thrombosis. Pooling is accentuated in the presence of an incompetent valve, and such dysfunctional leaflets with resultant varicosity formation have been described in ovarian vein specimens and in radiographic studies of the pelvic veins (56, 57, 64–66).

Both ovarian veins have minimal adventitial sheaths, unlike the veins of the lower extremities. Although this lack of a restrictive fibrous sheath permits the veins to enlarge their capacity during pregnancy, it also makes them vulnerable to compression from external forces. There is good evidence that the right ovarian vein is particularly susceptible to wide fluctuations in flow rates due to external compression (56, 67, 68). The right ovarian vein crosses the right ureter at the pelvic brim. Both the vein and ureter are vulnerable to compression at this point from one another and from the dextrorotated uterus.

Pelvic vein thrombophlebitis may lead to serious complications, including septic pulmonary emboli (67). In two reported series, 32–38% of patients with pelvic vein thrombophlebitis had clinical and laboratory evidence of pulmonary embolization (58, 66). Major sequelae of septic pulmonary embolization include lung abscess, lung infarction, bronchopleural fistula, and empyema. In addition, emboli from infected pelvic veins may precipitate acute endocarditis, primarily affecting the right side of the heart, and cause disseminated abscesses in other organ systems.

Clinical Presentation

Pelvic vein thrombophlebitis appears to occur in two distinct clinical forms. The most commonly described disorder is that of acute thrombosis of one or both ovarian veins. Since such large-scale thrombus formation occurs most commonly on the right side, many authors have referred to this disease process as the right ovarian vein syndrome (57, 64, 69, 70).

Patients with acute ovarian vein thrombophlebitis usually have distinct clinical findings. Although not all individuals are febrile, most will have a mild to moderate temperature elevation in the first 48–96 hr postoperatively and experience lower abdominal pain. The initial physical examination usually is consistent with endomyometritis or pelvic cellulitis, and the attending physician quite properly initiates antibiotic therapy. Despite administration of systemic antibiotics, however, the patients do not improve. Temperature elevations may persist, often accompanied by shaking chills. Subjectively, patients experience steadily worsening adominal pain which is constant and localized to the side of the affected vein. The pain may radiate into the groin, upper abdomen, or flank.

Gastrointestinal symptoms such as nausea, vomiting, and distention also may be present.

On physical examination, patients usually are febrile and appear acutely ill. The pulse rate usually is elevated, often disproportionately so as compared with the actual temperature. Tachypnea, stridor, and other signs of respiratory distress may be present when pulmonary embolization has occurred. Changing cardiac murmurs suggest acute endocarditis.

The most striking findings are demonstrable on abdominopelvic examination. Bowel sounds usually are normoactive, but may be diminished to absent in the presence of a paralytic ileus. Patients usually have direct tenderness on the affected side in association with both voluntary and involuntary guarding. The most definitive sign on physical examination is the detection of a rope-like, tender abdominal mass. Such a mass will be palpable in one-half to two-thirds of patients and usually originates centrally near the uterine cornua and extends laterally and cephalad toward the upper abdomen (56, 70).

The second presentation of pelvic vein thrombophlebitis is less distinct and has been called "enigmatic fever" (71, 72). Initially, patients demonstrate many of the same clinical manifestations as the individuals described previously. They have evidence of operative site infection following surgery and are begun on antibiotic therapy. Unlike the patients with acute ovarian vein thrombosis, however, these women usually experience definite improvement in all clinical parameters with the singular exception of spiking temperatures. Patients do not appear to be critically ill, and positive physical findings usually are absent except for recurrent temperature elevations, often as high as 103–104°F, and associated tachycardia. Whereas the majority of patients with acute ovarian vein thrombosis have palpable abdominal masses, very few of the patients with this second syndrome have demonstrable masses.

Diagnosis

The diagnosis of pelvic vein thrombophlebitis should be suspected in any patient with an antecedent soft tissue pelvic infection and an elevated temperature that persists despite appropriate broad spectrum antibiotic therapy.

The disorder most likely to be confused with the right ovarian vein syndrome is acute appendicitis (56). Other common disorders that should be considered are broad ligament cellulitis or hematoma, torsion of the adnexa, uretherolithiasis, pyelonephritis, degenerating pedunculated leiomyoma, pelvic cellulitis, and pelvic or abdominal abscess (65, 66). The disorders most likely to be confused with the second clinical syndrome are drug fever, collagen vascular disease, coexisting viral illness, and pelvic abscess (71, 72).

The diagnosis of pelvic vein thrombophlebitis must be made largely on the basis of the patient's clinical history and physical examination. A pattern of persistent fever in association with lower abdominal pain and a palpable mass in either or both mid quadrants is highly suggestive that a thrombotic disorder is present. Laboratory data will be of aid in excluding other diagnoses. In isolated instances, intravenous pyelography has been of value in confirming the suspected diagnosis of acute ovarian vein thrombosis. Derrick and co-workers (57) and Darney and Wilson (73) have described the presence of a distinct concentric narrowing of the proximal right ureter in two patients with unilateral right ovarian vein thrombophlebitis. Similarly, Maull and colleagues noted the presence of ureteral compression in association with right ovarian vein thrombosis (66). Dykhuizen and Roberts also have stressed the value of excretory urography in patients suspected of having thrombosis of one of the ovarian vessels (64). In their evaluation of 15 patients with the right ovarian vein syndrome, they noted that caliectasis, pyeloectasis, and ureterectasis were common findings on excretory urograms. It is essential to remember, however, that many normal puerperal patients may have mild degrees of hydroureter as a consequence of the normal physiologic changes of pregnancy.

Although the presence of an abnormal excretory urogram may be helpful in making the diagnosis of pelvic vein thrombophlebitis, the finding of a normal study does not mean that the clinical diagnosis is incorrect. In fact, when multiple small pelvic vein emboli are present, as appears to be the case in patients with the clinical syndrome of enigmatic fever, it may be the exception rather than the rule to have an abnormal excretory urogram.

Venography may be of assistance in establishing the diagnosis of ovarian vein thrombosis. Both Jacobs (67) and Munsick and Gillanders (70) have described techniques for selected radiographic study of the gonadal veins. Similarly, Salzer and Abas have described an interesting technique for ovarian vein phlebography in postpartum patients (74). Also, Allan and associates recently performed an inferior vena cavagram to document the presence of a large thrombosis at the junction of the inferior vena cava and the right ovarian vein (59). However, there is no study that has evaluated the accuracy of venography in confirming the diagnosis of ovarian vein thrombophlebitis.

Other diagnostic studies that may be of help in evaluating the patient with suspected pelvic vein thrombophlebitis include gallium scan, computerized axial tomography (CT scan), sonogram, and ventilation-perfusion scan of the lung. When indicated clinically, the gallium scan and sonogram may be useful in excluding the presence of a pelvic abscess. Ventilation-perfusion scan of the lung may be indicated to determine whether pulmonary embolization has occurred as a result of pelvic vein thrombophlebitis. CT scan may be helpful in delineating an intravascular thrombus in patients with ovarian vein thrombophlebitis, but there is no prospective study that systematically has investigated the efficacy of these tests in confirming the diagnosis of pelvic vein thrombophlebitis.

Conventional chest radiographs are usually normal but may demonstrate evidence of pulmonary embolization. However, the classic wedge-shaped defect associated with noninfected pulmonary emboli is rarely seen, and more commonly there will be multiple small nodular densities in both lower lobes that may, with time, become confluent and progress to actual abscess formation. The conventional electrocardiogram may demonstrate changes consistent with acute pulmonary embolization such as ST-T wave changes, acute right heart strain, and right axis deviation.

Treatment

Several surgical and medical approaches have been utilized in the treatment of pelvic vein thrombophlebitis. (Please see Table 17.3.) In considering these treatment schemes proposals, it must be remembered that the diagnosis has not always been confirmed by laparotomy or radiographic study. In many cases, the diagnosis was one of exclusion, based upon a clinical response to administration of heparin. In such circumstances, it often is difficult to determine whether the clinical response was due to the cumulative effect of long-term antibiotic administration or due specifically to the institution of heparin therapy. Moreover, therapy was instituted in an uncontrolled fashion. Few of the studies provide for long-term follow-up of patients undergoing either medical or surgical therapy.

Based upon the retrospective data presented by various investigators, it still is possible to establish certain general principles for the management of patients with suspected pelvic vein thrombophlebitis. First, because bacterial injury to the venous endothelium has been an important mechanism in initiating the thromboembolic process in most patients, we believe that broad spectrum antibiotics should be administered.

Second, therapeutic anticoagulation should be initiated when the diagnosis of pelvic vein thrombophlebitis is made. Intravenous heparin is the anticoagulant of choice (58). The proper length of therapy has not been determined, although most investigators have utilized a course of 7-10 days. In most cases, long-term anticoagulation with oral agents does not appear to be necessary. Some favor extended anticoagulation when there has been documentation of septic pulmonary emboli, but there are no data regarding the need for this.

Antibiotic and heparin administration should be the initial therapy in all patients with suspected pelvic vein thrombophlebitis. There are several well-documented reports in the literature of patients who underwent exploratory laparotomy for presumed ruptured appendix, pelvic abscess, or torsed ovary and were found to have only large thrombi in one or both ovarian veins (75–77). In each instance, the operative procedure was terminated without ligation of either ovarian vessel or the inferior vena cava. Heparin therapy was initiated, and the patient experienced complete recovery without need for additional surgery.

Moreover, the extensive experience of Josey and Staggers with medical therapy of pelvic vein thrombophlebitis is a persuasive argument in favor of selecting anticoagulation as the initial treatment (58). In their series of 46 patients with pelvic vein thrombophlebitis, 42 responded completely to anticoagulation alone. Significantly, 7 of 28 obstetric patients were thought to have acute ovarian vein thrombosis, and 15 of the total group of 46 had documented septic pulmonary emboli. Two of the 4 patients who did not respond to medical therapy had both pelvic vein thrombophlebitis and a pelvic abscess. The additional experience of Dunn and VanVorrhis (71) and Schulman (72) also attests to the efficacy of anticoagulation as the initial therapy in patients with suspected pelvic vein thrombophlebitis.

Table 17.3
Summary of Reported Treatments for Pelvic Vein Thrombophlebitis[a]

Author	Year	No. of cases	Treatment
Austin (81)	1976	1	ROV resection and IVC ligation
Collins (83)	1941–58	140	Bilateral OV and IVC ligation
Sanders (80)	1964	2	1—IVC ligation, LOV ligation, ROV and partial excision, postoperative antibiotics, and heparin 1—Bilateral OV ligation, IVC ligation, and heparin
Lotze (65)	1962–64	6	1—ROV resection, RSO, antibiotic, and Coumadin 1—ROV resection, RSO, and antibiotics 1—Bilateral OV and IVC ligation, antibiotics, heparin, and Coumadin 1—Bilateral OV ligation, partial resection of left renal vein, antibiotics, and heparin
Brown (56)	1971	16	2—Unilateral OV ligation, antibiotics, and heparin 1—Bilateral OV ligation, antibiotics, and heparin 10—Antibiotics and heparin 1—Prednisone and heparin 1—Phenylbutazone 1—Antibiotics
Gardstein (82)	1971	1	TAH, BSO, bilateral hypogastric artery ligation
Josey (58)	1965–73	46	42—Heparin and antibiotics 2—Heparin, antibiotics, TAH and BSO 2—Heparin, antibiotics, TAH, BSO, and IVC ligation
Allan (59)	1976	6	1—ROV excision, TAH, BSO, bilateral hypogastric artery ligation, antibiotics, and heparin 2—Antibiotics and heparin 1—ROV excision, LOV ligation, and antibiotics 1—Antibiotics, intraoperative death during IVC ligation 1—Bilateral OV and IVC ligation, right renal vein thrombectomy, and antibiotics 1—TAH, BSO, appendectomy, heparin, and antibiotics
O'Lane (77)	1965	2	1—Heparin 1—Subtotal hysterectomy
Dunn (71)	1962–65	6	Heparin and antibiotics
Schulman (72)	1965	7	Heparin and antibiotics
Robinson (79)	1960–69	4	1—ROV resection and heparin 1—ROV resection 1—ROV resection, RSO, and IVC thrombectomy 1—ROV resection, RO artery resection, and RSO
Montalto (69)	1969	1	IVC plication, ROV excision, and antibiotics

[a] Legend: OV, ovarian vein; ROV, right ovarian vein; LOV, left ovarian vein; IVC, inferior vena cava; RSO, right salpingo-oophorectomy; TAH, total abdominal hysterectomy; BSO, bilateral salpingo-oophorectomy; RSO, right salpingo-oophorectomy; TAH, total abdominal hysterectomy; BSO, bilateral salpingo-oophorectomy.

Table 17.3—*continued*

Author	Year	No. of cases	Treatment
McElin (60)	1970	1	TAH, BSO, IVC resection, and antibiotics
Collins (78)	1970	202	IVC and bilateral OV ligation with concurrent TAH in 22 cases
Huntsinger (75)	1970	1	Heparin
Ledger (76)	1970	4	Heparin antibiotics
Darney (73)	1977	1	Antibiotics and heparin
Maull (66)	1978	4	1—ROV ligation, excision, and antibiotics 1—ROV ligation and biopsy 1—Antibiotics, heparin, and IVC ligation

Surgery should be reserved for those patients who remain clinically ill despite effective antimicrobial and anticoagulant therapy (58, 66, 71). Almost all of these patients will ultimately be proved to have the ovarian vein syndrome rather than the enigmatic fever syndrome. The critical question is what procedure should be performed in patients who do not respond to medical therapy. Multiple surgical procedures have been proposed as the optimal technique, including bilateral ovarian vein ligation and inferior vena cava ligation (75, 76, 78–80), unilateral ovarian vein ligation with and without vena cava ligation (56), and excision of the infected vein ligation with and without ligation of the contralateral vein and vena cava (60, 65, 76, 81). The most reasonable approach would seem to be that advocated by Brown and Munsick who propose ligation of the infected vein(s) and concurrent ligation of the vena cava only when the ovarian vein thrombolus extends into this large vessel (56). Ligation of the vena cava also is indicated in patients who have experienced pulmonary embolization while on therapeutic doses of anticoagulants and in patients who have not responded to more conservative surgical measures (65, 66, 79). Renal vein thrombectomy is indicated when the thrombosis has extended into either renal vein (56).

When ovarian vein and vena cava ligation is performed, it is not necessary to perform concurrent hysterectomy and bilateral salpingoophorectomy unless there is coexisting disease in these organs. Gardstein and colleagues reported bilateral ovarian infarction as a complication of ovarian vein thrombophlebitis and removed both ovaries in conjunction with administration of anticoagulants (82). Collins performed concurrent hysterectomy in 22 of 202 patients with suppurative pelvic vein thrombophlebitis. The most common indication for hysterectomy was the presence of an adnexal, intramyometrial, or pelvic abscess (78). Similarly, Joscy and Staggers, although major proponents of medical ther-

apy for pelvic vein thrombophlebitis, have acknowledged the occasional need for more extensive surgery when both venous thrombosis and localized pelvic abscess are present concurrently (58).

Although a well-defined collateral circulation develops following ligation of the vena cava and ovarian vessels, patients treated surgically may develop lower extremity edema. Although this usually is transient, it may evolve into a definite postphlebitic syndrome (56). Patients also may experience impaired fertility following surgery. For example, Collins has described 47 pregnancies in 23 patients who underwent vena cava and ovarian vein ligation. Only 30 of the 47 pregnancies progressed beyond 28 weeks gestation, and only 22 of these 30 continued to term (83). A more worrisome aspect of Collins' study is the lack of information about the reproductive performance of the other 117 of the original 140 patients treated surgically for septic pelvic vein thrombophlebitis. In a more recent report, Allan and co-workers described a patient who experienced four spontaneous abortions and then a premature delivery at 24 weeks of a stillborn infant following ovarian vein and vena cava ligation (59).

The procedure for ligation of the vena cava and ovarian vein also may be associated with major intra- and perioperative complications. In the preantibiotic era, Miller described 50% mortality in patients undergoing surgery for suppurative pelvic vein thrombophlebitis (84). More recently, Allan and Maull with their co-workers (59, 66) have described perioperative mortalities secondary to cardiac arrest during vena cava ligation.

For a thorough review of this topic, please see reference (85).

References

1. Filer R, Monif GRG: The significance of temperature during the first 24 hours postpartum. *Obstet Gynecol* 53:358, 1979.

2. Gibbs RS, Blanco JD: Asymptomatic parturients with high virulence bacteria in the amniotic fluid. *Soc Gynecol Invest*, abstract. San Francisco, 1984.
3. Vital Statistics of the U.S. 1973, vol II, *Mortality*, Part A, Tables 1–15. Cited in Huff RW, Pauerstein CJ: *Human Reproduction Physiology and Pathophysiology*. New York, J. Wiley & Sons, 1979.
4. Stevenson CS, Behney CA, Miller NF: Maternal death from puerperal sepsis following cesarean section. *Obstet Gynecol* 29:181, 1967.
5. Stevenson CS: Maternal death from puerperal sepsis following vaginal delivery. *Am J Obstet Gynecol* 104:699, 1969.
6. Schaffner W, Federspiel CF, Fulton ML, et al: Maternal mortality in Michigan: an epidemiologic analysis, 1950–1971. *Am J Public Health* 67:821, 1977.
7. Gibbs RS, Weinstein AJ: Puerperal infection in the antibiotic era. *Am J Obstet Gynecol* 124:769, 1976.
8. Gibbs RS, Blanco JD: Streptococcal infections in pregnancy, a study of 48 bacteremias. *Am J Obstet Gynecol* 140:405, 1981.
9. Pezzlo MT, Hesser JW, Morgan T, et al: Improved laboratory efficiency and diagnostic accuracy with new double-lumen-protected swab for endometrial specimens. *J Clin Microbiol* 9:56, 1979.
10. Knuppel RA, Scerbo JC, Mitchell GW, et al: Quantitative transcervical uterine cultures with a new device. *Obstet Gynecol* 57:243, 1981.
11. Duff WP, Gibbs RS, Blanco JD, et al: Endometrial culture techniques in puerperal patients. *Obstet Gynecol* 61:217, 1983.
12. Gibbs RS: Clinical risk factors for puerperal infection. *Obstet Gynecol* 55(S):178, 1980.
13. Gibbs RS, Rodgers PJ, Castaneda YS, et al: Endometritis following vaginal delivery. *Obstet Gynecol* 56:555, 1980.
14. Gibbs RS, Jones PM, Wilder CJ: Antibiotic therapy of endometritis following cesarean section. *Obstet Gynecol* 52:31, 1978.
15. diZerega G, Yonekura L, Roy S, et al: A comparison of clindamycin-gentamicin and penicillin-gentamicin in the treatment of post cesarean section endomyometritis. *Am J Obstet Gynecol* 134:238, 1979.
16. Frigoletto FD Jr, Ryan KJ, Philippe M: Maternal mortality rate associated with cesarean section: an appraisal. *Am J Obstet Gynecol* 136:969, 1980.
17. Gilstrap LC, Cunningham FG: The bacterial pathogenesis of infection following cesarean section. *Obstet Gynecol* 53:545, 1979.
18. Blanco JD, Gibbs RS, Castaneda YS, et al: Correlation of quantitative fluid cultures with endometritis after cesarean section. *Am J Obstet Gynecol* 143:897, 1982.
19. Blanco JD, Gibbs RS: Infections following classical cesarean section. *Obstet Gynecol* 55:167, 1980.
20. D'Angelo LJ, Sokol RJ: Time-related peripartum determinants of postpartum morbidity. *Obstet Gynecol* 55:319, 1980.
21. Gibbs RS, Listwa HM, Read JA: The effect of internal fetal monitoring on maternal infection following cesarean section. *Obstet Gynecol* 48:653, 1976.
22. Bobitt JR, Ledger WJ: Amniotic fluid analysis. Its role in maternal and neonatal infection. *Obstet Gynecol* 51:56, 1978.
23. Gibbs RS, Jones PM, Wilder CJY: Internal fetal monitoring and maternal infection following cesarean section: a prospective study. *Obstet Gynecol* 52:193, 1978.
24. Rehu M, Nilsson CG: Risk factors for febrile morbidity associated with cesarean section. *Obstet Gynecol* 56:269, 1980.
25. Nielsen TF, Hokegard KH: Postoperative cesarean section morbidity: a prospective study. *Am J Obstet Gynecol* 146:911, 1983.
26. Hawrylyshyn PA, Bernstein P, Papsin FR: Risk factors associated with infection following cesarean section. *Am J Obstet Gynecol* 139:294, 1981.
27. Ott WJ: Primary cesarean section: factors related to postpartum infection. *Obstet Gynecol* 57:171, 1981.
28. Hagglund L, Christensen KK, Christensen P, et al: Risk factors in cesarean section infection. *Obstet Gynecol* 46:145, 1983.
29. Hagen D: Maternal febrile morbidity associated with fetal monitoring and cesarean section. *Obstet Gynecol* 46:260, 1975.
30. Perloe M, Curet LB: The effect of internal fetal monitoring on cesarean section morbidity. *Obstet Gynecol* 53:354, 1979.
31. Anstey JT, Sheldon GW, Blythe JG: Infectious morbidity after primary cesarean sections in a private institution. *Am J Obstet Gynecol* 136:205, 1980.
32. Gassner CB, Ledger WJ: The relationship of hospital-acquired maternal infection to invasive intrapartum monitoring techniques. *Am J Obstet Gynecol* 126:33, 1976.
33. Minkoff HL, Sierra MF, Pringle GF, et al: Vaginal colonization with group B beta-hemolytic streptococcus as a risk factor for post-cesarean section febrile morbidity. *Am J Obstet Gynecol* 142:992, 1982.
34. Minkoff HL, Henry V, Decrease R, et al: The relationship of amniotic fluid phosphate-to-zinc ratios to post-cesarean section infection. *Am J Obstet Gynecol* 142:988, 1982.
35. Gibbs RS, Blanco JD, Castaneda YS, et al: A double-blind, randomized comparison of clindamycin-gentamicin versus cefamandole for treatment of post-cesarean endomyometritis. *Am J Obstet Gynecol* 144:261, 1982.
36. McCormack WM, Lee Y, Lin J, et al: Genital mycoplasmas in postpartum fever. *J Infect Dis* 127:193, 1973.
37. Wallace RJ, Alpert S, Browne K, et al: Isolation of *Mycoplasma hominis* from blood cultures in patients with postpartum fever. *Obstet Gynecol* 51:181, 1978.
38. Lamey JR, Eschenbach DA, Mitchell SH, et al: Isolation of mycoplasmas and bacteria from the blood of postpartum women. *Am J Obstet Gynecol* 143:104, 1982.
39. Platt R, Lin JL, Warren JW, et al: Infection with *Mycoplasma hominis* in postpartum fever. *Lancet* 2:1217, 1980.
40. Wager GP, Martin DH, Koutsky L, et al: Puerperal infectious morbidity: relationship to route to delivery and to antepartum *Chlamydia trachomatis* infection. *Am J Obstet Gynecol* 138:1028, 1980.
41. Cunningham FG, Hauth JC, String JD, et al:

Infectious morbidity following cesarean section: comparison of two treatment regimens. *Obstet Gynecol* 52:656, 1978.

42. Weinstein WM, Onderdonk AB, Bartlett JG, et al: Experimental intra-abdominal abscesses in rats: development of an experimental model. *Infect Immun* 10:1250, 1974.

43. Weinstein WM, Onderdonk AB, Bartlett JG, et al: Antimicrobial therapy of experimental intraabdominal sepsis. *J Infect Dis* 132:282, 1975.

44. Gibbs RS, Blanco JD, Duff P, et al: A double-blind, randomized comparison of moxalactam versus clindamycin-gentamicin in treatment of endomyometritis after cesarean section. *Am J Obstet Gynecol* 146:769, 1983.

45. Zaske DE, Cipolle RJ, Strate RG, et al: Rapid gentamicin elimination in obstetric patients. *Obstet Gynecol* 56:559, 1980.

46. Duff WP, Jorgensen JH, Alexander G, et al: Serum gentamicin levels in patients with post-cesarean endomyometritis. *Obstet Gynecol* 61:723, 1983.

47. Blanco JD, Gibbs RS, Duff P, et al: Serum tobramycin levels in puerperal women. *Am J Obstet Gynecol* 147:466, 1983.

48. Deveraux WP: Acute puerperal mastitis. *Am J Obstet Gynecol* 108:78, 1970.

49. Niebyl JR, Spence MR, Parmley TH: Sporadic (nonepidemic) puerperal mastitis. *J Reprod Med* 20:97, 1978.

50. Thomsen AC, Hansen KB, Moller BR: Leukocyte counts and microbiologic cultivation in the diagnosis of puerperal mastitis. *Am J Obstet Gynecol* 146:938, 1983.

51. Stamm WE, Counts GW, Running KR, et al: Diagnosis of coliform infection in acutely dysuric women. *N Engl J Med* 307:463, 1982.

52. Dripps RD, Vandam LD: Long term follow-up of patients who received 10,098 spinal anesthetics. *JAMA* 156:1486, 1954.

53. Male CG, Martin R: Puerperal spiral epidural abscess. *Lancet* 1:608, 1973.

54. Hibbard LR, Snyder EN, McVann RM: Subgluteal and retropsoal infection in obstetric patients. *Obstet Gynecol* 39:137, 1972.

55. Wenger DR, Gitchell RG: Severe infections following pudental block anesthesia: need for orthopedic awareness. *J Bone Joint Surg (Am)* 55A:202, 1973.

56. Brown TK, Munsick RA: Puerperal ovarian vein thrombophlebitis: a syndrome. *Am J Obstet Gynecol* 109:263, 1971.

57. Derrick FC, Turner WR, House EE, et al: Evidence of right ovarian vein syndrome in pregnant females. *Obstet Gynecol* 35:37, 1970.

58. Josey WE, Staggers SR: Heparin therapy in septic pelvic vein thrombophlebitis: a study of 46 cases. *Am J Obstet Gynecol* 120:228, 1974.

59. Allan TR, Miller GC, Wabrek AJ, et al: Postpartum and postabortal ovarian vein thrombophlebitis. *Obstet Gynecol* 47:525, 1976.

60. McElin TW, Lapata RE, Westenfelder GO, et al: Postpartum ovarian vein thrombophlebitis and microaerophilic streptococcal sepsis. *Obstet Gynecol* 35:632, 1970.

61. Pechet L, Alexander B: Increased clotting factors in pregnancy. *N Engl J Med* 265:1093, 1961.

62. Ratnoff OD, Holland TR: Coagulation components in normal and abnormal pregnancies. *New York Acad Sci* 75:626, 1959.

63. Hodgkinson CP: Physiology of the ovarian veins during pregnancy. *Obstet Gynecol* 1:26, 1953.

64. Dykhuizen RF, Roberts JA: The ovarian vein syndrome. *Surg Gynecol Obstet* 130:443, 1970.

65. Lotze EC, Kaufman RH, Kaplan AL: Postpartum ovarian vein thrombophlebitis. *Obstet Gynecol Surv* 21:853, 1966.

66. Maull KI, VanNagell JR, Greenfield LJ: Surgical implications of ovarian vein thrombosis. *Am Surg* 44;727, 1978.

67. Jacobs JB: Selective gonadal venography. *Radiology* 92:885, 1969.

68. Reynolds SRM: Right ovarian vein syndrome. *Obstet Gynecol* 37:308, 1971.

69. Montalto NJ, Bloch E, Malfetano JH, Janelli DE: Postpartum thrombophlebitis of the ovarian vein. *Obstet Gynecol* 34:867, 1969.

70. Munsick RA, Gillanders LA: A review of the syndrome of puerperal ovarian vein thrombophlebitis. *Obstet Gynecol Surv* 36:57, 1981.

71. Dunn LJ, VanVorrhis LW. Enigmatic fever and pelvic thrombophlebitis. *N Engl J Med* 276:265, 1969.

72. Schulman H: Use of anticoagulants in suspected pelvic infection. *Clin Obstet Gynecol* 12:240, 1969.

73. Darney PD, Wilson EA: Intravenous pyelography in the diagnosis and management of postpartum ovarian vein thrombophlebitis: a case report. *Am J Obstet Gynecol* 127:439, 1977.

74. Salzer RB, Abas S: Ovarian vein phlebography in postpartum patients. *Obstet Gynecol* 35:270, 1970.

75. Huntsinger LA, Good DC: "Atypical" puerperal ovarian vein thrombophlebitis. *Am J Obstet Gynecol* 106:309, 1970.

76. Ledger WJ, Peterson EP: The use of heparin in the management of pelvic thrombophlebitis. *Surg Gynecol Obstet* 131:1115, 1970.

77. O'Lane JM, Lebherz TB: Puerperal ovarian thrombophlebitis. *Obstet Gynecol* 26:676, 1965.

78. Collins CG: Suppurative pelvic thrombophlebitis. *Am J Obstet Gynecol* 108:681, 1970.

79. Robinson DW: Postpartum ovarian vein thrombophlebitis. *Am J Obstet Gynecol* 113:497, 1972.

80. Sanders JG, Malinak LR, Gready TG: Ovarian vein thrombosis: a postpartum surgical emergency. *Obstet Gynecol* 24:903, 1964.

81. Austin OG: Massive thrombophlebitis of the ovarian vein. *Am J Obstet Gynecol* 47:525, 1976.

82. Gardstein HF, Ferenczy A, Richart RM: Asymptomatic bilateral ovarian infarction and venas thrombosis. *Am J Obstet Gynecol* 116:1154, 1973.

83. Collins JH, Cohen CJ: Pregnancy subsequent to ligation of the inferior vena cava and ovarian vessels. *Am J Obstet Gynecol* 77:760, 1959.

84. Miller CF: Ligation or excision of the pelvic veins in the treatment of puerpheral pyemia. *Surg Gynecol Obstet* 25:431, 1917.

85. Duff P, Gibbs RS: Pelvic vein thrombophlebitis: diagnostic dilemma and therapeutic challenge. *Obstet Gynecol Surv* 38:365, 1983.

CHAPTER 18

Urinary Tract Infection

URINARY TRACT INFECTION

Urinary tract infections (UTI) are extremely frequent, exceeded only by infections of the respiratory tract (1). Kass has suggested that bacteriuria is the most common bacterial infection in Western industrialized nations (2). Urinary tract infections are 14 times more common in females than in males (3). Stamey has suggested that this observed sexual differential is due to: (a) a short urethra in women; (b) the external one-third of the urethra is continuously contaminated by pathogens from the vagina and rectum; (c) women do not empty their bladder as completely as men; and (d) massage of bacteria into the bladder with sexual intercourse (4, 5). Thus it is not surprising that clinicians providing health care for women are frequently called upon to diagnose and treat the major forms of UTI: (a) asymptomatic bacteriuria; (b) cystitis; (c) pyelonephritis; and (d) acute urethral syndrome. Not only do UTIs occur commonly in outpatients, they are also important causes of nosocomial infections. Charles estimated that 10–20% of women have at least one episode of infection (6).

Epidemiology

The introduction into clinical practice of quantitative urine culture by Kass has led to a total reevaluation of the concepts of etiology, pathogenesis, and treatment of UTIs (1). The investigative work of Kass showed that significant bacteriuria can occur in the absence of clinical symptoms or signs of urinary tract infection and established quantitative microbiology as the indispensable laboratory aid for the diagnosis, follow-up, and confirmation of cure for urinary tract infection (1, 7). These studies demonstrated that urinary bacterial counts on midstream voided urine specimens distinguished between contamination and infection with a high degree of accuracy. If two consecutive midstream specimens contain greater than 100,000 colonies/ml of a bacterial pathogen, there is greater than a 95% chance that a third specimen would also have more than 100,000 colonies/ml of the same organism. From this work evolved the accepted definition of asymptomatic bacteriuria, the presence of 100,000 or more colonies of a bacterial pathogen per milliliter of urine on two consecutive clean catch midstream voided specimens in the absence of signs or symptoms of urinary tract infection. A single catheterized specimen revealing greater than 100,000 colonies/ml of a pathogen is sufficient to make such a determination. Because of the difficulty in obtaining clean voided specimens, suprapubic bladder aspiration has been recommended by some investigators to confirm the presence of bacteriuria (4, 8).

There is a trend for an increasing prevalence of bacteriuria with increasing age (9, 10). Kunin and co-workers reported an incidence of bacteriuria of 1.2% in early schoolhood children (11). By the time of high school graduation at least 5% of young women have had bacteriuria (12). There is a significant increase in the rate of asymptomatic bacteriuria following the onset of sexual activity, and the prevalence of bacteriuria in females rises with age at a rate of approximately 1% for each decade of life (10). Nicolle and colleagues documented the importance of sexual intercourse as a precipitating factor for urinary tract infections in sexually active women (13). Fully 75% of UTI episodes in women with a history of recurrent urinary infections occurred within 24 hr of coitus. The incidence of asymptomatic bacteriuria is comparable for pregnant and nonpregnant women of the same socioeconomic group (3). Turck and co-workers noted that the socioeconomic status of patients influenced the prevalence of bacteriuria (14). While bacteriuria was present in only 2% of nonindigent patients, it was detected in 6.5% of indigent patients. Additional studies have confirmed this inverse relationship between socioeconomic status and prevalence of bacteriuria (15, 16).

Etiology

Most of the organisms responsible for urinary tract infections are considered part of the normal fecal flora. *Escherichia coli* is the etiologic agent in approximately 80–90% of acute infections (3, 5, 6). Other gram-negative facultative bacteria such as *Klebsiella*, *Proteus*, *Enterobacter*, and *Pseudomonas* and the enterococcus are responsible for the remainder. Recently, *Staphylococcus saprophyticus* has been demonstrated to be the second most common cause of UTI in young sexually active women (17, 18). In the study by Latham et al, this organism accounted for 11% of UTIs seen in college women (18).

In patients who have received antibiotics, undergone urologic instrumentation, or have chronic recurrent infections, the causative organism is more likely to be *Klebsiella*, *Enterobacter*, *Proteus*, *Pseudomonas*, *Serratia*, or the enterococcus. Surprisingly, despite their predominance in the fecal and probably vaginal flora, anaerobic bacteria are not common pathogens in UTI.

This association between the enteric flora and urinary pathogens has led to the hypothesis that the mechanism of acquiring UTIs is by an ascending route of infection from the bowel to the vaginal vestibule and then to the urethra and ultimately the bladder (5, 19, 20, 21). A number of factors predispose to development of UTIs. These include: (a) age-UTIs are more common in older patients; (b) sex-UTIs are more frequent in females; (c) obstruction; (d) instrumentation; (e) pregnancy; (f) vesicoureteral reflux; and (g) diabetes mellitus.

Stamey and Sexton noted that the vaginal vestibule of women with recurrent bacteriuria had a higher incidence of colonization by Enterobacteriaceae between episodes than the vestibule of women without recurrent urinary tract infection (22). Subsequently, Fowler and Stamey demonstrated that *E. coli* adheres more readily to introital epithelial cells in women with recurrent urinary tract infection (23). Lastly, Stamey and co-workers reported that colonization of the vaginal introitus with gram-negative enteric bacteria was associated with absence of antibody in the cervicovaginal secretions (24).

Diagnosis

The absolute criteria for the diagnosis of UTI is microbiologic confirmation of pathogenic bacteria in the urinary tract above the urethra. The presence of pyuria suggests infection but is not diagnostic of UTI.

As described above, asymptomatic bacteriuria is diagnosed on the basis of quantitative cultures with greater than 100,000 colonies of a pathogen/milliliter of clean voided urine specimens in asymptomatic patients. In women with lower urinary tract infection, urethral catheterization is associated with a 90% or greater accuracy. However, the procedure has the risk of introducing infection and should not be indiscriminately utilized. Direct suprapubic bladder aspiration is an excellent technique for obtaining meaningful urine cultures. The presence of any bacterial pathogen in a suprapubic aspirate is indicative of a UTI. Stamey and colleagues claim to have had no complications occur in over 2500 bladder aspirations (4). These authors noted with suprapubic bladder aspiration that one-third of urinary infections were associated with bacterial counts of less than 10^5 bacteria/ml. Recently Stamm and co-workers proposed new diagnostic criterion for UTI in acutely dysuric females (25). While the classic studies by Kass (1) demonstrated the appropriateness of using the criterion of $\geq 10^5$ bacteria/ml in women with acute pyelonephritis and for asymptomatic bacteriuria, 30–50% of patients with acute lower tract infection characterized by dysuria, urgency, and frequency do not meet the $\geq 10^5$ bacteria/ml criterion for infection. These investigators noted that the traditional diagnostic criterion of $\geq 10^5$ bacteria/ml of midstream urine identified only 51% of women whose bladder urine (obtained by catheterization or suprapubic aspirate) contained coliforms. They found the best diagnostic criterion to be $\geq 10^2$ bacteria per ml with a sensitivity of 0.95, specificity of 0.85, and a high predictive value (0.88) among symptomatic women.

Once a sample of urine is obtained to confirm a diagnosis of UTI, the specimen must be rapidly brought to the microbiology laboratory or refrigerated. A delay of greater than 2 hr will result in an erroneous high bacterial count (26). The urine should be cultured on blood agar as well as desoxycholate, eosin-methylene, or MacConkey agar for gram-negative rods. Quantitation of bacteria can be accomplished by means of standard dilutions, using either the pour plate or the streak spread plate technique. There are available for office use commercially prepared diagnostic aids for the detection of urinary tract infections. An example is the dip slide technique which has overcome the problem of transport of the urine sample and keeps costs down (27). One surface of the slide is plain soy agar which will grow gram-negative as well as gram-positive organisms. The other side contains an agar only capable of growing gram-negative bacteria (i.e., MacConkey agar or eosin-methylene blue). Other available office diagnostic aids include Microstix or Uricult (28).

Frequency, urgency, and dysuria are usually associated with cystitis, whereas fever, chills, and flank pain are associated with pyelonephritis. However, these signs and symptoms are not specific for the localizing site of infection (i.e., bladder or kidney). This has led to attempts at localizing the site to the bladder or kidney.

Various methodologies have been employed in the localization of urinary tract infection(s) (3, 29). Direct methods include ureteric catheterization for culture. However, most investigators have relied on indirect methods such as measurement of maximum urinary concentrating ability (30, 31), serum antibody titers against infecting organisms (32–34), pattern of response to therapy (3, 33) β-glucoronidase excretion in urine (31), bladder washout techniques (35), and antibody-coated bacteria in the urinary sediment (36, 37).

Recently, the role of antibody-coated bacteria in localization of urinary tract infection site has received the most attention. Thomas and co-workers demonstrated that bacteria from the kidney are coated with antibody, while organisms limited to the bladder or urethra are not (36). Jones et al have documented the clinical value of this test (37). In general, 40–50% of bacteriuria is believed to be of renal origin.

URINARY TRACT INFECTION IN PREGNANCY

Urinary tract infections are the most common medical complications of pregnancy. These may be either asymptomatic (asymptomatic bacteriuria of pregnancy) or they may be symptomatic (cystitis or acute pyelonephritis).

Epidemiology

Obstetricians have recognized the frequency and the seriousness of symptomatic urinary tract infections in pregnancy for a long time. In the mid-1950s the investigative work of Kass documented that significant bacteriuria can occur in the absence of symptoms or signs of urinary tract infections (1). Kass identified persistent asymptomatic bacteriuria in 6% of prenatal patients (7, 38). Acute pyelonephritis developed in 40% of these patients receiving a placebo; when bacteriuria was eliminated, pyelonephritis did not occur. He noted that neonatal death rates and prematurity rates were 2 to 3 times greater in bacteriuric women receiving placebo than in nonbacteriuric women or bacteriuric patients in whom bacteriuria was eliminated (39, 40). He concluded that detection of maternal bacteriuria would identify a group of patients at risk for pyelonephritis and premature delivery. He maintained that pyelonephritis in pregnancy could be prevented by detection and treatment of bacteriuria in early pregnancy and with treatment of bacteriuria 5–10% of premature deliveries could be prevented.

It has long been recognized that symptomatic urinary tract infection is more frequently encountered in pregnant women. This suggests that factors are present during gestation that allow bacteria to replicate in the urine and ascend to the upper urinary tract. Several findings support this view. The normal female urinary tract undergoes dramatic physiologic changes during pregnancy (3). There is decreased ureteric muscle tone and activity that results in a reduced rate of passage of urine throughout the urinary collecting system. The upper ureter and renal pelvices become dilated, resulting in a physiologic hydronephrosis of pregnancy. This hydronephrosis is a result of the effects of progesterone on muscle tone and peristalsis, and most importantly, mechanical obstruction by the enlarging uterus. Vesicle changes also occur in pregnancy. These include decreased tone, increased capacity, and incomplete emptying. These findings predispose to vesicoureteric reflux. Hypotonia of the vesicle musculature, vesicle ureteral reflux, and dilatation of the ureter and renal pelvis result in a static column of urine in the ureter which facilitates the ascending migration of bacteria to the upper urinary tract after bladder infection is established. The hypokinetic collecting system reduces urine flow. And as a result, the ability of the kidney to clear itself of infection is diminished.

It is also possible that alterations in the physical/chemical properties of urine during pregnancy can result in exacerbations of bacteriuria, thus predisposing the ascending infection. Urinary pH is elevated during pregnancy, partly because of the increased excretion of bicarbonate, and a high urine pH encourages bacterial growth. Glycosuria, which is common in pregnancy, may favor an increase in the rate of bacterial multiplication. The increased urinary excretion of estrogens may be a factor in the pathogenesis of symptomatic urinary tract infection during pregnancy. It has been demonstrated by means of animal experiments that estrogen can enhance the growth of strains of *Escherichia coli* that cause pyelonephritis and also predispose the animal to the development of renal infection (41, 42). In addition, the renal medulla is particularly susceptible to infection because its hypertonic environment inhibits leukocyte migration, phagocytosis, and complement activity (41, 43, 44).

The cumulative effect of these physiologic factors is an increased risk for ascending infection from the bladder, colonized with bacteria, to the kidneys. What role, if any, pregnancy itself plays in the acquisition of asymptomatic bacteriuria must be evaluated. The bulk of investigations have shown that the vast majority of patients with asymptomatic bacteriuria of pregnancy will be detected at the initial prenatal visit and that relatively few pregnant women acquire bacteriuria after the initial visit (1, 7, 45). There is no evidence that bacteriuria is acquired between the time of conception and the first antenatal visit. In fact, there is good evidence that in many instances the bacteriuria antedates the pregnancy. The prevalence of asymptomatic bacteriuria in school girls is approximately 1%. There is a considerable increase in the rate of asymptomatic bacteriuria following the onset of sexual intercourse, and the prevalence of bacteriuria in females increases with age at a rate of about 1% for each decade of life. Several investigations have shown that nonpregnant populations had an incidence of asymptomatic bacteriuria comparable to that found in pregnant women in the same locale. It appears that the major source of patients with bacteriuria first discovered during pregnancy are those women who acquired asymptomatic bacteriuria early in life and in whom the incidence of bacteriuria increased as a result of sexual activity. Although pregnancy per se does not cause any major increase in bacteriuria, it does predispose to the development of acute pyelonephritis in these patients. The physiologic changes which occur with pregnancy permit bacterial colonization of the bladder to ascend and invade the kidney (32, 46).

Asymptomatic Bacteriuria

As a result of Kass' initial observations, considerable interest has focused on asymptomatic bacteriuria in pregnant women (7). It is generally accepted that untreated asymptomatic bacteriuria during pregnancy often leads to acute pyelonephritis. For this reason, it is clear that bacteriuria must be viewed with concern. How-

ever, other claims, such as those that asymptomatic bacteriuria predisposes the patient to anemia, preeclampsia, and chronic renal disease are controversial and unproved. Even more controversial is the association between bacteriuria and prematurity and low birth weight infants.

The prevalence of asymptomatic bacteriuria in pregnant women ranges from 2 to 11% (Table 18.1); a majority of investigations report an incidence between 4 and 7% (7, 46–68). An increased prevalence of bacteriuria in pregnant females has been associated with the presence of sickle cell trait, lower socioeconomic status, reduced availability of medical care, and increased parity.

As in nonpregnant women, *E. coli* has been the predominant pathogen isolated in each study of asymptomatic bacteriuria and was present in 60–90% of the cases. The next most common are *Proteus mirabilis*, *Klebsiella pneumoniae*, and the enterococcus. Group B β-hemolytic streptococci are also recognized as potential pathogens in the urinary tract during pregnancy (69).

Bacteriuria and Pyelonephritis

Acute pyelonephritis, one of the most frequent medical complications of pregnancy, is a serious threat to maternal and fetal well-being (70, 71). The association between acute pyelonephritis of pregnancy and preterm delivery was appreciated in the preantibiotic era with prematurity rates of 20–50% being reported (72–75). Subsequent studies in the postantibiotic era have confirmed this association between acute pyelonephritis and an increased risk of premature delivery (2, 7, 10, 14, 15, 55, 57, 76–78). Several mechanisms have been proposed to explain this association: pyrogens given pregnant women cause increased myometrial activity (79); ureteric contractions result in reflex myometrial contractions (72); the endotoxin of gram-negative organisms, often associated with pyelonephritis, may have an oxytocic-like effect on the myometrium (78, 80); and the endotoxin of gram-negative organisms may in fact cross the placenta and produce fetal effects resulting in premature labor.

The concept of quantitative urine cultures which made it possible to determine when infection of the urinary tract was present in individuals without symptoms or signs of urinary tract infection was a major contribution to the understanding of the pathogenesis of pyelonephritis. Even though the physiologic changes in the urinary tract during pregnancy predispose to stasis

Table 18.1
Prevalence of Bacteriuria in Pregnancy

Study	Total no. of patients	No. of patients with bacteriuria	% Bacteriuria
Blunt and Williams (60)	1,055	27	2.5
Gruneberg et al (49)	8,907	392	3.5
Stuart et al (57)	2,713	95	3.5
Pathak et al (64)	7,602	288	3.8
Williams et al (59)	5.542	211	3.8
Gower et al (62)	5,000	265	4.4
Kaitz and Holder (83)	616	27	4.4
Condie et al (48)	4,590	210	4.6
Little (53)	5,000	265	5.3
Eykin and McFadyen (68)	1,000	59	5.9
Kincaid-Smith (93)	4,000	240	6.0
Robertson et al (65)	8.275	511	6.2
Carrol et al (61)	5,200	331	6.4
Sleigh et al (86)	1,684	111	6.4
LeBlanc and McGanity (63)	1,325	87	6.5
Norden and Kilpatrick (55)	1,703	111	6.5
McFadyen et al (54)	2,000	132	6.6
Layton (84)	1,000	67	6.7
Savage et al (66)	6.202	431	6.9
Turner (67)	1,500	108	7.0
Bryant et al (47)	448	32	7.1
Monson et al (85)	1,400	102	7.3
Patrick (102)	2,521	219	8.7

and set the stage for ascending infection to the kidneys, Kass' initial studies identified that it was the presence of asymptomatic bacteriuria that was the significant factor associated with the development of acute pyelonephritis of pregnancy (1, 7). Kass noted that 20–40% of pregnant women with asymptomatic bacteriuria receiving a placebo developed pyelonephritis subsequently during the pregnancy. However, when the bacteriuria was treated and eliminated with antimicrobials, pyelonephritis did not occur. Subsequent studies have confirmed that detection of asymptomatic bacteriuria in pregnant women does identify a group of patients at high risk to develop acute pyelonephritis during pregnancy (Table 18.2). In these studies, 13.5–65% of pregnant women with asymptomatic bacteriuria not treated went on to develop acute pyelonephritis during pregnancy (10, 40, 47, 51, 53, 55, 63, 64, 67, 81–87). Detection and treatment of pregnant women with asymptomatic bacteriuria significantly reduce the risk of developing pyelonephritis. Initially Kass maintained that pyelonephritis, with its attendant maternal and fetal morbidity and/or mortality, could be completely prevented by detecting and treating bacteriuria early in pregnancy. In contrast, most investigators have found that a small proportion

of women without bacteriuria at the first antenatal visit will develop pyelonephritis. The explanation for this phenomenon is that approximately 1% of pregnant women who do not have bacteriuria at the first antenatal visit acquire asymptomatic bacteriuria later in pregnancy (2). These women are then at risk for developing pyelonephritis. In pregnant women whose bacteriuria was treated, the reported incidence of pyelonephritis ranged from 0 to 5.3%, with an average of 2.9%. Although detection and eradication by treatment of bacteriuria early in pregnancy will not completely eliminate pyelonephritis, it should prevent at least 70 to 80% of the cases of pyelonephritis in pregnancy (2, 30, 46, 88). The prevention rate could be raised still higher if screening for bacteriuria was performed at several intervals throughout the duration of pregnancy rather than only at the initial prenatal visit. However, it should be recognized that there will always be a small group of women who develop their pyelonephritis prior to their initial prenatal visit.

Multiple studies have attempted to identify those pregnant patients with bacteriuria who are at the greatest risk for developing acute pyelonephritis. It has been recognized that asymptomatic renal infection may occur in pa-

Table 18.2
Relationship between Asymptomatic Bacteriuria and Pyelonephritis in Pregnancy

Study		Patients with bacteriuria		Patients without bacteriuria	
		Total	Pyelonephritis	Total	Pyelonephritis
Kass and Zinner (10)	Placebo-	95	18 (19.0%)		
	treated	84	0		
Kincaid-Smith and Bullen (51)	Placebo-	60	19 (31.0%)	4000	48 (1.2%)
	treated	64	1 (1.5%)		
LeBlanc and McGanity (63)	Placebo-	41	8 (19.5%)	1028	21 (2.0%)
	treated	69	3 (4.3%)		
Little (53)	Placebo-	52	19 (36.5%)	1916	9 (0.5%)
	treated	57	3 (5.3%)		
Pathak et al (64)	Placebo-	49	17 (22.0%)	729	8 (1.0%)
	treated	75	3 (4.0%)		
Brumfitt (81)		179	55 (31.0%)		
Bryant et al (47)		32	8 (25.0%)	44	6 (13.6%)
Dixon and Brandt (82)		71	14 (19.7%)	1238	28 (2.3%)
Elder et al (40)			57 (16.0%)		
Kaitz and Holder (83)		17	3 (18.0%)	573	9 (1.6%)
Layton (84)		67	42 (65.0%)	118	2 (1.7%)
Monson et al (85)		115	35 (30.0%)		
Norden and Kilpatrick (55)		111	25 (23.0%)	1592	16 (1.0%)
Sleigh et al (86)		100	43 (43.0%)	100	14 (14.0%)
Turner (67)		79	49 (62.0%)	64	1 (1.6%)
Whalley (87)		179	46 (26.0%)	179	0

tients with bacteriuria and that the classical distinctions between infection limited to the bladder and pyelonephritis based on localization of symptoms are of limited value (27, 89). Possibly the group of bacteriurics with renal involvement may be at high risk for acute pyelonephritis and other associated complications of bacteriuria (58, 77).

Localization of urinary infection has been attempted using various methodologies (26). Direct methods include ureteric catheterization for culture and renal biopsy. Indirect measures include ureteric catheterization for culture and renal biopsy. Indirect measures include maximum urinary concentrating ability, serum antibodies against infecting organisms, antibody-coated bacteria in urinary sediment, pattern of response to therapy, β-glucoronidase excretion in urine, and bladder washout techniques. The results of these investigations suggest that renal involvement already exists in many pregnant women with bacteriuria, despite lack of clinical evidence for upper urinary tract and/or kidney infections. Based on these attempts to localize the site of asymptomatic urinary tract infection, it has been suggested that 25–50% of pregnant women with asymptomatic bacteriuria have renal tissue involvement and silent pyelo-

nephritis (50, 80, 89). It is this group of bacteriuric women with subclinical renal involvement who are at high risk to develop symptomatic pyelonephritis during pregnancy. Stamey and co-workers, in nonpregnant women with bacteriuria, using ureteral catheters noted that 60% of patients had infection involving the upper urinary tract (4). Similarly, in nonpregnant infections, studies with antibody-coated bacteria have confirmed a high rate of renal involvement (33, 34).

BACTERIURIA AND ANEMIA

Several studies have noted an association between bacteriuria in pregnant women and the presence of anemia (56, 65, 81, 84, 91). However, other studies have failed to document such an association (46, 48, 53, 66, 83). Little, in a study of 5,000 pregnant women of whom 265 had bacteriuria, found no significant difference in hemoglobin concentration in the women with renal and urinary tract infection and the other prenatal patients (53). The experience of Whalley and co-workers at Parkland Hospital with asymptomatic bacteriuria in pregnant women indicates that there is no cause and effect between this condition and anemia (92). Moreover, in 553 women with acute pyelonephritis, they found there is no difference in the incidence of anemia in these women when compared to controls with no urinary tract infection.

It is difficult to reconcile these opposing views and results. It seems reasonable that those bacteriuric women with subclinical renal disease would have a greater risk of developing anemia. However, with the use of antibody-coated bacteria the Parkland group has failed to demonstrate this association (92). The relation between bacteriuria and low socioeconomic status might explain the propensity for anemia to be more prevalent in pregnant women with bacteriuria. Socioeconomic deprivation, bacteriuria, and anemia are features common to prenatal clinic patients. However, before any relationship between bacteriuria and anemia can be substantiated, large prospective longitudinal, epidemiologic surveys are required.

BACTERIURIA AND HYPERTENSION

An increased incidence of hypertensive disease of pregnancy has been alleged to exist in pregnant women with asymptomatic bacteriuria; such a relationship has been the subject of much controversy. Although some investigations have confirmed this postulate (51, 54, 55, 64, 93), in general, most workers have failed to document any association between bacteriuria and hypertension (47, 48, 53, 63, 65, 81). Moreover, the studies supporting an association between bacteriuria and gestational hypertension have reported conflicting results as to whether or not eradication of bacteriuria by antimicrobial treatment reduces the incidence of hypertensive disease of pregnancy among bacteriuric women (40, 51, 53, 63, 64, 65). The Parkland Group has noted that there was no relationship between asymptomatic bacteriuria in pregnant women and pregnancy-induced hypertension (92). Moreover, when they looked at the pregnancy outcomes of 553 women with acute pyelonephritis, they found there was no difference in the presence of pregnancy-induced hypertension in this group versus their controls with no urinary tract infection. The presence of antibody-coated bacteria identifying the asymptomatic bacteriuric patients with renal infection did not show an association with hypertensive disease of pregnancy as compared to just those with bladder infection or to the control population.

At the present time the presence of an asso-

ciation between bacteriuria and hypertensive disease of pregnancy is questionable. No standardization was present for the diagnosis of hypertensive disease of pregnancy among the multitude of studies. Thus it is difficult to interpret these conflicting views. In addition, hypertensive disease may be a reflection of the socioeconomic status of the patients studied. Any definite conclusion as to the role of bacteriuria in the development of hypertensive disease of pregnancy must await future well controlled prospective studies. At present such a relationship seems unlikely.

BACTERIURIA AND CHRONIC RENAL DISEASE

Although urinary tract infections are interrelated, the factors that determine their frequency in the etiology of chronic renal disease have not been defined. Zinner and Kass estimated that 10–15% of bacteriuric pregnant women are destined to have evidence of chronic pyelonephritis 10–12 yr following delivery (94). Kass and Zinner estimate that renal failure will ultimately develop in 1 of 3000 pregnant women with bacteriuria (10). Several groups of investigators have reported that women with bacteriuria who were not treated during pregnancy continue to have persistent bacteriuria over the year postdelivery in 35 to 80% of cases (58, 85, 94–96). Other groups have noted that bacteriuria still persisted in 20–30% of patients, even when the bacteriuria had been treated in pregnancy (10, 62, 93, 94). Zinner and Kass reported that 20% of women with bacteriuria during pregnancy had persistent bacteriuria at follow-up examination 10–12 yr postdelivery (94). In contrast, only 5% of women who were not bacteriuric during pregnancy had significant bacteriuria at the follow-up exam. Interestingly, the rate of bacteriuria was similar whether the patient had been treated or received a placebo. It has been suggested that the patients with evidence of underlying renal involvement are the group at high risk to have persistent bacteriuria following delivery.

The evaluation of renal function in follow-up studies of bacteriuric patients confirms this suggestion; patients with bacteriuria at follow-up have lower maximal urine osmolality and decreased creatinine clearance of less than 80 ml/min over the 1st year after delivery. Cobbs et al noted that one-third of pregnant women with untreated bacteriuria had a creatinine clearance of less than 80 ml/min at 3 months to 1 yr postpartum (96). Both Monson and colleagues (85) and Zinner and Kass (94) reported that bacteriuric women were more likely to have impaired urinary concentrating ability.

Follow-up investigations with intravenous pyelography have disclosed that women with pregnancy bacteriuria have an 8–33% incidence of radiologic changes consistent with pyelonephritis (48, 51, 54, 58, 62, 64, 85, 94–96). In addition, these authors have found a high incidence of other abnormalities, such as congenital anomalies of the urinary tract, renal calculi, and ureteric dilatation. The highest incidence of radiologic evidence of chronic pyelonephritis was noted in those patients who had infection localized in the upper urinary tract or in whom bacteriuria during pregnancy was difficult to eradicate.

It is clear from these follow-up studies of bacteriuria in pregnancy that a significant number of women have abnormal renal function and radiological evidence of pyelonephritis. However, the relationship between bacteriuria during pregnancy and the renal lesions or decreased renal function detected subsequently is not clear. Perhaps pregnancy is only an opportunity for detecting a chronic renal condition that was present long before the pregnancy started. Bacteriuria in pregnancy may be part of a continuous infection of the renal tract starting in childhood and not infrequently associated with renal abnormalities. Perhaps serious renal compromise results from recurrent infections from childhood through later life.

Because of the incidence of persistent bacteriuria, abnormal renal function, and radiologic evidence of chronic pyelonephritis which has been documented in follow-up studies of patients with asymptomatic bacteriuria of pregnancy, long-term follow-up of mothers with bacteriuria is essential. They should be closely followed with periodic urine cultures, treatment if bacteriuria persists or recurs, and intravenous pyelograms to detect urinary tract abnormalities that may be correctable or chronic pyelonephritis. With such close surveillance and management the progression to end stage renal disease may hopefully be delayed or prevented.

BACTERIURIA AND PREMATURITY AND LOW BIRTH WEIGHT INFANTS

It is well documented that pregnant women who develop acute pyelonephritis are at a significantly increased risk for preterm labor and delivery. In contrast, the relationship of asymptomatic bacteriuria to preterm delivery, low birth weight, small for gestational age babies, and fetal mortality remains a controversial subject. Kass initially reported that there was an association between asymptomatic bacteriuria and prematurity and that eradication of bacteriuria with antimicrobial therapy significantly reduced the rate of premature delivery (7, 38). He noted that the prematurity rate was two to three times greater in bacteriuric women receiving a placebo than in nonbacteriuric women or patients whose bacteriuria had been eliminated. Kass initially suggested that early detection and treatment of bacteriuria would prevent 10–20% of prematurity. It should be pointed out that the term "prematurity" in the initial study was based entirely on a birth weight of 2500 g or less. Kass noted that more than one-fifth of women with bacteriuria at Boston City Hospital gave birth to infants weighing less than 2500 g and that adequate therapy for bacteriuria reduced the incidence of low birth weight to 10%, a figure comparable to that for their nonbacteriuric pregnant women. Over the past 2 decades numerous studies have concerned themselves with the role asymptomatic bacteriuria plays in the develoment of preterm labor and delivery or low birth weight infants (Table 18.3). Many workers have confirmed the original finding by Kass of an increased risk for preterm delivery or low birth weight infants in women with bacteriuria (48, 51, 56, 57, 63–66, 78, 81, 84). Conversely, many investigators have failed to confirm a relationship between asymptomatic bacteriuria and preterm delivery or low birth weight infants (15, 46, 47, 53, 55, 62, 83, 85, 87, 97). The Parkland Group has reported that their experience with asymptomatic bacteriuria in pregnant women indicates there is no cause and effect between this condition and the incidence of prematurity and/or low birth weight infants. Moreover, they have been unable to document an influence on the incidence of preterm delivery or low birth weight infants in the subgroup of asymptomatic bacteriuric women with evidence of renal infection based on antibody-coated bacteria (98). Among women with bacteriuria the mean gestational age of 39.9 weeks, incidence of preterm delivery of 8%, and incidence of low birth weight of 13% were not significantly different from the rate among controls—38.5 weeks, 4% and 12%, respectively (98). In women with pyelonephritis, although the <2500 g weight rate of 15% was significantly ($p < 0.05$)

Table 18.3
Bacteriuria and Prematurity

Study	Patients with bacteriuria		Nonbacteriuric patients	
	Total	Premature	Total	Premature
Brumfit (81)	413	39 (9.4%)	477	32 (6.7%)
Gower et al (62)	265	23 (8.7%)	4735	360 (7.6%)
Gruneberg et al (49)	266	19 (7.2%)	507	28 (5.5%)
Kass (38)	179	32 (17.8%)	1000	88 (9.0%)
Kincaid-Smith and Bullen (51)	240	32 (13.3%)	500	25 (5.0%)
Layton (84)	63	10 (17.0%)	114	10 (9.0%)
Little (53)	265	23 (8.7%)	4735	360 (7.6%)
Pathak (64)	129	20 (15.5%)	729	83 (11.4%)
Robertson et al (65)	365	16 (4.4%)	1980	62 (3.0%)
Savage et al (66)	203	32 (15.7%)	5771	779 (13.5%)
Stuart et al (57)	88	20 (23.0%)	729	83 (11.0%)
Wilson et al (97)	230	26 (11.0%)	6216	606 (10.0%)
Wren (78)	173	18 (10.4%)	3000	140 (4.6%)
Bryant et al (47)[a]	32	2 (6.0%)	44	2 (10.0%)
Norden and Kilpatrick (55)[a]	114	17 (15.0%)	109	14 (13.0%)
Sleigh et al (86)[a]	100	7 (7.0%)	100	7 (7.0%)
Whalley (87)[a]	176	24 (14.8%)	176	21 (11.9%)
Condie et al (48)[a]	180	23 (12.8%)	180	9 (5.0%)
Leveno et al (98)[a]	138	11 (9.0%) (preterm)	125	5 (4.0%)
		18 (13.0%) (2500 g)		16 (12.0%)

[a] Studies with matched controls.

greater than the 10% incidence in the uninfected controls, there were no significant differences in mean birth weight (3,044 ± 210) or the incidence of perinatal mortality of 2.7 versus 2.5%. When bacteriuric patients were compared to matched nonbacteriuric women in control studies (Table 18.3), the majority of investigators have not found a significant association between bacteriuria and prematurity (45, 47, 55, 86, 99). The exception was Condie and associates who noted a two-fold increase in the premature delivery rate of the bacteriuric infections (48).

In controlled trials in which treatment of bacteriuria was compared with treatment with placebo, the results are also conflicting (Table 18.4). While some workers noted that antibiotic treatment of bacteriuria did not significantly reduce the rate of occurrence of low birth weight infants (51, 53), others have reported a significant reduction in the incidence of premature births when bacteriuria was eradicated with antimicrobial therapy (38, 63, 64, 66, 68, 78, 81). These conflicting studies on the efficacy of treatment have further confused the issue on the role of bacteriuria in preterm labor.

Kincaid-Smith and Bullen first suggested that underlying renal disease was the major cause for the excess risk of prematurity or low birth weight among the infants of the bacteriuric women (51). The hypothesis has evolved that those bacteriuric women with subclinical renal involvement are the population at risk to deliver premature or low birth weight infants. Gruneberg and co-workers noted that an increased rate of prematurity and a decrease in their infants' birth weight occurred in those bacteriuric women who were either refractory to treatment or in whom bacteriuria had recurred (49). Previous investigations had reported that bacteriuric patients who do not respond to treatment are likely to have subclinical renal involvement (28, 30, 100). These data have been used to support the hypothesis that those women with subclinical renal involvement are the population at risk to deliver premature or low birth weight infants. The varying definitions for prematurity used in the literature have contributed to the confusion that exists. Unfortunately, the majority of the studies have used a definition of prematurity based on a weight of less than 2500 g. Prematurity is a reflection of gestational age and should be applied to those infants delivered at less than 37 weeks of gestation. Kass suggested that the increased incidence of prematur-

Table 18.4
Effect of treatment for Bacteriuria on Preterm Delivery

Study	Bacteriuric patients treated		Bacteriuric patients placebo		Nonbacteriurics	
	Total	Preterm	Total	Preterm	Total	Preterm
Kincaid-Smith and Bullen (51)	52	9 (17.3%)	56	12 (21.5%)		
Little (53)	57	7 lb. 6 oz.	52	7 lb. 4 oz		
Kass (38)	84	6 (7.0%)	95	26 (27.0%)	1000	188 (9.0%)
Brumfitt (81)	235	18 (7.6%)	78	21 (11.8%)	477	32 (6.7%)
LeBlanc and McGanity (63)	101	7 (6.9%)	27	6 (22.1%)	1141	133 (11.6%)
Pathak et al (64)	80	10 (12.5%)	49	10 (20.4%)	729	83 (11.4%)
Robertson et al (65)	160	3 (2.0%)	204	13 (6.0%)	1980	62 (3.0%)
Savage et al (66)	103	8 (7.5%)	100	24 (24.0%)	5771	779 (13.5%)
Wren (78)	83	4 (5.0%)	90	14 (15.5%)	3000	140 (4.6%)

ity may be due to a bacterial endotoxin that either stimulates uterine contractions or causes decidual placental hemorrhage, thrombosis, and necrosis. Another possible mechanism for initiating premature labor could be the release of prostaglandins as a result of decidual necrosis. Recent work by Gluck and his co-workers has noted that certain bacteria, including the gram-negative facultatives, such as *E. coli*, commonly found in urinary tract infections, can produce an enzyme, phospholipase α-2, which can initiate the prostaglandin cascade.

The relationship between bacteriuria and preterm and small for gestational age infants remains controversial. Many variables comprise the etiology of prematurity, and bacteriuria is only one of the many factors which may influence the onset of premature labor. As the incidence of both pregnancy bacteriuria and prematurity increases with decreasing socioeconomic status, any relationship between bacteriuria and gestational length and birth weight may be complex and difficult to establish. The design of the majority of studies can be justly criticized on account of the paucity of bacteriuric and nonbacteriuric patients studied. No study has yet been able to furnish statistically significant data. Beard and Roberts reviewed the data from the major studies and demonstrated that the mean incidence of low birth weight infants among women without bacteriuria was 9.5% and among bacteriuric women was 13.5% (101). These authors considered that with such an incidence of bacteriuria in pregnancy 6000 patients would have to be screened to demonstrate a 95% probability that bacteriuria was a significant factor in the etiology of low birth weight infants. To attain a 99% probability 13,000 prenatal patients would have to be screened. It seems obvious that the question will not be

settled until a large scale, collaborative study with a well designed protocol is accomplished. If asymptomatic bacteriuria during pregnancy is related to prematurity, it accounts for only 5–10% of preterm births, and eradication of bacteriuria would only minimally reduce the overall rate of prematurity.

BACTERIURIA AND FETAL LOSS, FETAL INFECTION, AND CONGENITAL ANOMALIES

An increased frequency of abortions and/or stillbirths in pregnant women with bacteriuria has been reported by several investigators (48, 51, 78, 81, 84). In addition, Wren (78) and Gruneberg et al (49) reported a significant decrease in the incidence of spontaneous abortions and stillbirths when bacteriuria was successfully eradicated with antimicrobial therapy. However, although Kincaid-Smith and Bullen noted that bacteriurics had an increased frequency of abortions, they could show no significant difference in the abortion and stillbirth rates between treated and untreated women with bacteriuria (51). Moreover, no increase in the frequency of abortions or stillbirths has been noted in other studies (68, 102).

An association between maternal bacteriuria and congenital abnormalities has also been proposed. Patrick noted an increased incidence of dorsal midline fusion defects in the offspring of women with asymptomatic bacteriuria (102). Savage et al (66) and Kincaid-Smith and Bullen (51) also noted an increase in congenital abnormalities in the newborns of bacteriuric women. Evidence has been put forth by Patrick suggesting that UTI pathogens (i.e., *E. coli*) are present in neonates of bacteriuria pregnant women (102). He noted that 22% of the neonates of bacteriurics had neonatal bacteriuria, as compared to no cases among newborns of nonbacteriuric women (102). However, the failure to use suprapubic taps rather than bag collection techniques leaves this study open to criticism. In addition, Gower et al were unable to confirm the presence of neonatal bacteriuria in the offspring of bacteriuric women (62). Establishment of a causal relationship between pregnancy bacteriuria and congenital anomalies must await further investigations.

TREATMENT OF ASYMPTOMATIC BACTERIURIA IN PREGNANCY

Since at a minimum bacteriuria predisposes the pregnant woman to acute pyelonephritis, it is a potential hazard to the fetus. Thus, detection and treatment of asymptomatic bacteriuria provides the obstetrician an ideal opportunity to prevent a significant medical complication of pregnancy. Screening at the original antenatal visit in combination with appropriate treatment and eradication of bacteriuria will result in prevention of 70–80% of all antenatal acute pyelonephritis (3). Such a reduction, with its attendant decline in risk to mother and fetus is, by itself, sufficient justification for such a screening program.

Treatment should be designed to maintain a sterile urine throughout pregnancy, with the shortest possible course of antimicrobial agent(s) in order to minimize the toxicity of these drugs on mother and fetus. The majority of antibacterial agents are excreted by glomerular filtration, and, as a result, therapeutic concentrations are readily achieved in the urine. In fact, the concentrations of these drugs in the urine greatly exceeds that required for the treatment of most urinary tract infections. Even those drugs that do not have a therapeutic concentration in the serum, such as nitrofurantoin, are present in significant concentrations in urine. Ideally, treatment should be confined to those women with bacteriuria who are high risk for developing acute pyelonephritis, or the other complications reported to exist in bacteriuric patients. However, until convenient and reliable techniques for identifying this high risk group are available, it will remain necessary to treat all pregnant patients with asymptomatic bacteriuria.

Early studies advised continuous therapy until delivery because of the high rate of recurrence with short courses of treatment and with such an approach documented eradication of bacteriuria in 60–82% of pregnant women (38, 48, 53,

65). More recent investigations have indicated that short courses of treatment (1–3 weeks) with sulfonamides, ampicillin, or nitrofurantoin are as effective as continuous therapy in eradicating bacteriuria and eliminate the bacteriuria in 79–90% of patients (48, 49, 59, 61, 64, 68, 88). No single agent seems uniquely better than any other.

In a recent collaborative study at Parkland Memorial Hospital and Wilford Hall Air Force Base, the investigators reported that both renal bacteriuria (positive fluorescent antibody test) and those with bladder bacteriuria (negative fluorescent antibody test) responded to a single course of therapy with eradication of bacteriuria despite the regimen employed (98). At Parkland Memorial Hospital women were given Macrodantin, 100 mg at bedtime for 10 days; while patients at Wilford Hall Hospital either received Macrodantin, ampicillin, Keflex, or Gantrisin four times a day for 21 days. Despite initial success with either a 10-day course of an antimicrobial given at bedtime or a 21-day course of antimicrobials given four times a day, an interesting pattern of recurrence was noted. With either treatment, approximately one-third of the women had recurrent bacteriuria during the index pregnancy. At Parkland Memorial nearly 70% of the women with recurrences had a relapse (i.e., due to same organism which possibly was not eradicated from upper tract sites). Moreover, those women with renal asymptomatic bacteriuria tested with the 10-day single dose approach were three times more likely to have a relapse than the group with bladder bacteriuria. On the other hand, while the recurrence rate at Wilford Hall was identical to that at Parkland Memorial, these recurrences were due to reinfection. There was no difference for the reinfection rate noted for the renal bacteriurics as compared to bladder bacteriurics. Because of the high rate of recurrence among women with treated asymptomatic bacteriuria, some form of surveillance for recurrent urinary infection must be employed in order to detect and eradicate recurrent UTI. At present, it is generally accepted that short courses of treatment are preferable, because the duration of initial therapy does not effect the recurrence rate, a short course minimizes the adverse drug effects on mother and fetus, emergence of resistant bacteria is discouraged and costs kept to a minimum.

When the presence of asymptomatic bacteriuria is detected, treatment should be instituted with a 10- to 14-day course of a short acting sulfonamide, nitrofurantoin, or ampicillin (Fig.

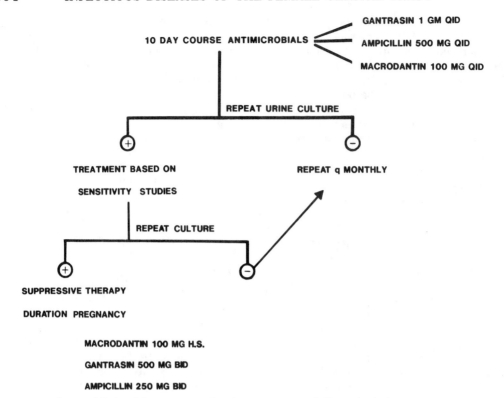

Figure 18.1.   Management plan for asymptomatic bacteriuria in pregnancy.

18.1). Our preference has been the short acting sulfonamide, Gantrisin. *E. coli* has been the offending organism in the vast majority of bacteriuric patients, and most strains of nonhospital-acquired *E. coli* are sensitive to the urinary levels obtained with this agent. In the last trimester, we prefer ampicillin, because of the potential risk of hyperbilirubinemia in the newborn, with competition between the sulfa drugs and bilirubin for binding on albumin.

However, if infection recurs, the patient should be maintained on suppressive antimicrobials for the remainder of the pregnancy. When short courses of therapy are prescribed for asymptomatic bacteriuria during pregnancy, continuous surveillance of the patients for recurrent bacteriuria by repeated urine cultures is essential. Relapse, however, is not uncommon. A second course of treatment often proves effective. Localization of bacteriuria has been shown to correlate with the pattern of recurrence after treatment. Leveno et al noted that the incidence of renal bacteriuria was 42% regardless of the site of infection, and after one course of short-term (10-day) or long-term (21-day) antimicrobial therapy, almost two-thirds of these women

were abacteriuric for the remainder of gestation (98). Although the timing of recurrence varied significantly in relation to duration of treatment and site of infection, the ultimate risk of recurrence was not related to either. These investigators concluded that the localization of asymptomatic bacteriuria does not contribute to the management of asymptomatic bacteriuria in pregnant women, since the overall recurrence rates are independent of the site of infection. Persistent asymptomatic bacteriuria is frequently, although by no means invariably, associated with excretion-urinographic evidence of some abnormality. Persistent asymptomatic bacteriuria may necessitate continuous antimicrobial therapy for the duration of pregnancy. A single daily dose of nitrofurantoin (100 mg), preferably after the evening meal, is recommended. Alternatively, a short acting sulfonamide preparation may be prescribed.

General consensus is that short-term therapy is effective management when combined with surveillance for recurrent bacteriuria. This initial therapy is empiric based on the recognition of the frequency with which *E. coli* is recovered in initial bacteriurias. Two to three days posttherapy a urine culture is repeated. The recurrence of bacteriuria during the same pregnancy has been detected in 16–33% of women. It is our policy that patients with recurrent asymptomatic bacteriuria are treated with antimicrobials on the basis of the microorganism's sensitivities and then remain on suppressive antimicrobial therapy for the remainder of the pregnancy and for 2 weeks postpartum. Others have treated recurrence with a second short period of therapy with favorable results. The effectiveness of therapy for asymptomatic bacteriuria is best documented by Harris' report of a decrease in the incidence of pyelonephritis in their institution once a screening program has been implemented (103). The incidence of acute pyelonephritis was reduced from 2.5% of all obstetrics admissions in 1974 to 0.5% in December of 1978. The Parkland group has similarly noted a dramatic decrease in their incidence of pyelonephritis in pregnancy following the introduction of a routine screening program for asymptomatic bacteriuria (95); this occurred despite no decrease in the incidence of bacteriuria.

The duration of therapy for urinary tract infection remains a subject of considerable debate. Although 7–14 days is still the usual and the approved duration of therapy, recent observation suggests that it is probably not suitable for all infections. An increasing number of reports have confirmed that an uncomplicated urinary tract (i.e., localized to the bladder) infection can be treated as well with a single day of therapy as with a 10- or 14-day course, especially if the bacteria are not antibody-coated (104–106).

Souney and Polk have reviewed the results of 19 prospective studies of single dose therapy for urinary tract infections (106). In 80% of the controlled trials there was no difference in outcome observed between single dose and traditional therapy patients in whom infection was localized to the bladder or localization studies were not performed. As Souney and Polk described, the potential benefits of single dose therapy are several fold (108); (a) reduction in cost of therapy; (b) less toxicity than traditional therapy; (c) noncompliance minimized; (d) earlier identification of patients who fail therapy results in prolonged therapy and/or urologic investigations being instituted sooner; and (e) reduced rate of emergence of resistant bacteria.

However, it has been suggested in several early studies that single dose therapy may be less effective in pregnant patients than in the nonpregnant population (107, 108). More recently, Harris and co-workers reported their results in the treatment of asymptomatic bacteriuria in pregnant women with four single dose regimens (ampicillin, cephalexin, nitrofurantoin, and sulfisoxazole) (109). Among the 86 women treated with one of the single-dose regimens there was a 31% failure rate and a 3.5% recurrence rate. The results with ampicillin, nitrofurantoin, and sulfisoxazole were relatively good with failure rates of 29, 27, and 25%, respectively. On the other hand, results with cephalexin were poor, and the failure rate was 45%. Additional studies have also demonstrated poor results with the use of cephalosporins for single dose therapy of UTI (108, 110). At the present time, single dose therapy for asymptomatic bacteriuria in pregnancy should not be utilized. Bacteriuria is associated with more serious complications during pregnancy and as Williams and Smith (107) and Harris et al (109) noted UTI are usually more difficult to eradicate in pregnant women (111). Before such therapy can be recommended, the efficacy of single dose antimicrobial therapy for asymptomatic bacteriuria must be demonstrated in controlled clinical trials.

Although it has been suggested that localization of bacteriuria is helpful in predicting which patients will be successfully treated by a single dose regimen, no method of localization clinically available is reliable enough to determine the proper duration of therapy in a particular patient (106).

CYSTITIS IN PREGNANCY

Acute cystitis during pregnancy is a distinct clinical entity. Acute cystitis is a syndrome characterized by urinary urgency and frequency, dysuria, and suprapubic discomfort in the absence of systemic symptoms, such as fever and costovertebral angle tenderness. Gross hematuria may be present; the urine culture is invariably positive for bacterial growth at greater than 100,000 colonies/ml. It is important to recognize that only approximately 50% of women presenting with dysuria or other lower urinary tract symptoms will have bacteriologic confirmation of a urinary tract infection (112). Those cases with symptoms of urinary infection but without bacteriologic evidence of infection are called the acute urethral syndrome, which is in many instances associated with chlamydial infection. Thus, bacterial confirmation is crucial to establishing a diagnosis of acute cystitis. Traditionally, quantitative urine cultures were the "gold standard" and greater than 100,000 colonies/ml the significant count. Recently, Stamm and co-workers suggested that in acutely dysuric patients a count greater than or equalling 100 colonies/ml was significant (25). Multiple dipstick culture and/or nitrite test techniques have been used to simplify and decrease the cost of screening urine for bacteria.

Harris and Gilstrap reported an incidence of 1.3% for cystitis during pregnancy (113). Although the increased diagnosis and treatment of asymptomatic bacteriuria resulted in a decreasing incidence of pyelonephritis at their institution, the incidence of acute cystitis has remained constant. On initial screening of urine cultures 64% of the cystitis patients had negative cultures. This is in contrast to the patients with asymptomatic bacteriuria and acute pyelonephritis, in which only a minority had negative initial screening cultures. These authors noted that the recurrence pattern of patients with acute cystitis is also different from patients with either bacteriuria or acute pyelonephritis. While 75% of patients with acute pyelonephritis developed a recurrence if not given suppressive antimicrobial therapy and one-third of patients with ASB subsequently developed positive urine cultures as evidence of recurrence, only 17% of patients with acute cystitis developed subsequent positive cultures. They reported that only 6% of patients with acute cystitis had a positive fluorescent antibody test, suggesting upper urinary tract involvement; this is in comparison to the nearly 50% of patients with asymptomatic bacteriuria and the two-thirds of the patients with acute pyelonephritis that had positive FA tests and, presumably, renal bacteriuria. This low incidence of renal involvement may well explain the decreased likelihood for recurrence among acute cystitis patients.

Interestingly, the cases of acute cystitis tended to occur in the second trimester (113). This is in contrast to reports which put the majority of cases of acute pyelonephritis in the first and third trimester and almost all cases of asymptomatic bacteriuria in the first trimester. Harris and Gilstrap did not have a single case of acute pyelonephritis following acute cystitis in their series (113).

Pregnant patients with acute cystitis should begin on immediate therapy, either nitrofurantoin macrocrystals, Gantrisin, or ampicillin. The recommended dosage schedules for these agents are: (1) nitrofurantoin (100 mg, four times a day,

for 10–14 days); (2) Gantrisin (1 g, four times a day, for 10–14 days); and (3) ampicillin (500 mg, four times a day, for 10–14 days). While combinations of sulfa with trimethoprim have been proven very effective in nonpregnant women, this combination is not recommended for use in pregnancy because of the theoretic teratogenic potential. Although cephalexin is effective, it is expensive and only in rare instances (i.e., Klebsiella UTI) does it possess a demonstrated advantage over the less expensive antimicrobial regimens.

The most commonly isolated microorganisms from the urine in patients with acute cystitis have been *E. coli* and other gram-negative facultative organisms, such as *Klebsiella*, *Proteus*, or *Enterobacter*; less commonly, group B streptococcus and *Staphylococcus saprophyticus*. These organisms are equally sensitive to these antimicrobial agents. Either a catheterized specimen, or a clean catch midstream urine should be obtained, prior to the institution of antibiotics, for urinalysis and urinary culture and sensitivities. The duration of therapy of cystitis remains a subject of considerable debate. Although 7–14 days is still the usual approved duration of therapy, recent observation suggests that it is probably not necessary in all infections. As discussed in the section on treatment of asymptomatic bacteriuria, it is likely that an uncomplicated urinary tract infection can be treated as well with even one day of therapy, especially if FA tests are negative. Because of the symptomatology associated with acute cystitis, it is not possible to await the results of culture; therefore, the constellation of symptoms and a urinalysis revealing white cells and bacteria should be sufficient to initiate therapy. It is important that the physician obtain follow-up culture for examination of the urine to determine the effectiveness of therapy. It is important to realize that immediate therapy is necessary for acute cystitis, to prevent upward extension of the infection to the kidney.

ACUTE PYELONEPHRITIS IN PREGNANCY

Acute pyelonephritis is one of the most frequent medical complications of pregnancy. The overall incidence is reported to be between 1–2.5% of all obstetric patients, with an estimated recurrence rate of 10–18% during the same gestation. Predisposing factors include obstructive and neurologic diseses of the urinary tract, ureteral, or renal calculi, and asymptomatic bacteriuria of pregnancy, which is the major predisposing factor. As screening for and treatment of asymptomatic bacteriuria increases, the incidence of pyelonephritis decreases (103). Diagnosis of pyelonephritis is based on a history of shaking chills, fever, and flank pain, symptoms and signs of nausea and vomiting, frequency, urgency, and dysuria, and physical findings showing costovertebral angle tenderness and fever, and laboratory reports revealing pyuria and bacteriuria. The pregnant woman with pyelonephritis generally presents clear-cut signs and symptoms that allow one to easily make the diagnosis (92). The majority of women will have chills, documented fever, and will complain of back pain (85%). A significant number (40%) have symptoms of lower urinary tract infection, e.g., dysuria, frequency. Almost one of four have nausea and vomiting. Fever is universal, and the diagnosis should be suspect if this is not present. Gilstrap and colleagues (92) noted a temperature greater than 38.4°C was present in 84% of their patients, while it was greater than 40°C in 12%. Costovertebral angle (CVA) tenderness was demonstrated in 97% of pregnant women with pyelonephritis; right-sided CVA tenderness predominated.

Pyelonephritis poses a serious threat to maternal well-being. Obstetric patients with acute pyelonephritis require hospitalization for vigorous treatment with intravenous fluids and parenteral antimicrobial agents and close monitoring of renal function. Nausea, vomiting, anorexia, and pyrexia frequently result in severe dehydration. An indwelling Foley catheter should be placed to obtain urine for microscopic examination and culture and to closely monitor urine output. (Once the patient is stable and has adequate urine output the Foley can be discontinued.) Intravenous fluids are instituted promptly, and fluid replacement with isotonic crystalloid solutions should be given until adequate urine flow is established. Either Ringer's lactate or normal saline is used, and 2000 cc often must be administered before adequate hydration is evident (i.e., improved urine output). If septicemia with shock is present the amount of fluids required to restore isovolemia may be considerably larger. Moreover, approximately 20% of the pregnant women with pyelonephritis have transient renal dysfunction as documented by decreased creatinine clearance (89). This factor is especially important when the antimicrobial agent(s) used is nephrotoxic, eliminated by the kidney, or both. Important management points include hydration and lowering of the elevated temperature monitoring of the renal function with intake and output, and close attention to the possibility of gram-negative shock. Approximately 10% of pregnant women with acute pyelonephritis will have bacteremia if appropriate blood cultures are taken; moreover, indirect evidence of endotoxin is frequently apparent in many of these women. In addition to diminished glomerular infiltration, these effects include: hypothermia, relative hypotension, although despite these findings, they clinically look and feel well. Cunningham and colleagues recently reported the occurrence of adult respiratory distress syndrome or "shock lung" in pregnant women with acute pyelonephritis but without full blown evidence of septic shock (114).

The initial choice of antimicrobial agent(s) for the treatment of acute pyelonephritis is empiric. This choice should be based on knowledge of the common etiologic agents and recognition of the need for bactericidal agents. The most common isolates recovered from pregnant women with pyelonephritis are *E. coli* rather than organisms of the *Klebsiella-Enterobacter* group and *Proteus* species. Both the enterococcus and group B streptococcus are increasingly recognized as pathogens in acute pyelonephritis of pregnancy. In the past empiric therapy with ampicillin 1 to 2 g intravenously every 6 hr or cephalothin in similar doses was sufficient. With these drugs, the total daily dosage could be increased to 12 g if necessary. More recently, we have recommended that empiric therapy for acute pyelonephritis during pregnancy be instituted using a combination of either ampicillin or a first generation cephalosporin (i.e., cephalothin or cefazolin) with an aminoglycoside (i.e., gentamicin or tobramycin). This combination is preferred for the following reasons: (a) there has been a steadily increasing pattern of resistance by *E. coli* to ampicillin and first generation cephalosporins; (b) women with recurrent infections (or occasionally initial infections) are more likely to have microorganisms resistant to ampicillin or first generation cephalosporins (i.e., *Enterobacter* or *Klebsiella*); and (c) the high probability for bacteremia and/or endotoxin sepsis argues for inclusion of a bactericidal agent that is effective against a wide range of gram-negative facultative bacteria including resistant organisms such as *Klebsiella*, *Enterobacter*, *Pseudomonas*, or *Seratia*. Because either group B streptococcus or the enterococcus are responsible for a small percentage of acute pyelonephritis in pregnancy, we prefer the ampicillin plus aminoglycoside combination which covers these two pathogens as well.

Either gentamicin or tobramycin is the aminoglycoside employed; because their antimicrobial susceptibility patterns are so similar, the choice of agent is usually determined by cost. It has been suggested that tobramycin use is associated with a lower incidence of nephrotoxicity and/or ototoxicity, but this is not well substantiated. The dose recommended for these aminoglycosides is 3–5 mg/kg/24 hr in 3 divided doses. We recommend that pregnant women receiving aminoglycosides be monitored with serum levels to ensure adequate dosage and prevention of toxicity. Intravenous antibiotics are continued until the patient is afebrile and can tolerate oral medications; ideally a minimum of 5 days of parenteral therapy is necessary. On the 3rd day of treatment a repeat culture is done. Using sensitivity as a basis, we would switch antimicrobial agents if necessary, and the patient is not responding. With prompt treatment a rapid clinical response occurs, and the majority of patients are afebrile and asymptomatic within 48 hr. Monitoring of serum levels is crucial in pregnancy where the associated increase in vascular volume and glomerular filtration rate result in a high prevalence of subtherapeutic serum levels with aminoglycosides (116). Peak levels of gentamicin and tobramycin should be <10 μg/ml and the trough level <2 μg/ml. We recommend obtaining peak and trough serum levels approximately 24 hr after initiation of therapy, and if they are in the normal range and the serum creatinine is normal, they should be repeated every 3 days. Following intravenous antimicrobial therapy, 85% of patients become afebrile within 48 hr, and nearly 100% of patients do so within 4 days (92). If this does not occur and the patient continues to be febrile, it must be assumed that resistant organisms are present or obstructive uropathy exists. A change or an addition of antimicrobial agent(s)) may be necessary as based upon the sensitivities of the microorganisms recovered on urine culture.

Although we initiate therapy with an ampicillin plus aminoglycoside combination, if the pretreatment urine culture discloses an organism sensitive to ampicillin, we discontinue the aminoglycoside and treat solely with ampicillin.

The incidence of recurrence for acute pyelonephritis during the same gestation is reported to be between 10 and 18% for all patients with pyelonephritis. In a retrospective analysis Harris and Gilstrap reported that patients with acute pyelonephritis who did not receive suppressive antimicrobial therapy for the remainder of gestation had a 60% incidence of recurrence requiring rehospitalization (117). This was in contrast to the low incidence (2.7%) of recurrence and rehospitalization in patients who were maintained on suppressive antimicrobial therapy for the duration of the gestation. Cunningham and co-workers had noted a similar high incidence of recurrence among patients not receiving suppressive therapy (71). Suppression is accomplished with 100 mg nitrofurantoin each night before bed. Other alternatives are short acting sulfonamides or ampicillin given in similarly small dosages. An acceptable alternative to suppressive therapy is the continued examination every 2 weeks of urine cultures for the detection of and prompt treatment of recurrent bacteriuria. We feel that the risk of recurrence of pyelonephritis is too great not to suppress the urinary tract infection with antimicrobial therapy following an acute episode of pyelonephritis.

Acute pyelonephritis may complicate as many as 2% of all pregnancies, unless asymptomatic bacteroides are eradicated. It is apparent that even if a bacteriuria screen is employed in the first prenatal visit, only two-thirds of the cases of pyelonephritis can be prevented. The majority of the nonpreventable cases occur prior to the initial prenatal visit. Only a small percent of acute pyelonephritis will occur among the patients whose initial bacteriuria screen was negative. These data demonstrate the importance of early prenatal care and initial screening for bacteriuria. Almost one-third of the women with acute pyelonephritis during pregnancy will have recurrent urinary tract infections and/or radiographic renal abnormalities, either during a subsequent pregnancy or when studied after the initial episode. This acute pyelonephritis during pregnancy warrants close follow-up and investigation following pregnancy in order to detect recurrent bacteriuria and/or the need for therapeutic intervention of upper urinary tract disease.

Nosocomial Urinary Tract Infection

Epidemiology

Hospital-acquired urinary tract infections are among the most frequent of nosocomial infections. An exact prevalence for nosocomial urinary tract infections is difficult to come by because of various surveillance systems and different definitions (i.e., clinically manifest infection versus laboratory evidence of significant bacteriuria). Based on data obtained from surveillance studies of nosocomial infections, approximately one-third of these hospital-acquired infections involve the urinary tract (118–122). Sixty percent of the nosocomial infections occurring in gynecologic patients involve the urinary tract (123). Current estimates are that approximately 500,000 patients per year acquire urinary tract infections in acute care hospitals in the United States (124, 125). The majority of these urinary tract infections are associated with usage of indwelling urethral catheterization or other types of urinary instrumentation (126, 127). Turck and Stamm suggested that female sex, advanced age, and debilitating underlying illness are associated with an increased risk of nosocomial urinary tract infections (128).

It has been estimated that 1% of nosocomial urinary tract infections (i.e., 5000 cases) are associated with bacteremia and potentially life-threatening illness (128). Platt and co-workers report that the acquisition of urinary tract infection during indwelling bladder catheterization is associated with nearly a three-fold increase in mortality among hospitalized patients (129). These investigators concluded that 14% of the deaths among the catheterized patients represented the excess mortality that was associated with acquisition of infection. Based on estimates that nearly 400,000 deaths per year occur in the approximately 7.5 million persons catheterized annually in the United States, they estimated that the excess mortality associated with catheter-related infection is 56,000 patients per year.

ETIOLOGY AND PATHOGENESIS

As in other urinary tract infections, *E. coli* is the most common etiologic agent in nosocomial infections involving the urinary tract; it accounts for approximately 50% of nosocomial bacteriuria (130). The *Klebsiella-Enterobacter* group of organisms are recovered in 13–15% (130–132), *Proteus* species in 3–13% (130–132) and *Pseudomonas aeruginosa, Serratia*, enterococci, staphylococci, and yeast make up the remainder of etiologic agents (128, 130–133). *E. coli* and the *Klebsiella-Enterobacter* group tend to occur among patients who have not received antimicrobial therapy. Among patients who are debilitated, immunosuppressed, or on antibiotic therapy organisms such as *Proteus, Pseudomonas, Serratia*, enterococcus, and yeasts are recovered with greater frequency. Stamm and co-

workers reported that *Serratia* and *Klebsiella* are associated with an inordinate frequency of bacteremia (122).

It has been estimated that 75–80% of nosocomial bacteriuria follows urinary tract catheterization (122, 127). Certain risk factors have been identified which are unavoidable; these include increasing age, debilitating illness, and female sex. Turck and Stamm have also described additional factors involved in the risk of acquiring bacteriuria which are alterable (128). These factors relate to both the method and duration of catheterization. Thus a single in and out catheterization is associated with an incidence for infection of less than 1% while 100% of patients with indwelling urethral catheters draining into an open system for more than 4 days develop bacteriuria (1, 133). Garibaldi et al noted that, even with use of a closed drainage system, the risk of infection increased 5–10% per day of catheterization (130).

Bacteria that cause catheter-associated urinary tract infection gain access to the urinary tract by three major routes. The first is introduction of microorganisms from the external genitalia and/or distal urethra into the bladder at the time of catheterization. In general, bacteria introduced in this way are well tolerated and controlled by voiding and the antibacterial defense mechanism of the bladder (128). A second mechanism by which bacteria gain access to the bladder is via a thin film of urethral fluid on the outside of the catheter (134). Thirdly, once the drainage system has been contaminated bacteria may migrate up inside the catheter lumen (130, 131). Turck and Stamm believe that the intraluminal ascending route accounted for the majority of nosocomial urinary tract infections (128). Such contamination may be due to failure to use sterile technique in disconnecting the catheter and drainage tube to obtain a specimen or to irrigate the catheter (123). Also inadvertent disconnection occurs and frequently results in contamination. An additional important factor in the pathogenesis of catheter-associated urinary tract infection is cross-contamination of catheters by transmission of bacteria from patient to patient on the hands of hospital personnel (123).

TREATMENT AND PREVENTION

In general, we do not treat with antimicrobial agents those patients in whom bacteriuria occurs during catheterization but who remain asymptomatic. This concern relates to the risk of persistent colonization and/or emergence of more resistant nosocomial organisms. Fortunately, in the large majority of such situations, removal of the catheter results in eradication of the bacteriuria. If signs and symptoms of cystitis or acute pyelonephritis occur with the presence of an indwelling catheter, systemic antimicrobial therapy should be administered for 10–14 days. Regimens similar to what is used in treating acute cystitis are appropriate for this situation.

The most important and effective method for prevention of nosocomial urinary tract infections is to limit the use of indwelling catheters only to instances where they are necessary. Additional preventive measures have been recommended (123). These include: (a) urinary catheters should be removed as soon as possible; (b) only adequately trained hospital personnel should insert urinary catheters; (c) use of aseptic technique in inserting catheters so as to avoid introducing bacteria; (d) cleansing the meatal-catheter junction with soap and water once or twice a day to reduce periurethral bacterial contamination; (e) maintain unobstructed "downhill" flow in a closed drainage system; (f) disconnect the drainage system only to irrigate an obstructed catheter, not to obtain specimens or to routinely irrigate; and (g) whenever feasible separate catherized patients from each other in order to prevent cross-contamination.

Measures which have been proposed as adjuncts in prevention attempts, but for which supporting data are lacking to demonstrate an advantage over a closed drainage system include: (a) a flutter valve to prevent reflux of urine from the collection bag to the drainage tube; (b) continuous bladder irrigation via a triple lumen catheter with either acetic acid or a neomycin-polymixin solution; (c) use of suprapubic catheterization; and (d) prophylactic systemic antibiotics.

The final aspect of catheter care is to obtain a follow-up culture after the catheter is removed and to institute appropriate antimicrobial therapy if significant bacteriuria persists following removal of the catheter.

References

1. Kass EH, Finland M: Asymptomatic infections of the urinary tract. *Trans Assoc Am Phys* 69:56–64, 1956.
2. Kass EH: Should bacteriuria be treated? *Med J Aust* 1(suppl):38–43, 1973.
3. Sweet RL: Bacteriuria and pyelonephritis during pregnancy. *Semin Perinatol* 1:25–40, 1977.
4. Stamey TA, Goven DE, Palmer JM: The localization and treatment of urinary tract infections: the role of bactericidal urine levels as opposed to serum levels. *Medicine (Baltimore)* 44: 1–36, 1965.
5. Stamey TA, Timothy M, Millar M, et al: Recurrent urinary infections in adult women. The role of introital enterobacteria. *Calif Med* 115:1–19, 1971.
6. Charles D: Infections in Obstetrics and Gynecology, Philadelphia, WB Saunders, 1980, p 323.
7. Kass EH: The role of asymptomatic bacteriuria in the pathogenesis of pyelonephritis. In Quinn EL, Kass EH (eds): *Biology of Pyelonephritis*. Boston, Little, Brown, 1960, pp 399–412.
8. Paterson L, Miller A, Henderson A: Suprapubic aspiration of urine in diagnosis of urinary tract infection during pregnancy. *Lancet* 2:1195–1196, 1970.
9. Sabath LD, Charles D: Urinary tract infections in the female. *Obstet Gynecol* 55(suppl):162–169, 1980.
10. Kass EH, Zinner SH: Bacteriuria and pyelonephritis in pregnancy. In Charles D, Finland M (eds): *Obstetric and Perinatal Infections*. Philadelphia, Lea & Febiger, 1973, pp 407–446.
11. Kunin CM, Zacha E, Paquin AJ: Urinary tract infections in school children. I. Prevalence of bacteriuria and associated urologic findings. *N Engl J Med* 266:1287–1296, 1962.
12. Kunin CM: The natural history of recurrent bacteriuria in school girls. *N Engl J Med* 282:1443–1448, 1970.
13. Nicolle LE, Harding GKM, Preiksaitis J, Ronald AR: The association of urinary tract infection with sexual intercourse. *J Infect Dis* 146:579–583, 1982.
14. Turck M, Goffe BS, Petersdorf RG: Bacteriuria of pregnancy: relationship to socioeconomic status. *N Engl J Med* 266:857–860, 1962.
15. Henderson M, Entwiste G, Tayback M: Bacteriuria and pregnancy outcome: preliminary findings. *Am J Public Health* 52:1887–1893, 1962.
16. Williams JD, Reeves DS, Condie AP, et al: The treatment of bacteriuria in pregnancy. In O'Grady F, Brumfitt W (eds): *Urinary Tract Infection*. London, Oxford University Press, 1968, pp 160–169.
17. Jordan PA, Iravani A, Richard GA, Baer H: Urinary tract infection caused by *Staphylococcus saprophyticus*. *J Infect Dis* 142:510–515, 1980.
18. Latham RH, Runing K, Stamm WE: Urinary tract infections in young adult women caused by *Staphylococcus saprophyticus*. *JAMA* 250:3063–3066, 1983.
19. Cox CE, Lacey SS, Hinman F Jr: The urethra and its relationship to urinary tract infection. The urethral flora of the female with recurrent urinary tract infection. *J Urol* 99:632–638, 1968.
20. Brumfitt W, Hamilton-Miller JMT, Bakhtiar M, et al: New technique for investigating bacterial flora of female periurethral area. *Br Med J* 2:1471–1472, 1976.
21. Lidin-Janson G, Lindberg U: Asymptomatic bacteriuria in school girls. VI. The correlation between urinary and faecal *Escherichia coli*. Correlation of the relation of bacteriuria and the sampling technique. *Acta Paediatr Scand* 66:349–354, 1977.

22. Stamey TA, Sexton CC: The role of vaginal colonization with Enterobacteriaceae in recurrent urinary infections. *J Urol* 113:214–217, 1975.

23. Fowler JE, Stamey TA: Studies of introital colonization in women with recurrent urinary infection. VII. The role of bacterial adherence. *J Urol* 117:472–473, 1977.

24. Stamey TA, Wehner N, Mihara G, et al: the immunologic basis of recurrent bacteriuria: role of cervicovaginal antibody in enterobacterial colonization of the introital mucosa. *Medicine* 57:47–56, 1978.

25. Stamm WE, Counts GW, Running KR, et al: Diagnosis of coliform infection in acutely dysuric women. *N Engl J Med* 307:463–468, 1982.

26. Hindman R, Tronic B, Bartlett R: Effect of delay on culture of urine. *J Clin Microbiol* 4:102–103, 1976.

27. Guttmann D, Naylor GRE: Dip slide: an aid to quantitative urine culture in general practice. *Br Med J* 3:343–345, 1967.

28. Hamilton-Miller JMT, Brooks SJD, Brumfitt W, et al: Screening for bacteriuria: microstix and dipslides. *Postgrad Med J* 53:248–250, 1977.

29. Boutros P, Mourtada H, Ronald AR: Urinary infection localization. *Am J Obstet Gynecol* 112:379–381, 1972.

30. Kaitz AL: Urinary concentrating ability in pregnant women with asymptomatic bacteriuria. *J Clin Invest* 40:1331–1338, 1961.

31. Clark H, Ronald AR, Cutler RE, et al: The correlation between site of infection and maximal concentrating ability in bacteriuria. *J Infect Dis* 120:47–51, 1969.

32. Percival A, Brumfitt W, Delouvois J: Serum antibody level as an indication of clinically inapparent pyelonephritis. *Lancet* 2:1027–1033, 1964.

33. Brumfit W, Reeves DS: Recent developments in the treatment of urinary tract infection. *J Infect Dis* 120:61–81, 1969.

34. Vinacur JC, Casellas JM, Rubi RA, et al: Serum anti-Escherichia coli antibodies and urinary B-g lucuronidase for the diagnosis and control of evolution of urinary infection during pregnancy. *Am J Obstet Gynecol* 120:812–816, 1974.

35. Heineman HS, Lee JH: Bacteriuria in pregnancy. A heterogeneous entity. *Obstet Gynecol* 41:22–26, 1973.

36. Thomas V, Shelokov A, Farland M: Antibody coated bacteria in the urine and the site of urinary tract infection. *N Engl J Med* 290:588–590, 1974.

37. Jones SR, Smith JW, Sanford JP: Localization of urinary tract infections by detection of antibody-coated bacteria in urine sediment. *N Engl J Med* 290:591–593, 1974.

38. Kass EH: Bacteriuria and pyelonephritis of pregnancy. *Arch Intern Med* 205:194–198, 1960.

39. Elder HA, Kass EH: Renal function in bacteriuria of pregnancy: its relationship to prematurity, acute pyelonephritis and excessive weight gain. In Kass EH (ed): *Progress in Pyelonephritis.* Philadelphia, FA Davis, 1965, pp 81–86.

40. Elder HA, Santamarina BAG, Smith S, et al: The natural history of asymptomatic bacteriuria during pregnancy: the effect of tetracycline on the clinical course and the outcome of pregnancy.

Am J Obstet Gynecol 111:441–462, 1971.

41. Andriole V, Cohn GL: The effect of diethylstilbesterol on the susceptibility of rats to hematogenous pyelonephritis. *J Clin Invest* 43:1136–1145, 1964.

42. Harle EMJ, Bullen JJ, Thompson DA: Influence of estrogen on experimental pyelonephritis caused by *Escherichia coli. Lancet* 2:283–286, 1975.

43. Braude AI: Current concepts of pyelonephritis. *Medicine (Baltimore)* 52:257–264, 1973.

44. Fass RJ, Klainer AS, Perkins RL: Urinary tract infection. Practical aspects of diagnosis and treatment. *JAMA* 225:1509–1513, 1973.

45. Kass EH: Bacteriuria and pyelonephritis of pregnancy. *Arch Intern Med* 105:194–198, 1960.

46. Whalley P: Bacteriuria of pregnancy. *Am J Obstet Gynecol* 97:723–738, 1967.

47. Bryant RE, Windom RE, Vineyard JP, et al: Asymptomatic bacteriuria in pregnancy and its association with prematurity. *J Lab Clin Med* 63:224–231, 1964.

48. Condie AP, Williams JD, Reeves DS, et al: Complications of bacteriuria in pregnancy. In O'Grady F, Brumfitt W (eds): *Urinary Tract Infection.* London, Oxford University Press, 1968, pp 148–159.

49. Gruneberg RN, Leigh DA, Brumfitt W: Relationship of bacteriuria in pregnancy to acute pyelonephritis, prematurity and fetal mortality. *Lancet* 2:1–3, 1969.

50. Harris RE, Thomas VL, Shelokov A: Asymptomatic bacteriuria in pregnancy: antibody-coated bacteria, renal function and intrauterine growth retardation. *Am J Obstet Gynecol* 126:20–25, 1976.

51. Kincaid-Smith P, Bullen M: Bacteriuria in pregnancy. *Lancet* 1:395–399, 1965.

52. Kunin CM: Asymptomatic. *Annu Rev Med* 17:383–406, 1966.

53. Little PJ: The incidence of urinary infection in 5000 pregnant women. *Lancet* 4:925–928, 1966.

54. McFadyen IR, Eykyn SJ, Gardner NHN, et al: Bacteriuria in pregnancy. *J Obstet Gynaecol Br Commonw* 80:385–405, 1973.

55. Norden CW, Kilpatrick WH: Bacteriuria of pregnancy. In Kass EH (ed): *Progress in Pyelonephritis.* Philadelphia, FA Davis, 1965, pp 64–72.

56. Norden CW, Kass EH: Bacteriuria of pregnancy—a critical appraisal. *Annu Rev Med* 19:431–470, 1968.

57. Stuart KL, Cummins GT, Chin WA: Bacteriuria, prematurity and the hypertensive disorders of pregnancy. *Br Med J* 1:554–556, 1965.

58. Whalley P, Martin F, Peters P: Significance of asymptomatic bacteriuria detected during pregnancy. *JAMA* 193:879–881, 1965.

59. Williams GL, Campbell HM, Davies KJ: The influence of age, parity and social class on the incidence of asymptomatic bacteriuria in pregnancy. *J Obstet Gynaecol Br Commonw* 76:229–239, 1969.

60. Blunt A, Williams RH: Asymptomatic bacteriuria in pregnancy. *Aust NZ J Obstet Gynecol* 9:196–198, 1969.

61. Carrol R, MacDonald D, Stanley JC: Bacteriuria in pregnancy. *Obstet Gynecol* 32:525–527, 1968.

62. Gower PE, Haswell B, Sidaway ME, et al: Fol-

low-up of patient with bacteriuria of pregnancy. *Lancet* 2:990–994, 1968.

63. LeBlanc AL, McGanity WJ: The impact of bacteriuria in pregnancy—a survey of 1300 pregnant patients. *Tex Rep Biol Med* 22:336–347, 1964.

64. Pathak UN, Tang K, Williams LL, et al: Bacteriuria of pregnancy: results of treatment. *J Infect Dis* 120:91–95, 1969.

65. Robertson JG, Livingstone JRB, Isdale MH: The management and complications of asymptomatic bacteriuria in pregnancy. *J Obstet Gynaecol Br Commonw* 75:59–65, 1968.

66. Savage WE, Hajj SN, Kass EH: Demographic and prognostic characteristics of bacteriuria in pregnancy. *Medicine (Baltimore)* 46:385–407, 1967.

67. Turner GC: Bacilluria in pregnancy. *Lancet* 2:1062–1064, 1967.

68. Eykin SJ, McFadyen IR: Suprapubic aspiration of urine in pregnancy. In O'Grady F, Brumfitt W (eds): *Urinary Tract Infection*. London, Oxford University Press, 1968, pp 141–147.

69. Wood EG, Dilllon HC Jr: A Prospective study of group B streptococcal bacteriuria in pregnancy. *Am J Obstet Gynecol* 140:515–520, 1981.

70. Andriole VT: Bacterial infections. In Burrow GN, Ferris TF (eds): *Medical Complications during Pregnancy*. Philadelphia, WB Saunders, 1975, pp 382–394.

71. Cunningham FG, Morris GB, Mickal A: Acute pyelonephritis of pregnancy: a clinical review. *Obstet Gynecol* 42:112–117, 1973.

72. Baird D: The upper urinary tract in pregnancy and the puerperium with special reference to pyelitis of pregnancy. *J Obstet Gynaecol Br Emp* 43:1–59, 1936.

73. Dodds GH: Bacteriuria in pregnancy, labor and puerperium. *J Obstet Gynaecol Brit Emp* 38:773–787, 1931.

74. Crabtree E: Urological Diseases in Pregnancy. Boston, Little, Brown, 1942.

75. McLane CM: Pyelitis of pregnancy. *Am J Obstet Gynecol* 38:117–123, 1939.

76. Hibbard L, Thrupp L, Summeril S, et al: Treatment of pyelonephritis in pregnancy. *Am J Obstet Gynecol* 98:609–615, 1967.

77. Kass EH: Pregnancy, pyelonephritis and prematurity. *Clin Obstet Gynecol* 13:239–254, 1973.

78. Wren BG: Subclinical renal infection and prematurity. *Med J Aust* 2:956–600, 1969.

79. Calderyo-Barcia R: In Kowlessor M (ed): *Physiology of Prematurity*, Fifth Conference, Josiah Macy Jr. Foundation, 1960, p 105.

80. Wiederman J, Stone ML, Pataki R: Urinary tract infections and uterine activity. Effect of *Escherichia coli* endotoxins on uterine motility in vitro.

81. Brumfitt W: The effects of bacteriuria in pregnancy on maternal and fetal health. *Kidney Int* 8(suppl):113–119, 1975.

82. Dixon HG, Brandt HA: The significance of bacteriuria in pregnancy. *Lancet* 1:19–20, 1967.

83. Kaitz AL, Holder EW: Bacteriuria and pyelonephritis of pregnancy. *N Engl J Med* 265:667–672, 1961.

84. Layton R: Infection of the urinary tract in pregnancy: an investigation of a new routine in antenatal care. *J Obstet Gynaecol Br Commonw* 71:927–933, 1964.

85. Monson OT, Armstrong D, Pion RJ, et al: Bacteriuria during pregnancy. *Am J Obstet Gynecol* 85:511–518, 1963.

86. Sleigh JD, Robertson JG, Isdale MH: Asymptomatic bacteriuria in pregnancy. *J Obstet Gynecol. Br Commonw* 71:74–81, 1964.

87. Whalley PJ: Bacteriuria in pregnancy. In Kass EH (ed): *Progress in Pyelonephritis*. Philadelphia, FA Davis, 1965, pp 50–57.

88. Norden CW: Significance and management of bacteriuria of pregnancy. In Kaye D (ed): *Urinary Tract Infection and Its Management*. St Louis, CV Mosby, 1972, pp 171–187.

89. Fairley KF, Whitworth JA, Radford HJ, et al: Pregnancy bacteriuria. The significance of site of infection. *Med J Aust* 2:424–427, 1973.

90. Thrupp LD, Cotron RS, Kass EH: Relationship of bacteriuria in pregnancy to pyelonephritis. *JAMA* 189:899–902, 1964.

91. Giles C, Brown JAH: Urinary infection and anemia in pregnancy. *Br Med J* 2:10–13, 1962.

92. Gilstrap LC, Cunningham FG, Whalley PJ: Acute pyelonephritis in pregnancy: an anterospective study. *Obstet Gynecol* 57:409–413, 1981.

93. Kincaid-Smith P: Bacteriuria in pregnancy. In Kass EH (ed): *Progress in Pyelonephritis*. Philadelphia, FA Davis, 1965, pp 11–26.

94. Zinner SH, Kass EH: Longterm (10–12 years) follow up of bacteriuria of pregnancy. *N Engl J Med* 285:820–824, 1971.

95. Leigh DA, Gruneberg RN, Brumfitt W: Long term follow up of bacteriuria in pregnancy. *Lancet* 2:603–605, 1968.

96. Cobbs CG, Stickler JC, McGovern JH, et al: The postpartum renal status of women with untreated asymptomatic bacteriuria during pregnancy. *Am J Obstet Gynecol* 99:221–227, 1967.

97. Wilson MG, Hewitt WL, Monzon OT: Effect of bacteriuria on the fetus. *N Engl J Med* 274:1115–1118, 1966.

98. Leveno KJ, Harris RE, Gilstrap LC, et al: Bladder versus renal bacteriuria during pregnancy: recurrence after treatment. *Am J Obstet Gynecol* 139:403–406, 1981.

99. Whalley PJ: Bacteriuria in pregnancy. In Kass EH (ed): *Progress in Pyelonephritis*. Philadelphia, FA Davis, 1965, pp 50–57.

100. Norden CW, Levy PS, Kass EH: Predictive effect of urinary concentrating ability and hemagglutinating antibody titer upon response to antimicrobial therapy in bacteriuria of pregnancy. *J Infect Dis* 121:588–596, 1970.

101. Beard RW, Roberts AP: Asymptomatic bacteriuria during pregnancy. *Br Med Bull* 24:44–49, 1968.

102. Patrick MJ: Renal infection in pregnancy. The natural development of bacteriuria in pregnancy. *J Obstet Gynaecol Br Commonw* 73:973–976, 1966.

103. Harris RE: the significance of eradication of bacteriuria during pregnancy. *Obstet Gynecol* 53:71–73, 1979.

104. Fang LST, Tolkoff-Rubin NE, Rubin RH: Efficacy of a single dose and conventional amoxicillin therapy in urinary tract infection localized by the antibody-coated bacteria technic. *N Engl J Med* 298:413–416, 1978.

105. Buckwold FJ, Ludwig P, Harding GKM, et al:

Therapy for acute cystitis in adult women. Randomized comparison of single-dose sulfisoxazole vs Trimethoprim-Sulfamethoxazole. *JAMA* 247:1839–1842, 1982.

106. Souney P, Polk BF: Single-dose antimicrobial therapy for urinary tract infections in women. *Rev Infect Dis* 4:29–34, 1982.

107. Williams JD, Smith EK: Single-dose therapy with streptomycin and sulfametopyrazine for bacteriuria during pregnancy. *Br Med J* 4:651–653, 1970.

108. Brumfitt W, Faiers MC, Franklin INS: The treatment of urinary infection by means of a single dose of cephaloridine. *Postgrad Med J* 46(suppl):65–69, 1970.

109. Harris RE, Gilstrap LC, Petty A: Single-dose antimicrobial therapy of asymptomatic bacteriuria in pregnancy. *Obstet Gynecol* 59:546–549, 1982.

110. Greenberg RN, Sanders CV, Lewis AC: Single dose therapy for urinary tract infection with cefaclor. *Am J Med* 71:841–845, 1981.

111. Williams JD, Reeves DS, Condie AP, et al: The treatment of bacteriuria in pregnancy. In O'Grady F, Brumfitt W (eds): *Urinary Tract Infection.* London, Oxford University Press, 1968, pp 160–169.

112. Gallagher DJA, Montgomerie JZ, North JDK: Acute infections of the urinary tract and the urethral syndrome in general practice. *Br Med J* 1:622–626, 1965.

113. Harris RE, Gilstrap LC: Cystitis during pregnancy: a distinct clinical entity. *Obstet Gynecol* 57:578–580, 1981.

114. Cunningham FG, Leveno KJ, Hankins GDV, Whalley PJ: Respiratory insufficiency associated with pyelonephritis during pregnancy. *Obstet Gynecol* 63:121–125, 1984.

115. Smith CR, Lipsky JJ, Laskin OL, et al: Double-blind comparison of the nephrotoxicity and auditory toxicity of gentamicin and tobramycin. *N Engl J Med* 302:1106–1109, 1980.

116. Zaske DE, Cipolle RJ, Strate RG, et al: Rapid gentamicin elimination in obstetric patients. *Obstet Gynecol* 56:559, 1980.

117. Harris RE, Gilstrap LC: Prevention of recurrent pyelonephritis during pregnancy. *Obstet Gynecol* 44:637–641, 1974.

118. Kislak JW, Eickhoff TC, Finland M: Hospital-acquired infection and antibiotic usage in the Boston City Hospital. *N Engl J Med* 271:834–835, 1964.

119. Barrett FF, Casey JI, Finland M: Infections and antibiotic use among patients at Boston City Hospital. *N Engl J Med* 278:5–9, 1968.

120. Moody ML, Burke JP: Infections and antibiotic use in a large private hospital. *Arch Intern Med* 130:261–266, 1972.

121. McNamara MJ, Hill MC, Balows A, et al: A study of bacteriologic patterns of hospital infections. *Ann Intern Med* 66:486–488, 1967.

122. Stamm WE, Martin SM, Bennett JV: Epidemiology of nosocomial infections due to gram-negative bacilli. Aspects relevant to development and use of vaccines. *J Infect Dis* 136(suppl):151–160, 1977.

123. American College of Obstetricians and Gynecologists: Prevention of Hospital Acquired Urinary Tract Infections in Gynecologic Patients. *ACOG Technical Bulletin,* no 46, May 1977.

124. Centers for Disease Control: *National Nosocomial Infections Study Report, Annual Summary 1979.* Atlanta, GA: Centers for Disease Control. Issued March 1982.

125. *American Hospital Association Guide to the Health Care Field.* Chicago: American Hospital Association, 1980.

126. McGowan JE Jr, Finland M: Infection and antibiotic usage at Boston City Hospital: changes in prevalence during the decade 1964–1973. *J Infect Dis* 129:421–428, 1974.

127. Martin CM, Bookrajian EN: Bacteriuria prevention after indwelling urinary catheterization: a controlled study. *Arch Intern Med* 110:703–711, 1962.

128. Turck M, Stamm W: Nosocomial infection of the urinary tract. *Am J Med* 70:651–654, 1981.

129. Platt R, Polk BF, Murdock B, Rosner B: Mortality associated with nosocomial urinary-tract infection. *N Engl J Med* 307:637–642, 1982.

130. Garibaldi RA, Burke JP, Lickman ML, Smith MD: Factors predisposing to bacteriuria during indwelling urethral catheterization. *N Engl J Med* 291:214–219, 1974.

131. Kunin CM, McCormack RC: Prevention of catheter-induced urinary tract infections by sterile closed drainage. *N Engl J Med* 274:1155–1161, 1966.

132. Buddington WT, Graves RC: Management of catheter drainage. *J Urol* 62:387–393, 1949.

133. Turck M, Goffe B, Petersdorf RG: The urethral catheter and urinary tract infection. *J Urol* 88:834–837, 1962.

134. Kass EH, Schneiderman LJ: Entry of bacteria into the urinary tract of patients with inlying catheters. *N Engl J Med* 282:33–35, 1970.

CHAPTER 19

Antimicrobial Agents

Because bacterial infections play a prominent role in obstetrics and gynecology, antimicrobial agents are among the most frequently administered drugs. Confronted with a seemingly incomprehensible array of antibiotics, the clinician must be well-versed in use of antibiotics in the day to day care of patients.

MODE OF ACTION OF ANTIBIOTICS (1, 2)

Antibiotics exert inhibitory effects on bacteria by interfering with their metabolic activities or the function of their structural components. This inhibition is dose-related and requires the administration of effective inhibitory concentrations of the agent without reaching toxic levels. A bacterial species is considered sensitive to an antimicrobial agent if the organism is inhibited by concentrations of the antibiotic that can be obtained without harm to the host. Ideally, the action of an antibiotic should be directed against bacterial, not human, processes, thus avoiding toxicity for the host. This search for selective antimicrobial toxicity has been the impetus for the development of antibiotics that affect bacterial characteristics and physiologic attributes that differ from those of human cells.

Antimicrobial agents may interfere with bacterial metabolism, the synthesis or integrity of structural components, such as cell wall or plasma membrane, and biosynthesis of proteins and nucleic acids. In general, the metabolic activities of bacteria are similar to those of mammalian cells. However, in some cases, the bacteria synthesize certain compounds that animal cells must obtain as preformed molecules. Folic acid is an example of such a compound. Thus, the inhibition of folate biosynthesis affects bacterial cells selectively. In addition, bacteria require a cell wall that serves to protect them from osmotic damage and provides them with a characteristic shape. Because a cell wall is not present in mammalian cells, it is a selective target for antibiotic action. The cell membrane, which

lies inside the cell wall, represents another site where antibiotic action may be demonstrated. The bacterial plasma membrane has essentially the same structure as the cell membrane of mammalian cells. As a result, antibiotics which are active against the bacterial cell membrane are usually quite toxic for the host. Bacterial protein synthesis occurs on 70-S ribosomes within the cell. Mammalian ribosomes (except in mitochondria) are 80-S entities, and this difference may account for some selective action of antibiotics that inhibit protein synthesis. Nucleic acid synthesis by bacteria also offers a possible site for antibiotic action.

Antibiotics are classified as bactericidal or bacteriostatic on the basis of their mode of action. Bactericidal drugs produce a change in the bacterial cell that is incompatible with survival. Examples of such changes include disruption of the cell wall structure or disorganiztion of the cell membrane. Drugs are considered bacteriostatic if they inhibit certain metabolic events and thus cause suspension of bacterial growth. This blockade of metabolic activity is not immediately lethal, and if the antibiotic is removed from the environment resumption of growth may recur. The multitude of sites in bacteria where antibiotics can exert their action is summarized in Table 19.1.

PHARMACOKINETIC CONSIDERATIONS IN OBSTETRIC PATIENTS

Pertinent to this chapter are two general pharmacokinetics considerations: the effect of pregnancy upon serum antibiotic levels and distribution of antibiotics into the fetal compartment and into breast milk.

Effect of Pregnancy upon Serum Antibiotic Levels (3, 4)

Administration of antimicrobials during pregnancy may be used to treat a coincidental ma-

Table 19.1
Mechanism of Action of Antimicrobial Agents

Inhibition of synthesis of essential metabolites
  Sulfonamides   Para-aminosalicylic acid
                      (PAS)
  Trimethropim   Isoniazid (INH)

Inhibition of cell wall synthesis
  Penicillins   Bacitracin
  Cephalosporins   Cycloserine
  Cephamycins   Ristocetin
  Vancomycin

Inhibition of protein synthesis
  Bactericidal   Bacteriostatic
    Streptomycin   Erythromycin
    Neomycin   Lincomycin
    Kanamycin   Clindamycin
    Gentamicin   Chloramphenicol
    Tobramycin   Tetracyclines
    Amikacin   Spectinomycin

Alteration of cell membrane
  Polymyxin B   Amphotericin B
  Colistin   Nystatin

Interference with nulceic acid synthesis
  Rifampin   Actinomycin D

ternal infection, such as pneumonia or pyelonephritis, to treat a maternal-fetal infection, such as syphilis or chorioamnionitis, or to treat a predominantly fetal infection, such as some cases of toxoplasmosis.

Physiologic changes occurring in pregnancy may have important influences upon serum concentrations of antibiotics. The relevant changes include:

1. A marked increase in the volume of distribution (vascular and interstitial fluid volumes and the fetal compartment)
2. A marked increase in cardiac output
3. A large increase in renal blood flow and glomerular filtration
4. A fall in plasma protein concentrations by about 1 g/100 ml.

In addition, technical and ethical problems may make the studies of antibiotic kinetics more difficult in pregnant than in nonpregnant women.

Present data regarding serum antibiotic levels in pregnancy are subject to many criticisms. First, in many studies, patients were given a

single dose of drug, and only one maternal sample was obtained, usually during labor or delivery. Consequently, there are widely varying times, with each patient being represented by only one point. Second, circulatory adjustments of delivery may itself influence levels. In only rare studies have healthy prenatal patients been available. Third, in nearly all studies, levels in pregnant women have been compared to levels measured in nonpregnant adults from different populations and in different laboratories. In the occasional study in which the pregnant woman has been her own control, levels were determined before and a few weeks after delivery. Fourth, there may be important differences between early and late gestations; few investigations have reported serum levels in the same woman at varying stages of gestation.

Despite these limitations, lower serum or plasma levels are suspected for a number of antibiotics, and for ampicillin serum levels have been documented to be lower in pregnancy. Table 19.2 summarizes the effect of pregnancy on antibiotic concentration. Overall, the percent decrease in levels ranges from 10 to 50%. Decreases in serum ampicillin concentrations have been observed after both oral and intravenous administration. Reasons for the lower levels of antibiotics in pregnant women may be more rapid excretion, a larger volume of distribution, or perhaps sequestration of the drug in the fetal compartment.

Table 19.2
Effect of Pregnancy on Serum Antibiotic Levels

Antibiotics for which levels are clearly lower in pregnancy
  Ampicillin

Antibiotics for which levels are suspected of being lower in pregnancy
  Methicillin   Gentamicin
  Cephalexin   Kanamycin
  Cephalothin   Amikacin
  Cephazolin   Tobramycin (?)
  Erythromycin   Nitrofurantoin

Antibiotics for which levels are probably unchanged in pregnancy
  Cephaloridine
  Clindamycin
  Thiamphenicol
  Trimethoprim-sulfamethoxazole

The therapeutic implication of these findings is not altogether clear, however, as peak blood levels even in pregnancy are usually many times greater than minimal inhibitory or minimal bactericidal concentrations. Further, in pregnant women given standard doses, there have been few documented cases of antibiotic failure due soley to subtherapeutic levels. Accordingly, it would seem wise to proceed as follows. With agents with wide margins of safety (such as ampicillin and cephalosporins), use dosages in the upper ranges. For agents with narrower margins of safety such as the aminoglycosides, use standard doses (on a milligram/kilogram bases). Then, if therapy does not appear adequate, determine antibiotic levels. It seems important to point out, however, that more common causes of antibiotic failure include resistant organisms, abscesses, and septic pelvic thrombophlebitis.

Distribution of Antibiotics

Distribution of drugs into various body fluids depends upon whether the mechanism of transfer is active or passive. Passive mechanisms are probably more important for antibiotic transfer, and this mechanism (i.e., mainly diffusion) is influenced by the concentration gradient, molecular weight, binding to protein, and ionization of the drug. In general, rapid transfer is favored by large concentration gradients, small molecular weight, and low protein binding. The effect of ionization is more complex; only an unionized, nonprotein-bound drug engages in diffusion across membranes. If all other factors were equivalent, drugs which are weak bases will have a higher concentration in a more acid medium, and drugs which are weak acids will have a greater concentraion in a more alkaline medium.

Placental Transfer of Antibiotics (5)

Available clinical experiments of placental transmission of antibiotics have shown that all antibiotics pass into the fetal circulation. Many of the criticisms offered on antibiotic levels in pregnant women apply even more so to placental transmission. Of special importance is the relative inaccessibility of the fetal circulation and, to lesser extent, the amniotic fluid. Consequently, much of the information comes from "single dose, single determination" studies. This is an important limitation because levels of antibiotics in the fetal compartment should increase after repeated, regular maternal dosing. In addition, there are likely to be marked differences in transmission at different gestational ages. Thus, data obtained from mid-trimester pregnancies may not be directly applicable to term pregnancies. This entire topic has been comprehensively reviewed recently.

Although there is wide variation, placental transfer of many antibiotics including ampicillin, cephalothin, clindamycin, carbenicillin, and the aminoglycosides follows a similar pattern. After an *intravenous* injection, maternal levels achieve peak concentrations within 15 min and then fall exponentially. Umbilical blood concentrations also peak rapidly (within 30–60 min) and also fall exponentially. Infant to maternal peak serum level ratios for the above antibiotics range from 0.3 to 0.9. Levels in amniotic fluid at term are usually not detectable for a few hours and then gradually increase. Amniotic fluid levels of antibiotics are dependent to a large extent upon the excretion of the antibiotic(s) in fetal urine. Thus, obtaining therapeutic levels of antibiotic(s) in the amniotic fluid at term requires a live fetus. For some antibiotics including erythromycin and dicloxacillin, placental transmission is more limited. Infant to maternal peak level ratios for these are 0.1.

Antibiotic Excretion in Breast Milk (6)

Excretion of antibiotics in breast milk is governed by the same principles which regulate placental transmission. In addition to the influence of concentration gradient, molecular weight, and protein binding, differences in pH between breast milk and serum may be especially important. Because the pH of milk (range 6.4–7.6) is usually lower than that of plasma, antibiotics which are weak bases tend to have higher concentrations in the milk. Conversely, antibiotics which are weak bases tend to have higher concentrations in serum. In addition to the concentration of an antibiotic in breast milk, it is necessary to consider the amount of antibiotic consumed by the newborn (i.e., concentration in milk X volume consumed).

Some antibiotics achieve concentrations in breast milk that are from 50 to 100% of serum concentrations. These antibiotics include erythromycin, lincomycin, tetracycline, sulfonamides, chloramphenicol, and NIH. More commonly used antibiotics such as penicillin G and oxacillin achieve milk levels which are a smaller percentage of maternal serum concentrations (generally, 2–20%). Of the aminoglycosides, data are available for the oldest preparation, streptomycin, which is excreted in small amounts in breast milk for some time after IM administration to the mother.

INTERPRETATION OF CLINICAL TRIALS

Many antibiotic trials in obstetric and gynecologic patients have been reported in the last years, but caution must be used in interpreting the results. Although antibacterial spectrum of the drug being tested is important, at least four other factors influence the results. Of these, perhaps the most important is the type of infection studied. Clearly, patients with tuboovarian abscess will have a poorer immediate response to antibiotics than will patients with acute, uncomplicated salpingitis. Similarly, a better cure rate is expected in endometritis after vaginal delivery than after cesarean, regardless of antibiotic tested. Second, with some newer antibiotics, with minimal inhibitory concentration (MIC_{90}) values near achievable serum levels, dose of the antibiotic is important. Third, the investigator's criteria for an unsatisfactory response will determine the failure/cure proportion. There is no agreed upon time limit beyond which a response is considered unsuccessful, but most investigators use 48–72 hr. Approximately 15% of patients who have not responded by 48 hr will respond later. Thus in studies in which failure is determined after 48 hr, one would expect a higher failure rate. Fourth, most comparative studies are relatively small (less than 100 patients total). Thus there is a strong possibility that a true difference in cure rates will not be detected because the sample size is too small. In general, it would take a total sample size of 150–200 subjects to show a statistically significant effect when the difference in cure rates is 15%. Such "oversights" are called β errors. Finally, the cure rate is dependent upon the antibiotics' spectra, but organisms of special interest (*Staphylococcus aureus*, enterococci, *Bacteroides fragilis* group, etc.) are each present in a minority of patients. Further, there is often a poor correlation between *in vitro* activity and *in vivo* effect. Accordingly, it is entirely possible that drugs with moderately different in vitro activities will result in similar cure rates, especially in smaller studies.

PENICILLINS

Penicillin was initially isolated from the mold *Penicillium notatum* by Fleming in 1929. However, it was not introduced into clinical medicine until 1941 by the efforts of Florey, Chain and colleagues. The penicillin used by these early workers was actually a mixture of several penicillin compounds, of which penicillin G (benzylpenicillin) was found to be the most satisfactory. The basic chemical structure of penicillin consists of three components—a thiazolidine ring, the β-lactam ring, and a side chain which largely determines the antibacterial spectrum and pharmacologic properties of each penicillin (1).

In 1959 the penicillin nucleus, 6-amino-penicillanic acid, was isolated (2). It is from this compound that the wide variety of semisynthetic penicillins are derived. As suggested by Neu (1), the penicillins can be divided into six major classes on the basis of their antibacterial activities (Table 19.3).

Natural Penicillins

The natural penicillins include penicillin G, penicillin V (phenoxymethylpenicillin), and three additional phenoxypenicillins—phenethicillin, propicillin, and phenbenicillin—which are not commonly used. Penicillin G is available as potassium penicillin G, sodium penicillin G, procaine penicillin G, and benzathine penicillin G.

SPECTRUM OF ACTIVITY

The penicillins are bactericidal antibiotics that act by interfering with cell wall formation, by affecting the formation of the mucopeptide portion of the cell wall. Penicillin G is active against a wide range of bacteria, predominantly gram-positive organisms. Among the gram-positive, facultative or aerobic cocci, penicillin G is highly active against group A streptococci. While the majority of *Streptococcus pneumoniae* strains remain extremely sensitive, relatively resistant pneumococcal strains requiring higher penicillin concentrations have appeared (3) and more recently, pneumococci completely resistant to penicillin have been reported in South Africa (4). Group B β-hemolytic streptococci are sensitive to penicillin G, but are approximately 10-fold less sensitive than the group A streptococci. In addition, groups C and G β-hemolytic streptococci and the α-hemolytic streptococci such as *Streptococcus viridans* and nonenterococcal group D streptococci are sensitive to penicillin G. The anaerobic gram-positive cocci such as *Peptococcus* and *Peptostreptococcus* species are highly susceptible to penicillin G. On the other hand, enterococcal group D streptococci are resistant to penicillin G, as are the majority

Table 19.3
Classification of Penicillins

1. Natural penicillins Penicillin G Penicillin V Phenethicillin	4. Antipseudomonas penicillins Carbenicillin Indanylcarbenicillin Ticarcillin Azlocillin

2. Penicillinase-resistant penicillins
Methicillin
Nafcillin
Isoxazolyl penicillins
    Cloxacillin
    Dicloxacillin
    Flucloxacillin[a]
    Oxacillin
	5. Extended-spectrum penicillins
	Mezlocillin
	Piperacillin

3. Aminopenicillins Ampicillin Amoxicillin Bacampicillin Cyclacillin[a] Epicillin[a] Hetacillin[a] Pivampicillin[a]	6. Amidino penicillins Mecillinam[a] Pivmecillinam[a]

[a] Not available in the United States.

of *S. aureus* strains whose resistance is due to β-lactamase (penicillinase) production.

Among gram-positive bacilli, *Corynebacterium diptheriae*, *Bacillus anthracis*, and many strains of *Listeria monocytogenes* are sensitive to penicillin G. Anaerobic gram-positive spore-forming bacilli such as *Clostridium perfringens* and other *Clostridium* species are penicillin G-sensitive. In addition, penicillin G is active against most anaerobic nonspore-forming bacilli such as *Actinomyces*, *Eubacterium*, *Bifidobacterium*, *Propionibacterium*, and *Lactobacillus* species.

In the gram-negative cocci group of bacteria, *Neisseria meningitidis* remains very sensitive to penicillin G. However, *Neisseria gonorrhoeae* susceptibility has dramatically changed from the situation where the gonococcus was always highly sensitive to penicillin G. Relatively resistant gonococcal strains are now recognized (5), and recently β-lactamase-producing strains of *N. gonorrhoeae* (PPNG), which are completely penicillin-resistant, have occurred (6, 7). Gram-negative anaerobic cocci such as *Veillonella* species are also sensitive to penicillin G.

Among gram-negative bacilli, the Enterobacteriaceae such as *Escherichia coli*, *Proteus*, *Klebsiella*, *Enterobacter*, *Serratia*, *Salmonella*, *Shigella*, and *Citrobacter* spp. are resistant to penicillin G. In addition, *Pseudomonas aeruginosa* and other *Pseudomonas* species are resistant to penicillin G. While penicillin G is active against many gram-negative anaerobes such as *Fusobacterium* and most *Bacteroides* species, *B. fragilis*, *Bacteroides bivius*, and *Bacteroides disiens* are generally resistant. Recently, increasing resistance to penicillin G has been noted among strains of *Bacteroides melaninogenicus*.

Treponema pallidum is sensitive to penicillin G. The mycoplasmata, rickettsiae, fungi, and Protozoa are completely penicillin-resistant, while chlamydiae are relatively resistant.

The spectrum of activity of the phenoxypenicillins—penicillin V, phenethicillin, propicillin, and phenbenicillin—is generally similar to that described above for penicillin G. However, penicillin G is more active against streptococci, pneumococci, *N. gonorrhoeae*, and *N. meningitidis*.

DOSAGE AND ROUTE

Penicillin G is largely destroyed by acid in the stomach with only about one-third of orally administered penicillin G being absorbed. Thus, when oral therapy with penicillin is desired penicillin V (phenoxymethyl penicillin) because of its greater acid stability is the usual choice in a dosage of 250–500 mg (400,000–800,000 units) every 6 hr. Penicillin V may be given with meals.

Crystalline penicillin G is available to be administered either intramuscularly or intravenously. When administered intramuscularly, crystalline penicillin G reaches peak serum concentrations 15–30 min after injection; a 1,000,000-unit dose results in a peak serum level of 12 μg/ml. By 3–4 hr serum concentrations are negligible. Crystalline penicillin G is usually given in dosages ranging from 300,000 to 1,000,000 units every 6 hr by the intramuscular route, but can be given as frequently as every 2 hr. Crystalline penicillin G may be administered intravenously by either intermittent bolus infusion or continuous infusion. The intermittent infusion of high concentrations of penicillin G is generally preferred. A rapid infusion of 5 million units of crystalline penicillin G results in peak serum concentrations of 400 μg/ml within a few minutes. By 4 hr after injection the serum concentration falls to 3 μg/ml. Intravenous therapy is administered in a dose of 1–5 million units every 2–6 hr, depending on the severity of the clinical infection.

Repository penicillins for intramuscular injection are also available; these are procaine penicillin G and benzathine penicillin G. With procaine penicillin peak serum levels occur 1–3 hr after injection, and detectable levels are usually present for up to 24 hr. The standard dose of procaine penicillin is 600,000–1,200,000 units intramuscularly every 6–12 hr. Benzathine penicillin when injected intramuscularly results in a slow release of penicillin which lasts over a 2- to 4-week period of time. Following injection of 2.4 million units of benzathine penicillin, 0.12 μg/ml of penicillin can be detected at 14 days postinjection. The usual dose is 1,200,000–2,400,000 units, and the interval of dosing is dependent upon the clinical indication.

SIDE EFFECTS

Penicillin G is associated with a wide variety of side effects. Although penicillin is one of the least toxic antimicrobial agents, it is commonly responsible for hypersensitivity reactions. These hypersensitization reactions include skin rash, urticarial reactions, anaphylactic reactions, serum sickness, contact dermititis, and angioedema. Local reactions may occur such as swelling, pain, and redness at the site of injection or phlebitis after intravenous infusion.

Direct penicillin toxicity may occur with massive doses (60–100 million units daily). Neurologic toxicity with convulsions and coma may result, especially in patients with renal insufficiency, underlying central nervous system disease, or hyponatremia. Interstitial nephritis or hemolytic anemia may occur with large doses of penicillin G. Rarely administration of penicillin G has been associated with development of thrombocytopenic purpura, glossitis, and stomatitis.

Penicillin V may result in gastrointestinal side effects such as nausea, vomiting, and diarrhea. Hypersensitivity reactions may occur as noted for penicillin G.

COST

Pencillin G and penicillin V are inexpensive antimicrobial agents. Thus, for microorganisms susceptible to these agents, the penicillins remain the drug of choice.

USE IN PREGNANCY

Penicillin G rapidly crosses the placenta and achieves levels in cord blood and amniotic fluid. To date no adverse effects on the fetus have been demonstrated with the use of penicillin G, and this drug is considered safe to use during pregnancy. Similarly penicillin V has not been linked with adverse fetal effects.

METABOLISM

Penicillin G is primarily excreted in the urine. In patients with normal renal function, over 70% of the injected dose is excreted within 6 hr. Ninety percent of penicillin G excretion occurs by tubular excretion and 10% by glomerular filtration. This renal tubular secretion can be partly blocked by probenecid, resulting in a doubling of serum levels of penicillin. Approximately 5% of penicillin G is excreted in the bile. The penicillin not excreted in urine or bile is inactivated in the liver, with penicilloic acid as the major end product.

The phenoxypenicillins are also excreted in urine and bile. During the first 6 hr after oral intake, 20–40% of the dose of penicillin V can be recovered from urine.

Penicillin G is widely distributed in the body. High concentrations of penicillin G are present in blood, liver, bile, skin, intestines, and kidneys. Low concentrations occur in joint fluid, pericardial fluid, and pleural fluid. Peritoneal fluid contains high concentrations. Small amounts of penicillin G are distributed to brain, nerve, dura, bone marrow, bone, pancreas, adrenal glands, or spleen. While penicillin G poorly penetrates the blood-brain barrier in the presence of normal meninges, when the meninges are inflamed, cerebrospinal fluid levels of penicillin G are adequate.

INDICATIONS IN OBSTETRICS AND GYNECOLOGY

Penicillin G remains one of the most effective antibiotics. Because of its activity against a wide spectrum of bacteria and its safety, penicillin G remains the preferred agent for many clinical infections.

Penicillin G is the drug of choice for infections due to group A β-hemolytic streptococci or group B β-hemolytic streptococci. In addition, penicillin G is very effective against pneumonococcal pneumonia. Because of its activity against aerobic and anaerobic streptococci, *Clostridium* species, and many of the *Bacteroides* species, penicillin G was commonly employed in combination with an aminoglycoside as initial therapy for mixed aerobic-anaerobic soft-tissue pelvic infections. However, recognition of the role of penicillin-resistant anaerobes such as *B. fragilis* and *B. bivius* has resulted in a diminished role for penicillin G in such infections.

When enterococcal infection is a concern, penicillin G may be added to the clindamycin-aminoglycoside regimen because penicillin plus an aminoglycoside have a synergistic effect on the enterococcus.

As described in Chapter 3, penicillin G is the drug of choice for the treatment of syphilis. In addition, it remains a very effective agent for the treatment of nonpenicillinase-producing gonococci.

Penicillin G is the drug of choice for the treatment of actinomycosis infections which are associated with IUD usage. Similarly it is the drug of choice for clostridial infections. In combination with an aminoglycoside, penicillin G is recommnded for prophylaxis against bacterial endocarditis.

Penicillinase-Resistant Penicillins

The emergence of β-lactamase producing *S. aureus* led to major efforts for the development of antimicrobial compounds resistant to the hydrolysis of β-lactame enzymes. This resulted in a large variety of semisynthetic penicillins derived from 6-aminopenicillanic acid. The narrow-spectrum penicillinase-resistant penicillins include methicillin, oxacillin, nafcillin, cloxacillin, dicloxacillin, and flucloxacillin.

SPECTRUM OF ACTIVITY

Methicillin was the first antistaphylococcal penicillin introduced into clinical medicine. Although it is active against pneumococci and streptococci, its efficacy against these organisms is many fold less than that of penicillin G. Methicillin is active against the majority of strains of *S. aureus*, but increasingly methicillin-resistant *S. aureus* has been reported. These methicillin-resistant staphylococci are also resistant to penicillin G, the cephalosporins, and other penicillinase-resistant penicillins such as nafcillin, oxacillin, cloxacillin, and dicloxacillin.

The isoxazolyl penicillins—oxacillin, cloxacillin, and dicloxacillin— have a spectrum of activity similar to methicillin. Nafcillin also has a similar antibacterial spectrum. Its stability in the presence of staphylococcal penicillinase is comparable to that of methicillin but greater than that of the isoxazolyl penicillins (8).

DOSAGE AND ROUTE

Methicillin is administered only by the intravenous route. The dosage can be varied depending upon the site and severity of the infection. For infections of moderate severity 1 g every 4 hr is generally used, and for serious infections such as endocarditis a dose of 2 g every 2–3 hr may be given. After an intravenous injection of 1 g methicillin, a peak serum level of 60 μg/ml is obtained. There is a rapid fall in serum levels to 7 μg/ml by 1 hr and less than 1 μg/ml by 2–3 hr. The peak level can be doubled by doubling the dose.

Although oral oxacillin is available it is absorbed erratically. Oxacillin may be given in a dose of 250–500 mg every 4–6 hr, intravenously or intramuscularly for mild to moderate infections. The dose for severe infections is 1 g intravenously every 4–6 hr. Peak serum levels after a single intramuscular injection of oxacillin (500 mg) is 14–16 μg/ml.

Cloxacillin and dicloxacillin are analogues of oxacillin. They are acid stable and thus well absorbed after oral ingestion. Following an oral dose of 500 mg of cloxacillin a peak serum level of 8 μg/ml is reached in 30–60 min. Dicloxacillin produces serum levels that are twice as high as those of cloxacillin. Serum levels of flucloxacillin are similar to those seen with dicloxacillin.

The usual oral adult dose of these penicillins is 500 mg every 6 hr. For dicloxacillin a dose of 125–250 mg every 6 hr may suffice.

Oxacillin, cloxacillin, and flucloxacillin can be given intramuscularly or intravenously, while dicloxacillin can be given intramuscularly. For mild injections 250 mg every 6 hr is recommended. For moderate infections the usual dose is 1 g every 4 hr, and in severe infections this is increased to 2 g every 4 hr.

Nafcillin is poorly absorbed and is unreliable when used orally. It can be given either intramuscularly or intravenously. The usual adult dose is 1 g every 4 hr, but this dose can be increased to 2 g every 4 hr for severe infections. Following a 1-g intramuscular injection, a peak serum level of 8 μg/ml of nafcillin is reached in about 1 hr. By 6 hr the level is 0.5 μg/ml.

SIDE EFFECTS

Methicillin, isoxazolyl penicillins, and nafcillin are contraindicated in penicillin-allergic patients because they can produce any of the hypersensitivity reactions described for penicillin G. Methicillin has been associated with drug fever and leukopenia (9). In addition, interstitial nephritis may result from the use of large doses of intravenous methicillin (10). Most patients recover from the methicillin interstitial nephritis after stopping the agent.

The isoxazolyl penicillins may produce nausea and diarrhea with oral administration. Oxacillin may cause fever, nausea, and vomiting in association with abnormal liver function tests (11). Neutropenia has been noted as well. With very large doses neurotoxicity occurs, especially in patients with impaired renal function.

Nafcillin has been reported to cause nephropathy and neutropenia on rare occasion.

COST

The penicillinase-resistant group of penicillins are relatively expensive drugs. They should be used only in the treatment of staphylococcal strains resistant to penicillin G.

USE IN PREGNANCY

All the penicillinase-resistant penicillins are capable of crossing the placenta. No untoward effects on the fetus have been described.

METABOLISM

Methicillin is excreted in urine, both by glomerular filtration and tubular secretion. Up to 80% of an injected dose can be recovered from urine (12). A small percentage (2–3%) of the administereed drug is excreted in bile. The unexcreted methicillin is inactivated in the body by the liver. Methicillin is widely distributed thoughout the body.

Isoxazolyl penicillins are mainly excreted in the urine with dicloxacillin and flucloxacillin present in larger amounts than cloxacillin where 30% of an oral dose is excreted in the urine. Oxacillin is excreted in smaller amounts than cloxacillin. Excretion occurs by glomerular filtration and tubular secretion. These penicillins are also excreted in the bile to a small extent. Inactivation of the isoxazolyl penicillins probably occurs in the liver.

Following administration of nafcillin, 30% of the dose can be recovered from the urine. Between 5–10% of a dose is excreted in bile. The remainder of the nafcillin is inactivated in the liver. Nafcillin reaches high concentrations in the CSF of patients with normal meninges as well as in those with inflamed meninges.

INDICATIONS IN OBSTETRICS AND GYNECOLOGY

The penicillinase-resistant penicillins are indicated solely for the treatment of infections due to *S. aureus*. Examples include mastitis, endocarditis, osteomyelitis, and toxic shock syndrome.

Aminopenicillins

The aminopenicillins are semisynthetic derivatives of 6-aminopenicillanic acid and include ampicillin and antibiotics structurally related to ampicillin - amoxicillin, epicillin, cyclacillin, hetacillin, pivampicillin, talampicillin, bacampicillin, and metampicillin.

SPECTRUM OF ACTIVITY

Ampicillin is active against most of the bacteria which are sensitive to penicillin G. However, it is also active against some of the gram-negative bacteria that are penicillin G-resistant. Similar to penicillin G, it is a bactericidal antibiotic that inhibits cell wall synthesis.

Against aerobic gram-positive cocci ampicillin is generally as effective as penicillin G. Thus, group A and group B β-hemolytic streptococci, most *S. pneumoniae*, and the α-hemolytic streptococci of the viridans groups are susceptible. Nearly all *S. aureus* are resistant to ampicillin.

Unlike penicillin G, ampicillin is effective against enterococcal strains of the group D streptococci. The anaerobic gram-positive cocci such as *Peptococcus* and *Peptostreptococcus* species are almost always sensitive to ampicillin.

Among gram-positive aerobic bacilli, *C. diptheriae*, *B. anthracis*, and *L. monocytogenes* are generally susceptible to ampicillin. Ampicillin is active against anaerobic gram-positive spore-forming bacilli such as *Clostridia* and anaerobic gram-positive nonspore-forming bacilli such as *Actinomyces*, *Eubacterium*, *Bifidobacterium*, *Propionibacterium*, and *Lactobacillus* species.

Unlike penicillin G, ampicillin is effective against some of the enterobacteriaceae. Although *E. coli* is often sensitive, increasing resistance by this organism to ampicillin has occurred (13). Unless it is a betalactamase-producing strain, most *Proteus mirabilis* is susceptible to ampicillin. *Enterobacter, Klebsiella, Serratia, Citrobacter*, and indole-positive *Proteus* strains are generally resistant to ampicillin. Salmonellae are usually sensitive, but resistant strains have occurred. On the other hand, *Shigella* species tend to be resistant.

Among the other gram-negative aerobic bacteria, *P. aeruginosa* is always resistant to ampicillin. *Haemophilus influenzae* type b was generally sensitive to ampicillin, but recently plasmid-mediated ampicillin resistance has occurred. *N. gonorrhoeae* is generally susceptible to ampicillin, but gonococcal strains with relative resistance to penicillin G also show ampicillin resistance. In addition PPNG strains are completely ampicillin-resistant. *N. meningitidis* remains sensitive. Similar to the pattern with penicillin G, many of the *Bacteroides* species and *Fusobacterium* are ampicillin-sensitive. The notable exceptions are *B. fragilis* group, *B. bivius*, and *B. disiens*. Mycoplasmas and rickettsiae are ampicillin-resistant, while chlamydiae are relatively resistant.

DOSAGE AND ROUTE

The usual oral dosage of ampicillin is 250–500 mg every 6 hr. Following oral administration of 500 mg, peak serum levels of 3 μg/ml are obtained at approximately 2 hr, and drug is still detectable at 6 hr. Doubling the dose results in a doubling of the serum level. Oral absorption of ampicillin is significantly lowered if it is taken with meals.

An intramuscular preparation of ampicillin is available, but rarely is necessary. The usual dose is 0.5–1.0 g every 6 hr. Following a 500-mg injection a peak serum level of 10 μg/ml is achieved in 1 hr, and levels persist for 4 hr.

The usual intravenous dosage is 1–2 g every 4–6 hr by intermittent infusion, depending upon the severity of the clinical infection.

Amoxicillin is significantly better absorbed than ampicillin when given orally, and peak serum levels are approximately 2–2½ times those achieved with a similar dose of ampicillin. The usual adult dose of amoxicillin is 250–500 mg every 6–8 hr. A similar dose schedule is recommended for epicillin, cyclacillin, hetacillin, or metampicillin.

Bacampicillin when administered orally is totally hydrolyzed to free ampicillin. It is absorbed better than ampicillin in the presence of food. Peak serum levels of 1½–2 times greater are achieved with bacampicillin as compared to a similar dose of ampicillin. The usual adult dose is 200 mg, 400 mg, or 800 mg every 8–12 hr.

The adult dose of pivampicillin is 350–700 mg every 6 hr (this is comparable to 250–500 mg of ampicillin), and for talampicillin the adult dose is 375–750 mg every 8 hr (equal to 250–500 mg of ampicillin).

SIDE EFFECTS

Ampicillin and the other aminopenicillins may cross-react with other penicillins and should, therefore, not be used in patients with a history of penicillin allergy. Any of the hypersensitivity reactions described for penicillin G may occur with ampicillin. The incidence of skin rash in ampicillin users is much greater than that reported with use of penicillin G. Five to seven percent of patients treated with ampicillin develop a diffuse macular rash (14, 15). However, these rashes are specific for ampicillin and do not represent a true penicillin allergy.

Gastrointestinal side effects such as nausea and diarrhea occur commonly but are generally not serious. Because of their enhanced gastrointestinal absorption, the aminopenicillins other than ampicillin are associated with less gastrointestinal side effects. More rarely *pseudomembranous colitis* has been reported with ampicillin use. Unusual side effects noted in ampicillin treatment include nephropathy, agranulocytosis, and encephalopathy.

Ampicillin may impair the absorption of oral contraceptives and, thus, can be associated with breakthrough bleeding. Monilia vaginitis may develop secondary to ampicillin suppression of the normal vaginal microflora.

COST

Ampicillin is a relatively inexpensive antibiotic, both in oral and parenteral forms. The other aminopenicillins are more costly than ampicillin and the additional cost may limit their use.

USE IN PREGNANCY

Ampicillin has been used extensively in pregnancy. No adverse fetal effects have been associated with ampicillin, and thus the drug is considered safe for use in pregnancy. In pregnant women serum levels of ampicillin are approximately 50% of those obtained in nonpregnant women (16). This is the result of the significant increase in plasma volume and renal clearance of ampicillin which occur in pregnancy.

Ampicillin rapidly crosses the placenta and following a single maternal dose, peak cord blood levels are achieved that are 40% of the peak maternal levels. In turn, amniotic fluid levels are lower than those in the umbilical cord.

Experience with the other aminopenicillins in pregnancy is limited to date and are not generally recommended for use in pregnant women.

METABOLISM

Similar to penicillin G, ampicillin is largely excreted in urine as the result of glomerular filtration and tubular secretion. Following oral administration 30% of a dose appears in urine, while with parenteral administration 75% of a dose is excreted in the urine. The remainder of an ampicillin dose is either excreted in the bile or inactivated in the liver.

Ampicillin is evenly distributed throughout body tissues with levels in the kidneys and liver being significantly greater than serum levels. While only very low levels can be detected in normal CSF, with inflamed meninges high levels of ampicillin are achieved in the CSF.

INDICATIONS IN OBSTETRICS AND GYNECOLOGY

Ampicillin is widely employed in the therapy of asymptomatic bacteriuria, acute cystitis, and acute pyelonephritis in pregnant and nonpregnant women. Because of increasing resistance of *E. coli* to ampicillin, we combine an aminoglycoside with ampicillin in the empiric treatment of acute pyelonephritis of pregnancy. For pyelonephritis, ampicillin is used in a dose of 4–8 g/day.

While in the past ampicillin alone or in combination with an aminoglycoside was commonly used for the treatment of mixed aerobic-anaerobic soft tissue pelvic infections such as endomyometritis, pelvic cellulitis or pelvic inflammatory disease, the recognition of the need to provide therapy against *B. fragilis*, *B. bivius*, and *B. disiens* in such infections has resulted in a significant decrease in the use of ampicillin on obstetric and gynecologic services.

For uncomplicated lower genital tract gonorrhea, oral ampicillin may be used as a single dose (3.5 g) plus probenecid (1.0 g); amoxicillin (3.0 g) may be alternately used. Recent recommendations by the Centers for Disease Control (CDC) urge that therapy for gonorrhea also include an agent to treat any concomitant chlamydial infection such as tetracycline HCl (500 mg four times a day for 7 days) or doxycycline (100 mg two times a day for 7 days).

Ampicillin is the drug of choice for group B streptococcus and is included in the treatment of intraamniotic infection (chorioamnionitis) in combination with agent(s) effective against anaerobes including *B. fragilis* and *B. bivius* and gram-negative aerobes such as *E. coli*. Ampicillin is also the optimal drug for the treatment of *L. monocytogenes* infections.

Lastly ampicillin has been effectively used as a prophylactic antibiotic with cesarean sections and vaginal hysterectomy. Because the other aminopenicillins have a similar antibacterial spectrum to ampicillin, the indication for their use are similar to those for ampicillin. Because of enhanced oral absorption amoxicillin may replace oral ampicillin in the treatment of UTI and gonorrhea.

Antipseudomonas Penicillins

The antipseudomonas group of penicillins include the carboxypenicillins, carbenicillin, and ticarcillin, and the ureidopenicillin, azlocillin. The major importance of these antimicrobial agents is their activity against *Pseudomonas*. However, they are all susceptible to β-lactamase enzymes produced by gram-negative and gram-positive organisms.

SPECTRUM OF ACTIVITY

Carbenicillin's spectrum of activity is similar to that of ampicillin. However, it does possess activity against *P. aeruginosa* and certain indole-positive *Proteus* species. Carbenicillin is less active than ampicillin against the facultative streptococci, while its activity against *N. gonorrhoeae*, *N. meningitidis*, and *Haemophilus* is similar to ampicillin. *Klebsiella pneumoniae* is resistant.

In addition, at high concentrations carbenicillin is active against anaerobic bacteria including *B. fragilis*, although not to the extent of clindamycin, chloramphenicol, metronidazole, or cefoxitin. Carbenicillin acts synergistically with aminoglycosides to inhibit *P. aeruginosa*. This was clinically important because resistance to carbenicillin often developed among *P. aeruginosa* during therapy.

The antibacterial spectrum of ticarcillin is similar to that of carbenicillin with the exception that it is two to four times more active against *P. aeruginosa*. However, these strains of *P. aeruginosa* which are highly resistant to carbenicillin are also resistant to ticarcillin.

Azlocillin is a ureidopenicillin whose main advantage is its significantly enhanced activity against *P. aeruginosa* as compared to carbenicillin or ticarcillin.

All three of these agents are ineffective against β-lactamase producing *S. aureus*.

DOSAGE AND ROUTE

Carbenicillin is not orally absorbed and is available in intramuscular or intravenous forms. An oral form, carbenicillin indonyl sodium, is available but is useful only for UTI because adequate serum concentrations are not acheived. For the treatment of systemic pseudomonas infections or anaerobic infection, intravenous intermittent doses of carbenicillin 5 g every 3–4 hr is required (total 30–40 g daily). Parenteral carbenicillin for *Pseudomonas* urinary tract infection (UTI) requires 1 to 2 g every 4–6 hr. The usual adult dose for oral indanylcarbenicillin is 0.5–1.0 g every 6 hr.

Following an intramuscular dose of 1 g, peak carbenicillin serum levels of 20 μg/ml are achieved in 1 hr, and no drug is detectable by 4 hr. While these serum levels are inadequate for *Pseudomonas* or anaerobic infections in soft tissue, the urine levels reach 2000–4000 μg/ml, which are sufficient for the treatment of *Pseudomonas* UTI. With an intravenous infusion of 70–100 mg/kg carbenicillin serum levels of 150–200 μg/ml can be obtained; these levels are sufficient, in many instances, for the treatment of soft tissue *Pseudomonas* or anaerobic infections.

With ticarcillin an adult dose of 18–24 g per 24 hr is recommended for systemic *Pseudomonas* infections or anaerobic infections; this is given as a 3 g dose every 3–4 hr. For treatment of UTI a dose of 1 g every 6 hr is recommended. After a 1 g dose intramuscularly of ticarcillin, a mean peak serum level of 35 μg/ml is achieved in 1 hr, and by 6 hr it is 6 μg/ml. Following a 3 g intravenous infusion, mean serum levels postinfusion are 239 μg/ml, and at 4 hr they are 94 μg/ml (18).

Azlocillin is administered intravenously in a dose of 12–16 g per day divided into four doses. Administration of a 2 g dose of azlocillin results in peak serum levels of 60 μg/ml at 1 hr.

SIDE EFFECTS

Carbenicillin, ticarcillin, and azlocillin may provoke any of the hypersensitivity reactions which occur with penicillin G. High doses of carbenicillin may result in neurotoxicity. Each gram of carbenicillin contains 4.7 meq of sodium. With the use of the required large dose of 30–40 g per day the potential for sodium overload may occur in patients with cardiac or renal disease. In addition, hypokalemia may occur as a result of this sodium overload. Finally, carbenicillin rarely is associated with bleeding as the result of diminished platelet adhesiveness (17).

Ticarcillin, in high doses, also may result in neurotoxicity, electrolyte disturbances similar to that described with carbenicillin, and altered platelet function. The lower required dose of ticarcillin as compared to carbenicillin is associated with a lower sodium load and less platelet dysfunction.

COST

The antipseudomonal penicillins are relatively costly antimicrobial agents because of the large doses required.

USE IN PREGNANCY

Carbenicillin, ticarcillin, and azlocillin have not been used extensively during pregnancy. As like other penicillins, they are most likely safe to use during pregnancy. However, they should only be used in pregnant women when no safe alternative choice is available.

METABOLISM

Carbenicillin is excreted via the kidney with about 95% of a parenteral dose excreted into the urine during the first 6 hr after administration. It is excreted via glomerular filtration and tubular secretion. A small amount (<1%) of carbenicillin is excreted in the bile or inactivated in the liver. Similarly ticarcillin and azlocillin are also primarily excreted via the kidneys.

INDICATIONS IN OBSTETRICS AND GYNECOLOGY

The clinical role for carbenicillin and ticarcillin in obstetrics and gynecology are now very limited. While clinical studies have demonstrated relatively good efficacy with these agents (as single agents or in combination with aminoglycosides) in the treatment of mixed aerobic-anaerobic soft tissue infections of the pelvis (19, 20), the introduction of the ureidopenicillins, mezlocillin, and piperacillin into clinical practice has significantly reduced their usefulness.

While *Pseudomonas* infections of soft tissue are rare on obstetric and gynecologic services, when present, azlocillin is an appropriate therapeutic agent. Its major advantage over aminoglycosides is a decreased potential for nephrotoxicity or ototoxicity. For serious *Pseudomonas* infection azlocillin should be combined with an aminoglycoside.

Extended Spectrum Penicillins

The new ureidopenicillins, such as mezlocillin (Mezlin) and piperacillin (Piperacil), have replaced the carboxypenicillins, carbenicillin, and ticarcillin. As compared with carbenicillin and ticarcillin, they have an extended coverage against the enterobacteriaceae, a diminished sodium load, and an increased bioavailability in CSF, amniotic fluid, and cord blood.

SPECTRUM OF ACTIVITY

Mezlocillin is fairly similar to carbenicillin and ticarcillin in its antibacterial spectrum with several important differences (21). It is more active against *Proteus* and *Enterobacter* strains. Mezlocillin is significantly more active than carbenicillin or ticarcillin against *K. pneumoniae* with nearly 75% of *Klebsiella* species susceptible. Mezlocillin is more active against enterococci and somewhat more active against *B. fragilis*. However, the majority of *S. aureus* strains are resistant.

Piperacillin demonstrates a wide spectrum of antibacterial activity (22, 23). Piperacillin is ac-

tive against most clinically important gram-negative facultative bacteria, especially indole-positive *Proteus* sp., *Klebsiella*, many *Serratia marcescens*, and *Pseudomonas aeruginosa*; *E. coli*, *Proteus mirabilis*, *Enterobacter*, *Citrobacter*, *Salmonella*, and *Shigella* species are sensitive to low concentrations of piperacillin. Piperacillin demonstrates activity against gram-positive aerobic bacteria, including the enterococcus. In addition, virtually all clinically important anaerobes, including *B. fragilis* and *B. bivius*, are sensitive to piperacillin. The drug is very active against *N. gonorrhoeae* (not PPNG strains).

The major defect in the spectrum of these agents is lack of coverage for *S. aureus*, 10% of *E. coli*, and some *Klebsiella* (especially with piperacillin which covers only half of *Klebsiella* strains).

DOSAGE AND ROUTE

Mezlocillin (Mezlin) may be administered intramuscularly or intravenously (preferred). The recommended adult dosage is 200–300 mg/kg/day which is usually given as 3 g intravenously every 4 hr (18 g/day). Up to 24 g/day may be given for severe infections. A 30-minute infusion of 3 g of mezlocillin results in peak serum concentrations of about 260 μg/ml, and by 1 hr and 4 hr the serum levels are 57 μg/ml and 4.4 μg/ml, respectively.

Piperacillin (Piperacil) is available for intramuscular or intravenous (preferred) administration. The usual adult dose is 3–4 g every 4–6 hr as an intravenous infusion (total 12–18 g/day). Following a 30-min intravenous infusion of 4 g piperacillin, peak serum levels of 215 μg/ml are reached; by 1 hr the level is 105 μg/ml, and it falls to 15 μg/ml by 4 hr.

SIDE EFFECTS

As with other penicillins, mezlocillin and piperacillin have been associated with hypersensitivity reactions, nausea, diarrhea, CNS irritability with large doses, and local reactions such as phlebitis.

A major advantage of mezlocillin and piperacillin over carbenicillin and ticarcillin is a significant decrease in sodium load. The ureidopenicillins contain 1.85 mEq/g of sodium compared to the 5.23 mEq/g for carbenicillin and 5.20 mEq/g for ticarcillin. This dramatically reduces the risk for congestive heart failure in patients with cardiovascular compromise.

COST

Both mezlocillin and piperacillin are expensive antimicrobial agents due to the need for large doses, frequent intravenous administration, and a moderately expensive per gram cost.

USE IN PREGNANCY

Because of altered protein binding, the ureidopenicillins are able to enter cord blood and amniotic fluid in therapeutic concentrations. The experience with these agents in pregnancy is very limited. In theory their broad spectrum of activity against Enterobacteriaceae, group B streptococcus and anaerobic bacteria including *B. bivius* make them excellent candidates for the treatment of chorioamnionitis. Being penicillins they are probably safe for use during pregnancy, but long-term follow-up studies are as of yet unavailable.

METABOLISM

As are other penicillins, both mezlocillin and piperacillin are primarily excreted by the kidneys. This is accomplished by both glomerular filtration and tubular secretion. Approximately 55% of a mezlocillin dose appears in urine within 6 hr and 26% is excreted in the bile. For piperacillin nearly 80% of a dose is excreted in urine within 24 hr. Excretion also occurs via the biliary route for piperacillin.

Both mezlocillin and piperacillin are widely distributed throughout body tissues. While little of either drug penetrates the CSF in normal patients, mezlocillin and piperacillin both achieve satisfactory levels in the CSF with inflamed meninges.

INDICATIONS IN OBSTETRICS AND GYNECOLOGY

The in vitro studies reviewed above suggested that mezlocillin or piperacillin might be effective single agents for the treatment of mixed aerobic-anaerobic soft tissue infection in the female pelvis. Preliminary clinical investigations have confirmed the efficacy of these agents in the treatment of such infections.

Sorrell and co-workers reported that mezlocillin cured 30 (91%) of 33 patients with postpartum endomyometritis compared to 30 (81%) of 37 patients treated with ampicillin (24). Sweet et al noted that piperacillin resulted in a clinical cure in 21 of 23 (91%) pelvic infections versus 23 of 25 (92%) of pelvic infections treated with cefoxitin; this study included patients with pelvic inflammatory disease (PID), endomyometritis, pelvic cellulitis, and tuboovarian abscess (23). Recently Eschenbach and co-workers, in a collaborative study, reported that 156 of 168 (93%) patients treated with piperacillin and 156 of 164 (95%) treated with a clindamycin plus gentamicin regimen were clinically cured (25). This study included patients with a variety of pelvic infections, such as endomyometritis, pelvic cellulitis, PID, tuboovarian abscess, and septic abortion.

While these preliminary studies are encouraging, they include a limited number of patients. More experience is required to determine if the use of mezlocillin or piperacillin as single agent therapy of mixed aerobic-anaerobic infections will be as equally efficacious as current standard single agent therapy, such as cefoxitin, or combination therapy, such as clindamycin plus aminoglycoside, in the treatment of such infections.

Both these agents have been used as prophylactic antibiotics in patients undergoing cesarean section or hysterectomy. The coverage of enterococcus and *P. aeruginosa* is a theoretic advantage for mezlocillin or piperacillin over commonly used cephalosporins or ampicillin in prophylactic attempts. However, they are significantly more costly than older drugs.

Amidino Penicillins

Mecillinam, although derived from the penicillin nucleus, 6-aminopenicillanic acid, is actually a new class of penicillins. Pivmecillinam is an ester of mecillinam, which is orally administered. These drugs are available in Europe, but at this date are undergoing clinical investigation in the United States.

SPECTRUM OF ACTIVITY

Mecillinam differs from most penicillins in its spectrum of activity. Unlike other penicillins, mecillinam has poor activity against gram-positive bacteria and is much more active against gram-negative organisms (26). Thus it is highly active against most Enterobacteriaceae including *E. coli*, *Klebsiella*, *Enterobacter*, *P. mirabilis*, *Proteus vulgaris*, and *Citrobacter*. Most *Serratia marcescens* are resistant, as are almost all *P. aeruginosa* and *B. fragilis*. Both *N. gonorrhoeae* and *H. influenzae* are significantly less susceptible to mecillinam than ampicillin. Interestingly, mecillinam acts synergistically with other β-lactam antibiotics—penicillins and cephalosporins—against most enterobacteriaceae.

DOSAGE AND ROUTE

Mecillinam is adminstered intramuscularly or intravenously. The dosage is 200–400 mg every 6 hr, but can be increased to 600 mg. Peak serum levels after 200 mg intravenous dose is 6.5 μg/ml which falls to 2 μg/ml by 1 hr.

Pivmecillinam is usually administered in 400-mg doses every 6 hr orally. Mean peak serum levels of 2.5 μg/ml are achieved 1.5 hr after administration of a 400 mg dose.

SIDE EFFECTS

Mecillinam use is associated with few toxic effects. Gastrointestinal side effects are uncommon, as are the penicillin-type hypersensitivity reactions.

COST

Not clinically available in the United States.

USE IN PREGNANCY

The use of mecillinam in pregnancy is not clear at this time. Animal studies suggest that it achieves low levels in the fetus.

METABOLISM

Mecillinam is excreted in the urine; 60% of parenterally administered and 40% of orally administered drug appear in the urine within 24 hr. The drug is also excreted in bile, where levels greater than those in serum are obtained.

INDICATIONS IN OBSTETRICS AND GYNECOLOGY

Little available information on the use of mecillinam in obstetrics and gynecology exists. Its major appeal would be as a safe β-lactam agent in the treatment of infections due to Enterobacteriaceae such as pyelonephritis as a single agent or in combination with drugs effective against gram-positive aerobes and anaerobic bacteria in mixed infections. The final answer must await such clinical trials.

CEPHALOTHIN, CEFAZOLIN, AND OTHER FIRST GENERATION CEPHALOSPORINS

The cephalosporin antibiotics make up an extensive group, all of which are comprised of a seven-aminocephalosporanic acid with a D-aminodipic acid side chain. Changes in the side chain of this molecule have led to the development of cephalothin (Keflin), cefazolin (Kefzol, Ancef), cephapirin (Cefadyl), cephalexin (Keflex), and other so called first generation cephalosporins. Because of similar properties, these antibiotics will be discussed as a group (1–3).

Spectrum of Activity

The cephalosporins are active against a wide variety of aerobic gram-positive organisms (including *S. aureus* but excluding the enterococcus) and *L. monocytogenes*. They also possess activity against *N. gonorrhoeae* and some aerobic gram-negative rods, including many strains of *E. coli*, most strains of *P. mirabilis* and *K. pneumoniae*, and some strains of *Salmonella*, *Shigella*, and *H. influenzae*. Resistant aerobic gram-negative organisms include *Enterobacter*, *Pseudomonas*, and *Serratia* species. Although many anaerobes are susceptible to older cephalosporins, other antibiotics are preferable because of their broader activity especially against the *Bacteroides* group.

The mechanism of action of cephalosporin antibiotics is quantitatively and qualitatively similar to that of penicillin. Cephalosporins interfere with the cell wall synthesis, resulting in the accumulation of nucleotides in the cell and the development of protoplasts.

Cephalothin, the first commercially available cephalosporin, is highly resistant to penicillinase, but a number of gram-negative organisms produce a cephalosporinase. *Chlamydia trachomatis* and the genital mycoplasms are resistant.

Dosage and Route

Four cephalosporin antibiotics, cephalexin (Keflex), cephradine (Cefadyl), cefaclor (Ceclor), and cefadroxil (Duracef) are absorbed orally. For adults, the usual dosage is 250 mg every 6 hr for cephalexin and cephradine and 1 g twice daily for cefadroxil. For cefaclor, the newest of these four agents, the dosage is 250 mg three times daily.

When parenteral cephalosporins are administered by either the intramuscular or intravenous route, they are readily absorbed and widely distributed. Cephalosporins are detectable in ascitic, synovial, and pericardial fluids.

Cephalothin (Keflin) may be administered intramuscularly or intravenously. After a 0.5-gm intramuscular injection, caphalothin achieves peak serum concentrations of approximately 20 μg/ml in 30 min. Within 4 hr, the serum concentration falls to 4 μg/ml. After a 2-gm intravenous injection, concentrations exceed 100 μg/ml within a few minutes, but are undetectable within 4 to 6 hr. Its serum half-life is 37 min. Susceptible organisms generally have MICs of less than 4 μg/ml. Depending on the type of infection, the dose of cephalothin may vary from 2 to 12 g/day.

Cefazolin (Ancef, Kefzol) may be administered by the intramuscular or intravenous route. Since serum concentrations of cefazolin are significantly higher than those of cephalothin, the usual dose is lower; namely, 1.5–6.0 g/day.

Cephradine (Anspor, Velosef) and cephapirin (Cefadyl) are administered by parenteral routes. Serum concentrations and doses are similar to those of cephalothin.

Since excretion of most cephalosporins is delayed in patients with diminished renal function, the dose should be decreased modestly for these persons. For example, for patients with moderate renal failure (creatinine clearance of 10–50 ml/min), the dose of cephalothin should be reduced to 1 g q 6–12 h. In severe renal failure (creatinine clearance < 10 ml/min), the dose should be 1 g q12h. Similar dosage adjustments should be made for related antibiotics. The "first generation" parenteral cephalosporins (cephalothin, cephaloridine, cefazolin, cephradine, and cephapirin) have similar antibacterial spectra. While slight differences may be observed in the activity of these antibiotics against particular strains, these differences appear not to be clinically significant. Although cefazolin achieves serum concentrations that are significantly higher than those of the other cephalosporins, all these compounds achieve concentrations adequate to inhibit most cephalosporin susceptible bacteria. It has been difficult to discern significant microbiologic or pharmacologic differences between these five parenteral cephalosporin compounds.

Side Effects

The cephalosporins are generally very well tolerated. Fever, eosinophilia, serum sickness, and skin rashes occur rarely, and transient neutropenia has been observed. Although Coombs positivity is commonly observed in patients receiving cephalosporins, particularly cephalothin, hemolytic anemia is extremely uncommon.

Pain on intramuscular injection is common with cephalothin, but uncommon with other cephalosporins. Phlebitis has been observed with intravenous administration of all the ceph-

alosporins. Cephaloridine is the only member of the "first generation" cephalosporins that may be associated with the production of significant nephrotoxicity. This occurs most commonly when the total daily dose of the drug exceeds 4 g but may be observed at lower dosage levels. For this reason, cephaloridine has been removed from most hospital formularies. Nephrotoxicity has been very rarely observed after administration of the other cephalosporins.

Cross-reactivity may exist between penicillins and cephalosporins (4). Although precise incidence data are not available, it has been observed that persons who have had an immediate hypersensitivity reaction to penicillin, as manifest by urticaria, wheezing, or anaphylaxis, are at greater risk for the development of similar reactions after cephalosporin administration. Cephalosporins are contraindicated in such individuals.

Cost

Although this group of antibiotics had been available for a number of years, there has been little reduction in price, and cephalosporin antibiotics remain costly, compared to penicillin and ampicillin.

Use in Pregnancy

To date, no adverse fetal effects have been reported for this group of antibiotics.

Placental Transfer

Cephalothin crosses the placenta rapidly after intravenous injection to the mother, attaining peak cord levels equal to approximately one-half of the maternal peak. As with ampicillin, detectable concentrations of cephalothin are not achieved in the amniotic fluid for a few hours.

Metabolism

Cephalosporins are excreted by the renal route. For cephalothin, the primary mode of excretion is tubular excretion, and excretion is delayed in the presence of diminished renal function. Approximately 55–65% of cephalothin is bound to protein. Cephalothin is also metabolized by esterases in the liver and other organs to a relatively inactive metabolite, desacetylcephalothin. Cephalothin may be removed by peritoneal dialysis in 48 hr.

Indications in Obstetrics and Gynecology

The cephalosporins have gained an important role in the practice of medicine, and they are the most commonly used group of antibiotics in hospitals in this country. In other specialties, they have been frequently used as prophylactic agents in cardiac, orthopedic, vascular, and gastrointestinal surgery. They are also active and effective agents in the treatment of staphylococcal and a limited number of gram-negative infections.

Yet, there are no situations in which they are clearly the drugs of choice. In most situations, other antibiotics are clearly preferable. Thus, for a penicillin-sensitive organism, penicillin should be used, and for treating infections caused by *S. aureus*, a penicillinase-resistant penicillin should be used.

In a number of situations, however, the "first generation" cephalosporin antibiotics are valuable. The first of these is in the patient with delayed typed penicillin hypersensitivity. A cephalosporin may be used safely in most of these patients in place of penicillin, ampicillin, or methicillin, oxacillin, cloxacillin, and nafcillin. The second situation is for prophylaxis in obstetric and gynecologic surgery. The rationale for using a cephalosporin antibiotics may be used in treating some urinary tract infections. Depending upon the susceptibility pattern of causative microorganism, a first generation cephalosporin may be a good choice for the empiric treatment of pyelonephritis in pregnancy. With rising resistance of bacteria to ampicillin, cephalosporins may offer a high degree of both efficacy and safety. In patients with severe pyelonephritis and shock or with multiple previous infections, a broader spectrum of therapy is indicated. Finally, a cephalosporin may be used in the initial treatment (with or without an aminoglycoside) of *postoperative* (or other hospital-acquired) pneumonia, since it may be caused by either gram-positive cocci or by gram-negative aerobes, particularly *Klebsiella* species.

CEFOXITIN AND CEFAMANDOLE— THE SECOND GENERATION CEPHALOSPORINS

These two agents became available in late 1978. Both have an extended spectrum of activity compared with previous cephalosporins. To be exact, cefoxitin is a cephamycin antibiotic, whereas cefamandole is a cephalosporin.

Spectrum of Activity (5, 6)

Like the penicillins and other cephalosporins, cefoxitin (Mefoxin) and cefamandole (Mandol) are bactericidal, inhibiting cell wall synthesis. For gram-positive aerobic organisms, the in vitro activity of both agents is equal to or less than that of older cephalosporins. In standard doses, both drugs inhibit most gram-positive organisms including *S. aureus*, but not enterococci.

Cefamandole and cefoxitin have wider activity against gram-negative aerobes than previous cephalosporins. *E. coli*, *Klebsiella* species, and *P. mirabilis* have usually been susceptible to cephalothin (Keflin), and these species show greater susceptibility to cefamandole and cefoxitin. Other *Proteus* and *Enterobacter* species have typically been resistant to older cephalosporins. Now many of these *Proteus* species are susceptible to both new antibiotics, and *Enterobacter* species are generally susceptible to cefamandole, but not to cefoxitin. However, emergence of resistance during therapy of organisms to cefamandole has been noted. In addition, *Pseudomonas* species are highly resistant to both of these new agents. *H. influenzae*, an organism rarely seen in obstetric and gynecologic infections, is inhibited by cefamandole. *N. gonorrhoeae*, including penicillinase-producing strains, are susceptible to cefoxitin.

Gram-positive anaerobic organisms are susceptible to both the agents as well as to penicillin and older cephalosporin antibiotics.

Against gram-negative anaerobes, cefoxitin clearly has better activity than older cephalosporins. Indeed, *in vitro* it inhibits 95% of strains of *B. fragilis* and has a resistance rate equivalent to clindamycin (7). Cefamandole is *not* so active against *B. fragilis* group as is cefoxitin, but in high dosages (12 g/day), it is possible to achieve levels of cefamandole that inhibit the majority of strains (8). This antibiotic is generally active against other strains of *Bacteroides*, as are other cephalosporins.

Susceptible organisms have MICs of less than 16 μg/ml, whereas intermediate organisms have MICs of 32 μg/ml.

As with older cephalosporins, *C. trachomatis* and the genital mycoplasmas are resistant.

Dosage and Route

Both these antibiotics are administered parenterally. For initial treatment of most infections with cefoxitin, the dosage is 1–2 g every 6 hr intravenously. For cefamandole, the comparable dose would be 2–3 g every 6 hr. At the lower range of these dosage ranges, these agents can be given intramuscularly.

Because both these agents are excreted mainly in the urine, the dose should be reduced somewhat in patients with renal impairment. For example, the dose for a patient with moderate renal failure (creatinine clearance of 10–50 ml/min) should be reduced to 1 g every 6–12 hr, and for a patient with severe renal failure (creatinine clearance < 10 ml/min) 1 g every 24 hr.

After a 1-g intravenous injection of either drug, peak levels average approximately 100 μg/ml in 0.5 hr, and concentrations fall to 1 μg/ml in about 3–4 hr.

Side Effects

Cefamandole and cefoxitin, like other cephalosporins, are generally well tolerated. (Please see above for comments on hypersensitivity, renal, liver, and hematologic effects of the cephalosporins.) One of the problems with some antibiotics in this class is local irritation on intramuscular or intravenous injection. In clinical trials, pain on intramuscular injection and thrombophlebitis on intravenous injection were reported infrequently (approximately 5 to 6% of the cases) with cefamandole. Pain on intramuscular injection is more common with cefoxitin, although it can be decreased by diluting the drug with 0.5% lidocaine solution.

Cost

Both agents are expensive and are considerably more costly per gram than old cephalosporins.

Use in Pregnancy and Placental Transfer

In patients undergoing midtrimester abortion, Giamarellou and colleagues studied the pharmacokinetics of cefoxitin (9). They noted that 1 hr after a 2-g IV infusion, mean maternal serum levels averaged 30 μg/ml, and by 6 hr after the infusion, the levels had fallen to 0.6 μg/ml. These levels were reported to be similar to those noted in nonpregnant women. Amniotic fluid of cefoxitin were 2–6 μg/ml between 1 and 5 hr after infusion.

Metabolism

As with other cephalosporins, these antibiotics are excreted mainly by the kidney. Approxi-

mately 75% of an intravenous dose can be recovered in the urine within 8 hr. Probenecid inhibits tubular secretion and results in higher blood levels.

Indications in Obstetrics and Gynecology

Because of its broader spectrum including many anaerobic gram-negative rods, cefamandole has been evaluated as a single agent for the treatment of a variety of polymicrobial obstetric-gynecologic infections. Using 12 g/day, Gibbs and Huff evaluated cefamandole in 43 cases of endomyometritis after cesarean section and found an 85% cure rate (8). Cunningham et al used the same dose in 95 women with various pelvic infections and reported a cure rate of 90% (10). In a small series of 20 cases, Gall and Hill found an overall cure of 85% in cases of endomyometritis or pelvic inflammatory disease (11).

In 1982, Gibbs and colleagues repeated a double-blind comparison of clindamycin-gentamicin versus cefamandole (8 g/day) in 198 patients with endomyometritis after cesarean section (12). If one excluded the side effect failures, the cure rate for cefamandole was 85% (76/89), which was less than the 93% (93/99) cure rate for clindamycin-gentamicin (p = 0.06).

In view of its moderate activity against the *B. fragilis* group and its modest record in clinical trials, cefamandole cannot be recommended for single agent therapy in polymicrobial, pelvic infections.

The extended activity of cefoxitin to include 95% of *B. fragilis* group isolates has made it more attractive for single agent therapy. In 1979, Sweet and Ledger evaluated use of 2 g q8H in 109 patients with genital infection (13). The overall cure rate was 92% (100 of 109). Included were seven patients with pelvic abscess, only three of which were cured. For salpingitis, endomyometritis and pelvic abscess, cure rates were 97%, 92%, and 89%, respectively. In a similar report, Ledger and Smith noted a 94% cure rate in 178 patients treated with cefoxitin for a variety of genital tract infections (14). Recently, Sweet and colleagues compared cefoxitin (2 g IV q6h) to piperacillin (4.5 g IV q6h) in a total of 48 pateints (15). Of the 25 treated with cefoxitin, 23 (92%) were cured; both failures resulted from tuboovarian abscess. The cure rate in the piperacillin group was 91% (21 of 23).

However, cefoxitin has not led to high cure rates in other studies. Duff and co-workers compared cefoxitin (2 g IV q8h) to penicillin plus gentamicin (16). For cefoxitin, the cure rate was only 61% (19/31), and for penicillin-gentamicin it was 63% (27/43). In this study, the authors used a lower dose of cefoxitin, encountered a large number of abscesses, and decided upon success or failure of therapy at 48 hr. An intermediate cure rate was reported by Hager and McDaniel who treated 25 cases of pelvic infection with cefoxitin (2 g IV q6h) (17). The response rate was 84% (21 of 25). Of the four failures, three required surgical drainage, and the fourth showed a response to clindamycin plus gentamicin.

Because of its activity against *N. gonorrhoeae*, including penicillinase-producing species, cefoxitin has been recommended by the Centers for Disease Control as part of combination therapy for pelvic inflammatory disease (18).

Although cefoxitin has been shown to be effective for prophylaxis, it has no advantage compared to older, less expensive agents such as cefazolin (19). Because cefoxitin may be used for therapy and it is more expensive than older agents, its use for prophylaxis is not recommended.

In summary, cefoxitin has an excellent spectrum for treating pelvic infections. It is well tolerated and achieves high concentrations in serum. In most clinical trials, its efficacy has been good, except in cases of pelvic abscess, but results have not been uniform. Overall, though, cefoxitin when used in a dose of 8 g/day would seem to be a reasonable initial choice for pelvic infections such as endomyometritis, salpingitis, and cuff cellulitis after hysterectomy.

THE THIRD GENERATION CEPHALOSPORINS

This new group of antibiotics is made up for a number of parenteral agents with an even more extended spectrum of activity (20). Technically, not all of these agents are true cephalosporins. For example, moxalactam has an oxygen atom in place of the sulfur in dihydrothiazolidine ring. Yet, in common usage, the term cephalosporins is applied to the entire group. Modification of the side chains provides these new antibiotics with changes in spectrum and alterations in metabolism.

Spectrum of Activity

Although all these new compounds possess very broad activities, they should not be considered to be interchangeable. Especially in regard to the array of organisms involved in pelvic infections, there are important in vitro differences in activity.

For aerobic streptococci, these agents have activity which is inferior to penicillin G or ampicillin. Within the group of third generation cephalosporins, cefotaxime has greater intrinsic activity than do cefoperazone and ceftazidime, which, in turn, have somewhat better activity than moxalactam. Yet, with usual doses, all of these agents provide sufficient coverage for all aerobic streptococci except enterococci.

For *S. aureus*, an antistaphlylococcal penicillin (such as nafcillin) or a first generation cephalosporin (cephalothin or cefazolin) would be preferable, as the newer agents have 10- to 80-fold less activity. The MIC_{90} values for these new agents range from 2 to 16 $\mu g/ml$, compared to 0.2 $\mu g/ml$ for cefazolin, but satisfactory coverage is still supplied by usual doses of the new antibiotics. Methicillin-resistant staphylococci are not susceptible to the new agents.

Activity against *N. gonorrhoeae* is excellent with MIC_{90} values less than 0.1 $\mu g/ml$ for cefotaxime, ceftazidime, cefoperazone, and moxalactam. All of these inhibit penicillinase-producing species.

Activity of these agents against aerobic gram-negative rods is impressive. MIC_{90} values of most of these agents for *E. coli*, *K. pneumoniae*, and *P. mirabilis* are less than 0.5 $\mu g/ml$, but for cefoperazone the MIC_{90} is 16 $\mu g/ml$ for the first two species. *Enterobacter* species have higher MIC_{90} values, but these are generally within the susceptible range. The exception is that for *E. cloacoe* the MIC_{90} of cefoperazone is 32 $\mu g/ml$. Many of aminoglycoside-resistant strains are susceptible to low concentrations of these new cephalosporins. *P. aeruginosa* occurs infrequently in pelvic infections, and activity of these new agents varies widely. Ceftazidime is the most active ($MIC_{90} = 8$ $\mu g/ml$), with cefoperazone and moxalactam having moderate activity ($MIC_{90} = 32$ $\mu g/ml$). For cefotaxime, the MIC_{90} is 64 $\mu g/ml$. Other *Pseudomonas* species are likely to be resistant.

Gram-positive anaerobes are inhibited by these new agents. MIC_{90} values for anaerobic staphylococci and streptococci were less than 1 $\mu g/ml$ (22, 22). Clostridial species usually have low MICs (28).

Among the anaerobic gram-negative species, *B. bivius* and *B. disiens* are inhibited by 4–8 $\mu g/ml$ of moxalactam, cefoperazone, and cefotaxime, but the *B. fragilis* group has a more variable response. Tally and co-workers found that only 65% of stains were inhibited by 32 μg cefotaxime and cefoperazone (7). For moxalactam, 88% of strain were inhibited by 32 $\mu g/ml$. For comparison, clindamycin, metronidazole, and chloramphenicol inhibited 90% of *B. fragilis* group strains with 2, 8, and 1 μg/ml, respectively. Tally and colleagues found that cefoxitin inhibited 92% of these strains at 16 μg/ml and 98% at 32 μg/ml (7).

Susceptibility testing of anaerobes may vary with inoculum size and media used, however. Jorgensen and colleagues used a medium proposed by the National Committee for Clinical Laboratory Standards and found moxalactam to have greater activity than cefoxitin against *B. fragilis* group isolates and considerably greater activity than cefotaxime and cefoperazone (22).

In general the activity of these new drugs versus anaerobes may be summarized as follows:

1. Moxalactam and cefoxitin, a second generation cephalosporin, have the best activity against the *B. fragilis* group;
2. All possess good activity against anaerobic cocci and *Bacteroides* species other than *B. fragilis*;
3. Clindamycin, metronidazole, and chloramphenicol have superior intrinsic activity against anaerobes

None of these agents are active against either *C. trachomatis* or the genital mycoplasmas.

Dosage, Route, and Metabolism

These drugs are available only for parenteral administation. They possess different routes of metabolism and different half-lives.

Cefotaxime has a relatively short half-life of 1 hr and should be administered every 6–8 hr. After a 2 g infusion over 30 min, peak levels of 80–90 μg/ml are attained. By 6 hr, the levels are approximately 5 μg/ml. It is excreted mainly in the kidney, by tubular excretion as well as glomerular filtration. In renal insufficiency, cefotaxime does not accumulate, but the desacetyl derivative which is not active biologically has a longer half-life.

Cefoperazone has a longer half-life of 1.6–2.4 hr. After a 2-g IV dose, serum levels equal 250 μg/ml. At 12 hr, levels are 1–2 μg/ml. Accordingly, cefoperazone has been used with dosing every 8 or 12 hr. In contrast to most cephalosporins, this agent is cleared mainly by biliary excretion and does not accumulate in patients with renal failure.

Moxalactam's pharmacokinetics are similar to those of cefoperazone. For moxalactam, the serum half-life is approximately 2 hr. After a 2-g infusion, the peak serum level is approximately 200 μg/ml, and at 12 hr the level is still 2–4 μg/ml. Unlike cefoperazone, however, moxalactam is cleared by the kidney. In patients with renal impairments excretion is decreased. For example, with a creatinine clearance of 10–30 ml/min, the half-life is 8.5 hr. Dosing should be decreased accordingly. Moxalactam should be administered every 8 to 12 hr.

Cost

All of these new agents have a high direct cost per gram. However, because of less frequent doses and safety, they probably have lower indirect costs (pharmacy and nursing time, tests to monitor safety, etc.). Total cost of antibiotic administration varies widely.

Use in Pregnancy and Placental Transfer

Data are becoming available. Bawdon and colleagues performed a study of placental transfer of moxalactam in 28 women undergoing cesarean section (23). In this single dose, single measurement experiment, they measured antibiotic levels by high pressure liquid chromatography and found that maternal levels at a mean of 48 min after infusion were 62 μg/ml. Corresponding cord levels were 22 μg/ml (36% of the maternal level). Evaluating placental transfer of cefotaxime, Kafetzis and colleagues repeated serum levels in women undergoing midtrimester abortion of 8.2 μg/ml at 1 hr after a 1-g IV infusion and 0.9 μg/ml at 3 hr after infusion (24). The corresponding mean cord level at 1 hr was 1.9 μg/ml (23% of maternal levels). The serum levels were less than expected for a nonpregnant woman. Cefotaxime was also found in breast milk in low concentrations (mean 0.35 μg/ml) (24). In midtrimester patients, Giamarillou and co-workers studied the kinetics of moxalactam and ceftazidime (2 g and 1 g infusion, respectively) (15). For moxalactam the mean serum level 1 hr after infusion was 38 μg/ml, and at 6 hr after infusion it was 2.7 μg/ml. These levels are lower than expected in nonpregnant women. Moxalactam was detectable within the amniotic fluid within 2 hr after the infusion (range 3–15 μg/ml), and after 6 hr, levels were in therapeutic range for many bacteria (range 1.5–6.5 μg/ml). For ceftazidime, peak values occurred 2 hr after the infusion and were equal to 13.2 μg/ml. At 6 hr after infusion, the serum levels averaged 1.9 μg/ml. In amniotic fluid, ceftazidime levels ranged from 1–4 μg/ml from 2 to 6 hr after infusion.

Side Effects

In general, adverse effects with these new agents are similar to those seen with older cephalosporins, but there have been several special problems (20). Allergic reactions, skin rashes, and local pain have been reported infrequently. They probably occur in a similar frequency as seen with first generation cephalosporin, but comparative studies have not been performed.

Diarrhea has been observed in 1–7% of patients receiving these compounds. Enterocolitis due to *Clostridium difficile* has been reported (20). Because cefoperazone is mainly excreted into the bile, it might be anticipated that it would cause diarrhea more often, but this has not been the case.

Two special adverse effects have been seen with some of these new antibiotics (25). Bleeding has been reported in patients receiving moxalactam or cefoperazone. In preclinical trials, 2.5% of patients treated with moxalactam developed clinical bleeding. Extensive evaluation led to recognition of three mechanisms. The most common was hypoprothrombinemia, which is preventable by a weekly injection of vitamin K (10 mg) during therapy. A platelet dysfunction and rarely an immune thrombocytopenia may also occur. Bleeding due to moxalactam developed generally in patients with the following risk factors: renal or liver disease, poor nutrition, use of anticoagulants or aspirin, or thrombocytopenia. Obstetric-gynecologic patients would rarely have any of these risk factors. In addition, it has been observed that bleeding could be prevented by avoiding use of more than 4 gm/day for *more than* 3 days. The package insert for moxalactam carries a warning regarding these measures.

Also seen with moxalactam and cefoperazone has been a disulfiram reaction (25), i.e., acute alcohol intolerance due to inhibition of acetaldehyde dehydrogenase. This reaction has been seen in patients taking the antibiotics before alcohol, but not in intoxicated individuals who are treated with these antibiotics.

Other adverse effects including mild elevation of liver enzymes and neutropenia have occurred infrequently and have been mild and transient.

Because of their very broad spectra, superinfection may result. Enterococcal and candidal infections have been reported, but the incidence is low. In obstetric-gynecologic patients, especially those who develop infection after prophylaxis with a first-generation cephalosporin, enterococci are isolated frequently, usually in mixed culture. Nevertheless, most of these patients respond promptly to these new antibiotics. Development of resistance during therapy has been seen with *P. aeruginosa* and *E. cloacae*. In debilitated patients, this has led to failure of therapy. In obstetric-gynecologic patients, colonization with resistant organisms has been noted with other antibiotics, but in healthy patients receiving short courses of therapy, poor clinical response has not been attributed to development of resistance. When response has not been satisfactory and when enterococci are present, it is appropriate to use antibiotic therapy active against this organism.

Indications in Obstetrics and Gynecology

In view of their broad in vitro activity, these agents have been used in a number of trials as single agent therapy in pelvic infections.

Of these newer compounds, the one most thoroughly evaluated in obstetrical-gynecological infections is moxalactam. As shown in Table 19.4, reported experience includes over 200 cases in which a consistent cure rate of approximately 90% has been achieved (26–28). It is of special interest that Cunningham and colleagues evaluated both 3 and 6 g/day. Among 36 patients treated with the lower dose (1 g IV q8h), there were 5 failures (14%), four of which required laparotomy. In view of this experience and the relatively high MIC_{90} values for *B. fragilis*, it seems wise to initiate therapy with greater than 3 g/day when moxalactam is used. In a double-blind comparison of moxalactam (6 g/day) to clindamycin-gentamicin, Gibbs and colleagues found the regimens to be equivalent (28).

Cefotaxime has been evaluated by Hemsell and colleagues (29). As with moxalactam, a higher cure rate has been seen with 6 than with 3 g/day (97 versus 84%, $p < 0.05$). Of the total of 143 women treated with the larger doses, there were 5 failures. Of these, two responded to the addition of other antibiotics, and three required surgical drainage. In one phase of these studies, cefotaxime was compared to clindamycin plus gentamicin. No difference in rates was found.

This same group of investigators have evaluated cefotaxime in 53 cases of pelvic inflammatory disease and 21 posthysterectomy infections.

Table 19.4
Clinical Trials with Newer Cephalosporin Antibiotics

Drug	Author, references	No.	Dose (g/day)	Kind of infection	Cure rate (%)	Comment
Cefoxitin	Sweet and Ledger (13)	109	6	Various	92	
	Ledger and Smith (14)	178	—[a]	Various	94	
	Duff and Keiser (16)	31	6	Various	61	Comparison to penicillin-gentamicin
	Hager and McDaniel (17)	25	8	Various	84	
	Sweet et al (15)	25	8	Various	92	
Moxalactam	Gibbs et al (26)	62	6	Endometritis	90	
	Cunningham et al (27)	36	3	Various	86	
		43	6		91	
	Gibbs et al (28)	56	6	Endometritis	96	Comparison to clindamycin-gentamicin
Cefotaxime	Hemsell et al (29)	55	3	Endometritis	84	
		143	6	Endometritis	97	Comparison to clindamycin-gentamicin in part
Cefoperazone	Strausbaugh and Llorens (31)	107	4	Various	91	
Ceftazidime	Blanco et al (32)	38	6	Endometritis	90	Comparison to clindamycin-gentamicin

[a] Not stated.

The cure rate was 96% for PID and 100% for the 21 other infections (30).

Cefoperazone has been reported in the therapy of 107 obstetric-gynecologic infections (31). It had a very good overall cure rate (91%), and adverse effects were infrequent (4%).

Ceftazidime has been compared to clindamycin-gentamicin in treatment of 77 cases of endometritis after cesarean section (32). The cure rates were 90 and 87% respectively (32).

As noted earlier in this chapter, there are other determinants of the outcome of a clinical study besides the spectra of activity of the drugs tested. Accordingly, it it not surprising that the overall cure rates for all of these agents are closely lumped together at approximately 90–95%.

In general, none of these agents has so extensive a spectrum of activity to warrant its use in septic shock or similar serious infections. When the organism is known, other antibiotics would often be preferable as in staphylococcal or streptococcal wound infections. Although these agents may be effective for prophylaxis, there is no evidence that they are more effective than older, less expensive antibiotics. Indeed, it seems unwise to use them for prophylaxis.

Accordingly, some of these agents would seem to be reasonable choices in the moderate, polymicrobial infections commonly seen on obstetric-gynecologic services. These infections would include endometritis after cesarean section and pelvic cellulitis after hysterectomy.

For PID, all of these agents yield a high immediate cure rate especially in patients without a tuboovarian abscess. Yet, because none of these antibiotics is active against *C. trachomatis*, other agents would be needed in addition. Although it is not possible to discern a differential effect from clinical studies, the newer cephalosporins with somewhat better spectra are cefoxitin and moxalactam in preference to cefotaxime and cefoperazone. Side effects in obstetric and gynecologic patients are seen infrequently and are mild, by and large.

Cost of these agents is considerable. Decisions regarding use of these versus a more familiar combination with an excellent efficacy (such as clindamycin-gentamicin) must take this aspect into consideration.

MONOBACTAMS (AZTREONAM AND RELATED ANTIBIOTICS)

This class of new antibiotics resembles the cephalosporins, but has only one ring. Aztreonam, a representative member, has an unusual spectrum. It is mainly active against the aerobic gram-negative rods. Yet, like the cephalosporins and penicillins, it has a wide margin of safety and readily achieves therapeutic levels. Hence, the potential advantage of these antibiotics would be to provide an alternative to the aminoglycosides as drugs of choice in treating gram negative infections. In the empiric treatment of pelvic infections, however, aztreonam must be combined with an agent such as clindamycin to provide anaerobic and gram-positive activity.

Clinical trials were reported in 1984. In treating endometritis, Gibbs and colleagues compared aztreonam (2 g IV q8h) with gentamicin (1.5 mg/kg IV q8h), each given with clindamycin (33). Both regimens were highly efficacious and well tolerated. Yet, it should be remembered that obstetric and gynecologic patients are usually at low risk for aminoglycoside toxicity, and that new antibiotics are likely to be considerably more expensive than the aminoglycosides. Potential benefits of the monobactams will have to be weighed against their cost and the risks of other antibiotics used along with them.

THIENAMYCIN (IMIPEMIDE)

At this writing, this is an investigational antibiotic, but it has an extraordinary antibacterial spectrum. Previously known as MK0787, it has been recognized for its activity for a number of years but has been unstable. A new derivative N-formimidoyl thienamycin has resolved this problem.

At low concentrations, this compound is active against gram-positive cocci including S. aureus (even methicillin-resistant isolates), S. pneumoniae, and groups A and B streptococci. The MIC_{90} values for enterococci was only 1 μg/ml. Against aerobic gram-negative rods, it has a very broad activity including Enterobacter, S. marcescens, and P. aeruginosa (MIC_{90} of 4 μg/ml) (34). Against B. fragilis isolates, its in vitro activity was similar to that of clindamycin (35).

Its clinical efficacy has been reported in abstracts in 1983. Initial doses in obstetric-gynecologic infection is 500 mg IV q6h. In a preliminary series, Berkeley and colleagues presented data on 24 cases collected at three institutions. There were 22 complete cures (92%), and 1 patient was improved and discharged on oral antibiotics. The one patient who had a nonsuccessful response to thienamycin did respond to a combination antibiotic regimen (36).

More complete clinical trials will be welcome in view of the activity of this antibiotic.

TETRACYCLINE

Since the introduction of chlortetracycline in 1944, numerous tetracycline compounds have been developed. These agents have a similar molecular structure consisting of four benzene rings and, generally, the same spectrum of activity. The tetracyclines are primarily bacteriostatic. There are two major groups of tetracycline which are based on pharmacokinetic properties: short acting compounds of which tetracycline HCl is the prototype and long acting compounds, doxycycline and minocycline.

Spectrum of Activity

Tetracyclines have a broad spectrum of activity that includes gram-positive, gram-negative, aerobic and anaerobic bacteria, spirochetes, chlamydiae, mycoplasmas, rickettsiae, and even some protozoa. The antimicrobial spectra of all tetracyclines are similar. However, some differences do exist in the degree of activity against these microorganisms. In general, the MIC of tetracycline HCl is two- to four-fold higher against many bacteria than those of doxycycline or minocycline (1).

Tetracyclines are active against S. pneumoniae, many H. influenzae and S. pyogenes. With the exception of minocycline, tetracyclines are not very effective against S. aureus. None of the tetracyclines is effective against the enterococci.

N. gonorrhoeae and N. meningitidis are generally susceptible to tetracyclines. However, gonococci resistant to penicillin are likely to be resistant to tetracyclines; approximately 50% of penicillinase-producing N. gonorrhoeae are resistant to tetracycline as well (2). Tetracyclines are active against Enterobacteriaceae such as E. coli (especially community acquired), Enterobacter, and Klebsiella.. However, many Enterobacteriaceae acquire tetracycline resistance.

While the tetracyclines inhibit the growth of many anaerobic bacteria, their activity is not comparable to agents such as clindamycin, chloramphenicol, or metronidazole. In particular, less than half of B. fragilis are sensitive to tetracycline; doxycylcine and minocycline are somewhat more active (3). Tetracyclines (tetracycline HCl, doxycycline, and minocycline) are the drugs of choice against C. trachomatis, mycoplasmas (both Mycoplasma hominis, Ureaplasma urealyticum, and M. pneumoniae), and rickettsia.

Tetracyclines enter the bacterial organism where they bind reversibly to the 30-S ribosomal unit of susceptible organisms. As a result polypeptide synethesis is inhibited.

Dosage and Route

Tetracycline HCl, doxycycline, and minocycline are available for administration by the oral, intramuscular, and intravenous routes. The tetracyclines are most commonly administered orally. The available oral preparations include: (a) the short acting drugs chlortetracycline (Aureomycin), oxytetracycline (Terramycin), and tetracycline (Achromycin); (b) the intermediate drugs methacycline (Rondomycin) and demeclocycline (Declomycin); and (c) the long acting forms doxycycline (Vibramycin) and minocycline (Minocin).

Of the short acting forms the most commonly used agent is tetracycline, which is the one that is best absorbed, obtains the highest serum levels and is the least costly. The usual adult oral dose is 500 mg every 6 hr. Absorption takes place in the proximal small bowel. Peak serum levels of 4 μg/ml are reached 1–3 hr after oral administration of a 500-mg dose of tetracycline (4). Following a 500-mg oral dose, oxytetracycline reaches a peak serum level of 2–3 μg/ml and chlortetracycline, 1–2 μg/ml.

For doxycycline the usual adult oral dosage is a single dose of 200 mg (or 100 mg every 12 hr) on day one of treatment, followed by a maintenance dose of 100 mg/day. A commonly used alternative is to use 100 mg every 12 hr as the maintenance dose. Doxycycline is almost completely absorbed in the proximal bowel following oral administration. The serum half-life is 18–22 hr. Following an oral dose of 200 mg, peak serum levels of 2–4 μg/ml are attained. Minocycline, like doxycycline, is basically completely absorbed after oral administration, and after a loading dose of 200 mg reaches peak serum levels of 2–4 μg/ml.

Although available, intramuscular forms of the tetracyclines are irritating and rarely used. After intravenous administration of 500 mg of tetracycline, serum levels reach about 8 μg/ml at 30 min and decrease to 2–3 μg/ml by 5 hr. Intravenous doxycycline or minocycline in a dose of 200 mg produces a serum level of 4 μg/ml at 30 min.

Food of any type markedly reduces the absorption of tetracycline, oxytetracycline, or chlortetracycline. These short-acting agents also have a marked affinity for divalent cations (calcium, magnesium, aluminum) to which they bind and chelate and thus are excreted in the feces.

Side Effects

The tetracyclines are relatively safe agents, but may be associated with local and systemic untoward effects. Allergic reactions including rash, urticaria, and anaphylaxis occur but are uncommon. Photosensitivity reactions associated with onycholysis occur in areas exposed to sunlight. These drugs are irritating and frequently oral administration produces gastrointestinal symptoms such as nausea, vomiting, and epigastric distress. Diarrhea (including pseudomembranous colitis) may develop, especially with the forms which are poorly absorbed (i.e., chlortetracycline and oxytetracycline).

Secondary infection with *Candida albicans* is a frequent complication of tetracycline treatment. Tetracycline is deposited in the deciduous teeth of children early in life or if they were exposed as a fetus. The period of mineralization of the decidual teeth commences during the midtrimester of pregnancy and ends at 2–3 months after birth. Exposure to tetracycline during this time period results in yellow discoloration of the "baby" teeth. If tetracyclines are administered to children less than age 6, a lifelong discoloration of the permanent teeth may occur. The deposition of tetracycline in the bones of infants causes temporary inhibition of bone growth.

A dose-related hepatotoxiticy occurs, especially during the third trimester of pregnancy, with doses greater than 2 gm intravenously of tetracycline. It appears pathologically as "fatty liver" of pregnancy and is associted with a high mortality rate (5). Tetracycline therapy may result in nephrotoxicity as well, either as a result of "acute fatty liver" or by a direct toxic renal effect that aggravates preexisting renal failure. The latter phenomenon results from tetracycline's ability to inhibit protein synthesis, which increases the azotemia from amino acid metabolism.

Minocycline, but not the other tetracyclines, can cause vestibular disturbances with dizziness, ataxia, vertigo, and tinnitus. It is reversible when the drug is stopped. This side effect is much more common in women than men, occurring in 50–70% of women receiving minocycline.

Cost

Tetracycline is a relatively inexpensive antibiotic. Chlortetracycline, oxytetracycline, doxycycline, and minocycline are considerably more costly for a 7- to 10-day oral course of treatment.

Use in Pregnancy and Placental Transfer

Tetrcyclines cross the placenta and are deposited in decidual teeth and growth centers of long bones with resultant discoloration of decidual teeth and inhibition of bone growth. Thus tetracyclines are best not used in pregnancy unless alternative drug(s) are not available.

Metabolism

All the tetracyclines are excreted by the kidneys via glomerular filtration. Nearly 20% of an orally administered dose of tetracyclines is excreted in the urine, while about 50% of a parenterally administered tetracycline is excreted in the urine within 24 hr. Tetracyclines are also excreted in the bile, but a large proportion of this is reabsorbed from the intestine. Except for doxycycline and minocycline, tetracyclines are incompletely absorbed from the gastrointestinal tract, and this unabsorbed drug is excreted in the feces.

Indications in Obstetrics and Gynecology

As a general rule tetracyclines should not be administered to pregnant or lactating women. The major indication for tetracycline in gynecology practice is the treatment of *C. trachomatis* infections, either singly or in combination with other agents depending upon the clinical setting (see Chapters 3, 4, and 8). In nonpregnant patients allergic to penicillin, it is the alternative drug for the treatment of syphilis and/or gonorrhea.

Tetracyclines are the drug of choice against *M. hominis* and ureaplasma, but their role as pathogens in nonpregnant patients remains unclear (see Chapter 7).

CLINDAMYCIN

Clindamycin (Cleocin) which is derived from lincomycin, is a macrolide antibiotic. Because of its spectrum of activity, clindamycin is important in treating pelvic infections.

Spectrum of Activity

Clindamycin attaches to the 50-S ribosome and inhibits bacterial protein synthesis. It is bacteriostatic. Against gram-positive aerobic organisms, clindamycin has wide activity, including *S. aureus*, but excluding enterococci (*Strep-

tococcus faecalis). *N. gonorrhoeae* is often resistant, and the entire group of aerobic gram-negative bacilli is also highly resistant.

Its activity against the anaerobic organisms provides clindamycin with its main value. With the exception of a very few strains of *Clostridium* sp., and a few percent of strains of *Bacteroides* species, anaerobic organisms are susceptible to this antibiotic. Clindamycin is one of the few drugs to which *B. fragilis* and related species are highly sensitive. Approximately 7% of strains had MIC values in the resistant range (4 μg/ml), and there has been little change in recent years (1). Clindamycin is active against *M. hominis* but not *U. urealyticum*. Although erythromycin, another macrolide antibiotic, is active against *C. trachomatis*, clindamycin in relatively low doses has not been effective clinically. However, in vitro testing demonstrates good efficacy.

The minimal inhibitory concentration for susceptible organisms varies from 0.01 to 4 μg/ml.

Dosage and Route

Clindamycin may be administered intravenously, intramuscularly, or orally. For intravenous or intramuscular administration, clindamycin phosphate is used. For initial treatment of serious infections, the dosage for intravenous injection is usually 600 mg every 6–8 hr by "piggyback" injection with an infusion over 30 min. After a 300-mg infusion over 30 min, serum levels peak at 12–15 μg/ml and fall to 5 μg/ml in 2–3 hr. For intramuscular injection, the maximum dosage is 300–600 mg every 8 hr. For oral administration, clindamycin hydrochloride is used, in a dosage of 150–300 mg every 6 hr. Gastrointestinal absorption is impaired with food in the stomach. No reduction is necessary for patients in renal failure, unless it is severe. For patients with liver disease, the dose should be decreased, however.

Side Effects

GASTROINTESTINAL SYMPTOMS

Nausea, vomiting, and particularly diarrhea occur fairly commonly during clindamycin therapy. The incidence of diarrhea varies widely in large series but in obstetric-gynecologic patients the incidence has been from 2 to 6%.

PSEUDOMEMBRANOUS COLITIS

Pseudomembranous colitis (PMC) is suggested when diarrhea, abdominal cramps, and fever develop. Using clinical criteria only, however, it is not possible to distinguish PMC from nonspecific colitis, antibiotic-associated diarrhea, or other diarrheal disorders. The diagnosis of PMC is made by proctoscopic examination during which typical raised, yellow-white plaques ("pseudomembranes") are observed in an edematous, erythematous mucosa. Microscopically, the plaques consist of mucin, fibrin, white blood cells, and epithelial cells. The proctoscopic examination is so characteristic that biopsy and histologic examination are usually unnecessary.

Much attention has been directed at the association of PMC and clindamycin usage (2–6). Yet, pseudomembranous enterocolitis was first reported in the 1890s in postoperative patients, many of whom had developed hypotension. PMC has been reported as a complication with a variety of broad spectrum antibiotics, including tetracycline, ampicillin, and the cephalosporin antibiotics in addition to clindamycin. In 1975 two deaths from pseudomembranous colitis were reported in obstetric and gynecologic patients, neither of whom had received clindamycin when their symptoms developed (7).

The frequency of pseudomembranous colitis may be greater with clindamycin than with other antibiotics. The ranges are highly variable, with a reasonable estimate being 1 in 10,000. Pseudomembranous colitis may develop more commonly after oral administration.

The occurrence of cases in conjunction with clindamycin has prompted an intense effort to uncover the mechanism. Based on a hamster model, investigators have shown that pseudomembranous colitis may be caused by a toxin elaborated by *C. difficile*, an infrequent organism of the human gut. This species is resistant to clindamycin and many other antibiotics. Thus, a variety of antibiotics may eliminate susceptible intestinal organisms and allow *C. difficile*, if present, to proliferate and to elaborate its toxin. *C. difficile* may be isolated from stool culture, and an assay for the toxin is available in many hospital laboratories. The assay is positive in nearly all patients with *C. difficile* enterocolitis, but may also be positive in some patients with nonspecific colitis (i.e., without pseudomembranes) or in a small percent of patients with simple antibiotic-associated diarrhea. The organism is susceptible to vancomycin.

If a patient develops diarrhea (more than four or five loose stools per day) while receiving antibiotics, especially clindamycin, she is evaluated closely. We stop suppositories and laxatives and next discontinue clindamycin. If treatment of the *B. fragilis* group is still needed, we will empirically replace it with an alternative agent such as metronidazole or chloramphenicol. Lomotil and related compounds should be avoided. If the diarrhea does not stop within 24 hr proctoscopy is in order.

If pseudomembranous colitis is then diagnosed on proctoscopic examination, antibiotic therapy must be discontinued promptly. Continued use of antibiotics has been shown to prolong the course of the colitis and to worsen the prognosis. Vigorous supportive therapy is essential, but use of Lomotil is dangerous. Oral vancomycin appears to alleviate acute symptoms, but recurrences may develop.

OTHER SIDE EFFECTS

For the most part, other adverse reactions to clindamycin are rare. Minor elevations in liver function tests (particularly SGOT) occur in a small percent of patients.

Cost

Both the oral and parenteral preparations of clindamycin are expensive agents.

Use in Pregnancy

Although clindamycin carries the standard FDA warning that safety of the use of this drug in pregnancy has not been established, there is indirect evidence, that it is probably safe. In a long-term, prospective evaluation of lincomycin in pregnancy, no adverse fetal effects were noted (8). In view of the close structural similarity of lincomycin and clindamycin, the latter is probably also a relatively safe agent. Thus, pregnancy should not be considered a contraindication to the appropriate use of clindamycin, but there are few infections requiring clindamycin with an intact pregnancy.

Placental Tranfer

After intravenous administration to the mother at term, clindamycin rapidly appears in the cord blood (9). Peak levels are achieved within 20 min and are approximately 40% of peak maternal levels. Clindamycin did not appear in the amniotic fluid in detectable concentrations during the 1st hour after maternal injection. In studies of midtrimester pregnancies, oral clindamycin when given to the mother resulted in detectable levels in a variety of fetal tissues and in amniotic fluid (10). The liver showed the highest clindamycin concentration.

Metabolism

Clindamycin is removed from the body largely by direct excretion in the bile. A smaller amount is excreted by the kidney, and some is also inactivated in the body, probably in the liver.

Indications in Obstetrics and Gynecology

Clindamycin is a potent and valuable antibiotic, but its use has been accompanied on rare occasion by serious adverse effects. Parenteral clindamycin is indicated in the initial treatment (before cultures are available) of pelvic infections such as endometritis, pelvic cellulitis after hysterectomy, tuboovarian abscess, and pelvic abscess. Because these infections are polymicrobial, clindamycin should be used initially in combination with other agents such as aminoglycoside.

Because of widespread clinical use and consistently high cure rates in many studies, clindamycin and an aminoglycoside is usually considered the standard against which other antibiotics are measured (11–16). Excluding side effect failures, cure rates with this combination are generally from 90–97%.

Oral clindamycin may be used to *continue* therapy for 3 or 4 days in a patient who has shown a response to parenteral clindamycin, but there is little reason to *initiate* a course of clindamycin in an outpatient.

Although *S. aureus* is susceptible to clindamycin, it is not the drug of choice for infections caused by these organisms. Penicillinase-resistant penicillins (methicillin, etc.) are preferred, and the cephalosporin antibiotics would be the alternative in most patients with a penicillin allergy. In the rare patient with anaphylaxis to penicillin or a cephalosporin, clindamycin may be used to treat infections with *S. aureus*.

ERYTHROMYCIN

Erythromycin is a macrolide antibiotic and is comprised of a many membered lactone ring with one or more deoxy sugars attached. Erythromycin is most active in an alkaline medium and is primarily bacteriostatic.

Spectrum of Activity

The antibacterial spectrum of erythromycin is limited. It is active against a variety of aerobic gram-positive cocci and possesses activity against some *Neisseria* species, *C. diptheriae, L. monocytogenes, Treponema pallidum, Mycoplasma pneumoniae,* and *Legionella pneumophila.* Many gram-positive and gram-negative anaerobic bacteria are inhibited, but by relatively high concentrations. Erythromycin also is active against *C. trachomatis* and *M. hominis* but not *U. urealyticum.*

Erythromycin is bound to the 50-S ribosomal unit of susceptible microorganisms and inhibits polypeptide synthesis in ribosomal complexes. The drug accumulates 100 times more in grampositive than in gram-negative bacteria.

Dosage and Route

Erythromycin preparations are available for administration by the oral, intramuscular, and intravenous routes. Oral preparations of erythromycin include erythromycin base (E-Mycin), erythromycin stearate (Bristamycin, Ethril, Pfizer, SK-Erythromycin, Erypar, Erythrocin Stearate), erythromycin estolate (Ilosone), and erythromycin ethyl succinate (Pediamycin, Wyamicin) (1).

Erythromycin base is a very bitter, weak base (pk = 8.8). In order to make it tolerable, enteric coatings have been applied. In some preparations of erythromycin base, gastrointestinal absorption has been erratic, but E-Mycin (Upjohn) is well absorbed in both the fasting and nonfasting state. Mean peak serum levels of E-Mycin are 0.73 μg/ml 5 hr after a single 250-mg dose. Similar levels are achieved in nonfasting subject. After multiple doses of 250 mg q.i.d., peak levels of 1.5 μg/ml are achieved.

Erythromycin stearate hydrolyzes to erythromycin base in the duodenum, where absorption takes place. After a 250-mg dose in a fasting subject, levels of 0.82 μg/ml are achieved 2 hr later. Multiple doses every 6 hr lead to levels of 1.0–1.5 μg/ml in fasting state. This preparation should be given 1 hr before or 2 hr after meals. When given with meals, erythromycin is destroyed considerably because of longer periods in the stomach and greater exposure to acid. Acceptable bioavailability of this preparation also depends upon administration with adequate amounts of water.

Erythromycin estolate is acid stable, and its absorption is unaffected by food. Although this preparation achieves higher levels than do erythromycin base or stearate esters, erythromycin estolate is apparently absorbed primarily as the proprionate ester, which is not active until hydrolyzed to the base.

Erythromycin ethyl succinate is tasteless and is reported to be stable in acid. The usual adult dosage is 250–500 mg orally every 6 hr.

Because intramuscular administration of erythromycin is associated with extreme pain, the antibiotic should not be administered by this route. Intravenous administration of erythromycin is associated with a significant incidence of thrombophlebitis at the intravenous site. The dosage for this route is usually 500 mg every 6 hr.

Side Effects

The erythromycins have a good safety record, but may be associated with both local and systemic untoward effects. Epigastric distress and gastrointestinal upset occur often after oral administration. Individuals experiencing these symptoms at 500 mg q6h are often able to tolerate 250 mg q6h. Pseudomembranous enterocolitis has rarely been observed. Pain may develop after intramuscular administration and phlebitis after intravenous administration. Hypersensitive reactions, manifest by fever, eosinophilia, and skin eruption may occur.

The only major adverse effect is hepatotoxicity which has been seen with the estolate and ethylsuccinate esters. This syndrome is not dose related and usually does not occur after the first exposure to the drug. After 1–3 weeks of therapy, patients may develop abdominal cramps, nausea, vomiting, jaundice, fever, leukocytosis, and abnormal liver function. All manifestations usually resolve when administration of the drug has been discontinued.

Cost

As an older preparation, erythromycin is a relatively inexpensive antibiotic.

Use in Pregnancy and Placental Transfer

Erythromycin has not been associated with adverse effects on the fetus, but the estolate salt may cause mild hepatotoxicity more commonly in pregnant women than in other adults (2). Approximately 10% of 161 women treated with the estolate ester in the second trimester had elevated SGOT levels. These returned to normal after the antibiotic was discontinued. Erythromycin crosses the placenta, but achieves cord blood concentrations of only 6–20% of maternal levels (3). Like many other antibiotics, erythromycin may lower urinary estriol levels (36).

Metabolism

When erythromycin is administered orally, 2–5% of the antibiotic is excreted in active form in the urine. After intravenous administration, 12–15% is excreted in the urine. Erythromycin is concentrated in the liver and is excreted primarily in the active form in the bile.

Indications in Obstetrics and Gynecology

Erythromycin has been indicated for the treatment of staphylococcal and streptococcal infections in penicillin-allergic patients. In recent years, recognition of the importance of infections due to the *C. trachomatis* may serve to broaden the clinical indications for the use of this antibiotic, especially in pregnancy (when tetracycline is contraindicated). Erythromycin is also an alternative agent to tetracycline for the treatment of ureaplasma, but clinical indications for treating this organism are not clear.

M. pneumoniae is among the microorganisms most frequently responsible for the production of lower respiratory infection ("walking pneumonia") in people 20–40 yr of age. *L. pneumophila* has been recognized as an important cause of sporadic pneumonia ("Legionnaires' disease"). Erythromycin is the agent of first choice for the treatment of these two organisms.

Furthermore, erythromycin is an alternative agent for treating syphilis in penicillin-allergic patients, but is no longer recommended for treatment of gonorrhea (24).

LINCOMYCIN

Lincomycin (Lincocin) is active against gram-positive bacteria, clostridia, *C. diptheriae*, and some strains of *B. fragilis*. It binds to the 50-S subunit of ribosomes and suppresses protein synthesis by inhibition of peptide synthesis.

Toxic effects are common after administration of lincomycin. Approximately 20% of the people receiving this antibiotic develop diarrhea after oral administration. A variety of gastrointestinal disturbances, including glossitis, stomatitis, nausea, vomiting, enterocolitis, and pruritis ani may develop. Skin rashes, urticaria, general pruritis, and vaginitis have been observed. Allergic reactions, such as angioedema, serum sickness, and anaphylaxis have been reported uncommonly. Reversible neutropenia, leukopenia, and thrombocytopenia have occasionally followed parenteral administration.

Because clindamycin appears to have superior antibacterial effectiveness, perhaps related to its increased solubility in cell-membrane lipid or because of an increased affinity of clindamycin for binding sites in the cell, this antibiotic has supplanted lincomycin in clinical practice. Clindamycin inhibits susceptible organisms at lower concentrations than lincomycin, and clinical indications for the use of lincomycin are rare.

AMINOGLYCOSIDES

The aminoglycoside-aminocyclitol antibiotics include streptomycin, kanamycin (Kantrex), gentamicin (Garamicin), tobramycin (Nebcin), and amikacin (Amikin). Streptomycin now has little utility, aside in the treatment of tuberculosis, and kanamycin has largely been replaced by newer members of this group. The remaining agents are the most effective ones against gram-negative aerobic organisms but have a relatively narrow margin of safety (1, 2).

Spectrum of Activity

The aminoglycoside antibiotics are bactericidal agents that induce defective protein molecules by inhibiting the 30-S subunit of the ribosome. Resistance to aminoglycosides may develop because (1) penetration of the antibiotic into the bacterial cell is prevented, (2) the bacterial ribosomes are modified to prevent binding of the aminoglycosides, and (3) bacterial enzymes destroy the antibiotics.

Gentamicin is the most widely used member of this group of antibiotics. Available for over 10 yr, it is active against nearly all strains of aerobic gram-negative bacteria, including *E. coli*, *Klebsiella* species, indole-positive and indole-negative *Proteus* species, *Enterobacter* species, and *P. aeruginosa*. Since the introduction of this antibiotic, it has gained a major place in the antibiotic armamentarium and is among the most frequently used antibiotics. This widespread use has led to development of strains of *P. aeruginosa* that are totally resistant to gentamicin. In view of the rarity of infections due to *P. aeruginosa* and other organisms uniquely susceptible to gentamicin (especially in obstetric and gynecologic patients) less toxic antibiotics can often be used.

Gentamicin is also active against some gram-positive organisms. It has a MIC of 1 μg/ml for *S. aureus* and acts synergistically with the penicillins against enterococci.

The antibacterial spectrum of tobramycin is similar to that of gentamicin, with two exceptions. Many strains of *P. aeruginosa* that are resistant to gentamicin are susceptible to tobramycin. On the other hand, *Serratia marcescens* is significantly more susceptible to gentamicin than to tobramycin.

Susceptible organisms have MICs of less than 4 μg/ml of gentamicin or tobramycin.

Amikacin is a recently introduced aminoglycoside antibiotic with activity against a wide range of gram-negative bacteria, including *P. aeruginosa*. At present, its use is restricted to the treatment of infections produced by organisms resistant to gentamicin and tobramycin.

Although kanamycin has been largely replaced by newer aminoglycoside antibiotics, it is still used in some nurseries. It is active against most strains of *E. coli*, *Klebsiella*, *Proteus*, and *Enterobacter* species, but in general, gentamicin has more extensive activity. Furthermore, kanamycin is not effective in treating infections caused by *Pseudomonas* or *Serratia* species.

Dosage and Route

Because their principal toxic effects are dose-related, dosages of aminoglycoside antibiotics should be based on the patient's weight. For gentamicin and tobramycin, the usual dosage is 1.0–1.5 mg/kg every 8 hr and for amikacin, either 7.5 mg/kg every 12 hr or 5.0 mg/kg every 8 hr. These preparations may be administered intravenously or intramuscularly in the same dosage. These are approximations only, and blood levels should be determined in patients with courses longer than 10 days, with renal disease, with use of other nephrotoxic agents, with marked obesity, and with poor clinical response.

After a 30-min intravenous infusion, a concentration of gentamicin or tobramycin of 6–10 μg/ml is achieved rapidly, and concentrations fall to 1–2 μg/ml within 6–8 hr.

Aminoglycosides are not absorbed after oral administration; oral preparations are intended only for bowel sterilization.

Determining the proper dose for very obese patients has been a problem (3). Until recently, it has been thought that aminoglycosides were distributed only in extracellular fluid and that dosages should, therefore, be calculated on lean body weight. Accordingly, when obese patients were given an aminoglycoside dose based on total body weight, then serum levels were higher than expected. Very recently, however, it has been recognized that obese patients, given a dose based on lean body weight, may have seriously low antibiotic levels since there is partial distribution into adipose tissue.

Based on recent pharmacokinetic study, it seems best to determine aminoglycoside doses in obese nonpregnant patients as follows:

1. For mildly obese patients (i.e., with less than 30% excess weight), use total body weight to calculate dose.
2. For moderately obese patients (i.e., with more than 30% excess weight), use lean body weight plus 40% of weight of adipose tissue.
3. For severely obese patients, do not exceed 150 mg every 8 hr for initial doses.
4. For moderately and severely obese patients, obtain antibiotic levels and adjust dose accordingly.

Pregnancy and the immediate puerperium represent additional situations when it is difficult to estimate the correct dose. Duff and colleagues and Blanco and co-workers found "subtherapeutic" peak levels (i.e., <5 μg/ml) in approximately one-third of postpartum women given 3.0 mg/kg/day of gentamicin and 4.5 mg/kg/day of tobramycin (4, 5). Zaske and co-workers found it necessary to use 3.0 to 11.6 mg/kg/day (in three divided doses) in pregnant women in order to achieve proper levels in 77 puerperal patients (6). These investigators emphasized the wide interpatient variation and the need to measure serum levels before employing these increased doses. A poor correlation was found between elimination rate of gentamicin and creatinine clearance, but a high correlation was noted between distribution volume and gentamicin elimination. The latter point suggested that changes in fluid volumes in pregnancy affected gentamicin kinetics. Zaske and colleagues also found widely ranging needs for gentamicin in gynecologic patients. In 249 patients with normal renal function (serum creatinine <1.5 mg/dl) the daily dose ranged from 1.9 to 14.0 mg/kg (in divided doses) (7).

Aminoglycosides are excreted by the kidney and must be used with caution in patients with renal disease. In such persons, adjustments in the dose of this antibiotic must be made; however, the formulas that have been used in the past are not reliable for determining dose modifications for these antibiotics. Serum concentrations must, therefore, be determined.

For gentamicin and tobramycin, desired peak levels are 5–10 μg/ml and trough levels are <2 μg/ml.

Side Effects

The principal toxic effects of all aminoglycoside agents are ototoxicity and nephrotoxicity. A relationship between gentamicin dose and the development of ototoxicity has been noted (1), but a recent analysis by Moore and colleagues found plasma aminoglycoside levels were not predictive of ototoxocity (8). Rather, they reported significant factors correlating with ototoxicity were: length of therapy, bacteremia, and higher temperature (8). Ototoxicity related to aminoglycoside administration may involve either the auditory or the vestibular portion of the eighth nerve. The ototoxicity may be uni or bilateral and is nearly always irreversible. It also tends to occur late in the course of therapy and may even develop or progress after the antibiotic has been stopped. Ototoxicity defined as greater than 15 dB loss of hearing has been reported in about 20% of patients (8) and is detected annually in about 2% (2).

Nephrotoxicity develops in approximately 2% of the patients who receive gentamicin (9). It ranges from minimal abnormalities of the urine sediment to frank renal failure. In the majority of patients who develop gentamicin-induced nephrotoxicity, renal function gradually returns to normal after the drug has been discontinued.

Neuromuscular blockade is a rare complication of all aminoglycosides. It is dose-related and is reversed by anticholinesterases and calcium salts.

Tobramycin possesses the potential for the production of both ototoxicity and nephrotoxicity, but a number of recent studies have suggested that the incidence of such untoward effects may be lower than with gentamicin. However, most obstetric patients are at low risk for aminoglycoside toxicity. Accordingly, potentially less nephrotoxicity is not a compelling reason to abandon gentamicin. Indeed, in studying over 200 women treated with gentamicin or tobramycin, in San Antonio, we found that none have a rise in creatinine greater than 0.5 mg/dl.

The experience with amikacin is too limited to allow an adequate assessment of the precise incidence of toxicity associated with its administration.

Cost

Cost of aminoglycoside agents vary widely. The price of gentamicin has fallen dramatically, and an 80-mg vial can be purchased for less than $1.00. The newer agents are more expensive.

Use in Pregnancy

In 1965, Conway and Birt reported the results of eighth nerve evaluation in 17 children born to women who received streptomycin in pregnancy for treatment of tuberculosis (10). Eight of these children, aged 6–13 yr, had detectable, but subclinical abnormalities.

Data are not available for other aminoglycosides, but the potential exists for fetal eighth nerve or renal toxicity. Although pregnancy should not be considered a contraindication to the use of aminoglycosides, alternative agents such as semisynthetic penicillins or a cephalosporins should be used, if possible.

Two studies have reported concentrations of kanamycin and gentamicin in pregnancy to be about 25% lower than expected, probably because of more rapid renal clearance (11, 12). Thus, for gentamicin or tobramycin in pregnant or immediately puerperal women, the initial dose should be 1.5 mg/kg q8H (provided there is normal renal function). If a pregnant patient does not respond to an aminoglycoside despite in vitro susceptibility, the antibiotic concentration should be determined.

Metabolism

As noted above, aminoglycoside antibiotics are excreted mainly by the kidneys, with a small amount being excreted in the bile.

Indications in Obstetrics and Gynecology

Because of their activity against aerobic gram-negative organisms, aminoglycoside antibiotics are widely used in genitourinary infections, usually in combination with other antibiotics.

SOFT TISSUE PELVIC INFECTIONS

In the treatment of serious infections of this kind, the combination of an aminoglycoside with other agents such as clindamycin (or less often metronidazole) is usually considered the standard. Yet, aerobic gram-negative organisms are isolated in perhaps only 25% of genital infections, and many of these are susceptible to less

toxic antibiotics. Thus, even in serious infections, therapy may be modified based on culture results and clinical response. Because of potential toxicity and difficulty in achieving the proper level of aminoglycosides as well as the expenses and toxicity of combination regimens, there has been a major stimulus to the search for newer, safe, single agents for therapy.

URINARY TRACT INFECTION

Although nearly all organisms causing urinary tract infection (except enterococci) are susceptible to gentamicin, other agents are usually indicated. Aminoglycosides should be used to treat infections caused by organisms with in vitro resistance to less toxic agents. Aminoglycoside antibiotics may also be used in the initial treatment (before cultures are available) of recurrent infection when highly resistant organisms are likely.

METRONIDAZOLE

Metronidazole is a nitroimidazole drug which was initially introduced for the treatment of trichomoniasis. Subsequently it was used extensively for infections due to *Giardia lamblia* and *Entamoeba histolytica*. Most recently, metronidazole has been recognized as an effective antimicrobial for the treatment of anaerobic infections and nonspecific vaginitis (vaginosis) (1).

Spectrum of Activity

The mode of action of metronidazole is not well understood. It is believed that the biologic activity of the drug is related to reduction of the nitro group at the S-position on the imidazole ring (2–4). O'Brian and Morris suggested that the reduction is most likely effected by electron-transport proteins of low redux potential such as ferredoxin or flavodoxin which play a major metabolic role in anaerobic microorganisms (5). This mode of action of metronidazole on anaerobic microorganisms requires four steps: (a) entry into the microorganisms; (b) reductive activation of the agent; (c) toxic effect of the reduced product(s) on microorganisms; and (d) release of inactivated end products (1).

The mechanism of the toxic action exerted by the reduced derivatives of metronidazole is not fully understood. It is generally assumed that this toxicity is due to unstable intermediate products (1). *N*-(-2-hydroxyethyl)-oxamic acid and acetamide form when metronidazole is reduced (6). It is possible that these partially reduced intermediates are also responsible for the mutagenicity and carcinogenicity associated with metronidazole (3). The intracellular targets(s) of the toxic action is unclear but believed to be an interaction with DNA or a degradation of DNA (1). This causes extensive damage to nucleic acids and destroys the organism (7).

Metronidazole is active against the anaerobic protozoa *Trichomonas vaginalis*, *Entamoeba histolytica*, and *Giardia lamblia*. Recently, metronidazole resistance in strains of *T. vaginalis* has been rarely reported (8, 9). Metronidazole is active against only those bacteria with primarily anaerobic metabolism (obligate anaerobes). Of the gram-negative anaerobic bacteria, *Fusobacterium* and *Bacteroides* species, especially *B. fragilis* and *B. melanogenicus*, are the most susceptible (10, 11, 12). Among the gram-positive anaerobes, the *Clostridium* species are the most sensitive; *Peptococcus*, *Peptostreptococcus*, and *Eubacterium* species are also frequently sensitive. However, *Actinomyces* species and *Bifidobacterium* species are less commonly sensitive. Metronidazole has no significant activity against aerobic or facultative anaerobes. In addition, it has less activity against microaerophillic streptococci. Other microaerophillic bacteria such as *Campylobacter fetus* and *Gardnerella vaginalis* are susceptible to metronidazole.

Dosage and Route

Metronidazole may be administered intravenously, orally or rectally. With oral adminstration metronidazole should be taken just after or during a meal. Oral doses range from 2–4 g as a single dose or 250–750 mg three times to four times a day. For treatment of trichomoniasis, the usual recommended dose is either a single 2-g regimen or 250 mg three times a day for 7–10 days. For giardiasis the dose is 250 mg three times a day for 7 days, for nondysenteric amebiasis 500 mg three times a day for 10 days, and for dysenteric amebiasis or amebic liver abscess 750 mg three times a day for 10 days. If oral dosing is used for the treatment of anaerobic soft tissue infections 500 mg three to four times a day are recommended. In nonspecific vaginitis the recommended dose is 500 mg twice a day for 7 days.

Intravenous administration of metronidazole is available as the hydrochloride salt in 100-ml bottles and buffered with sodium bicarbonate. It can be infused over a 20- to 30-min period.

The dosage varies from 250 to 750 mg three to four times a day. In general, intravenous metronidazole is reserved for the treatment of moderate to severe anaerobic infections, and the dose determined by the severity of the clinical infection. Intravenous administration of 2–4 gm of metronidazole has been used on occasion to treat resistant *T. vaginalis*.

In Europe, rectal administration of a 1-g metronidazole suppository has been used in a dosage regimen of 1 g every 8 hr.

Side Effects

When metronidazole has been used in relatively low doses for short periods of time, very few side effects occur. However, with administration of higher doses over a more prolonged period of time, side effects occur more frequently. The most common side effects are gastrointestinal disturbances such as nausea, an unpleasant metallic taste, a furred tongue, and abdominal cramps (13). Central nervous system symptoms with lower doses include headache, ataxia, vertigo, sleepiness, and depression (13). With larger doses reversible peripheral neuropathies have occurred (14) as well as myalgia, transient encephalopathies, and persistent paresthesia. Other side effects noted even at low dose therapy are vaginal burning, a disulfiram-like intolerance to alcohol, and the presence of dark red-brown urine. Transitory skin rashes and leukopenia have also occurred.

Concern has been voiced as to the safety of metronidazole because of reports suggesting that this agent may have mutagenic, carcinogenic, or teratogenic properties. Several reports have demonstrated that metronidazole and its metabolites are mutagenic in bacteria (3, 15, 16). However, as noted by Charles, metronidazole is not mutagenic under conditions where it is not reduced and mammalian cells are incapable of reducing the drug, and thus the mutagenic effect in bacteria may not be applicable to the use of the drug in humans (17). Chromosomal abnormalities have been described in the circulating lymphocytes of patients with Crohn's disease on long-term (1–24 months) therapy with metronidazole (18).

A carcinogenic effect has been reported with the use of very high doses of metronidazole in rodents (19, 20, 21). This effect has not been seen in other animal models (20). To date published studies have not found an association between previous exposure to metronidazole for treatment of clinical infections and an increased incidence of carcinoma (22, 23). However, as noted by Mirer and Silverstein, the follow up time in these clinical studies was shorter than the lag time required to demonstrate a carcinogenic effect (24). Thus, it seems apparent that the carcinogenic risk in humans is not yet known and its determination will require long-term follow-up of 20–25 yr. In addition, the use of multiple regimens and/or larger doses for longer periods of time must be considered.

Despite concern over a potential teratogenic effect, no teratogenicity has been demonstrated in animals or in humans. However, it is generally recommended that metronidazole be avoided during the first trimester and if possible during the entire pregnancy.

Recently, attention has been focused on the interaction of metronidazole with other drugs. The concomitant administration of metronidazole augments the hypoprothrombinemic effect of coumadin. On the other hand, diphenylhydantoin (dilantin) and phenobarbitol increase the metabolism of metronidazole.

Cost

Oral metronidazole is not under patent protection any longer and is thus relatively inexpensive. Intravenous metronidazole is a costly preparation.

Use in Pregnancy and Placental Transfer

Metronidazole passes across the placental barrier and can be found in fetal tissue, cord blood and amniotic fluid in high concentrations (25). As described above, metronidazole has been used extensively during pregnancy without apparent ill effects (13). Morgan recently reported no increased rate of stillbirths, small for age infants, preterm infants, or evidence of teratogenicity among 597 pregnant women with trichomoniasis (26). However, metronidazole should be avoided during the first trimester of pregnancy when major organogenesis is occurring. Indeed, when alternative agents are available, metronidazole is best avoided during the second and third trimester of pregnancy.

Metronidazole is excreted in breast milk and is present in breast milk in levels comparable to serum (13, 27). Thus it has been suggested that either lactating women should not receive metronidazole or that breast-feeding should be temporarily discontinued for 24 hr following a single oral dose of metronidazole.

Metabolism

Metronidazole is almost completely absorbed following oral administration (1, 28) and diffuses well into nearly all tissues, resulting in wide distribution throughout the body (1, 28). Following single oral doses of 250 and 500 mg, peak serum levels of 6 g and 12 μg respectively have been reported (28). Oral 500-μg doses of metronidazole administered four times daily resulted in peak serum levels of 20–50 μg/ml (28). The peak blood levels achieved with intravenous metronidazole approximate those of the oral route. After insertion of a 1-g suppository a mean serum level of 2.3 μg/ml was detected at 1 hr and 10.5 μg/ml at 4 hr.

Metronidazole binds to plasma protein in the range of 20% (29). In humans it is primarily eliminated through metabolism, which occurs mainly in the liver via oxidation, hydroxylation or conjugation of side chains on the imidazole rings (28, 29). Metronidazole is excreted primarily via the kidneys but is found in feces as well (29).

Indications in Obstetrics and Gynecology

Metronidazole is a potent antimicrobial agent against anaerobic protozoa and bacteria. In the United States, metronidazole is the only effective drug available for the treatment of *T. vaginalis*. Outside of the United States other nitroimidazoles are available. Both the 2-g single dose and 250-mg three times a day for 7 day regimens are very effective. Metronidazole is used for the treatment of amebiasis and giardiasis. It is the drug of choice for amebiasis, while metronidazole is an alternative therapy in giardiasis where quinacrine is the drug of choice.

Nonspecific vaginitis (NSV) (vaginosis) is a synergistic polymicrobial infection associated with *G. vaginalis* and anaerobic bacteria, especially *Peptococcus* species and *Bacteroides* species. Since the report by Pheifer et al (30), metronidazole has increasingly been used for the treatment of NSV.

The important role of anaerobic bacteria in soft tissue infections of the upper genital tract of female is well recognized with anaerobes recovered from approximately two-thirds of pelvic infection (31). With the recognition of metronidazole's excellent bactericidal activity against anaerobic bacteria, it has been used widely as a therapeutic agent in the treatment of infections associated with anaerobic bacteria. For this type of infection 250–750 mg three to four times a day is the recommended dosage. Because these infections are generally mixed infections involving facultative bacteria as well as anaerobes, metronidazole must be used in combination with an agent effective against gram-negative facultative bacteria such as aminoglycosides, second or third generation cephalosporins, or (when available) monobactam antimicrobial agents.

In the treatment of intraabdominal and pelvic infections, therapeutic trials comparing a metronidazole combination to a clindamycin combination have failed to demonstrate an enhanced clinical efficacy for metronidazole (32, 33). Because metronidazole has not resulted in an enhanced clinical efficacy over current standard therapies and because concern exists as to its carcinogenic potential, metronidazole should not be considered a first-line antimicrobial for treating mixed aerobic-anaerobic pelvic infections. Rather it should be used as a backup agent when other treatment regimens have failed or anaerobes resistant to clindamycin, chloramphenicol, or cefoxitin are present.

A multitude of inexpensive antimicrobial agents are available for use as prophylactic antibiotics in surgical procedures. These agents are not required for treating severe infection and make ideal prophylaxis choices. It seems inappropriate to use metronidazole as a prophylactic antibiotic at this time (1).

References

1. Moellering RC Jr: Mechanism of action of antimicrobial agents. *Clin Obstet Gynecol* 22:277, 1979.
2. Bennett N McK, Kucers A: *The Use of Antibiotics: A Comprehensive Review with Clinical Emphasis,* ed 3. Philadelphia, JB Lippincott, 1979.
3. Philipson A: Pharmacokinetics of ampicillin during pregnancy. *J Infect Dis* 136:370, 1977.
4. Philipson A: Pharmacokinetics of antibiotics in pregnancy and labor. *Clin Pharmacokinet* 4:297, 1979.
5. Charles D: Placental transmission of antibiotics. *Obstet Gynecol Annu* 8:19–86, 1979.
6. Knowles JA: Excretion of drugs in milk: a review. *J Pediatr* 66:1068, 1965.

Penicillins

1. Neu HC: Penicillins. In Mandell GL, Douglas RG, Bennett JE (eds): *Principles and Practice of Infectious Diseases.* New York, John Wiley & Sons, 1979, pp 218–238.
2. Batchelor FR, Doyle FP, Naylor JHC, et al: Synthesis of penicillin: 6-aminopenicillanic acid in penicillin fermentations. *Nature* 183:257, 1959.
3. Hansman D, Glasgow H, Sturt J, Devitt L, Douglas R: Increased resistance to penicillin of pneumococci isolated from man. *N Engl J Med* 284:175, 1971.

4. Applebaum PC, Scragg JN, Bowen AJ, et al: Streptococcus pneumoniae resistant to penicillin and chloramphenicol. *Lancet* 2:995, 1977.
5. Sparling PF: Antibiotic resistance in *Neisseria gonorrhoeae. Med Clin North Am* 56:1133, 1972.
6. Ashford WA, Golash RG, Hemming VG: Penicillinase-producing *Neisseria gonorrhoeae. Lancet* 2:657, 1976.
7. Siegel MS, Thornsberry C, Biddle JW, et al: Penicillinase producing *Neisseria gonorrhoeae*: results of surveillance in the United States. *J Infect Dis* 137:170, 1978.
8. Sabath LD, Garner C, Wilcox C, Finland M: Effect of inoculum and of beta-lactamase on the anti-staphylococcal activity of thirteen penicillins and cephalosporins. *Antimicrob Agents Chemother* 8:344, 1975.
9. Yow MD, Taber LH, Barrett FF, et al: A ten-year assessment of methicillin-associated side-effects. *Pediatrics* 58:329, 1976.
10. Schrier RW, Burger RJ, van Arsdel PP: Nephropathy associated with penicillin and homologues. *Ann Intern Med* 64:116, 1966.
11. Dismukes WE: Oxacillin induced hepatic dysfunction. *JAMA* 226:861, 1973.
12. Stewart GT: *The Penicillin Group of Drugs.* Amsterdam, Elsevier Publishing Company, 1965, p 70.
13. Yoshioka H, Rudoy P, Riley HD Jr, Yoshida K: Antimicrobial susceptibility of *Escherichia coli* isolated at a children's hospital. *Scand J Infect Dis* 9:207, 1977.
14. Shapiro S, Slone D, Siskind V, Lewis GP, Jick H: Drug rash with ampicillin and other penicillins. *Lancet* 2:969, 1969.
15. Arndt KA, Jick H: Rates of cutaneous reactions to drugs. A report from the Boston Collaborative Drug Surveillance Program. *JAMA* 235:918, 1976.
16. Philipson A: Pharmacokinetics of ampicillin during pregnancy. *J Infect Dis* 136:370, 1977.
17. McClure PD, Casserly JG, Monsier C, Crozier D: Carbenicillin induced bleeding disorder. *Lancet* 2:1307, 1970.
18. Parry MF, Neu HC: Ticarcillin for treatment of serious infections with gram-negative bacteria. *J Infect Dis* 134:476, 1976.
19. Harding GKM, Buckwold FJ, Ronald AR, et al: Prospective randomized comparative study of clindamycin, chloramphenicol and ticarcillin each in combination with gentamicin in therapy for intra-abdominal and female genital tract sepsis. *J Infect Dis* 142:384, 1980.
20. Faro S, Sanders CV, Aldridge KE: Use of single-agent antimicrobial therapy in the treatment of polymicrobial female pelvic infections. *Obstet Gynecol* 60:232–236, 1982.
21. Fu KP, Neu HC: Azlocillin and mezlocillin—new ureidopenicillins. *Antimicrob Agents Chemother* 13:930, 1978.
22. Winston DJ, Wang D, Young LS, Martin WJ, Hewitt WL: In vitro studies of piperacillin, a new semisynthetic penicillin. *Antimicrob Agents Chemother* 13:944, 1978.
23. Sweet RL, Robbie MO, Ohm-Smith M, Hadley WK: Comparative study of piperacillin versus cefoxitin in the treatment of obstetric and gynecologic infections. *Am J Obstet Gynecol* 145:342–349,

1983.

24. Sorrell TC, Marshall JR, Yoshimori R, Chow AW: Antimicrobial therapy of postpartum endomyometritis. II. Prospective, randomized trial of mezlocillin versus ampicillin. *Am J Obstet Gynecol* 141:246–251, 1981.

25. Eschenbach D, Faro S, Pastorek JH II, Gilstrap LC, Maier RC, Gibbs R, Gunning JE, Hemsell D: Treatment of patients with obstetric and gynecologic infections. A Scientific Exhibit presented at the Annual Meeting of the American College of Obstetricians and Gynecologists, San Francisco, May 7–10, 1984.

26. Neu HC: Mecillinam, a novel penicillanic acid derivative with unusual activity against gram-negative bacteria. *Antimicrob Agents Chemother* 9:793, 1976.

Cephalosporins

1. Moellering RC, Swartz MH: The newer cephalosporins. *N Engl J Med* 294:24, 1976.

2. Nightingale CH, Greene DS, Quintiliani R: Pharmacokinetics and clinical use of cephalosporin antibiotics. *J Pharm Sci* 64:1899, 1975.

3. Garrod LP: Choice among penicillins and cephalosporins. *Br. Med J* 3:96, 1974.

4. Grieco MH: Cross-allergenicity of the penicillins and the cephalosporins. *Arch Intern Med* 199:141, 1967.

5. Sutter VL, Kirby B, Finegold SM: *In vitro* activity of cefoxitin and parenterally administered cephalosporins against anaerobic bacteria. *Rev Infect Dis* 1(1):218, 1979.

6. Cefamandole and cefoxitin. *Med Lett* 12(3):13, 1979.

7. Tally FP, Cuchural GJ, Jacobus NV, et al: Susceptibility of the *Bacteroides fragilis* group in the United States in 1981. *Antimicrob Chemother* 23:536, 1983.

8. Gibbs RS, Huff RW: Cefamandole therapy of endomyometritis following cesarean section. *Am J Obstet Gynecol* 136:32, 1980.

9. Giamarellou H, Gazis J, Petrikkos G, et al: A study of cefoxitin moxalactam, and cefatazidime kinetics in pregnancy. *Am J Obstet Gynecol* 147:914, 1983.

10. Cunningham FG, Gilstrap LC III, Kappus SS: Treatment of obstetric and gynecologic infections with cefamandole. *Am J Obstet Gynecol* 133:602, 1979.

11. Gall SA, Hill GB: High-dose cefamandole therapy in obstetric and gynecologic infections. *Am J Obstet Gynecol* 137:914, 1980.

12. Gibbs RS, Blanco JD, Castaneda YS, et al: A double-blind, randomized comparison of clindamycin-gentamicin versus cefamandole for treatment of post-Cesarean section endomyometritis. *Am J Obstet Gynecol* 144:261, 1982.

13. Sweet RL, Ledger WJ: Cefoxitin: single-agent treatment of mixed aerobic-anaerobic pelvic infections. *Obstet Gynecol* 54:193, 1979.

14. Ledger WJ, Smith D: Cefoxitin in obstetric and gynecologic infections. *Rev Infect Dis* 1:199, 1979.

15. Sweet RL, Robbie MO, Ohm-Smith M, Hadley WK: Comparative study of piperacillin versus cefoxitin in the treatment of obstetric and gynecologic infections. *Am J Obstet Gynecol* 145:342,

1982.

16. Duff P, Keiser JF: A comparative study of two antibiotic regimens for the treatment of operative site infections. *Am J Obstet Gynecol* 142:996, 1982.

17. Hager WD, McDaniel PS: Treatment of serious obstetric and gynecologic infections with cefoxitin. *J Reprod Med* 28:337, 1983.

18. Centers for Disease Control: Sexually transmitted diseases treatment guidelines 1982. *MMWR* (suppl) 32(25:43(s), 1982.

19. Stiver HG, Forward KR, Livingstone RA, et al: Multicenter comparison of cefoxitin versus cefazolin for prevention of infectious morbidity after nonelective cesarean section. *Am J Obstet Gynecol* 145:158, 1983.

20. Neu HC: The new beta-lactamase-stable cephalosporins. *Ann Intern Med* 97:408, 1982.

21. Ohm-Smith MJ, Hadley WK, Sweet RL: *In vitro* activity of new B-lactam antibiotics and other antimicrobial drugs against anaerobic isolates from obstetric and gynecological infections. *Antimicrob Chemother* 17:711, 1982.

22. Jorgensen JH, Crawford SA, Alexander GA: Comparsion of moxalactam (LY127935) and cefotaxime against anaerobic bacteria. *Antimicrob Chemother* 17:901–904, 1980.

23. Bawdon RE, Cunningham FG, Quirk JG, Roark ML: Maternal and fetal pharmacokinetics of moxalactam given intrapartum. *Am J Obstet Gynecol* 144:546, 1982.

24. Kafetzis DA, Lazarides CV, Sifas CA, et al: Transfer of cefotaxime in human milk from mother to fetus. *J Antimicrob Chemother* (suppl A) 6:135, 1980.

25. Kammer RB: Moxalactam: clinical summary of efficacy and safety. *Rev Infect Dis* 4(S):712, 1982.

26. Gibbs RS, Blanco JD, Castaneda YS, ST Clair PJ: Therapy of obstetrical inections with moxalactam. *Antimicrob Chemother* 17:1004, 1980.

27. Cunningham FG, Hemsell DL, DePalma RT, et al: Moxalactam for obstetric and gynecologic infections in vitro and dose-finding studies. *Am J Obstet Gynecol* 139:915, 1981.

28. Gibbs RS, Blanco JD, Duff P: A double-blind, randomized comparison of moxalactam versus clindamycin-gentamicin in treatment of endomyometritis after cesarean section delivery. *Am J Obstet Gynecol* 146:769, 1983.

29. Hemsell DL, Cunningham FG, DePalma RT, et al: Cefotaxime sodium therapy for endomyometritis following cesarean section: dose-finding and comparative studies. *Obstet Gynecol* 62:489, 1983.

30. Hemsell DL, Cunningham FG: Combination antimicrobial therapy for serious gynecological and obstetrical infections-obsolete? *Clin Ther* 4:81, 1981.

31. Strausbaugh LJ, Llorens AS: Cefoperazone therapy for obstetric and gynecologic infections. *Rev Infect Dis* 5:S154, 1983.

32. Blanco JD, Gibbs RS, Duff P, et al: Randomized comparison of ceftazidime versus clindamycin-tobramycin in the treatment of obstetrical and gynecological infections. *Antimicrob Chemother* 24:500, 1983.

33. Gibbs RS, Blanco JD: A comparison of aztreonam plus clindamycin with gentamicin plus clindamycin in the treatment of endometritis after cesarean

section. *13th International Congress of Chemotherapy.* Abstract SS 4.1/3–11 Vienna, 1983.

34. Kesado T, Hashizume T, Asahi Y: Antibacterial activities of a new stabilized thienamycin, n-formimidoyl thienamycin, in comparison with other antibiotics. *Antimicrob Chemother* 17:912, 1980.

35. Kropp H, Sundelof JG, Kahan JS, et al: MK 0787 (N-formimidoyl thienamycin): evaluation of in vitro and in vivo activities. *Antimicrob Chemother* 17:993, 1983.

36. Berkeley AS, Strausbaugh LJ, Cohen AW, et al: Randomized comparative trial of theinamycin and moxalactam, 23rd ICAAC, 207, 1983.

Tetracyclines

1. Steigbigel NH, Reed CR, Finland M: Susceptibility of common pathogenic bacteria to seven tetracycline antibiotics in vitro. *Am J Med Sci* 255:179, 1968.

2. Centers for Disease Control: Penicillinase—(beta-lactamase-) producing *Neisseria gonorrhoeae*—worldwide. *MMWR* 27:10, 1978.

3. Sutter VL, Finegold SM: Susceptibility of anaerobic bacteria to 23 antimicrobial agents. *Antimicrob Agents Chemother* 10:736, 1976.

4. Finland M, Garrod LP: Demethylchlortetracycline. *Br Med J* 2:959, 1960.

5. Whalley PJ, Adams RH, Combes B: Tetracycline toxicity in pregnancy. *JAMA* 189:357, 1964.

Clindamycin

1. Tally FP, Cuchural GJ, Jacobus NV, et al: Susceptibility of the *Bacteroides fragilis* group in the United States in 1981. *Antimicrob Agents Chemother* 23:536, 1983.

2. George WL, Sutter VL, Finegold SM: Antimicrobial agent-induced diarrhea bacterial disease (editorial). *J Infect Dis* 136:822, 1977.

3. Bartlett JG, Onderdonk AB, Cisneros RL: Clindamycin-associated colitis in hamsters: protection with vancomycin. *Gastroenterology* 73:772, 1977.

4. Jenge WL, Rolfe PD, Mulligan ME, et al: Infectious diseases 1979—antimicrobial agent-induced colitis: an update (editorial). *J Infect Dis* 140:266, 1979.

5. Fekety R, Silva J, Armstrong J, et al: Treatment of antibiotic-associated enterocolitis with vancomycin. *Ref Infect Dis* 3(S):273, 1981.

6. Fekety R: Recent advances in management of bacterial diarrhea. *Rev Infect Dis* 5:246, 1983.

7. Ledger WJ, Puttler OL: Death from pseudomomembranous colitis. *Obstet Gynecol* 45:609, 1975.

8. Mickal A, Panzer JD: The safety of lincomycin in pregnancy. *Am J Obstet Gynecol* 121:1071, 1975.

9. Weinstein AJ, Gibbs RS, Gallagher M: Placental transfer of clindamycin and gentamicin in term pregnancy. *Am J Obstet Gynecol* 124:688, 1976.

10. Philipson A, Sabath LD, Charles D: Transplacental passage of erythromicin and clindamycin. *N Engl J Med* 288:1219, 1973.

11. Gibbs RS, Blanco JD, Castaneda YS, et al: A double-blind randomized comparison of clindomycin-gentamicin versus cefamandole for treatment of post-cesarean section endomyometritis. *Am J Obstet Gynecol* 144:261, 1982.

12. Gibbs RS, Blanco JD, Duff P: A double-blind, randomized comparison of moxalactam versus clindamycin-gentamicin in treatment of endomyometritis after cesarean section delivery. *Am J Obstet Gynecol* 146:769, 1983.

13. Hemsell DL, Cunningham FG, DePalma RT, et al: Cefotaxime sodium therapy for endomyometritis following cesarean section: dose-finding and comparative studies. *Obstet Gynecol* 62:489, 1983.

14. Gibbs RS, Blanco JD: A comparison of aztreonam plus clindamycin with gentamicin plus clindamycin in the treatment of endometritis after cesarean section. *13th International Congress of Chemotherapy.* Abstract SS 4.1/3–11 Vienna, 1983.

15. DiZerega G, Yonekura L, Roy S, et al: A comparison of clindamycin-gentamicin and penicillin-gentamicin in the treatment of post-cesarean section endomyometritis. *Am J Obstet Gynecol* 134:238, 1979.

16. Gall SA, Kohan AP, Ayers OM, et al: Intravenous metronidazole or clindamycin with tobramycin for therapy of pelvic infections. *Obstet Gynecol* 57:51, 1981.

Erythromycin

1. Frazer DG: Selection of an oral erythromycin product. *Am J Hosp Pharm* 37:1199, 1980.

2. McCormack WM, George H, Donner A, et al: Hepatotoxicity of erythromycin estolate during pregnancy. *Antimicrob Agents Chemother* 12:630, 1977.

3. Philipson A, Sabath LD, Charles D: Transplacental passage of erythromicin and clindamycin. *N Engl J Med* 288:1219, 1973.

4. Gallagher JD, Ismail MA, Aladjem S: Reduced urinary estriol levels with erythromycin therapy. *Obstet Gynecol* 56:381, 1980.

Aminoglycosides

1. Rosenthal SL: Aminoglycoside antibiotics. *NY State J Med* 75:535, 1975.

2. Torres-Rojas JR, Sander CV: Guidelines for using aminoglycosides. *Contemp Obstet Gynecol* 14:39, 1979.

3. Schwartz SN, Pazin GJ, Lyon JA, et al: A controlled investigation of the pharmacokinetics of gentamicin and tobramycin in obese subjects. *J Infect Dis* 138:499, 1978.

4. Duff P, Jorgensen JH, Alexander G, et al: Serum gentamicin levels in patients with post-cesarean endomyometritis. *Obstet Gynecol* 61:723, 1983.

5. Blanco JD, Gibbs RS, Duff P, et al: Serum tobramycin levels in puerperal women. *Am J Obstet Gynecol* 147:466, 1983.

6. Zaske DE, Cipolle RJ, Strate RG, et al: Rapid gentamicin elimination in obstetric patients. *Obstet Gynecol* 56:559, 1980.

7. Zaske DE, Cipolle RJ, Strate RG, et al: Increased gentamicin dosage requirements: rapid elimination in 249 gynecology patients. *Am J Obstet Gynecol* 139:896, 1981.

8. Moore RD, Smith CR, Lietman PS: Risk factors for the development of auditory toxicity in patients receiving aminoglycosides. *J Infect Dis* 149:23, 1984.

9. Appel GB, Neu HC: The nephrotoxicity of antimicrobial agents (second of three parts). *N Engl J Med* 296:722, 1977.

10. Conway N, Birt BD: Streptomycin in pregnancy:

effect on the foetal era. *Br Med J* 2:260, 1965.

11. Good RG, Johnson GH: Placental transfer of kanamycin during late pregnancy. *Obstet Gynecol* 38:60, 1971.

12. Weinstein AJ, Gibbs RS, Gallagher M: Placental transfer of clindamycin and gentamicin in term pregnancy. *Am J Obstet Gynecol* 124:688, 1976.

Metronidazole

1. Robbie MO, Sweet RL: Metronidazole use in obstetrics and gynecology: a review. *Am J Obstet Gynecol* 145:865–881, 1983.

2. Ingham HR, Selkon JB, Hale JH: The antibacterial activity of metronidazole. *J Antimicrob Chemother.* 1:355–361, 1975.

3. Lindmark DG, Muller M: Antitrichomonad action, mutagenicity and reduction of metronidazole and other nitroimidazoles. *Antimicrob Agents Chemother* 10:476–482, 1976.

4. Ings RMJ, McFadzean JA, Ormerod WE: The mode of action of metronidazole in *Trichimonas vaginalis*, other microorganisms. *Biochem Pharmacol* 23:1421–1429, 1974.

5. O'Brian RW, Morris JG: Effect of metronidazole on hydrogen production by *Clostridium acetobutylicum*. *Arch Microbiol* 84:225, 1972.

6. Ewan JTC, Koch RL, McLafferty MA, et al: Relationship between metronidazole metabolism and bactericidal activity. *Antimicrob Agents Chemother* 18:566, 1980.

7. Edwards DI: Mechanisms of selective toxicity of metronidazole and other nitroimidazole drugs. *Br J Vener Dis* 56:285–290, 1980.

8. Meingassner JG, Thurner J: Strain of *Trichomonas vaginalis* resistant to metronidazole and other 5-nitroimidazoles. *Antimicrob Agents Chemother* 15:254–257, 1979.

9. Muller M, Meingassner JG, Miller WA, Ledger WJ: Three resistant metronidazole-resistant strains of *Trichimonas vaginalis* from the United States. *Am J Obstet Gynecol* 138:808–812, 1980.

10. Chow AW, Patten V, Guze LB: Susceptibility of anaerobic bacteria to metronidazole: relative resistance of non-spore forming gram positive bacilli. *J Infect Dis* 131:182, 1975.

11. Sutter VL, Finegold SM: Susceptibility of anaerobic bacteria to 23 antimicrobial agents. *Antimicrob Agents Chemother* 10:736, 1976.

12. Sweet RL, Ohm-Smith M, Hadley WK: In vitro activity of N-formimidoyl thienamycin (MK0787) and other antimicrobials against isolates from obstetric and gynecologic infections. *Antimicrob Agents Chemother* 22:711–714, 1982.

13. Catterall RD: Fifteen years experience with metronidazole. In Finegold SM (ed): Metronidazole Proceedings, Montreal, Canada, May 26–28, 1976. *Excerpta Medica*, Amsterdam, 1977, pp 107–111.

14. Goldman P: Metronidazole. *N Engl J Med* 303:1212–12218, 1980.

15. Rosenkrantz HS, Speck WT: Mutagenicity of metronidazole activation by mammalian liver microsomes. *Biochem Biophys Res Commun* 66:520–522, 1975.

16. Voogd CE, Van Der Stel JJ, Jacobs JJJAA: The mutagenic action of nitroimidazoles. 1. Metronidazole, nimorazole, dimetridazole and ronidazole. *Mutat Res* 26:438, 1974.

17. Charles D: Chloramphenicol, clindamycin and metronidazole. In Ledger WJ (ed): *Antibiotics in Obstetrics and Gynecology*. The Hague, Martinus Nijhoff, 1982, pp 159–217.

18. Mitelman F, Hartley-Asp B, Ursing B: Chromosome aberration and metronidazole. *Lancet* 2:802, 1976.

19. Rustia M, Shubik P: Induction of lung tumors and malignant lymphomas in mice by metronidazole. *J Natl Cancer Inst* 48:721–729, 1972.

20. Roe FJC: Metronidazole: review of uses and toxicity. *J Antimicrob Chemother* 3:205–212, 1977.

21. Rustia M, Shubik P: Experimental induction of hepatomas, mammary tumors and other tumors with metronidazole in nonbred Sas:MRC (WI) BR rats. *J Natl Cancer Inst* 68:863, 1979.

22. Beard CM, Noller KL, O'Fallon M, et al: Lack of evidence for cancer due to use of metronidazole. *N Engl J Med* 301:519–522, 1979.

23. Friedman GD: Cancer after metronidazole. *N Engl J Med* 302:519, 1980.

24. Mirer FE, Silverstein MA: Letter. *N Engl J Med* 302:519, 1980.

25. Amon I, Amon K, Franke G, et al: Pharmacokinetics of metronidazole in pregnant women. *Chemotherapy* 27:73, 1981.

26. Morgan IFK: Metronidazole treatment in pregnancy. In Phillips I, Collier J (eds): *Metronidazole*. Proceedings, Geneva, April 25–27, 1979, Academic Press, pp 245–247.

27. Erickson SH, Oppenheim GL, Smith GH: Metronidazole in breast milk. *Obstet Gynecol* 57:48, 1981.

28. Bartlett JG: Metronidazole. *Johns Hopkins Med J* 149:89, 1981.

29. Andersson KE: Pharmacokinetics of nitroimidazoles. Spectrum of adverse reactions. *Scand J Infect Dis* (suppl) 26:60, 1981.

30. Pheiffer TA, Forsyth PS, Durfee MA, et al: Nonspecific vaginitis: role of *Haemophilus vaginalis* and treatment with metronidazole. *N Engl J Med* 298:1429–1434, 1978.

31. Sweet RL: Anaerobic infections of the female genital tract. *Am J Obstet Gynecol* 112:891, 1975.

32. Collier J, Calhoun EN, Hill PL: A multicenter comparison of clindamycin and metronidazole in the treatment of anaerobic infections. *Scand J Infect Dis* (suppl) 26:96, 1981.

33. Gall SA, Kohan AP, Ayers OM: Intravenous metronidazole or clindamycin with tobramycin for therapy of pelvic infection. *Obstet Gynecol* 57:51, 1981.

CHAPTER 20

Antibiotic Prophylaxis in Obstetrics and Gynecology

Because infections occur commonly after obstetric and gynecologic procedures, there has been great interest in antibiotic prophylaxis. In the last decade, there have been a large number of well designed studies, and present data allow conclusions regarding use of prophylaxis in many procedures.

It should be noted at the outset that there are special conditions regarding use of antibiotic prophylaxis in an obstetric-gynecologic population. First, nearly all obstetric and most gynecologic patients are healthy and free of serious, underlying disorders. Second, although the lower genital tract is a contaminated field, resistant gram-negative organisms are not found except under special circumstances. Third, operation through or adjacent to this contaminated field leads to a moderate to high incidence of infection, but serious infection measured by bacteremia, abscess, or death is unusual. Finally, use of certain antimicrobials for prophylaxis in pregnancy is often contraindicated because of the potential for adverse effects on the fetus, newborn, or mother.

In this chapter, *antibiotic prophylaxis* is defined as use of antibiotics for the prevention of infection in the absence of current signs or symptoms of infection.

USES IN OBSTETRICS

In obstetrical patients, most attention has been directed at prophylaxis of the patient undergoing cesarean delivery. Some interest has arisen for use in patients having premature or prolonged rupture of the fetal membranes.

Cesarean Delivery

Throughout the United States, there has been an unprecedented rise in the incidence of cesarean births within the last two decades. Recent data from the National Center for Health Statistics show that in 1979 and 1980 cesarean sections comprised 16.4% and 16.5%, respectively, of all deliveries (1). This rise has been largely due to use of cesarean delivery to avoid potentially traumatic forceps or breech deliveries. In some hospitals, the use of fetal monitoring has also led to a larger number of cesarean deliveries performed for fetal distress. A recent national conference has addressed many of the problems of the rise in cesarean birth rate (2).

As noted in Chapter 17, cesarean delivery is accompanied by more frequent and more serious puerperal infections (3). Indeed, cesarean delivery is probably the single most important risk factor for maternal postpartum infection. Patients undergoing cesarean delivery have a 5- to 20-fold greater risk for puerperal infection compared to patients having vaginal delivery (3).

Not all cesarean sections carry the same risk of puerperal infection. Many investigators have found that patients having nonelective cesarean delivery (i.e., in labor with or without membrane rupture) are at greater risk than patients having electively scheduled procedures (4). Especially among indigent populations, the risks in this subgroup have been reported as 45–85% (4, 5). Labor, membrane rupture, and vaginal examination increase postpartum infection probably because they allow ascent of bacteria into the amniotic cavity before surgery. One might consider this a subclinical infection established while the patient is in labor (5, 6).

Since 1968, over 30 studies have been reported on the use of prophylactic antibiotics in cesarean section. The results of randomized trials are shown in Table 20.1 (7–29). With few exceptions, prophylactic regimens have resulted in a statistically significant and clinically meaningful decrease in postoperative infection. In randomized clinical trials of primary cesarean deliveries, the infection rate in prophylaxis groups is 55% of the infection rate in placebo groups (30).

Table 20.1
Results of Randomized, Placebo-Controlled Trials of Antibiotic Prophylaxis in Patients Having Cesarean Section

Author, references	Antibiotic regimen	Number	Postoperative infection rate[a]	
			Placebo group (%)	Prophylaxis group (%)
Gibbs et al (7)	Ampicillin, kanamycin, methicillin, 3 doses	61	42	21
Gibbs et al	Ampicillin, kanamycin, 3 doses	68	64[b]	17[b]
Work (9)	Cephalothin, 3 doses	80	42.5[b]	20
Wong et al (10)	Cefazolin, 3 doses	93	58	35[b]
Kreutner et al (11)	Cefazolin, 3 doses	97	26	16
Gall (12)	Cefazolin, cephalothin, 4 doses	95	37[b]	13[b]
Phelan and Pruyn (13)	Cefazolin, 3 doses	122	16	11
Larson et al (14)	Cefoxitin, 3 doses	152	33[b]	19[b]
Kreutner et al (15)	Cephalothin, cefamandole, 2 doses	120	59[b]	30[b]
Duff and Park (16)	Ampicillin, 3 doses	57	42[b]	8[b]
McCowan and Jackson (17)	Metronidazole, 2 doses	73	31	37
Rehu and Jahkola (18)	Penicillin; clindamycin-gentamicin, 1 dose	147	33[b]	8[b]
Harger and English (19)	Cefoxitin, 3 doses	386	27.5[b]	11[b]
Polk et al (20)	Cefoxitin, 3 doses	266	20[b]	4[b]
Dillon et al (21)	Cefoxitin, 3 doses	101	29[b]	4[b]
Gibbs et al (22)	Cefamandole, 3 doses	100	52[b]	16[b]
Stiver et al (23)	Cefoxitin or cefazolin, 3 doses	354	24.3[b]	6[b]
Duff et al (24)	Ampicillin, 3 doses	82	15[b]	2.4[b]
Stage et al (25)	Cephradine, 2 doses	199	14[b]	0.75[b]
Apuzzio et al (26)	Ticarcillin, 1 or 2 doses	259	55[b]	32[b]
Hawrylyshyn et al (27)	Cefoxitin, 1 or 3 doses	189	29.8[b]	7.3[b]
Padilla et al (28)	Ampicillin, 1 dose	71	59.4[b]	14.7[b]
Hager and Williamson (29)	Cefamandole, 4 doses	90	27.7[b]	9.3[b]

[a] Infections noted are of the operative site, when provided by authors.
[b] Significant difference in infection rate, by χ^2 test.

These significant decreases in infection are attributed mainly to decreases in uterine and wound infections. Urinary tract infections, including both symptomatic and asymptomatic disorders, occurred less commonly in combined series (14% in controls versus 6% in the prophylactic group) (31), but in few individual studies were there significant decreases.

Four studies have compared the efficacy of antibiotics. Itskowitz et al compared ampicillin to cephalothin (32), Kreutner et al compared cephalothin to cefamandole (15), Vaughn compared cephadrine to metronidazole (33), and Rehu and Jahkola compared penicillin to clindamycin plus gentamicin (18). There were no statistically significant differences in infection rates, but there were relatively few patients in these studies (88 to 118) and the absolute differences in infection rate were small (3–8%). Recently, a group of Canadian investigators compared cefoxitin with cefazolin in nonelective cesarean sections and found no significant differences in rate of genital tract infection or in hospital stay (23).

There were few comparisons of short with long courses of prophylaxis. D'Angelo and Sokol carried out a randomized clinical trial of a 24-hr versus a 5-day regimen of cephalosporins (34) and found no significant difference in the rate of postoperative infection (29% in short course versus 20% in long course). Although Ayangade found that a 6–10-day-course was accompanied by less postoperative infection (10%) than was a 12-hr course (40%), this Nigerian study was not randomized (35). Swartz and Grolle have combined data from 26 studies and calculated that regimens of 12 hr or less are similarly effective compared to longer prophylactic courses (31). In a sequence of studies in patients at approximately 85% risk for uterine infection, investigators in Dallas showed that 4-day "early treatment" led to fewer cases of uterine infection than did a three-dose prophylactic regimen (12% versus 24%; p < 0.05). However, associated complications (parametrial phlegmon and wound abscess) occurred in 7% of both groups. Accordingly, the authors concluded that the three-dose course was preferable to the "early treatment" regimen. However, these were not blinded studies, and data from recent prospective studies at the same hospital were used for comparison (36–37).

Studies comparing administration of the prophylaxis before versus after cord clamping are also few in number. Gordon and colleagues found similar rates of postoperative infection whether they administered prophylactic ampicillin before or after cord clamping (11% versus 8%, not significant) (38). Swartz and Grolle's tabulation of 26 studies also showed similar effectiveness of antibiotic prophylaxis whether given before or after cord clamping (31).

Single dose prophylaxis has been compared to two doses (26) and to three doses (27). Appuzio and colleagues noted similar efficacy whether prophylaxis consisted of two doses of ticarcillin or one dose followed by a placebo (26). In the study of Hawrylyshyn and colleagues, there was no difference in the rate of endometritis whether one dose of cefoxitin or three doses were used for prophylaxis (9.4 and 5.0%, respectively) (27). Each regimen significantly reduced infection compared to placebo (Table 20.1).

As an alternative to parenteral administration of prophylactic antibiotics, Long and colleagues have reported excellent results by intraoperative irrigation of the uterus and peritoneal cavity with antibiotic solution (39, 40). In a double-blind study, they reported a decrease in endometritis from 26% (8/30) in those receiving saline to 0% (0/30) in those irrigated with cefamandole solution (2 g in 800–1000 ml) (39). In a third group receiving no irrigation, 23% (7/30) developed endometritis. In a subsequent study, authors at the same institution reported an overall rate of endometritis of 1.7% in a larger series of 298 patients (40). The potential advantages of this route include decreased cost and perhaps decreased toxicity.

However, Duff and co-workers found that there is appreciable absorption of cephalothin, cefamandole, and ampicillin when administered by this route (41). Although the levels were far below that achieved by IV administration, the concentrations exceeded the minimal inhibitory concentrations for many genital tract pathogens and were certainly high enough to elicit allergic reactions. More recent evaluations have reported that intraoperative prophylaxis is either equivalent to, or less effective than, IV prophylaxis.

QUESTIONS AND ADVERSE EFFECTS

First, are serious infections decreased? Whereas prophylaxis achieves a significant decrease in infections, nearly all of these infections are mild and respond promptly to antibiotic therapy. Mead has calculated that pelvic abscess or septic pelvic thrombophlebitis occurred in only 0.5% of 659 women receiving prophylaxis and in only 1.1% of 609 controls (42). In many series there are no serious infections or no significant decrease in hospital stay in patients given prophylaxis (9, 12, 13, 15, 19). This suggests that postoperative infection in the patients receiving placebo responds promptly to therapy. Second, are there neonatal sequelae? We note that antibiotics administered before cord clamping rapidly achieve measurable concentrations in the fetus. This may lead to possible direct adverse effect or sensitization. More commonly, though, it led the pediatrician to perform a sepsis workup and initiate antibiotic therapy for fear of overlooking a masked sepsis (43). Cunningham and co-workers found that sepsis evaluations were performed on 28% of neonates whose mothers received prophylactic antibiotics before cord clamping, whereas such evaluations were carried out in 15% of infants when prophylaxis was initiated after cord clamping (p < 0.001) (43). In view of the equivalent efficacy of prophylaxis administered after cord clamping, delayed injection would be favored to circumvent the problem for the neonate and pediatrician.

Also, untoward effects may accompany use of antibiotics for prophylaxis. These untoward effects consist of changes in flora and direct toxic reactions. Early studies of prophylaxis made no systematic attempt to identify bacteriologic shifts. With most studies recovering few organisms, there were no apparent shifts toward resistant organisms. However, four more recent studies have been more thorough and have detected significant changes (11, 15, 22, 43) (Table 20.2). Overall, there were decreases in highly

Table 20.2
Bacteriologic Effects of Prophylactic Antibiotic in Cesarean Section

Author, references	Prophylactic regimen	Effect on flora of prophylactic group	
		Increases	Decreases
Gibbs and Weinstein (43)	Clindamycin, gentamicin, 2 doses	*E. coli* enterococci	Anaerobes aerobic cocci
Kreutner et al (11)	Cefazolin, 3 doses	Enterobacteriaceae *Bacteroides* sp.	Staphylococci veillonella aerobes
Kreutner et al (15)	Cefamandole or cephalothin, 3 doses	Organisms resistant to prophylactic antibiotic	
Gibbs et al (22)	Cefamandole, 3 doses	Enterobacteriaeceae enterococci	Gram-positive anaerobes nonpathogens

susceptible organisms and increases in enterococci and Enterobacteriaceae. Although many of the Enterobacteriaceae were susceptible to the prophylactic agent, some isolates of *Pseudomonas* species also appeared. In these cases, the bacterial changes were without consequence. Yet, it would be unwise to ignore these shifts. In patients who develop infection after prophylaxis, it is essential to obtain appropriate cultures to guide antibiotic *therapy*. Routine continuation of the agent used for prophylaxis may lead to an unnecessary prolongation of illness and delayed recognition of the infecting organisms. For the environment, continued widespread use of prophylaxis may produce alarming effects, as Sack has noted recently in regard to use of antibiotics to prevent traveler's diarrhea (44).

Direct toxic effects are unlikely. No serious allergic or toxic reactions were noted among 1443 patients receiving prophylaxis in 26 studies (31). Less serious reactions such as skin rash were reported on occasion. However, several cases of fatal anaphylactic reaction to prophylactic antibiotics were reported in orthopedic patients (45), and two cases of fatal pseudomembranous enterocolitis have been attributed to a combination of prophylactic-therapeutic antibiotics (46).

ALTERNATIVES

In view of these adverse effects, we should consider alternatives to routine administration of prophylaxis. There is a need to develop better measures of target populations for prophylaxis. For example, Gilstrap and Cunningham have determined that their patients having cesarean birth more than 6 hr after membrane rupture encounter an 85% risk of postoperative infection (5). However, most others report the risk among patients having cesarean in labor and after membrane rupture to be considerably lower. In predominantly private patients, Harger and English (19) and Polk and colleagues (20) found the rate of endometritis with primary section to be 20 and 9%, respectively. In these lower risk populations, combinations of risk factors may allow determination of target groups, but equations to predict these groups would need to be simple.

Examination of amniotic fluid may improve precision in predicting infection. Recent investigations have noted an excellent correlation between positive amniotic fluid cultures collected at cesarean delivery and subsequent postoperative endometritis (6, 47). With rapid diagnostic techniques such as gas-liquid chromatography or counterimmunoelectrophoresis of amniotic fluid, it may be possible to identify with great specificity patients likely to develop endometritis. Thus, in these very high risk groups identified by clinical *and* laboratory techniques, prophylaxis might be used with a high degree of specificity. In groups at considerably lower risks, it may be wiser to treat infection as it becomes clinically evident.

A common concern about widespread use of prophylaxis is a dangerous relaxation of standard infection control measures. Clearly, hand washing, appropriate isolation techniques, proper disposal of infected materials and dressings, and changing of soiled scrub suits remain important elements in control of infections and cannot be replaced capriciously by antibiotic prophylaxis. Iffy et al noted a decrease in postoperative morbidity from 83–16% when these standard infection control measures were strictly enforced (48). As an important corollary, good intraoperative technique also remains essential.

As another alternative to prophylaxis, some have favored early treatment of clinically evident infection. This practice has generally been the norm in low risk populations (49). Because excellent cure rates are achieved with regimens such as clindamycin-gentamicin and newer penicillins and cephalosporins, it may be better to await clinical evidence of infection even among moderate risk groups. These *therapeutic* regimens have had a few clinical failures (5%), and few major infection-related complications. The postoperative hospital stay is often brief (50, 51).

RECOMMENDATIONS

The following conclusions are made by the author for patients undergoing cesarean delivery.

1. Prophylactic antibiotics for cesarean delivery should be restricted to patient groups with a moderate to high risk of postoperative infection.
2. When prophylaxis is used, a short course regimen of no more than three doses should be used.
3. Agents for prophylaxis should be shown effective, safe, and inexpensive. For obstetrical patients, possible choices are ampicillin and the "first generation" cephalosporins (including cephalothin, cefazolin, etc.).
4. Newer, broader spectrum antibiotics such as cefoxitin and cefamandole are no more effective as prophylactic agents. Since these agents are considerably more expensive, they should not be used for prophylaxis.
5. Administration of prophylaxis should be delayed until after cord clamping to avoid consequences to the fetus.
6. When prophylaxis is used, patients should be evaluated carefully when postprophylaxis fevers or other signs of infection develop. Appropriate cultures should be performed. When therapeutic antibiotics are necessary, initially use a broad spectrum regimen in view of changes in flora brought about by prophylactic antibiotics.

Finally, investigators need to identify better target populations and to evaluate alternatives to antibiotic prophylaxis.

Premature Rupture of the Membranes

Many recent studies have employed prophylactic antibiotics for either mothers or newborns, but few did so in a standardized fashion. Two recent studies evaluated prophylaxis among infants born after membranes had been ruptured for 24 hr or more. From a study of 100 such infants, Habel and colleagues concluded that prophylactic antibiotics were unnecessary because infections were few, and that they were potentially hazardous because fungal infections and colonization were increased (52). On the other hand, Wolf and Olinsky recommended use of prophylaxis until blood culture results were available (53).

Interest in prophylaxis among mothers with premature rupture of membranes (PROM) has been more limited than in the past, and usually reserved for patients undergoing cesarean delivery or receiving steroids. In the latter setting, Miller and colleagues found in a retrospective study a decrease (from 18–0%) in maternal infection when prophylactic ampicillin was used (54).

USES IN GYNECOLOGY

Studies in gynecologic patients have focused mainly upon vaginal and abdominal hysterectomy with a few additional studies of other procedures.

Vaginal Hysterectomy

The risk of postoperative infection in patients undergoing vaginal hysterectomy varies widely (Table 20.3). However, use of control patients from a comparative study may select patients in high risk groups. In the Professional Activities Study, it is noted that of 3500 patients having vaginal hysterectomy 38% had fever greater than 101°F (55). Patients at high risk for infection after vaginal hysterectomy are premenopausal women. Also, women with hysterectomy within 24–72 hr after cervical conization also encounter a higher rate of postoperative infection (56). There have been 15 double-blind placebo-controlled studies (25, 56–69). Twelve have shown statistically significant decreases in postoperative infection in patients receiving prophylactic antibiotics. Three others have shown de-

Table 20.3
Summary of Double-Blind, Placebo-Controlled, Randomized Studies of Prophylactic Antibiotics in Vaginal Hysterectomy

Author, references	Antibiotic regimen	Number	Postoperative infection rate[a]	
			Placebo group (%)	Prophylactic group (%)
Forney et al (56)	Cephaloridine-cephalexin, 5 days	32	43[b]	0[b]
Ledger et al (57)	Cephaloridine, 3 doses	100	34[b]	8[b]
Breedon and Mayo (58)	Cephaloridine, 3 doses	120	20[b]	3[b]
Bivens et al (59)	Cephalothin-cephalexin, 6 days	60	20	13
Ohm and Galask (60)	Cephaloridine-cephalexin, 5 days	48	34[b]	4[b]
Lett et al (61)	Cefazolin (1 dose) cephaloridine, 3 doses	153	61[b]	14[b]
Holman et al (62)	Cefazolin	84	23[b]	0[b]
Roberts and Holmesly (63)	Carbenicillin, 5 doses	52	12	0
Mendelson et al (64)	Cephradine, 1 and 4 doses	66	64[b]	2[b]
Grossman et al (65)	Cefazolin, penicillin, 48 hr	78	25[b]	6[b]
Mathews et al (66)	Trimethoprim-sulfa 1 dose	50	16	8
Polk et al (67)	Cefazolin, 3 doses	86	21[b]	2[b]
Hemsell et al (68)	Cefoxitin, 3 doses	99	57[b]	8[b]
Mickal et al (69)	Cefoxitin, 3 doses	125	30[b]	10[b]
Stage et al (25)	Cephradine, 2 doses	163	14[b]	1.9[b]

[a] Infections noted are of the operative site infection, when provided by authors.
[b] Significant difference in infection rate, by χ^2 test.

creases but not statistically significant ones (59, 63, 66). Polk has calculated that the overall preventative fraction is 82% in 11 studies of short course prophylaxis (30). Two studies have evaluated short course prophylaxis (single dose to 12 hours) versus long course (48 to 72 hours) (70, 71) and found no significant difference in infection rates.

Three studies compared the efficacy of different antibiotics for prophylaxis. No difference was found between cefazolin and penicillin (66), cefazolin (one dose) and cephaloridine (62) (three doses), or cephalothin and metronidazole (71).

The findings of these well designed studies are remarkably consistent in showing statistically significant and clinically impressive decreases in postoperative infection.

Abdominal Hysterectomy

There has been less interest in antibiotic prophylaxis for this operation perhaps because infection after abdominal hysterectomy may be less frequent than after vaginal hysterectomy. In four studies evaluating prophylaxis for both operations, the infection rate was 21% of 136 placebo patients undergoing vaginal hysterectomy and 14% of 367 placebo patients undergoing abdominal hysterectomy (30). Data from the Professional Activities Study show that, of 8400 patients having abdominal hysterectomy, infection appears to be less common than after vaginal hysterectomy, possibly due to less contamination from the vagina (55).

Double-blind studies of abdominal hysterectomy are summarized in Table 20.4 (25, 62, 63, 65, 67, 72–76). Only three of 10 observed significant differences, but in each study the infection rate was lower in the prophylaxis group. Polk has calculated that in studies using short course prophylaxis 49% of postoperative infections are prevented (30). Only one of these studies compared two agents. In Grossman's comparison of cefazolin and penicillin for prophylaxis, abdominal wound or vaginal cuff infections developed in 5% of 76 patients receiving penicillin and in 11% of 79 patients receiving

Table 20.4
Summary of Double-Blind, Placebo-Controlled, Randomized Studies of Prophylactic Antibiotics in Abdominal Hysterectomy

Author, references	Antibiotic regimen	Number	Postoperative infection rate[a]	
			Placebo group (%)	Prophylactic group (%)
Allen et al (72)	Cephalothin, 5 days	168	30[b]	14[b]
Ohm and Galask (73)	Cephaloridine, cephalexin, 5 days	93	15	6
Mathews et al (74)	Trimethoprim, sulfa	59	38	27
Holman et al (62)	Cefazolin, 3 doses	80	34[b]	5[b]
Roberts and Homesly (63)	Carbenicillin, 24 hr	47	14	4
Grossman et al (65)	Cefazolin, penicillin, 48 hr	239	11	8
Polk et al (67)	Cefazolin, 3 doses	429	13[b]	7[b]
Schepers and Merkus (75)	Cefoxitin	103	16	6
Duff (76)	Cefoxitin, 2 doses	91	24	18
Stage et al (25)	Cephradine, 2 doses	110	0	2.4

[a] Infections noted are of the operative site infection, when provided by authors.
[b] Significant difference in infection rate, by χ^2 test.

cefazolin (65). These differences were not significantly different from each other, nor from the placebo group (11% of 84).

ADVERSE EFFECTS OF PROPHYLAXIS IN HYSTERECTOMY

Ohm and Galask noted marked changes in flora in patients receiving 5-day cephalosporin prophylaxis for both abdominal and vaginal hysterectomy, as well as in patients receiving placebo. There was a shift toward more resistant isolates in patients receiving prophylactic antibiotics (77, 78). In patients receiving a 48-hr course of prophylaxis, Grossman and Adams noted changes in flora of patients who received short course prophylaxis for hysterectomy, but these changes were similar to those in patients who received placebo (79). Other adverse effects, including rashes and abnormalities in chemistry or hematology studies, have been reported infrequently. Some authors have noted difficulty identifying the source of fever after prophylaxis for 5 days (73).

ALTERNATIVE TO PROPHYLAXIS IN HYSTERECTOMY

In a retrospective study, Richardson and colleagues reported a decrease in postoperative morbidity and in hospital stay by using a nontraumatic technique (80). They avoided crushing tissue, heavy suture material, intraabdominal packs, and Foley catheters. Although the results of application of these prime surgical principles are encouraging, similar prospective studies have not been reported.

Another approach to decreasing postoperative infection has been special preparation of the lower genital tract. Immediately prior to vaginal hysterectomy, Osborne and colleagues performed hot conization of the cervix to eliminate the endocervical glands as a contaminated site and then performed a scrub of the vagina and perineum with an iodophore (81). In a retrospective study, they found that this preparation was as effective as antibiotic prophylaxis in reducing postoperative infection.

As another alternative, Swartz and Tanaree have demonstrated significant decreases in postoperative infections by use of suction drainage through a T-tube catheter (82). In abdominal prophylaxis, fever of more than 100.4°F developed in 26% of controls but in only 11% of patients with suction drainage, and pelvic infections were decreased from 7% of 100 controls to 9 of 100 with suction drainage. In vaginal hysterectomy, fever of more than 100.4°F developed in 32% of 50 controls and is 8% of 50 patients with suction drainage; there were 12 pelvic infections (24%) in the former group and only two (4%) in the latter. Further study has shown no further significant decrease in postoperative infection when antibiotic prophylaxis is combined with suction drainage (83).

RECOMMENDATION FOR HYSTERECTOMY

For vaginal hysterectomy, the author offers the following:

1. In premenopausal women and other groups at demonstrably high risk for postoperative infection, prophylactic antibiotics are indicated as they decrease the frequency and the severity of these infections.
2. A short course of prophylaxis involving no more than three doses should be used.
3. Agents which are reasonable choices are: "first generation" cephalosporins, penicillin G, ampicillin, or tetracycline. The latter two have been reported as effective in only nonblind studies of prophylaxis in hysterectomy.
4. Although newer agents are effective, they are probably not more effective, and they are more expensive.
5. Strict adherence to good surgical technique should not be compromised.

For abdominal hysterectomy:

1. Effectiveness of prophylaxis varies widely from institution to institution, perhaps depending upon background infection rates and definitions of infections.
2. Antibiotic prophylaxis would thus be best reserved for patients with a high risk of pelvic or abdominal wound infection.
3. In these circumstances, the recommendation should be the same as for vaginal hysterectomy.

Gynecologic Oncology

Antibiotic prophylaxis is widely used in major surgery for gynecologic cancer, but randomized trials have been limited. In a recent double-blind study, Creasman and colleagues reported that cefamandole significantly reduced pelvic or abdominal infection (from 36–4%, $p < 0.01$) in patients having *extended hysterectomy* for endometrial cancer (84). Using a prospective, randomized, but not placebo-controlled technique, Rosenshein and colleagues evaluated a single-dose doxycycline prophylaxis in 64 patients having radical abdominal hysterectomy (85). The fever index at 7 and at 14 days was significantly lower in patients getting doxycycline prophylaxis ($p < 0.02$ and 0.05, respectively). Eight patients (23.5%) in the control group and four patients (13.3%) in the doxycycline group developed cuff or pelvic cellulitis. This difference was not statistically significant, nor was the difference in postoperative hospital stay (15.6 in the control group and 16.1 in the doxycycline group).

Therapeutic Abortion

Use of prophylaxis for the first trimester abortion should be limited. Although Hodgson and co-workers reported prophylactic tetracycline decreased complications, the overall infection rate was low, and nearly all of them were "minor" or "minimal" (86). In a double-blind study, Sonne-Holm and colleagues have noted that prophylaxis for this procedure was effective only in patients with previous pelvic infection disease (87). Thus, except in truly high risk groups for infection after first trimester abortion, it would seem wiser to treat infection as it develops rather than using wide scale prophylaxis.

Uterine infection is more common after second trimester abortion. Spence and colleagues performed a randomized, blinded comparison of cephalothin versus placebo in 198 patients undergoing intraamniotic injection of hypertonic urea supplemented with prostaglandin F_2 (88). The prophylactic agent was given every 6 hr until the pregnancy aborted or until 48 hr. Endometritis developed in two patients (2%) receiving cephalothin and in nine patients (9%) receiving placebo ($p < 0.05$).

PROPHYLAXIS OF BACTERIAL ENDOCARDITIS

Bacteremia develops in perhaps 1% of women during delivery and in an undetermined percentage of women undergoing pelvic surgery. Bacteremia has been found in 3–20% of obstetric patients with infection. In 1977, the Committee on Prevention of Rheumatic Fever and Bacterial Endocarditis of the American Heart Association provided revised guidelines for antibiotic prophylaxis to prevent endocarditis (89).

Indications

Because endocarditis after "uncomplicated" vaginal delivery is extremely rare, the committee noted that the necessity for antibiotic prophylaxis has not been firmly established. Yet, in view of the possibility of endocarditis, we continue to use prophylaxis for vaginal delivery. For "complicated" deliveries, including cesarean section, prophylaxis is indicated in all patients with underlying heart disease.

Infective endocarditis rarely develops after dilation and curettage or uncomplicated insertion or removal of intrauterine devices. Thus, the committee suggested that antibiotic prophylaxis would not be required in most patients with underlying heart disease undergoing these procedures. However, they favored prophylaxis for patients with prosthetic values having either of the above procedures. For other gynecologic surgery such as hysterectomy, antibiotic prophylaxis is indicated in patients with heart disease.

Regimen

Endocarditis prophylaxis during pelvic procedures is directed primarily against enterococci (e.g., *Streptococcus faecalis*). Although gram-negative organisms are among the most common microbes causing bacteremia in this population, these organisms rarely cause endocarditis. Parenteral antibiotics are recommended as follows: aqueous crystalline penicillin G (2,000,000 units intramuscularly or intravenously) or ampicillin (1.0 g intramuscularly or intravenously) plus gentamicin (1.5 mg/kg intramusuclarly or intravenously) or streptomycin (1.0 g intramuscularly). Give initial doses 30 min to 1 hr before the procedure. If gentamicin is used, give a similar dose of gentamicin and penicillin (or ampicillin) every 8 hr for two additional doses. If streptomycin is used, give a similar dose of streptomycin and penicillin (or ampicillin) every 12 hr for two additional doses.

For those patients who are allergic to penicillin, give the regimen as follows: vancomycin (1.0 g intravenously, given over 30 min to 1 hr) plus streptomycin (1.0 g intramuscularly). A single dose of these antibiotics begun 30 min to 1 hr before the procedure is probably sufficient, but the same dose may be repeated in 12 hr.

In patients with significantly compromised renal function, it may be necessary to modify the dose of antibiotics used.

References

1. Placek PJ, Taffel SM: Trends in cesarean section rates for the United States, 1970–1978. *Public Health Rep* 95:540, 1980.
2. NIH consensus development task force statement on cesarean childbirth. *Am J Obstet Gynecol* 139:902, 1981.
3. Gibbs RS: Clinical risk factors for puerperal infection. *Obstet Gynecol* 55:178(S), 1980.
4. Gibbs RS, Jones PM, Wilder CJY: Internal fetal monitoring and maternal infection following cesarean section: a prospective study. *Obstet Gynecol* 52:193, 1978.
5. Gilstrap LC, Cunningham FG: The bacterial pathogenesis of infection following cesarean section. *Obstet Gynecol* 53:545, 1979.
6. Blanco JD, Gibbs RS, Casteneda YS, St. Clair PJ: Correlation of quantitative amniotic fluid cultures with endometritis after cesarean section. *Am J Obstet Gynecol* 143:897–901, 1982.
7. Gibbs RS, DeCherney AH, Schwart RH: Prophylactic antibiotics in cesarean section: a double-blind study. *Am J Obstet Gynecol* 114:1048, 1972.
8. Gibbs RS, Hunt JE, Schwarz RH: A follow-up study on prophylactic antibiotics in cesarean section. *Am J Obstet Gynecol* 117:419, 1972.
9. Work BA: Role of preventative antibiotics in patients undergoing cesarean section. *South Med J* 70(suppl):44, 1979.
10. Wong R, Gee CL, Ledger WJ: Prophylactic use of cefazolin in monitored obstetric patients undergoing cesarean section. *Obstet Gynecol* 51:407, 1978.
11. Kreutner AK, DelBene VE, Delamar D, et al: Perioperative antibiotic prophylaxis in cesarean section. *Obstet Gynecol* 52:279, 1978.
12. Gall SA: The efficacy of prophylactic antibiotics in cesarean section. *Am J Obstet Gynecol* 124:506, 1979.
13. Phelan JP, Pruyn SC: Prophylactic antibiotics in cesarean section: a double-blind study of cefazolin. *Am J Obstet Gynecol* 133:474, 1979.
14. Larson P, Nelson KE, Ismail M: Double-blind study of cefoxitin prophylaxis of post-cesarean section infection. In *Current Chemotherapy and Infectious Disease: Proc. 11th International Congress of Chemotherapy and the 19th Interscience Conference on Antimicrobial Agents and Chemotherapy.* Washington, D.C., American Society of Microbiology, 1980, p 1212.
15. Kreutner AK, DelBene V, Delmur D, et al: Perioperative cephalosporin prophylaxis in cesarean section: effect on endometritis in high risk patients. *Am J Obstet Gynecol* 134:925, 1979.
16. Duff P, Park RC: Antibiotic prophylaxis for cesarean section in a military population. *Milit Med* 145:377, 1980.
17. McCowan L, Jackson P: The prophylactic use of metronidazole in cesarean section. *N Z Med J* 92:153, 1980.
18. Rehu M, Jahkola M: Prophylactic antibiotics in cesarean section: effect of a short pre-operative course of benzylpenicillin or clindamycin plus gentamicin on postoperative infections morbidity. *Ann Clin Res* 12:45, 1980.
19. Harger JH, English DH: Selection of patients for antibiotic prophylaxis in cesarean sections. *Am J Obstet Gynecol* 141:752, 1981.
20. Polk BF, Krache M, Phillippe M, et al: Randomized clinical trial of perioperative cefoxitin in preventing infection after primary cesarean section. *Am J Obstet Gynecol* 142:983, 1982.
21. Dillon WP, Seigel MS, Lede AS, et al: Evaluation of cefoxitin prophylaxis for cesarean section. *Int J Obstet Gynecol* 19:133, 1981.
22. Gibbs RS, ST. Clair PJ, Castillo MS, et al: Bacteriologic effects of antibiotic prophylaxis high risk cesarean section. *Obstet Gynecol* 57:277, 1981.
23. Stiver HG, Forward KR, Livingstone RA, et al: Multicenter comparison of cefoxitin versus cefazolin for prevention of infectious morbidity after nonelective cesarean section. *Am J Obstet Gynecol* 145:158, 1983.

24. Duff P, Smith PN, Keiser JF: Antibiotic prophylaxis in low-risk cesarean section. *J Reprod Med* 27:133, 1982.
25. Stage AN, Glover DD, Vaughan JE: Low-dose cephradine prophylaxis in obstetric and gynecologic surgery. *J Reprod Med* 27:113, 1982.
26. Apuzzio JJ, Reyelt C, Pelosi M, et al: Prophylactic antibiotics for cesarean section: comparison of high- and low-risk patients for endomyometritis. *Obstet Gynecol* 59:693, 1982.
27. Hawrylyshyn PA, Bernstein P, Papsin FR: Short-term antibiotic prophylaxis in high-risk patients following cesarean section. *Am J Obstet Gynecol* 145:285, 1983.
28. Padilla SL, Spence MR, Beauchamp PJ: Single-dose ampicillin for cesarean section prophylaxis. *Obstet Gynecol* 61:463, 1983.
29. Hager WD, Williamson MM: Effects of antibiotic prophylaxis on women undergoing nonelective cesarean section in a community hospital. *J Reprod Med* 28:687, 1983.
30. Polk BF: Antimicrobial prophylaxis to prevent mixed bacterial infections. *J Antimicrob Chemother* 8(suppl):115, 1981.
31. Swartz WH, Grolle K: The use of prophylactic antibiotics in cesarean section, a review of the literature. *J Reprod Med* 26:595, 1981.
32. Itskowitz J, Paldi E, Katz M: The effect of prophylactic antibiotics on febrile morbidity following cesarean section. *Obstet Gynecol* 53:162, 1979.
33. Vaughn JE: Comparison of metronidazole and cephradine in the prevention of wound sepsis following cesarean section. In: Royal Society of Medicine International Congress and Symposium Series, No. 18:203, 1979.
34. D'Angelo LJ, Sokol RJ: Short-versus long-course prophylactic antibiotic treatment in cesarean section patients. *Obstet Gynecol* 55:583, 1980.
35. Ayangade O: Long- versus short-course antibiotic prophylaxis in cesarean section: a comparative study. *J Natl Med Assoc* 71:71, 1979.
36. De Palma RT, Leveno KJ, Cunningham FG, et al: Identification and management of women at high risk for pelvic infection following cesarean section. *Obstet Gynecol* 55:1855, 1980.
37. De Palma RT, Cunningham FG, Leveno KJ, et al: Continuing investigation of women at high risk for infection following cesarean section delivery. *Obstet Gynecol* 60:53, 1982.
38. Gordon JR, Phillips D, Blanchard K: Prophylactic cesarean section antibiotics: maternal and neonatal morbidity before or after cord clamping. *Obstet Gynecol* 53:151, 1979.
39. Long WH, Rudd EG, Dillon MB: Intrauterine irrigation with cefamandole nafate solution at cesarean section: a preliminary report. *Am J Obstet Gynecol* 138:755, 1980.
40. Rudd EG, Cobey EA, Long WH, et al: Prevention of endomyometritis following cesarean section. Armed Forces District Meeting of the American College of Obstetricians and Gynecologists, October, 1981, Phoenix, Arizona.
41. Duff P, Gibbs RS, Jorgensen JH, et al: The pharmacokinetics of prophylactic antibiotics administered by intraoperative irrigation at the time of cesarean section. *Obstet Gynecol* 60:409, 1982.
42. Mead PB: Prophylactic antibiotics and antibiotic resistance. Semin Perinatol 1:101, 1977.

43. Gibbs RS, Weinstein AJ: Bacteriologic effects of prophylactic antibiotics in cesarean section. *Am J Obstet Gynecol* 130:226, 1976.
44. Sack BB: Prophylactic antibiotics? The individual versus the community (editorial). *N Engl J Med* 300:1107, 1979.
45. Spruill FG, Minette LJ, Sturner WO: Two surgical deaths associated with cephalothin. *JAMA* 229:440, 1974.
46. Ledger WJ, Puttler OL: Death from pseudomembranous enterocolitis. *Obstet Gynecol* 45:609, 1975.
47. Cooperman NR, Kasim M, Rajashekaraiah KR: Clinical significance of amniotic fluid, amniotic membrane, and endometrial biopsy cultures at the time of cesarean section. *Am J Obstet Gynecol* 137:536, 1980.
48. Iffy L, Kaminestzky HA, Maidman JA, et al: Control of perinatal infection by traditional preventive measures. *Obstet Gynecol* 54:403, 1979.
49. Prophylactic antibiotics in cesarean section. *Br Med J* 2:675, 1973.
50. DiZerega G, Yonekura L, Roy S, et al: A comparison of clindamycin-gentamicin and penicillin-gentamicin in the treatment of post-cesarean endomyometritis. *Am J Obstet Gynecol* 134:238, 1979.
51. Gibbs RS, Blanco JD, Castaneda YS, St. Clair PJ: A double-blind, randomized comparison of clindamycin-gentamicin versus cefamandole for treatment of post-cesarean endomyometritis. *Am J Obstet Gynecol* 144:261, 1982.
52. Habel AH, Sandor GS, Conn NK, et al: Premature rupture of membranes and effects of prophylactic antibiotics. *Arch Dis Child* 47:401, 1972.
53. Wolf RL, Olinsky A: Prolonged rupture of fetal membranes and neonatal infections. *S Afr Med J* 50:574, 1976.
54. Miller JM, Brazy JE, Gall SA, et al: Premature rupture of the membranes. Maternal and neonatal infectious morbidity related to betamethasone and antibiotic therapy. *J Reprod Med* 25:173, 1980.
55. Ledger WJ, Child MA: The hospital care of patients undergoing hysterectomy: an analysis of 12,026 patients from the Professional Activities Study. *Am J Obstet Gynecol* 117:423, 1973.
56. Forney JP, Morrow CP, Townsend DE, et al: Impact of cephalosporin prophylaxis in conization—vaginal hysterectomy morbidity. *Am J Obstet Gynecol* 125:100, 1976.
57. Ledger WJ, Sweet RL, Headington JT: Prophylactic cephaloridine in the prevention of postoperative pelvic infection in premenopausal women undergoing vaginal hysterectomy. *Am J Obstet Gynecol* 115:766, 1973.
58. Breedon JT, Mayo JE: Low dose prophylactic antibiotics in vaginal hysterectomy. *Obstet Gynecol* 43:379, 1974.
59. Bivens MD, Neufeld J, McCarty WD: The prophylactic use of Keflex and Keflin in vaginal hysterectomy. *Am J Obstet Gynecol* 122:169, 1975.
60. Ohm MJ, Galask RP: The effect of prophylactic antibiotics in patients undergoing vaginal operations. I. Effect of morbidity. *Am J Obstet Gynecol* 123:590, 1975.
61. Lett WJ, Ansbacher R, Davison BL, Otterson WN: Prophylactic antibiotics for women undergoing vaginal hysterectomy. *J Reprod Med* 19:51, 1977.

62. Holman JF, McGowan JE, Thompson JD: Perioperative antibiotics in major elective gynaecologic surgery. *South Med J* 71:417, 1978.

63. Roberts JJ, Homesly HD: Low-dose carbenicillin prophylaxis for vaginal and abdominal hysterectomy. *Obstet Gynecol* 52:83, 1978.

64. Mendelson J, Portnoy J, DeSaint Victo JR, Gelfand MM: Effect of single and multidose cephradine prophylaxis on infectious morbidity of vaginal hysterectomy. *Obstet Gynecol* 53:31, 1979.

65. Grossman JH III, Greco TP, Minkin MJ, Adamas RL, Hierholzer WJ, Andriole VT: Prophylactic antibiotics in gynaecologic surgery. *Obstet Gynecol* 53:537, 1979.

66. Mathews DD, Agarwal V, Gordon AM, Cooper J: A double-blind trial of single-dose chemoprophylaxis with co-trimoxazole during vaginal hysterectomy and repair. *Br. J Obstet Gynaecol* 86:737, 1979.

67. Polk BF, Tager IB, Shapiro M, Goren-White B, Goldstein P, Schoenbaum SC: Randomized clinical trial of perioperative cefazolin in preventing infection after hysterectomy. *Lancet* 1:437, 1980.

68. Hemsell DL, Cunningham FG, Kappus S, Nobles B: Cefoxitin for prophylaxis in premenopausal women undergoing vaginal hysterectomy. *Obstet Gynecol* 56:629, 1980.

69. Mickal A, Curole D, Lewis C: Cefoxitin sodium: double-blind vaginal hysterectomy prophylaxis in premenopausal patients. *Obstet Gynecol* 56:222, 1980.

70. Ledger WJ, Gee C, Lewis CP: Guidelines for antibiotic prophylaxis in gynecology. *Am J Obstet Gynecol* 121:1038, 1975.

71. Hamod KA, Spence MR, Rosenshein MB, Dillon MB: Single-dose and multidose prophylaxis in vaginal hysterectomy: a comparison of sodium cephalothin and metronidazole. *Am J Obstet Gynecol* 136:976, 1980.

72. Allen JL, Rampone JF, Wheeles CR: Use of a prophylactic antibiotic in elective major gynecologic operations. *Obstet Gynecol* 39:218, 1972.

73. Ohm MJ, Galask RP: The effect of antibiotic prophylaxis on patients undergoing total abdominal hysterectomy. I. Effect on morbidity. *Am J Obstet Gynecol* 125:442, 1976.

74. Mathews DD, Ross H, Cooper J: A double-blind trial of single-dose chemoprophylaxis with co-trimoxazole during abdominal hysterectomy. *Br J Obstet Gynaecol* 86:894, 1979.

75. Schepers JP, Merkus FWHM: Cefoxitin sodium: a double-blind, placebo-controlled, prophylactic study in premenopausal patients undergoing abdominal hysterectomy. *Clin Pharmacol Ther* 29:281, 1981.

76. Duff P: Antibiotic prophylaxis for abdominal hysterectomy. *Obstet Gynecol* 60:25, 1982.

77. Ohm MJ, Galask RP: The effect of antibiotic prophylaxis on patients undergoing vaginal hysterectomy. II. Alterations of microbial flora. *Am J Obstet Gynecol* 123:597, 1975.

78. Ohm MJ, Galask RP: The effect of antibiotic prophylaxis on patients undergoing total abdominal hysterectomy. II. Alterations of microbial flora. *Am J Obstet Gynecol* 125:448, 1976.

79. Grossman JH, Adams RL: Vaginal flora in women undergoing hysterectomy with antibiotic prophylaxis. *Obstet Gynecol* 53:23, 1979.

80. Richardson AC, Lyon JB, Graham EE: Abdominal hysterectomy: relationship between morbidity and surgical technique. *Am J Obstet Gynecol* 115:953, 1973.

81. Osborne NG, Wright RC, Dubay M: Preoperative hot conization of the cervix: a possible method to reduce postoperative febrile morbidity following vaginal hysterectomy. *Am J Obstet Gynecol* 133:374, 1979.

82. Swartz WH, Tanaree P: Suction drainage as an alternative to prophylactic antibiotics for hysterectomy. *Obstet Gynecol* 45:305, 1975.

83. Swartz WH, Tanaree P: T-tube suction drainage and/or prophylactic antibiotics: a randomized study of 451 hysterectomies. *Obstet Gynecol* 47:665, 1976.

84. Creasman WT, Hill GB, Weed JC, et al: A trial of prophylactic cefamandole in extended gynecologic surgery. *Obstet Gynecol* 59:309, 1982.

85. Rosenshein NB, Ruth JC, Villar J, et al: A prospective randomized study of doxycycline as a prophylactic antibiotic in patients undergoing radical hysterectomy. *Gynecol Oncol* 15:201, 1983.

86. Hodgson JE, Major B, Portman K, et al: Prophylactic use of tetracycline for first trimester abortions. *Obstet Gynecol* 45:574, 1975.

87. Sonne-Holm S, Heisterbert L, Hebjorn S, et al: Prophylactic antibiotics in first trimester abortions: a clinical, controlled trial. *Am J Obstet Gynecol* 139:693, 1981.

88. Spence MR, King TM, Burkman RT, et al: Cephalothin prophylaxis for midtrimester abortion. *Obstet Gynecol* 60:502, 1982.

89. Kaplan EL, Anthony BF, Bisno A, et al: Prevention of bacterial endocarditis. *AHA News* 56:139A, 1977.

Index

Page numbers in *italics* denote figures; those followed by "t" or "f" denote tables or footnotes, respectively.